D1489203

Ostergard's Urogynecology and Pelvic Floor Dysfunction

Fifth Edition

Ostergard's Urogynecology and Pelvic Floor Dysfunction

Fifth Edition

Editors

Alfred E. Bent, M.D.
Associate Professor
Department of Gynecology and Obstetrics
Johns Hopkins School of Medicine
Chairman
Department of Gynecology
Greater Baltimore Medical Center
Baltimore, Maryland

Geoffrey W. Cundiff, M.D.
Associate Professor
Department of Obstetrics and Gynecology
Johns Hopkins School of Medicine
Chairman
Department of Obstetrics and Gynecology
Johns Hopkins Bayview Medical Center
Baltimore, Maryland

**Donald R. Ostergard, M.D.,
F.A.C.O.G.**
Professor
Department of Obstetrics and Gynecology
University of California, Irvine
Long Beach, California

Steven E. Swift, M.D.
Associate Professor
Department of Obstetrics and Gynecology
Division of Benign Gynecology
Medical University of South Carolina
Charleston, South Carolina

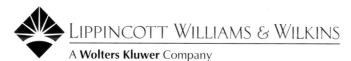

LIPPINCOTT WILLIAMS & WILKINS
A **Wolters Kluwer** Company
Philadelphia · Baltimore · New York · London
Buenos Aires · Hong Kong · Sydney · Tokyo

Acquisitions Editor: Lisa McAllister
Developmental Editor: Raymond E. Reter
Production Editor: Karina Mikhli
Manufacturing Manager: Colin Warnock
Cover Designer: Christine Jenny
Compositor: Lippincott Williams & Wilkins Desktop Division
Printer: Edwards Brothers

Previous edition published as: *Urogynecology and Urodynamics: Theory and Practice, Fourth Edition.*

Printed in the USA

Library of Congress Cataloging-in-Publication Data

Ostergard's urogynecology and pelvic floor dysfunction.—5th ed. / edited by Alfred E. Bent ... [et al.].
    p. ; cm.
    Rev. ed. of: Urogynecology and urodynamics / edited by Donald R. Ostergard, Alfred E. Bent. 4th ed. c1996.
    Includes bibliographical references and index.
    ISBN 0-7817-3384-7
    1. Urogynecology. 2. Urodynamics. I. Title: Urogynecology and pelvic floor dysfunction. II. Ostergard, Donald R., 1938– III. Bent, Alfred E.
IV. Urogynecology and urodynamics.
    [DNLM: 1. Genital Diseases, Female. 2. Pelvic Floor–physiopathology.
3. Urogenital Diseases. 4. Prolapse. 5. Urinary Incontinence. WJ 190 O85 2002]
RG484 .U76 2002
616.6–dc21

2002069531

10 9 8 7 6 5 4 3 2 1

I wish to dedicate this edition to my son, Nick (Nicholas Oliver Bent, June 5, 1975 to March 18, 2001), and his enduring memory. In the prior edition I recounted an appreciation to those special persons in my family and these remain—Mom, Dad, son Nate, and especially my wife, Callie. While we did not count on so short a journey for Nick, we feel blessed with knowledge of his intelligence and wit. May we draw strength from his memory as we press on in our journey until our paths meet once again.

A.E.B.

This special dedication is given to my wife and friend, Constance, for her encouragement in organizing and editing the fifth edition, and for her unselfish support in my academic pursuits and in the time commitments those involve. For these I am grateful.

D.R.O.

I dedicate this book to those who have facilitated my career; my mentors, Alf Bent, Rick Bump, and Al Addison, who focused and cultivated my interests; those I have mentored, who have kept me interested and challenged; and most importantly, my wife, Valerie, who is my eternal refuge of support and honesty in all things.

G.W.C.

I would like to dedicate this edition to those who are most important to me: my God, my wife Alisa, and my children Dylan, Brooks, and Taylor. In addition, I would like to thank my mentors, Robert Kirk, M.D. and Donald Ostergard, M.D., who took my interest in urogynecology and helped me turn it into a career.

S.E.S.

Contents

Section III. Pathology and Treatment

A. Urinary Tract Dysfunction

B. Colorectal Disorders

C. Pelvic Organ Prolapse

D. Urinary Incontinence

Contributing Authors

Rodney A. Appell, M.D., F.A.C.S.
Scott Department of Urology
Baylor College of Medicine
Houston, Texas

J. Thomas Benson, M.D.
Clinical Professor
Department of Obstetrics and Gynecology
Indiana University
Director
Department of Female Pelvic Medicine and
*   Reconstructive Surgery*
Methodist Hospital
Indianapolis, Indiana

Alfred E. Bent, M.D.
Associate Professor
Department of Gynecology and Obstetrics
Johns Hopkins School of Medicine
Chairman
Department of Gynecology
Greater Baltimore Medical Center
Baltimore, Maryland

Arieh Bergman, M.D.
Clinical Professor
Department of Obstetrics and Gynecology
University of Southern California
School of Medicine
Los Angeles, California

Narender N. Bhatia, M.D.
Professor
Department of Obstetrics and Gynecology
UCLA School of Medicine
Head
Division of Urogynecology
Harbor/UCLA Medical Center
Los Angeles, California

Joan Blomquist, M.D.
Greater Baltimore Medical Center
Towson, Maryland

Toby C. Chai, M.D., F.A.C.S.
Division of Urology
University of Maryland Medical Center
Baltimore, Maryland

Kimberly W. Coates, M.D.
Assistant Professor
Department of Obstetrics and Gynecology
Texas A&M University College of Medicine/Health
*   Science Center*
Assistant Professor
Department of Obstetrics and Gynecology
Scott & White Clinic
Temple, Texas

Geoffrey W. Cundiff, M.D.
Associate Professor
Department of Gynecology and Obstetrics
Johns Hopkins School of Medicine
Chairman
Department of Obstetrics and Gynecology
Johns Hopkins Bayview Medical Center
Baltimore, Maryland

John O. L. DeLancey, M.D.
Associate Professor
Department of Obstetrics and Gynecology
Chief
Division of Gynecology
University of Michigan Medical School
Ann Arbor, Michigan

R. Mark Ellerkmann, M.D.
Associate Director of the Obstetrics/Gynecology
*   Residency*
Department of Gynecology
Johns Hopkins School of Medicine
Attending Physician
Division of Urogynecology
Greater Baltimore Medical Center
Baltimore, Maryland

Scott A. Farrell, M.D.
Department of Obstetrics and Gynecology
Dalhouse University
Halifax, Nova Scotia
Canada

Rene Genadry, M.D.
Associate Professor
Department of Gynecology and Obstetrics
Johns Hopkins Medical Institutions
Baltimore, Maryland

Michelle M. Germain, M.D.
Greater Baltimore Medical Center
Towson, Maryland

Roger P. Goldberg, M.D., M.P.H.
Director
Division of Urogynecology
Evanston Continence Center
Northwestern University Medical School
Evanston, Illinois

Michael Gross, M.D.
Associate Professor
Department of Urology
Haifa University
Head of Female Urology and Voiding Dysfunction
  Unit
Department of Urology
Bnei Zion Medical Center
Haifa, Israel

Nicolette S. Horbach, M.D.
Associate Professor
Department of Obstetrics and Gynecology
George Washington University
Annandale, Virginia

W. Glenn Hurt, M.D.
Professor
Department of Obstetrics and Gynecology
Virginia Commonwealth University
School of Medicine
Medical College of Virginia Hospitals
Virginia Commonwealth University Health System
Richmond, Virginia

Mickey M. Karram, M.D., F.A.C.O.G.
Professor
Department of Obstetrics and Gynecology
University of Cincinnati
Director of Urogynecology
Department of Obstetrics and Gynecology
Good Samaritan Hospital
Cincinnati, Ohio

Howard Kaufman, M.D.
Department of Surgery
Johns Hopkins School of Medicine
Baltimore, Maryland

Vik Khullar, A.K.C., B.Sc., M.D., M.R.C.O.G.
Senior Lecturer
Faculty of Medicine
Imperial College School of Medicine
Honorary Consultant Urogynecologist
Department of Obstetrics and Gynecology
St. Mary's Hospital
London, England

Steven D. Kleeman, M.D.
Clinical Assistant Professor
Department of Obstetrics and Gynecology
Wright State University
Miami Valley Hospital
Dayton, Ohio
Clinical Instructor
Department of Obstetrics and Gynecology
Good Samaritan Hospital
Cincinnati, Ohio

John James Klutke, M.D.
Assistant Professor
Department of Obstetrics and Gynecology
University of Southern California-Keck School of
  Medicine
Los Angeles, California

Kari Kubic, M.D.
Department of Obstetrics and Gynecology
George Washington University
Annadale, Virginia

Kenneth S. Leffler, M.D.
Assistant Professor
Department of Gynecology and Obstetrics
Johns Hopkins Medical Institutions
Baltimore, Maryland

Lawrence R. Lind, M.D.
Clinical Instructor
Department of Obstetrics and Gynecology
Division of Urogynecology
North Shore-Long Island Jewish Health System
New York University School of Medicine
Manhasset, New York

Robert W. Lobel, M.D.
Assistant Professor and Director
Division of Urogynecology
Albany Medical College
Albany, New York

Mary T. McLennan, M.D., F.A.C.O.G.
Assistant Professor
Department of Obstetrics, Gynecology, and Women's
  Health
St. Louis University
Director of Urogynecology
Department of Obstetrics, Gynecology, and Women's
  Health
St. Louis University Hospital
St. Louis, Missouri

Joseph M. Montella, M.D.
Assistant Professor
Director of Urogynecology
Department of Obstetrics and Gynecology
Thomas Jefferson University Medical College
Director of Urogynecology
Department of Obstetrics and Gynecology
Thomas Jefferson University Hospital
Philadelphia, Pennsylvania

Mikio Albert Nihira, M.D., M.P.H.
Assistant Professor
Department of Obstetrics and Gynecology
Division of Urogynecology and Reproductive
  Pelvic Surgery
University of Texas Southwestern Medical Center
Dallas, Texas

Donald R. Ostergard, M.D., F.A.C.O.G.
Professor
Department of Obstetrics and Gynecology
University of California, Irvine
Long Beach, California

Harpreet Pannu, M.D.
Assistant Professor
Russell H. Morgan Department of Radiology
  and Radiology Sciences
Johns Hopkins Medical Institutions
Baltimore, Maryland

A. Cullen Richardson, M.D.
(Deceased)
Clinical Professor Emeritus
Department of Gynecology and Obstetrics
Emory University School of Medicine
Atlanta, Georgia

Robert M. Rogers, Jr., M.D.
Gynecologist
Department of Obstetrics and Gynecology
The Reading Hospital and Medical Center
West Reading, Pennsylvania

Peter K. Sand, M.D.
Associate Professor
Department of Obstetrics & Gynecology
Director
Division of Urogynecology
Northwestern University Medical School
Director
Evanston Continence Center
Evanston, Illinois

Bob L. Shull, M.D.
Department of Obstetrics and Gynecology
Texas A&M University College of
  Medicine/Health Science Center
Department of Obstetrics and Gynecology
Scott & White Clinic
Temple, Texas

Steven E. Swift, M.D.
Associate Professor
Department of Obstetrics and Gynecology
Division of Benign Gynecology
Medical University of South Carolina
Charleston, South Carolina

James Paul Theofrastous, M.D.
Clinical Associate Professor
Department of Obstetrics and Gynecology
University of North Carolina Chapel Hill School of
  Medicine
Chapel Hill, North Carolina
Director of Urogynecology and Reconstructive
  Pelvic Surgery
Mountain Area Health Education Center
Regional OB.GYN Specialists
Asheville, North Carolina

Marc R. Toglia, M.D.
Assistant Clinical Professor
Department of Obstetrics and Gynecology
Thomas Jefferson University Medical College
Philadelphia, Pennsylvania
Chief, Subdivision of Gynecology
Department of Obstetrics and Gynecology
Riddle Memorial Hospital
Media, Pennsylvania

Julia B. Van Rooyen, M.D.
Assistant Professor
Department of Gynecology and Obstetrics
Johns Hopkins School of Medicine
Baltimore, Maryland

Michael W. Weinberger, M.D.
Residency Program Director
Department of Obstetrics and Gynecology
Kaiser Permanente, Southern California
Director
Division of Urogynecology
Department of Obstetrics and Gynecology
Kaiser Permanente–Los Angeles Medical Center
Los Angeles, California

Preface

A few short years once again have changed the focus of the physician that deals with female urinary and pelvic floor disorders. Many urogynecologists see patients with predominant prolapse symptoms, rather than urinary incontinence. There continues to be patients with isolated urinary incontinence, but much more often patients present with multi-system problems involving urinary incontinence, disorders of pelvic prolapse, and fecal incontinence. In keeping with the change in focus, this book is renamed to honor the person responsible for so many trained physicians in this specialty, and to recognize the expanding emphasis placed on pelvic floor dysfunction.

The goal of this text is to promote the reader's understanding of lower urinary tract and pelvic floor dysfunction in the female patient. The chapters present a practical approach to problems, with the assistance of figures and tables, as well as with a concise number of references. Some chapters offer comprehensive opinions and extensive reference lists as in the previous edition. Information can now be obtained on virtually anything by consulting the Internet, and some links to these sites are provided.

This fifth edition has been shortened to present information without overlap, and yet includes new areas such as colorectal dysfunction and pelvic organ prolapse. There are sections on epidemiology and pathophysiology. The anatomy section has been expanded to include pelvic floor anatomy, as well as a chapter on clinical correlation and evaluation of support defects. Color photographs expand the view of cystourethroscopy. There is new material on evaluating colorectal dysfunction, imaging modalities, and sacral neuromodulation. Surgical sections on urinary incontinence have been condensed to reflect two major approaches to surgical intervention, as well as continued updates on periurethral injectables. There is extensive information presented on management of colorectal dysfunction, as well as surgical and nonsurgical approaches to pelvic prolapse. The Appendices contain important material on terminology as well as information for Internet users.

A brief look at the contents should point the reader to a specific section that will assist in the management of patients with a wide number of problems including the pelvic floor, urinary incontinence, colorectal dysfunction, and pelvic organ prolapse.

Alfred E. Bent

Introduction and Historical Perspectives: The Time Has Come

There is no more distressing lesion than urinary incontinence—A constant dribbling of the repulsive urine soaking the clothes which cling wet and cold to the thighs, making the patient offensive to herself and her family and ostracizing her from society.

Howard A. Kelly, M.D., 1928

It is a paradoxic that it has taken so long for the field of gynecologic urology, which gave birth to the greater discipline of gynecology, to become a science in its own right. In his book *Genitourinary Problems in Women*, Robertson discusses the ancient writing of the Kahun papyrus, written approximately 200 years B.C., which is devoted to diseases of women and includes a discussion of diseases of the urinary bladder. Indeed, the Ebers papyrus in 1550 B.C. classified diseases by systems and organs. Robertson states that Section 6 of this latter papyrus describes the cure for a woman suffering from diseases of the urine as well as the womb. Henhenit was one of six women attached to the court of Menuhotep II of the 11th dynasty, who reigned in Egypt about 2050 B.C. Her mummified body was found in 1955; radiographs of this mummy revealed that she had an extensive urinary fistula.

It was one of our own, Marion Sims, who is credited with the birth of modern gynecology through his pioneer work in the treatment of obstetrical urinary fistulas. Robertson writes that Marion Sims chose to study medicine, much to his father's disgust, as the elder had only contempt for the medical profession. Sims' father believed that there was no science in medicine, and that there was no longer honor in going from house to house with a box of pills in one hand and a squirt in the other. However, Marion Sims did enter the field of medicine and started his practice in Lancaster, South Carolina. His first two patients were infants who died from cholera. He was so disturbed by this that he moved to Mount Meigs, Alabama, where he earned the reputation as a great surgeon and married his childhood sweetheart, Eliza Theresa Jones, in December 1836. His practice had flourished at that point, and his income was a wholesome 3,000 dollars per year.

Robertson tells us of the birth of gynecology with a specific case. Evidently, Sims' settled life was changed by an event that eventually led to his great medical achievement. A Mrs. Merril was thrown from a horse, which resulted in an impacted retroverted uterus. She was brought to Sims after many other physicians had failed to help her. Although Sims did not like to examine women, he did recall the advice of one of his professors from medical school—he placed her in a knee-chest position and reluctantly applied pressure to the vagina. The impacted uterus suddenly yielded and Mrs. Merril had immediate relief. His success with this particular patient led him to examine several slave women with vesicovaginal fistulas, using the same advantageous knee-chest position. He found this position allowed careful examination of the vagina, which had hitherto been very difficult. When examining patients with a fistula, he was able to clearly see the opening, and he began thinking of methods for repair. As is well known, his first attempts at fistula repair used silk sutures, but the attempts failed.

Sims' first success was with a slave girl named Anarcha, whose fistula repair was accomplished with silver wire sutures. Her fistula first occurred at the age of 17 after childbirth, and she seemed doomed forever to be a disgusting object to herself and to everyone who came near her. This motivated her to submit to so many surgeries. Sims had convinced his jeweler to make the wire out of unalloyed silver drawn out as thin as horsehair. It was in May of 1849 when he prepared Anarcha for her 13th operation. He brought the edges of the fistula close together with four of his five flexible new silver wires, passing them through little strips of lead to keep them from cutting into the tissue and fastening them tightly by using, once again, his perforated lead shot. Then he introduced the essential catheter into the bladder and readied himself for the tedious week of waiting. On previous occasions he had been sure that he would witness a successful cure at the week's end; this time he was filled with anxiety. He thought he had played his last trump—if he failed to win now, the game was really lost. Even with this fanatical devotion, he could not keep on forever. At the end of the week, almost 4 years to the day when he had first seen those gaping, mocking holes that were Anarcha's souvenirs of childbirth, he had Anarcha placed again on the operating table. With pounding heart and fearful mind, he introduced the speculum. There lay the suture apparatus just as he had fixed it, quite undisturbed by swelling and inflammation. There was no longer any fistula; its edges had joined close in a perfect union. Anarcha's recovery with the silver sutures in place was uncomplicated, and she remained dry for the rest of her life. This was a great relief to her because her fistula not only opened into the bladder but into the rectum as well.

In 1852, Sims reported the cure of 252 fistulas out of 320 attempts. It was apparently the use of silver wire sutures that turned repeated failures into predictable successes. Shortly thereafter, Sims left Alabama for New York, where he became one of the founders of the Women's Hospital. He toured Europe and successfully operated on patients throughout the continent.

His success did not end with his accomplishments in fistula surgery. The Internal Medical Congress in London of 1881 was perhaps the most satisfactory medical meeting in the life of Marion Sims. This is where he delivered his thesis and his valedictory address as "Progress in Peritoneal Surgery." Dr. Sims began by saying that he was prompted to discuss the subject due to his observations in the surgical and obstetric sections at the International Medical Congress. His object was to lay before the Academy a synopsis of the progress of peritoneal surgery in his own pioneer practice. In his address, the physically afflicted 68-year-old pioneer surgeon was ardent in his plea for surgeons to adopt the new methods, aseptic technique in particular, in dealing with any wound that invaded the peritoneal cavity. He pleaded for the adoption of Lister's principle for preventing infection in all wounds, particularly in the abdomen. "Ovariotomy is the parent of peritoneal surgery," said Sims, and he gave credit to Ephraim McDowell and Washington Atlee, whom he called the "great ovariodomists".

Marion Sims died quietly in 1883 while working on his autobiography entitled *The Story of My Life*, a book that was to be released by his son, Harry Marion Sims, a year after his father's death.

The work of Marion Sims was assumed by Howard A. Kelly, who was appointed the first professor of gynecology at the Johns Hopkins Medical School. A decade later he relinquished his leadership in obstetrics to Dr. John Whitridge ("Bull") Williams and Kelly continued as professor of gynecology. Like Sims, Kelly believed that gynecology and urology were so closely related that they could not be separated. The American Urogynecologic Society is the fulfillment of the beliefs of Marion Sims and Howard Kelly.

In 1893, Kelly popularized the use of the cystoscope. According to Robertson, he used the so-called air cystoscope with the patient in the knee-chest position. Robertson relates that the cystoscope originally was a hollow tube with a handle and a glass partition that prevented water from running out of the bladder. The bladder had been distended with water before the insertion of the cystoscope, and light was reflected from a head mirror. One day, an assistant to Dr. Kelly dropped the scope and the glass shattered. Kelly had noticed that the vagina ballooned with air when the patient was in the knee-chest position and concluded that the bladder might be distended with air in a similar manner. He inserted the broken cystoscope, and when he removed the obturator, the bladder ballooned with air; he was able to satisfactorily inspect the bladder mucosa. Kelly's interest in urologic problems of the female intensified, and in 1919, he and Burnam coauthored a text entitled *Disease of the Kidney, Ureters and Bladder.* Kelly wrote, "The commonest form of incontinence is the result of childbirth, entailing an injury to the neck of the bladder; it is occasionally seen in elderly nullipara and is most common after the age of 40. It is usually progressive, beginning with an occasional dribble, later becoming more frequent and occurring on slight provocation. In its incipiency, a strain, cough, sneeze or stepping up to get on a tram car starts a little spurt of urine which, in the course of time, initiates the act which empties the bladder. The list of operations devised to overcome the incontinence is legion; most unsuccessful, but occasionally, temporarily at least, affording some control. The best plan, often successful, is to set free the thickened musculature (sphincter) at the neck of the bladder (Bell's muscle) and to suture it so as to overlap its ends, forming a good internal sphincter." This was to be the forerunner of Kelly's plication as a component of the anterior colporrhaphy.

Those that followed Kelly at the Johns Hopkins Medical School were similarly interested in female urology. Guy Hunner described the Hunner's ulcer, which today is called interstitial cystitis. Houston Everett, who succeeded Hunner, discovered the relationship of the urinary tract to cervical cancer. His concepts are fundamental in modern gynecologic oncology. Everett is the author of *Gynecologic and Obstetrical Urology* and coauthor of *Female Urology.*

In 1914, Latzko described a new operation for closure of the posthysterectomy vesicovaginal fistula. His simple method consisted of an upper vaginectomy and was easily applicable to a large number of patients in the United States with small fistula posthysterectomy. Many modifications of this technique have been proposed during the last several decades, but the fundamental methodology remains unchanged.

As stated earlier, a surgical approach to stress incontinence was begun by Howard A. Kelly, who reported on the successful outcome in 16 of 20 patients with incontinence who were treated by plication of the vesical neck. In 1949, Marshall, Marchetti, and Krantz reported on a new operation in which they treated 50 patients with stress incontinence; 25 of these patients had previous unsuccessful surgical procedures. Their overall success rate was 82%. This retropubic suspension of the bladder neck has been modified by many individuals over the past three decades. The procedure described by Burch in 1968 received great acceptance; it accomplishes the retropubic suspension by suturing the periurethral tissue to Cooper's ligament.

Over the last decades, the evaluation of bladder dynamics has been more carefully and scientifically approached. This began Robertson's report on the use of the modified culdoscope to accommodate the physician in his inspection of the bladder and urethra. The standard culdoscope, used for many years in gynecology, could not be used to visualize the vesical neck or the urethra because of the right angle of the lens and the heat from the bulb. Robertson modified the Kelly air cystoscope to overcome these obstacles. His urethroscope had optical glass fibers enclosed between double walls of a stainless steel barrel. An electric source in the handle transmitted cold light around the circumference at the distal end; this allowed magnification at the proximal end. An air vent allowed a closed system by the placement of a fingertip over the vent. The development of fiberoptic telescopes revolutionized endoscopy and has made many changes in the practice of gynecology. Robertson developed a female urethroscope with a direct view telescope that looks into an open barrel tube. The fiberoptic cord and the gas tubing are attached to the head, and carbon dioxide is used for distention of the urethra and bladder. This flexible system allows both thorough inspection of the urinary tract mucosa and the beginnings of bladder and urethral function analysis. Recently, by use of this instrument and modifications thereof, a more sophisticated system for dynamic assessment of bladder and urethral function has been pioneered that has resulted in a better understanding of the process of micturition.

It would appear that the discipline of urogynecology, which gave birth to the larger specialty of gynecology, has finally come of age. Many of us have been frustrated by the paucity of concrete knowledge in the area of stress incontinence and related problems. The number of surgical procedures that have been devised over the last century to accommodate and improve these afflicted patients is legion. Undoubtedly, the fundamental problem was a serious lack of understanding of the etiology. Developments in the last few years suggest that our understanding of the mechanisms involved in the proper function of the healthy and diseased bladder and urethra are at hand, as well as our understanding of the appropriate procedures to improve the well-being of this large group of afflicted patients.

The American Board of Obstetrics and Gynecology currently has a committee creating a subspecialty in urogynecology and reconstructive pelvic floor surgery; a subspecialty board will be announced soon. The committee has proceeded with the certification of a fellowship training program and expects there will be about 20 such programs by 2002. The process by which one would achieve subspecialty status would be analogous to that currently in place for gynecologic oncology, maternal fetal medicine, and reproductive endocrinology and infertility. The objective of this new entity would run parallel to the other subspecialties, and would hopefully create a cadre of academic teachers to educate young generalists and specialists in obstetrics and gynecology. The creation of formal fellowship programs and certification processes should encourage solidification of current centers of excellence and propagation of enhanced research activities in a field often neglected in the recent past. In addition, the creation of a subspecialty status will underscore that the historical roots for research and therapy into diseases of the female lower urinary tract truly rest in the field of gynecology.

Philip J. DiSaia

Normal Pelvic Floor, Epidemiology, and Pathophysiology

Ostergard's Urogynecology and Pelvic Floor Dysfunction, Fifth Edition. edited by A.E. Bent, et al. Lippincott Williams & Wilkins, Philadelphia © 2003.

1

Anatomy of the Female Bladder and Urethra

John O.L. DeLancey

Department of Obstetrics and Gynecology, and Division of Gynecology, University of Michigan Medical School, Ann Arbor, Michigan

Understanding the structure of the constituent parts of the lower urinary tract, how they are assembled, and how they function is fundamental to understanding the physiology and pathophysiology of this region. The following discussion of the urethra, bladder, and pelvic floor is intended to cover those aspects of the anatomy that are important to understanding dysfunctions of the lower urinary tract.

Many biologists have remarked on the intimate connection between form and function, and this is certainly true in the lower urinary tract. Its structure mirrors the dual activities of urine storage and evacuation. The bladder acts as a reservoir, relaxing to receive urine during the filling phase and contracting to evacuate it during the emptying phase. The urethra acts reciprocally by contracting during filling to maintain urine within the bladder and by relaxing during voiding to allow for micturition. Both the bladder and urethra contain several separate components within their walls, and these parts are described to the extent that they are functionally important.

The environment of the pelvic floor, where the urethra is located, is important to lower urinary tract function. One way in which the pelvic floor influences the bladder and urethra is in the support it provides for the vesical neck and proximal urethra. Although we usually think of parts of the urethra as above or below the pelvic floor, the urethra is actually a part of this structural unit. In fact, the relationship between genital support and urinary

incontinence was the genesis of the gynecologist's involvement with problems of lower urinary tract function. This remains one of the strongest arguments for our continued management of patients with lower urinary tract dysfunction.

ANATOMY OF THE LOWER URINARY TRACT

Several terms have been applied to parts of the lower urinary tract. Clinicians have traditionally divided the lower urinary tract into the bladder, vesical neck, and urethra. The bladder consists of the detrusor musculature and its underlining mucosa; it also contains the vesical trigone on its dorsal wall. The urethra is a multilayered muscular tube that extends below the bladder and has a specialized mucosal and vascular lining. The vesical neck represents that region of the bladder base where the urethral lumen traverses the wall of the bladder. In this area, therefore, the urethral lumen actually exists in a location surrounded by the bladder. Because the vesical neck has special functional characteristics, it is considered as a separate entity.

Bladder

The bladder is a hollow viscus whose wall consists of coarse bundles of smooth muscle. It is lined by a mucosa of transitional epithelium that rests on a loose submucosa. It can be further subdivided into a dome and a base roughly at the level of the ureteral orifices. The dome is a relatively thin portion of the bladder and is quite distensible, whereas the base has a thicker musculature and undergoes less distention during filling.

Detrusor Muscle

Although separate layers of the detrusor musculature are sometimes described, these are not nearly as well defined as the separate layers in the gut. This reflects the fact that the bladder needs to contract only periodically to increase intravesical pressure to evacuate urine, whereas the gut must work in a coordinated manner to propel its contents in a forward direction. In the dome, the layers are relatively indistinct, but near the base of the bladder, they become better defined. The outermost layer is primarily longitudinal in orientation. On the anterior surface of the bladder, longitudinal fibers continue past the vesical neck into the pubovesical muscles and insert into the tissues of the pelvic wall near the pubic symphysis (see later).

Within this outer longitudinal layer is an intermediate layer of oblique and circular fibers. The actual fiber directions in this portion of the dome are less well defined than those in the outer layer. The innermost layer is plexiform, as can be seen from the pattern of trabeculations visible during cystoscopy. A predominance of longitudinal fibers is usually described in this layer, but this is not striking when the bladder is viewed from its lumen.

In the region of the vesical neck, there are two U-shaped bands of fibers (with each U opening in opposite directions). The more prominent Heiss's loop (detrusor loop) passes anterior to the internal meatus and opens posteriorly. The second loop, which consists of that portion of the intermediate circular layer of the detrusor that lies under the trigone, opens anteriorly. The urethral lumen passes through the openings in these muscular loops (1). This arrangement may provide a sphincteric action when the two straps of muscle pull in opposite directions to close the ure-

thral lumen. However, this is somewhat illogical because these detrusor fibers are the ones that contract during micturition. This would therefore act to close the internal meatus and retard efficient emptying. If this area had a different autonomic innervation, however, reciprocal activity of the dome and base would be possible, and there is evidence that this is the case (2). Nevertheless, these fibers, along with the urinary trigone, form the thickened musculature described as the bladder base.

Trigonal Muscle

In the fetus, a separate trigonal primordium leads to a specialized smooth muscle body that exists in the base of the bladder and in the vesical neck and also extends down into the urethra (Fig. 1.1). It consists of three portions (3,4): the urinary trigone, the trigonal ring, and the trigonal plate. The urinary trigone is a triangular body of smooth muscle that has its

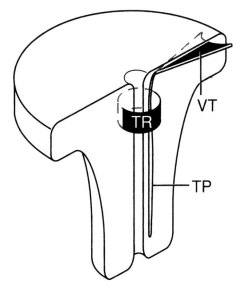

FIG. 1.1. Schematic diagram of the trigonal musculature within the bladder base and urethra (cut in sagittal section). TP, trigonal plate; TR, trigonal ring; VT, vesical trigone. (From DeLancey JOL. Anatomy and embryology of the lower urinary tract. *Obstet Gynecol Clin North Am* 1989;16:717–729, with permission.)

apices at the internal urinary meatus and the two ureteral orifices. It is slightly elevated above the rest of the detrusor musculature and can be seen cystoscopically, which aids in locating the internal orifices. At the level of the internal urinary meatus, this trigonal musculature spreads out to form a ring at the level of the internal urinary meatus. This ring can be seen surrounding the urethral lumen in the area of the vesical neck. Extending below the level of the trigonal ring is the trigonal plate, which is a column of trigonal tissue extending along the length of the urethra in its dorsal aspect. It lies between the ends of the striated urogenital sphincter.

The urinary trigone and trigonal ring lie within the area where α-adrenergically innervated muscle within the bladder base and vesical neck have previously been identified (2). It is anatomically plausible that this may be the α-adrenergically innervated tissue believed to be important to vesical neck closure, although large-section histochemistry has not been done to localize these receptors. That the trigonal ring might function to close the proximal urethra is suggested by its anatomic location in that area of the vesical neck that relaxes after denervation of this region. Such relaxation is seen in cases of myelodysplasia. This structure needs further study to confirm this functional association.

Urethra

The urethra is a complex muscular tube, and its structure has been described in detail by a number of authors (4–6). It extends below the lower border of the bladder base. As mentioned previously, the wall of the urethra begins some 15% of total urethral length below the beginning of the urethral lumen (7).

The urethra is a hollow tube, about 3 to 4 cm in length, whose wall comprises a series of layers (Fig. 1.2). The outermost layer is the striated urogenital sphincter muscle, which has sometimes been called the striated circular muscle, striated sphincter, or rhabdosphincter. This striated muscle surrounds a thin circular layer of smooth muscle that in turn surrounds a longitudinal layer of smooth muscle. Lying between the smooth muscle and the mucosa of the urethra is a submucosa that is unusually rich in its vascular supply.

Striated Urogenital Sphincter Muscle

Descriptions of the striated urogenital sphincter muscle in female patients have frequently been in error because the urethra had been removed to examine it. Studies by Oelrich (8), however, have corrected many previous misconceptions about this area and agree with functional observations of this region.

The striated urogenital sphincter has two different portions: an upper sphincteric portion and a lower archlike pair of muscular bands (Fig. 1.3). Fibers in the sphincteric portion are circular in orientation and occupy the upper two thirds of the body of this muscle, surrounding the urethral lumen in the region from about 20% to 60% of its length. This portion is called the sphincter urethrae and corresponds to the rhabdosphincter described by previous authors (9). Fibers in this region do not form a complete circle, and the gap between its two ends is bridged by the trigonal plate, which completes the circle. The defect in the muscular ring does not impair contraction because the trigonal ring functions as a tendon, bridging the gap between the muscles on its two ends.

The second portion of the striated urogenital sphincter occupies its distal one third, lying adjacent to the urethral lumen for about 60% to 80% of its length. It consists of two straplike bands of striated muscle, which arch over the ventral surface of the urethra. One of these bands originates in the vaginal wall and is called the urethrovaginal sphincter muscle. The other band of muscle, which originates near the ischiopubic ramus, is called the compressor urethrae. These two bands overlap around the ventral surface of the urethra and are separate only in their more lateral projections. In the past, this muscle was referred to as the deep transverse perineal muscle, and previous illustrations of this muscle have fre-

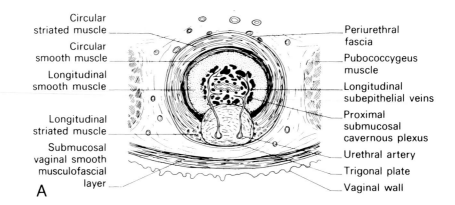

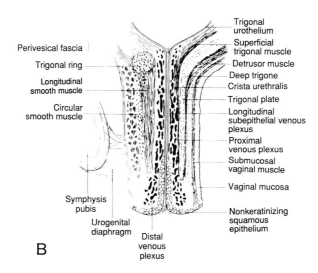

FIG. 1.2. Cross-sectional (**A**) and sagittal (**B**) schematic diagrams of the urethral structures. (From Asmussen M, Miller A. *Clinical gynaecological urology.* Oxford: Blackwell Scientific Publications, 1983:9, with permission.)

quently been inaccurate, leading to confusion about its role in continence.

All three portions of the striated urogenital sphincter muscle are part of the same muscle group and function as a unit. There has been considerable controversy over whether they are somatically or autonomically innervated, and evidence suggests that their innervation is complex. The fibers within this muscle are primarily slow-twitch muscle (10) and therefore are well suited to maintain constant tone while retaining the ability to contract when additional occlusive force is needed.

Contraction of the striated urogenital sphincter muscle would constrict the lumen of the urethra in its upper portion and compress its ventral wall in the lower one third. The importance of this muscle is that it provides the backup continence mechanism in 50% of continent women with an incompetent vesicle neck (11). It probably also functions during times when the bladder is full and detrusor pressure rises, when a woman must contract her pelvic floor until she can urinate. The importance of this muscle is demonstrated by the occurrence of stress

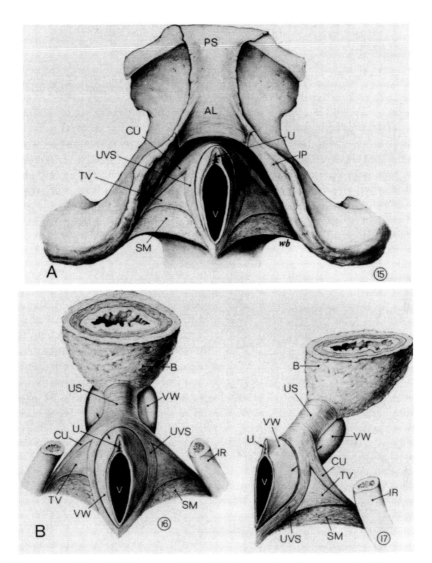

FIG. 1.3. Drawings of the striated urogenital sphincter muscle after removal of the perineal membrane. **A:** Pubic bones intact. **B:** Pubic bones removed. AL, arcuate pubic ligament; B, bladder; CU, compressor urethrae; IP, ischiopubic ramus; IR, ischial ramus; PS, pubic symphysis; SM, smooth muscle; TV, transverse vaginae muscle; U, urethra; US, urethral sphincter; UVS, urethrovaginal sphincter; V, vaginal orifice; VW, vaginal wall. (From Oelrich TM. The striated urogenital sphincter muscle in the female. *Anat Rec* 1983;205:223–232. Copyright © 1983 John Wiley & Sons, Inc. Reprinted with permission.)

urinary incontinence after radical vulvectomy, when the distal urethra containing the compressor urethra and urethrovaginal sphincter is excised. These patients have no change in resting urethral pressure or urethral support, but they develop stress or total incontinence after excision that includes this musculature (12).

Smooth Muscle

As previously mentioned, the smooth muscle of the urethra arises as a separate embryologic primordium (3). Although contiguous with the detrusor muscle, it is not, as is sometimes described, simply a downward extension of bladder muscle.

There are two distinct smooth muscle layers in the urethra (Fig. 1.4). The circular muscle of the urethra is poorly developed and difficult to identify. It is adjacent to the trigonal ring and extends below it, but as previously mentioned, the embryologic derivations of these two tissues seem different. The longitudinal muscle that lies inside this, however, is well developed and has considerable bulk. It is not continuous with the detrusor musculature as is sometimes described but does extend to the level of the trigonal ring (4). It

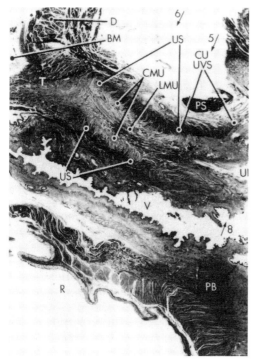

FIG. 1.4. Sagittal section from a 29-year-old cadaver. Cut just lateral to the midline and not quite parallel to it. The section contains tissue nearer the midline in the distal urethra, where the lumen can be seen, than at the vesical neck. BM, bladder mucosa; CMU, circular smooth muscle of the urethra; CU, compressor urethrae; D, detrusor muscle; LMU, longitudinal smooth muscles of the urethra; PB, perineal body; PS, pubic symphysis; R, rectum; T, trigonal ring; UL, urethral lumen; US, urethral sphincter; UVS, urethrovaginal sphincter; V, vagina. (From DeLancey JOL. Correlative study of paraurethral anatomy. *Obstet Gynecol* 1986;68:91–97, with permission.)

probably functions to shorten the urethra during micturition.

Submucosal Vasculature

The prominence of the submucosal urethral vasculature is remarkable (13). This has been studied by Huisman (4), who found it to be a highly organized arteriovenous complex capable of specific filling and emptying. Although it is difficult to study so small a vascular plexus, Rud and colleagues (14) found that clamping the arterial supply to the urethra significantly decreases resting urethral pressure. This vascular bed empties when the urethral pressure rises, and its function, therefore, might be to act like an inflatable cushion, filling the area within the urethral wall and the mucosa at rest and helping to form a hermetic seal. When the urethral musculature contracts, constricting the lumen, the vascular bed may empty as a result. At these times of increased muscular activity, the vasculature would be of less importance.

Glands

A series of glands is found in the submucosa, primarily along the dorsal (vaginal) surface of the urethra (15) (Fig. 1.5). These glands are concentrated mainly in the lower and middle thirds and vary in number. The location of urethral diverticula, which are derived from cystic dilation of these glands, follows this distribution, being most common distally and usually originating along the dorsal surface of the urethra. In addition, their origin within the submucosa indicates that the fascia of the urethra must be stretched and attenuated over a diverticulum. Reapproximation of this layer after removal of these lesions is therefore necessary.

Epithelium

The urethra is lined by hormonally sensitive epithelium (4,16). In the distal urethra, there is a stratified squamous epithelium; in

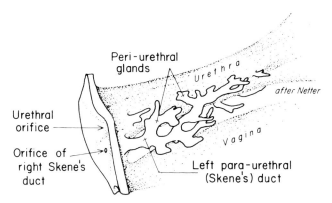

FIG. 1.5. The urethra and periurethral glands. (Redrawn with permission from *The Ciba collection of medical illustrations,* Vol. 6. Copyright © 1973.)

the bladder, as previously mentioned, the epithelium is a transitional type. The line of demarcation between these two epithelia varies depending on the hormonal status of the individual and other undefined factors. It can occur in the midurethra, as it does postmenopausally, or may extend well up into the bladder during the reproductive years. It is not uncommon during the reproductive years to have an area of stratified squamous epithelium covering the urinary trigone.

Topography

The continence mechanism consists of several structures, and their overall arrangement is displayed in Fig. 1.6. The first 15% of the urethra is that portion of the urethral lumen that passes through the bladder base. As previously mentioned, it is surrounded in this region by the trigonal ring and the detrusor musculature. Below this intramural region lies the midportion of the urethra that extends from 20% to 60% of the total urethral length. In this location is found the sphincteric portion of the striated urogenital sphincter muscle and the circular and longitudinal smooth muscle. Below this area (from 60% to 80%), the urethra encounters a region just above the perineal membrane (urogenital diaphragm) where the compressor urethrae and urethrovaginal sphincter portions of the striated urogenital sphincter

are found. The distal urethra includes the distal one fifth of the total urethral length, ending at the external urinary meatus. It is primarily fibrous and includes the urethral labia. It functions to aim the urine stream and therefore acts as a nozzle rather than as part of the continence mechanism.

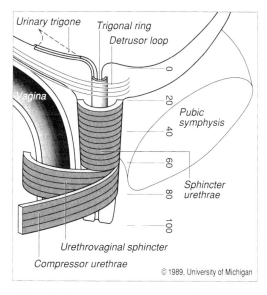

FIG. 1.6. Diagrammatic representation showing the component parts of the internal and external sphincteric mechanisms and their locations. The sphincter urethrae, urethrovaginal sphincter, and compressor urethrae are all parts of the striated urogenital sphincter muscle.

PELVIC FLOOR

Vesical Neck Support and Mobility

The previous sections of this chapter dealt with the components of the lower urinary tract. Studies of patients with stress incontinence revealed that this system cannot function optimally unless it is supported by the pelvic floor. The muscles and connective tissue of the pelvic floor must create an environment in which the urethra, vesical neck, and bladder can function effectively. Conversely, normal support alone is not enough to ensure continence. A woman's ability to remain continent, therefore, results from a combination of normal activity of the vesical neck and urethra and normal function of the pelvic floor. Neither of these two components alone can maintain continence. It has been shown that there is no one-to-one relationship between urethral support and stress continence (17) and that a patient with a poorly functioning vesical neck may have stress incontinence despite normal urethral support (18). Thus, urethral support is not the only factor involved in continence.

Previous studies based on anatomic dissection have emphasized an inert fibrous attachment of the urethra to the lower portion of the pubic bones, usually termed the posterior pubourethral ligaments (19). Such a ligamentous connection would imply that the urethra is firmly and immovably attached to the pubic bones. Further studies of the broader relationship between the urethra and the pelvic floor have shown, however, that it is only the distal one third of the urethra that is fixed in position; the upper two thirds are mobile. This distal portion is where the urethra is attached to the pubic bones by the perineal membrane (urogenital diaphragm) and by the lower portions of the striated urogenital sphincter.

Additionally, in normal, standing individuals (20), the vesical neck lies significantly above the level at which the posterior pubourethral ligaments insert into the pubic bones (Fig. 1.7), indicating that it would not be possible for these tissues to support the proximal urethra and vesical neck. Women

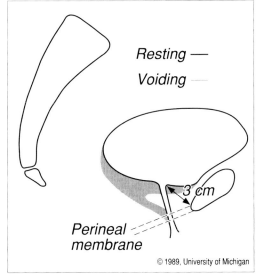

FIG. 1.7. Topography and mobility of the normal proximal urethra and vesical neck based on resting and voiding radiographs in normal women. (From Elbadawi A. Neuromuscular mechanisms of continence. In: Yalla SV, McGuire EJ, Elbadawi A, et al., eds. *Neurourology and urodynamics.* New York: Macmillan, 1989:3–35 and Noll LE, Hutch JA. The SCIPP line: an aid in interpreting the voiding lateral cystourethrogram. *Obstet Gynecol* 1969;33:680–689, with permission.)

can allow the vesical neck to descend at the onset of micturition by relaxing the levator ani muscles (21), thereby obliterating the posterior urethrovesical angle (2) and demonstrating that the position of the lower urinary tract is under voluntary control. Furthermore, recent electrophysiologic studies demonstrated that patients with stress incontinence have evidence of neuromuscular damage, again suggesting that the pelvic floor musculature plays a role in maintaining continence (22–25). Therefore, our understanding of urethral support must encompass more than the attachment of the endopelvic fascia to bone.

Urethra and Pelvic Floor

As previously mentioned, fluoroscopic examination of the urethra reveals that the distal portion is fixed in position and the proximal urethra is mobile (26). The point of inflection between these areas has been called the "knee" of the urethra. It lies at 56% of urethral length, at the point where the urethra comes into relation to the perineal membrane (7).

Perineal Membrane

The fixation of the distal urethra occurs because of its attachment to the pubic bones through the perineal membrane (urogenital diaphragm). The perineal membrane is a sheet of connective tissue that spans the region between the ischiopubic rami. It consists primarily of a sheet of fibrous connective tissue. The compressor urethrae and urethrovaginal sphincter muscles lie just above it, as does a variable amount of smooth muscle (8). The important attachments of the distal urethra occur immediately adjacent to the urethra and not posteriorly from the rest of the perineal membrane, as can be appreciated from the fact that the pubic bones can be easily palpated on either side of the urethra without any intervening connective tissue membrane. The pictures commonly used to illustrate the "urogenital diaphragm," which show two fascial layers separated by a transverse layer of muscle, are unfortunately incorrect. They have been copied without confirmation from a source more than 100 years old (27), despite a previous description that is more accurate (28).

Support of the Proximal Urethra

Because a woman can voluntarily control the position of her proximal urethra above the perineal membrane, one would expect that the support of the urethra includes voluntary muscle as well as inert connective tissue elements. This is, in fact, what examination of this region reveals. To understand this area, one must remember that the urethra and vagina are not separate structures. Because of their common derivation from the urogenital sinus (5), they are fused in the distal two thirds of the urethra. In this region, they are bound together by the endopelvic connective tissue so that the support of the urethra depends not only on the attachments of the urethra to adjacent structures but also on the connection of the vagina and periurethral tissues to the muscles and fasciae of the pelvic wall.

Some review of the anatomy of the space of Retzius is helpful in understanding urethral support (29). On either side of the pelvis, there is a band of fibers attached at one end to the lower one sixth of the pubic bone, 1 cm from the midline, and at the other to the ischial spine (Figs. 1.8 and 1.9). This is the arcus tendineus fasciae pelvis. In its anterior portion, this band lies on the inner surface of the levator ani muscles, which arise some 3 cm above the arcus tendineus fasciae pelvis. Posteriorly, the levator ani arises from a second arcus, the arcus tendineus fasciae levatoris ani, which fuses with the arcus tendineus fasciae pelvis near the spine. It is the lateral attachment of the endopelvic fascia that supports the urethra and bladder (pubocervical fascia). This structure, which has previously been described as the posterior pubourethral ligament, represents the most ventral portion of the arcus tendineus fasciae pelvis and the fascial attachment of the endopelvic fascia. It is also an attachment of the perineal membrane (30).

A number of structures, therefore, including both striated muscle and connective tissue, are important to urethral support. Because of this, we refer to the group of structures that collectively determine the position of the vesical neck as the urethral support system. This system includes the medial portion of the levator ani muscles, the arcus tendineus fasciae pelvis, and the endopelvic fascia.

The endopelvic fascia, in which the urethra and anterior vaginal wall are embedded, has two lateral attachments that participate in urethral support (Fig. 1.10), a fascial attachment and a muscular attachment. The fascial attachment of the urethral support connects the periurethral tissues and anterior vaginal wall to the arcus tendineus fasciae pelvis (Fig. 1.11) and has been called the paravaginal fas-

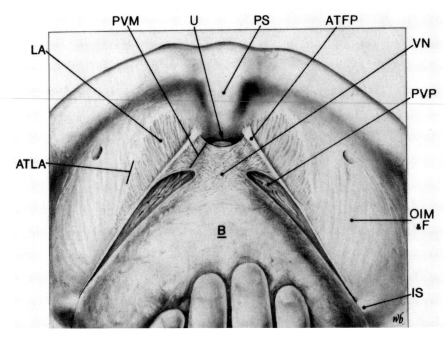

FIG. 1.8. Space of Retzius (drawn from cadaver dissection). Pubovesical muscle (PVM) can be seen going from vesical neck (VN) to arcus tendineus fasciae pelvis (ATFP) and running over the parau-rethral vascular plexus (PVP). ATLA, arcus tendineus levator ani; B, bladder; IS, ischial spine; LA, le-vator ani muscles; OIM&F, obturator internus muscle and fascia; PS, pubic symphysis; U, urethra. (From DeLancey JOL. Pubovesical ligament: a separate structure from the urethral supports [pubo-urethral ligaments]. *Neurourol Urodynam* 1989;8:53–61. Copyright © 1989 John Wiley & Sons, Inc. Reprinted with permission of Wiley-Liss, Inc., a division of John Wiley & Sons, Inc.)

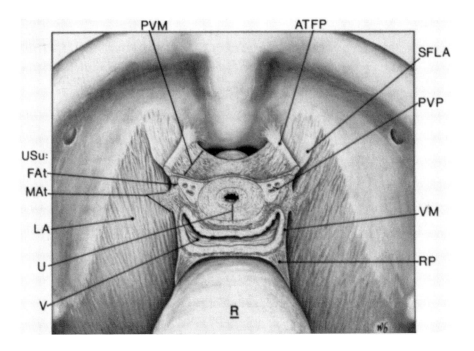

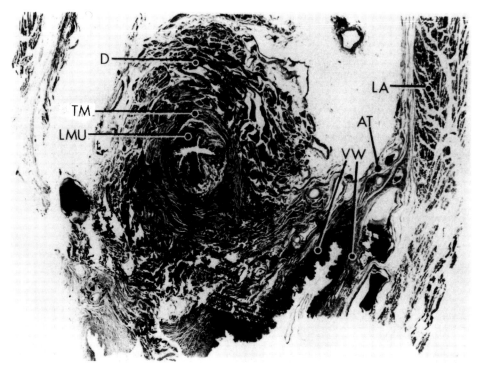

FIG. 1.10. Cross-section of the vesical neck and pelvic wall showing the connection of the vaginal wall (VW) and its surrounding endopelvic fascia to the arcus tendineus and thereby to the fascia over the levator ani (LA). AT, arcus tendineus fasciae pelvis; D, detrusor muscles; LMU, longitudinal smooth muscle; TM, trigonal muscle (trigonal ring portion).

cial attachment by Richardson and co-workers (31). The muscular attachments, on the other hand, connect this same periurethral endopelvic fascia to the medial border of the levator ani muscle (Fig. 1.11) (29). This attachment is primarily to the endopelvic fascia of the vagina, and that portion of the levator ani muscle between the pubic bone and vagina is called the pubovaginalis. [It was also referred to as the vaginolevator attachment in a previous work (7).]

This connection of the levator ani muscles to the endopelvic fascia surrounding the vagina and urethra allows the normal resting tone of the levators (32) to maintain the retropubic position of the vesical neck. When the muscle relaxes at the onset of micturition, this allows the vesical neck to rotate downward to the limit of the elasticity of the fascial attachments. Contraction at the end of urination allows the vesical neck to resume its normal position.

FIG. 1.9. Cross-section of the urethra (U), vagina (V), arcus tendineus fasciae pelvis (ATFP), and superior fascia of levator ani (SFLA) just below the vesical neck (drawn from cadaver dissection). Pubovesical muscles (PVM) lie anterior to urethra and anterior and superior to paraurethral vascular plexus (PVP). The urethral supports (USu) (the pubourethral ligaments) attach the vagina and vaginal surface of the urethra to the levator ani muscles (MAt, muscular attachment) and to the superior fascia of the levator ani (FAt, fascial attachment). R, rectum; RP, rectal pillar; VM, vaginal wall muscularis. (From DeLancey JOL. Pubovesical ligament: a separate structure from the urethral supports (pubo-urethral ligaments). *Neurourol Urodynam* 1989;8:53–61. Copyright © 1989 John Wiley & Sons, Inc. Reprinted with permission of Wiley-Liss, Inc., a division of John Wiley & Sons, Inc.)

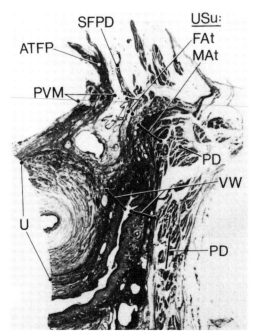

FIG. 1.11. Cross-section of the urethra (U), vaginal wall (VW), and pelvic diaphragm (levator ani) (PD) from the right half of the pelvis taken just below the vesical neck at approximately the same level shown in Fig. 1.9. The pubovesical muscles (PVM) can be seen anterior to the urethra and attach to the arcus tendineus fasciae pelvis (ATFP). Urethral supports (USu) run underneath (dorsal to) the urethra and vessels. Some of its fibers (MAt) attach to the muscle of the levator ani (LA), whereas others (FAt) are derived from the vaginal wall (VW) and vaginal surface of the urethra (U) and attach to the superior fascia of the levator ani (SFLA). (From Milley PS, Nichols DH. Relationship between the pubo-urethral ligaments and the urogenital diaphragm in the human female. *Anat Rec* 1971;170:281–283. Copyright © 1983 John Wiley & Sons, Inc. Reprinted with permission.)

The way in which the urethral support system contributes to stress continence can be understood best by viewing the supportive mechanism from the side (Fig. 1.12). The urethra can be seen to lie in a hammock-like layer composed of the endopelvic fascia and anterior vaginal wall. This layer is stabilized by its lateral attachments to the arcus tendineus fascia pelvic and to the medial margin of the levator ani muscles.

During increases in abdominal pressure, the downward force created by increased abdominal pressure on the ventral surface of the urethra compresses the urethra closed against the hammock-like supportive layer (Fig. 1.13). The stability of the fascial layer determines the effectiveness of this closure mechanism in opposing rises in abdominal pressure. If the layer is unyielding, it forms a firm backstop against which the urethra can be compressed closed, but if it is unstable, the effectiveness of this closure is compromised. The integrity of the attachment to the arcus tendineus and to the levator ani is critical to the stress continence mechanism. Kinesthesiologic electromyogram recordings of pelvic floor muscle timing showed that the levator ani muscles contract during a cough. This contraction would elevate the urethral supports, not only stabilizing the supportive hammock against abdominal pressure but also adding to the forces favoring urethral closure during times of increased abdominal pressure.

The muscular attachment between the levator ani muscle and the endopelvic fascia is responsible for the voluntary control of vesical neck position visible on vaginal examination or fluoroscopic visualization when the pelvic muscles are contracted and relaxed. Relaxation of these muscles with descent of the vesical neck is associated with the initiation of urination, and their contraction is associated with arrest of the urinary stream. The limit of downward vesical neck motion is determined by the limit of connective tissue elasticity in the attachments to the arcus tendineus fasciae pelvis.

Also embedded within the endopelvic connective tissue in this region are the pubovesical muscles, which are extensions of the detrusor muscle (29,33,34) (Figs. 1.9 and 1.11). They lie within some connective tissue, and when both muscular and fibrous elements are considered together, they are called the pubovesical ligaments in much the same way that the smooth muscle and connective tissue of the ligamentum teres is referred to as the round ligament. Although the terms pubovesical ligament and pubourethral ligament are

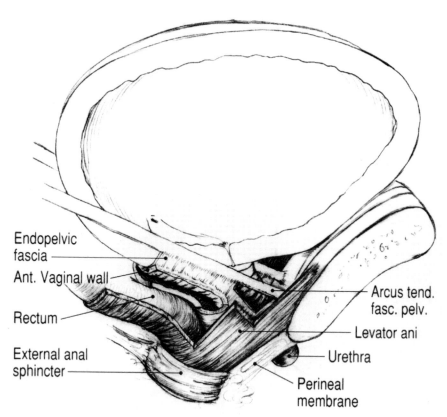

FIG. 1.12. Lateral view of the urethral supportive mechanism transected just lateral to the midline. The lateral wall of the vagina and a portion of the endopelvic fascia have been removed to see deeper structures. (From DeLancey JOL. Structural support of the urethra as it relates to stress urinary incontinence: the hammock hypothesis. *Am J Obstet Gynecol* 1994;170:1713–1720, with permission.)

sometimes considered to be synonymous, the pubovesical ligaments are only one aspect of the connective tissue and muscle that may influence continence, and they lie in a separate location from the rest of the urethral supportive tissues (29). It is not surprising, therefore, that these detrusor fibers found in the pubovesical muscles are no different in patients with stress incontinence than in those without this condition (35). The actual supportive tissues of the urethra, as described earlier, are easily separated from the pubovesical ligament by a prominent vascular plexus. Rather than supporting the urethra, the pubovesical muscles may be responsible for assisting in vesical neck opening, as some have suggested (36).

The relationship between urethral support and sphincteric function is a complex one. Miniaturized pressure transducers have permitted us to record highly localized pressures both at rest and during the rapid sequence of events that occur during a cough. A number of authors have noted that these recordings vary depending on which direction the transducer is oriented. Although this is usually considered to be artifact, it reflects the unequal forces that are applied by the supportive tissues of the urethra and the distal portion of the striated urogenital sphincter (37).

These pressure recordings also reveal a significant increase in intraurethral pressure during a cough. These urethral pressure responses have been ascribed to the transmis-

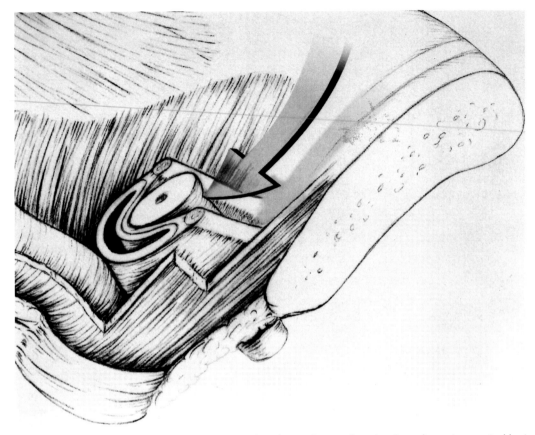

FIG. 1.13. The urethral support system seen after the urethra and vagina have been transected just below the vesical neck. The *arrow* represents the force generated by increased abdominal pressure. (From DeLancey JOL. Structural support of the urethra as it relates to stress urinary incontinence: the hammock hypothesis. *Am J Obstet Gynecol* 1994;170:1713–1720, with permission.)

sion of abdominal pressure to the intraabdominal portion of the urethra. Anatomically, it is not clear what separates the abdominal from the extraabdominal urethra. Examination of sagittal sections of the urethra (Fig. 1.4) reveals no structure that the urethra pierces to exit the abdomen, and the entire length of the urethra is separated from the visible lumen of the vagina only by the vaginal wall.

The several structures of the pelvic floor that surround the urethra and attach it to its surrounding bony and muscular supports are the active contracting floor that creates the environment of the urethra and vesical neck. Rather than an inert bottom of the abdominal cavity, they are a functioning unit that plays a role in continence. If the passive transmission of intraabdominal pressure to the urethra were the only factor involved in incontinence, pressures during a cough would be maximal in the proximal urethra. Measurements, however, reveal that the distal urethra has the highest-pressure elevations (38,39). This occurs from 60% to 80% of the urethral length in the region where the compressor urethrae and urethrovesical sphincter are located, suggesting that contraction of these muscles during a cough augments urethral pressure in this region. These pressures frequently exceed intraabdominal pressure, indicating that factors other than abdominal pressure play a role (40). In addition, these pressure rises precede the rise in cough pressure, demonstrating that

TABLE 1.1. *Hypotheses concerning function of the urinary continence mechanism elements*

Structure	Hypothetical function
Proximal urethral support	
Connection to levator ani	Tonic contraction maintains high position of vesical neck and contracts during cough to support vesical neck. Relaxes to change position of vesical neck to facilitate micturition.
Connection to arcus tendineus	Assists levators in support and limits the downward excursion of the vesical neck when the levators are relaxed or overcome during cough.
Pubovesical muscles	May facilitate vesical neck opening by pulling on vesical neck when levators relax.
Perineal membrane	Fixes distal urethra to pubic bones.
Internal sphincteric mechanism	
Trigonal ring, detrusor loop, and elastic tissue	Maintains vesical neck closure at rest and is necessary in addition to normal support for continence during cough.
Extrinsic sphincteric mechanism	
Striated urogenital sphincter and circular smooth muscle	Resting tone contributes to resting urethral pressure, and contraction prevents incontinence when marginally compensated proximal mechanism leaks.
Longitudinal smooth muscle	Contracts during micturition to shorten the urethra.
Submucosal vasculature	Fills the space within the muscular tube to maintain a watertight seal.

the pelvic floor muscles are contracting in preparation for the cough (40). This does not imply that abdominal pressure is an unimportant influence on urethral pressure during a cough, but it does raise the question of how the pelvic floor causes this to occur. The fact that stress incontinence persists in some patients despite adequate suspension of the urethra further supports the need to expand our concept of the urethra's response to a cough. Furthermore, recent studies demonstrated the importance of denervation of the pelvic floor to the problem of stress urinary incontinence and genital prolapse (23–25). This opens a new area of investigation that may prove helpful in further understanding the relationship of structure and function in the mechanism of urinary continence.

In summary, evolution has placed a number of structures in and around the lower urinary tract. Each may play some role in either storage or evacuation of urine (Table 1.1). Our understanding of lower urinary tract function depends on knowing the structure and function of each of these individual parts. No one structure is solely responsible for the proper functioning of this region, and future progress in better defining the exact nature of diseases of the lower urinary tract will come from ex-

amination of both the structures of this region and their function.

REFERENCES

1. Jeffcoate TNA, Roberts H. Observations on stress incontinence of urine. *Am J Obstet Gynecol* 1952;64: 721–738.
2. Elbadawi A. Neuromuscular mechanisms of continence. In: Yalla SV, McGuire EJ, Elbadawi A, et al., eds. *Neurourology and urodynamics.* New York: Macmillan, 1989:3–35.
3. Droes JTPM. Observations on the musculature of the urinary bladder and urethra in the human foetus. *Br J Urol* 1974;46:179–185.
4. Huisman AB. Aspects on the anatomy of the female urethra with special relation to urinary continence. *Contrib Gynecol Obstet* 1983;10:1–31.
5. Krantz KE. The anatomy of the urethra and anterior vaginal wall. *Am J Obstet Gynecol* 1951;62:374–386.
6. Ricci J, Lisa JR, Thom CH. The female urethra: a histologic study as an aid in urethral surgery. *Am J Surg* 1950;79:499–505.
7. DeLancey JOL. Correlative study of paraurethral anatomy. *Obstet Gynecol* 1986;68:91–97.
8. Oelrich TM. The striated urogenital sphincter muscle in the female. *Anat Rec* 1983;205:223–232.
9. Gosling JA. The structure of the female lower urinary tract and pelvic floor. *Urol Clin North Am* 1985;12: 207–214.
10. Gosling JA, Dixon JS, Critchley HOD, et al. A comparative study of the human external sphincter and periurethral levator ani muscles. *Br J Urol* 1981;53:35–41.
11. Versi E, Cardozo LD, Studd JWW, et al. Internal urinary sphincter in maintenance of female continence. *Br Med J* 1986;292:166–167.
12. Reid GC, DeLancey JOL, Hopkins MP, et al. Urinary

incontinence and radical vulvectomy. *Obstet Gynecol* 1990;75:852–858.

13. Berkow SG. The corpus spongiosum of the urethra: its possible role in urinary control and stress incontinence in women. *Am J Obstet Gynecol* 1953;65:346–351.

14. Rud T, Anderson KE, Asmussen M, et al. Factors maintaining the intraurethral pressure in women. *Invest Urol* 1980;17:343–347.

15. Huffman J. Detailed anatomy of the paraurethral ducts in the adult human female. *Am J Obstet Gynecol* 1948; 55:86–101.

16. Smith P. Age changes in the female urethra. *Br J Urol* 1972;44:667–676.

17. Fantl AJ, Hurt WG, Bump RC, et al. Urethral axis and sphincteric function. *Am J Obstet Gynecol* 1986;155: 554–558.

18. McGuire EJ. Urodynamic findings in patients after failure of stress incontinence operations. *Prog Clin Biol Res* 1981;78:351–360.

19. Zacharin RF. The anatomic supports of the female urethra. *Obstet Gynecol* 1968;21:754–759.

20. Noll LE, Hutch JA. The SCIPP line: an aid in interpreting the voiding lateral cystourethrogram. *Obstet Gynecol* 1969;33:680–689.

21. Muellner SR. Physiology of micturition. *J Urol* 1951; 65:805–810.

22. Snooks SJ, Swash M. Abnormalities of the innervation of the urethral striated sphincter in incontinence. *Br J Urol* 1984;56:401–406.

23. Snooks SJ, Badenoch DF, Tiptaft RC, et al. Perineal nerve damage in genuine stress urinary incontinence: an electrophysiological study. *Br J Urol* 1985;57: 422–426.

24. Smith ARB, Hosker GL, Warrell DW. The role of pudendal nerve damage in the aetiology of genuine stress urinary incontinence of urine. *Br J Obstet Gynaecol* 1989;96:29–32.

25. Smith ARB, Hosker GL, Warrell DW. The role of partial denervation of the pelvic floor in the etiology of genitourinary prolapse and stress incontinence of urine: a neurophysiological study. *Br J Obstet Gynaecol* 1989; 96:24–28.

26. Westby M, Asmussen M, Ulmsten U. Location of maximum intraurethral pressure related to urogenital di-

aphragm in the female subject as studied by simultaneous urethrocystometry and voiding urethrocystography. *Am J Obstet Gynecol* 1982;144:408–412.

27. Henle J. *Handbuch der systematischen Anatomie des Menschen.* Bd. II. Braunschweig: Friedrich Vieweg und Sohn, 1883.

28. Luschka H. *Die Anatomie des menschlichen Beckens.* Tubingen: Laupp and Siebeck, 1864.

29. DeLancey JOL. Pubovesical ligament: a separate structure from the urethral supports (pubo-urethral ligaments). *Neurourol Urodynam* 1989;8:53–61.

30. Milley PS, Nichols DH. Relationship between the pubourethral ligaments and the urogenital diaphragm in the human female. *Anat Rec* 1971;170:281–283.

31. Richardson AC, Edmonds PB, Williams NL. Treatment of stress urinary incontinence due to paravaginal fascial defect. *Obstet Gynecol* 1981;57:357–362.

32. Parks AG, Porter NH, Melzak J. Experimental study of the reflex mechanism controlling muscles of the pelvic floor. *Dis Colon Rectum* 1962;5:407–414.

33. Gil Vernet S. *Morphology and function of the vesico-prostato-urethral musculature.* Treviso: Edizioni Canova, 1968.

34. Woodburne RT. Anatomy of the bladder and bladder outlet. *J Urol* 1968;100:474–487.

35. Wilson PD, Dixon JS, Brown ADG, et al. Posterior pubo-urethral ligaments in normal and genuine stress incontinent women. *J Urol* 1983;130:802–805.

36. Power RMH. An anatomical contribution to the problem of continence and incontinence in the female. *Am J Obstet Gynecol* 1954;67:302–314.

37. DeLancey JOL. Structural aspects of the extrinsic continence mechanism. *Obstet Gynecol* 1988;72:296–301.

38. Constantinou CE. Resting and stress urethral pressures as a clinical guide to the mechanism of continence in the female patient. *Urol Clin North Am* 1985;12: 247–258.

39. Hilton P, Stanton SL. Urethral pressure measurement by microtransducer: the results in symptom-free women and in those with genuine stress incontinence. *Br J Obstet Gynaecol* 1983;90:919–933.

40. Constantinou CE, Govan DE. Spatial distribution and timing of transmitted and reflexly generated urethral pressures in healthy women. *J Urol* 1982;127:964–969.

Ostergard's Urogynecology and Pelvic Floor Dysfunction, Fifth Edition. edited by A.E. Bent, et al.
Lippincott Williams & Wilkins, Philadelphia © 2003.

2

Anatomy of Pelvic Support

Robert M. Rogers, Jr.

*Department of Obstetrics and Gynecolgy, The Reading Hospital and Medical Center,
West Reading, Pennsylvania*

The pelvic visceral support system is anatomically located between the parietal peritoneum and the parietal fascia covering the muscular basin of the female pelvis. The purpose of this support system is to maintain the spatial relationships of the cervix and vagina, bladder and urethra, and rectum and anal canal with each other within the confines of the pelvis. These organs primarily function in storage, distention, and evacuation and must maintain their normal anatomic relationships in order to sustain their normal physiologic functions.

In the normal nulliparous standing female patient, the bladder, the upper two-thirds of the vagina, and the rectum are oriented in a more horizontal axis, especially with increased pelvic pressures. The levator plate of the pelvic floor parallels these organs and provides a muscular dynamic backstop for them. This orientation is crucial in preventing pelvic organ prolapse. When the upper portion of the vagina is in its normal position, the cervix is found at the level of the ischial spines. The posterior vaginal fornix extends over the coccyx posteriorly, the lower sacrum medially, and the sacrospinous ligaments laterally.

In important contrast, the urethra, the distal one-third of the vagina, and the anal canal are more vertical in orientation. Each measures 3 to 4 cm in length. These lower pelvic structures are supported by the perineal body and the urogenital and anal triangles of the perineum. When these normal anatomic relationships are disrupted, physiologic dysfunction,

such as urinary and fecal incontinence and vaginal prolapse, occurs frequently (Fig. 2.1).

The pelvic visceral support system consists of visceral connective tissues that surround and mechanically support the pelvic viscera and their supplying vasculature, nerves, and lymph nodes and channels. These visceral supports form a network from the pelvic brim along the upper sidewalls and back wall of the pelvis to the anatomic level of the ischial spine, where the network then proceeds horizontally in the standing patient to the obturator internus muscles laterally and the pubic bones and perineal body inferiorly. This support network is continuous and interdependent within the three-dimensional muscular pelvic basin. However, these visceral connective tissues vary in composition, thickness, strength, and elasticity, depending on the mechanical and physiologic support requirements in each particular location within the network.

The upper visceral supports to the cervix and upper vagina (cardinal ligament–uterosacral ligament complexes) are flexible suspensory "leashes," also called sheaths. The midpelvic horizontal supports of the pubocervical fascia and rectovaginal septum are denser tissues, or septa, for the purposes of central hammock support and lateral attachments to the muscular sidewalls in order to support the bladder and rectum. The lower pelvic support tissues are very strong and fuse with the parietal fascia of the pubococcygeus muscle and perineal body in order to stabilize the urethra, the lower third of the vagina, and

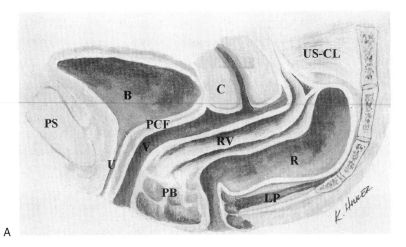

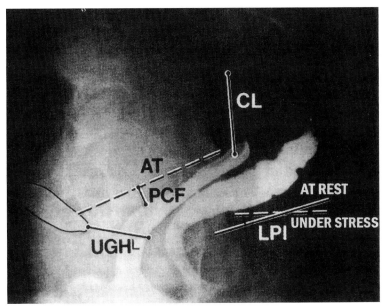

FIG. 2.1. A: Lateral view of pelvic structures. B, bladder; C, cervix; LP, levator plate; PB, perineal body; PCF, pubocervical fascia; PS, pubic symphysis; R, rectum; RV, rectovaginal septum (fascia); U, urethra; US-CL, uterosacral–cardinal ligament complex; V, vagina. **B:** Standing view of lateral radiograph of pelvis. AT, arcus tendineus fascia pelvis; CL, cardinal ligament; LPI, levator plate inclination (at rest—*solid line*; under stress—*dashed line*); PCF, pubocervical fascia; UGU^L, urogenital hiatus length. (**A** courtesy of Dr. Robert M. Rogers; **B** from DeLancey JOL. Vaginographic examination of the pelvic floor. *Int Urogynecol J Pelvic Floor Dysfunct* 1994;5:21, with permission.)

the anal canal. Ultimately, the visceral connective tissues and their leashes and septal attachments connect with the parietal fascia of the muscular pelvic basin, which is strongly attached to the bony pelvis (Fig. 2.2).

Parietal fascia is a mechanically dense matrix of connective tissue consisting of predominantly collagen fibers coalescing into thick bundles that are then interwoven into a strong, three-dimensional sheet (1). The vascular supply is limited, and active fibroblasts are few in number within this dense connective tissue. Parietal fascia covers the skeletal muscular basin within the pelvis.

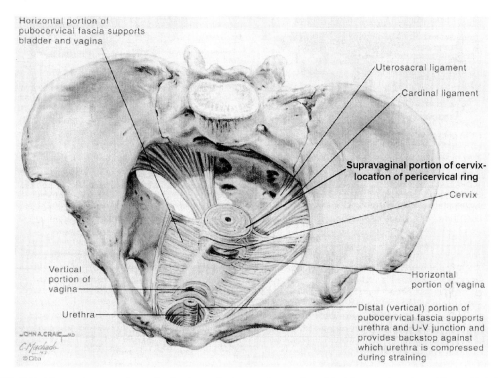

Horizontal portion of
pubocervical fascia supports
bladder and vagina

Uterosacral ligament

Cardinal ligament

**Supravaginal portion of cervix-
location of pericervical ring**

Cervix

Vertical
portion of
vagina

Horizontal
portion of vagina

Urethra

Distal (vertical) portion of
pubocervical fascia supports
urethra and U-V junction and
provides backstop against
which urethra is compressed
during straining

JOHN A. CRAIG

C. Machado

© Ciba

FIG. 2.2. Visceral supports and attachments to cervix, vagina, bladder, and rectum. (From Retzky SS, Rogers RM. Urinary incontinence in women. In: *Clinical symposia.* Summit, NJ: Ciba-Geigy Corp, 1995;47(3), adapted from Plate 3, p 7. Copyright © 1995 Icon Learning Systems, LLC. A subsidiary of MediMedia, USA, Inc. All rights reserved.)

In contrast, visceral fascia is a loose, three-dimensional meshwork of collagen, elastin, and smooth muscle with a richer vascular supply. This expansive meshwork contains a soft ground substance with different connective tissue cells deposited along its fibers. This visceral matrix surrounds and peripherally supports the viscera in both the abdominal and pelvic cavities. The visceral fascia is flexible and elastic, but only within limits. If this visceral connective tissue mechanically stretches beyond these limits, it breaks. Observations during reparative vaginal surgeries confirm the reality of these breaks. This finding of breaks in the pelvic visceral fascia is the key concept upon which our current understanding of pelvic support defects rests.

The pelvic visceral fascia, also known as endopelvic fascia, serves two important roles. The first is to suspend the viscera mechanically over the pelvic floor. In the standing female patient, the bladder, the upper two thirds of the vagina, and the rectum lie in a more horizontal axis over the muscular levator plate (2). This horizontal orientation creates a flap-valve mechanism that is critical for the prevention of vaginal prolapse (Fig. 2.1A). During increased intraabdominal pressure or Valsalva straining, the generated force pushes perpendicularly down against the longitudinal axis of the vagina and pelvic viscera. This force compresses these organs against the simultaneously contracting levator plate. The resulting entrapment, as well as contraction of the muscular levator hiatus, prevents organ prolapse.

The second purpose of the supporting visceral fascia is to function as flexible conduits and physical supports for the vasculature, visceral nerves, and lymph tissue that service the viscera. Function here can be divided into two broad categories: (a) the visceral fascial capsules, and (b) the supporting suspensory leashes and septal attachments (sheaths and septa) (3). Visceral fascial capsules envelop the bladder, urethra, cervix, vagina, rectum, and anal canal. They are intimately attached to the surrounding smooth muscle coat of each viscus. Within these capsules are contained the vasculature, visceral nerves, lymph nodes and channels, and adipose tissue (areolar tissue). The fascial covering of each hol-

low viscus provides support during storage, distention, and evacuation.

In addition, these visceral capsules serve as attachments for the visceral fascial sheaths and septa. These fascial structures envelop all the anatomic structures traveling to and from the pelvic viscera. In doing so, they connect

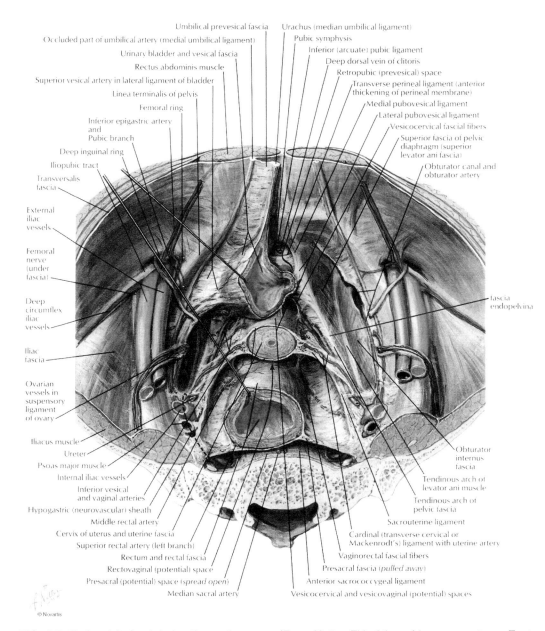

FIG. 2.3. Endopelvic fascial sheaths and spaces. (From Netter FH. *Atlas of human anatomy.* East Hanover, NJ: Novartis, 1997, Plate 341. Copyright © 1997 Icon Learning Systems, LLC. A subsidiary of MediMedia, USA, Inc. All rights reserved.)

the pelvic organs to the parietal fascia covering muscle and bone, anchoring them to the
pelvic walls—posterior, lateral, and anterior.
The endopelvic fascial sheaths and septa vary
in their strength, thickness, and composition,
depending on the support requirements of that
particular area within the pelvis (Fig. 2.3).

The integrity of the pelvic support network
is dependent on the elements that comprise
the pelvis: the bones, ligaments, muscles,
parietal fascia, and supporting visceral connecting tissue, as described (4). This chapter
first explains these elements individually. The
elements are then unified into the important
anatomic concepts that explain pelvic visceral
support. Mastery of this chapter will allow the
reader to evaluate pelvic support defects with
site-specific anatomic correlation. Peham and
Amreich stated in the preface to their book
published nearly 70 years ago, "It is recognized today, more than ever before, that a well
developed anatomic background is a requisite
for a successful operative experience" (5).

BONY PELVIS

The bony pelvis is the rigid outer shell
onto which the pelvic muscles and bony ligaments are attached. The hip bone, also
known as the coxal or innominate bone, ar-
ticulates posteriorly with the sacrum at the
sacroiliac joints and anteriorly with the other
pubic bone at the pubic symphysis. The
pelvis provides for weight bearing, locomo-
tion, and support for the pelvic organs and
accessory anatomic structures. In addition,
the pelvis provides for proper pressure transmission from the upper body through the
spine to the lower extremities. The coxal
bone is formed by the fusion of three smaller
bones: the ilium, the ischium, and the pubis.
The ilium is the superior portion of the
pelvis; the ischium forms the inferoposterior
portion; and the pubis forms the inferoante-
rior portion. These smaller bones fuse together at the acetabulum and articulate at the
pubic symphysis (Fig. 2.4).

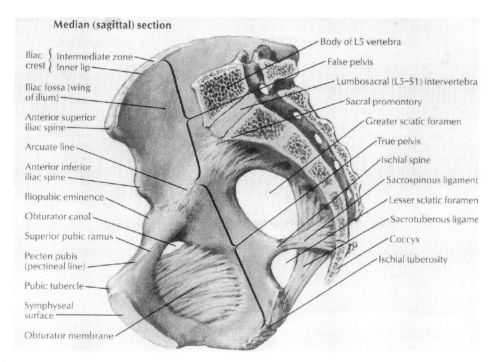

FIG. 2.4. Bones and ligaments of pelvis. (From Netter FH. *Atlas of human anatomy.* East Hanover, NJ: Novartis, 1997, Plate 330. Copyright © 1997 Icon Learning Systems, LLC. A subsidiary of Med-iMedia, USA, Inc. All rights reserved.)

The inlet to the true pelvis (linea terminalis) is formed bilaterally by the pubic symphysis, the superior pubic ramus, the arcuate line of the ilium, the alar or wing portion of the sacrum, and the promontory of the sacrum. In the standing female patient, this inlet forms a 60- to 65-degree angle with the horizontal plane or floor. The anterior border of the greater sciatic foramen is almost vertical in orientation. The internal iliac artery courses along this border and helps to establish the cardinal ligament sheath. This anterior border of the greater sciatic foramen ends in a blunt projection that is pointed medially, called the ischial spine. The ischial spine is about 2 to 3 cm above the level of the pubic crest. This orientation provides an almost horizontal relationship between the posterior aspect of the pubic bone and ischial spine. This relationship is critical for defining the horizontal axis of pelvic support in order to understand how the intact pubocervical fascia prevents cystoceles and anterior enteroceles (anterior vaginal wall prolapse) (Fig. 2.2) and how the intact rectovaginal septum prevents rectoceles and posterior enteroceles (posterior vaginal wall prolapse).

The sacrospinous ligament travels medially and posteriorly from the ischial spine to the lateral and anterior aspects of the lower portion of the sacrum and the coccyx. This ligament converts the greater sciatic notch into the greater sciatic foramen. On its pelvic surface, the sacrospinous ligament is covered by the thin coccygeus muscle. The coccygeus muscle becomes fibrotic and ligamentous in older women. Anatomically below the ischial spine is the lesser sciatic foramen, through which travels the tendon of the obturator internus muscle on its way to insert onto the greater trochanter of the femur.

The sacrotuberous ligament travels medially and superiorly from the ischial tuberosity to the lateral and posterior aspects of the lower half of the sacrum. This ligament forms the posterior border of the pelvic outlet and perineum.

The obturator foramen is a large oval window formed by the bodies and the rami of the pubis and ischium. The obturator membrane covers this opening. Anteriorly and laterally at the edge of the obturator foramen is a groove in the body of the pubis for the passage of the obturator vessels and nerve. The obturator internus muscle originates from the entire bony margin of the obturator foramen and from the pelvic side of the obturator membrane in order to form the lateral pelvic sidewall.

PELVIC MUSCULATURE

The female pelvis is a basin of skeletal muscles (Fig. 2.5). There is a front wall, a back wall, two sidewalls, and a floor. The top is open. The front wall is simply the back of the pubic symphysis. Each sidewall is formed by the obturator internus muscle. The back wall is formed by the sacrum centrally and the piriformis muscles laterally. Each piriformis muscle originates from the anterior and lateral aspect of the sacrum in its middle to upper portions. It then courses laterally through the greater sciatic foramen to insert upon the greater trochanter of the femur, along with the obturator internus tendon, which leaves the pelvis through the lesser sciatic foramen.

The floor is formed by the levator ani muscles as well as by the more posteriorly located coccygeus muscle. A curvilinear thickening of the parietal fascia covering the obturator internus muscle from the posterior and lateral aspect of the pubic bone toward the ischial spine gives rise to the levator ani muscles. This thickening is called the arcus tendineus levator ani or muscle white line. The anterior portion of each levator ani muscle arises from the superior ramus of the pubic bone and from the anterior end of the obturator internus muscle along this line. This is called the pubococcygeus portion of the levator ani muscles. Each pubococcygeus muscle surrounds the lower one-third of the vagina and inserts into the anococcygeal raphe and onto the coccyx.

The more inferior and more medial part of the pubococcygeus muscle arises from the lower part of the pubic body and passes pos-

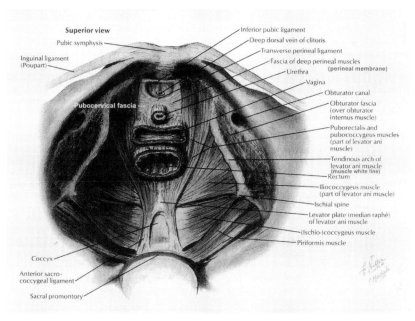

Superior view

Inferior pubic ligament
Pubic symphysis
Deep dorsal vein of clitoris
Transverse perineal ligament
Inguinal ligament (Poupart)
Fascia of deep perineal muscles (perineal membrane)
Urethra
Vagina
Obturator canal
Pubocervical fascia
Obturator fascia (over obturator internus muscle)
Puborectalis and pubococcygeus muscles (part of levator ani muscle)
Tendinous arch of levator ani muscle (muscle white line)
Rectum
Iliococcygeus muscle (part of levator ani muscle)
Ischial spine
Levator plate (median raphé) of levator ani muscle
(Ischio-)coccygeus muscle
Piriformis muscle
Coccyx
Anterior sacro-coccygeal ligament
Sacral promontory

FIG. 2.5. Muscles of the pelvis. (From Netter FH. *Atlas of human anatomy.* East Hanover, NJ: Novartis, 1997, Plate 333. Copyright © 1997 Icon Learning Systems, LLC. A subsidiary of MediMedia, USA, Inc. All rights reserved.)

teriorly around the rectum to form a sling in order to create the 90-degree rectoanal junction. This portion of muscle is called the puborectalis. The puborectalis muscle, when contracted, draws the rectoanal junction toward the pubic symphysis. This action is critical in the maintenance of solid fecal continence. The levator hiatus is the spatial separation of these muscles on one side from their sister muscles on the other side in the midline. This cleft allows passage of the urethra and vagina into the perineum.

The more posterior portion of the levator ani muscle is a thin, yet strong muscle only 3 to 4 mm in thickness, called the iliococcygeus muscle. It also originates from the muscle white line as it travels toward the ischial spine. This muscle slopes inferiorly toward the midline, sending off fibers that blend with the longitudinal coat of the rectum. It then fuses with its sister muscle from the opposite site just in front of the anococcygeal raphe and forms the levator plate, 3 to 4 cm long. In the standing female patient,

the levator plate is oriented in a horizontal plane from the rectoanal junction to the coccyx. The muscular levator plate is physiologically dynamic, constantly changing its tension in adjusting to changing intrapelvic pressures.

The muscles of the levator ani group are innervated on both sides. The pelvic surface is innervated by sacral efferents from the second, third, and fourth sacral nerves. The perineal or inferior surface receives its innervation from branches from each pudendal nerve.

Importantly, the parietal fascia of the levator ani muscles is thickened along a straight line from the pubic arch to the ischial spine on each side. This thickened line serves as the ultimate attachment of the horizontal supports of the pubocervical fascia and the rectovaginal septum. This linear structure is called the arcus tendineus fasciae pelvis (6) or fascial white line (Fig. 2.3).

Traveling obliquely posteriorly and inferiorly from the fascial white line on each side from the midpoint of the vagina is a thicken-

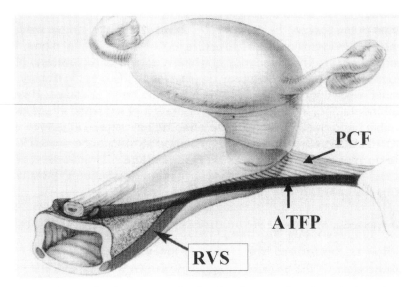

FIG. 2.6. Arcus tendineus fasciae rectovaginalis. Attachment of rectovaginal septum and arcus tendineus fascia pelvis to pelvic sidewall. Lateral defects in the rectovaginal septum should be sutured to the line of attachment at the pelvic sidewall. RVS, rectovaginal septum; ATFP, arcus tendineus fascia pelvis; PCF, pubocervical fascia. (From Leffler KS, Thompson JR, Cundiff GW, et al. Attachment of the rectovaginal septum to the pelvic sidewall. *Am J Obstet Gynecol* 2001;185:43, with permission.)

ing of parietal fascia over the iliococcygeus muscle. The lower portion of the rectovaginal septum inserts onto this new fascial line (Fig. 2.6), the tendinous arch of rectovaginal fascia, or the arcus tendineus fasciae rectovaginalis (7), which ends as the rectovaginal septum inserts onto the apex of the perineal body. Nearer to the ischial spine posteriorly, the arcus tendineus fasciae pelvis and the arcus tendineus fasciae rectovaginalis are the same linear thickening of parietal fascia, until the midportion of the vagina. Then, the arcus tendineus fasciae pelvis continues anteriorly toward the pubic arch, whereas the arcus tendineus fasciae rectovaginalis angles down with the rectovaginal septum toward the perineal body. The resultant sulci (anterolateral and posterolateral) are visible along each sidewall of the vagina.

PERINEUM

Just inferior to the levator ani muscles are the muscles of the perineum, which cover the outlet of the pelvis. This area is bounded anteriorly by the pubic arch and posteriorly by the tip of the coccyx. Laterally, the ischiopubic rami, ischial tuberosities, and sacrotuberous ligaments frame the perineum into a diamond shape. For descriptive purposes, the perineum can be further subdivided by drawing a line transversely just in front of the ischial tuberosities. Thus, the region is divided into two triangular parts. These two triangles are not in the same horizontal plane but are slightly angulated in relation to each other. The posterior division contains the anal canal and is known as the anal triangle.

The anterior portion contains the vagina and urethra and is called the urogenital triangle. The urogenital triangle is divided into superficial and deep compartments by the perineal membrane. These compartments are anchored to the perineal body between the vagina and anus. The key supporting structure in the urogenital triangle is the perineal membrane, which spans the gap between the two ischiopubic rami. The perineal membrane and the perineal body are important links in con-

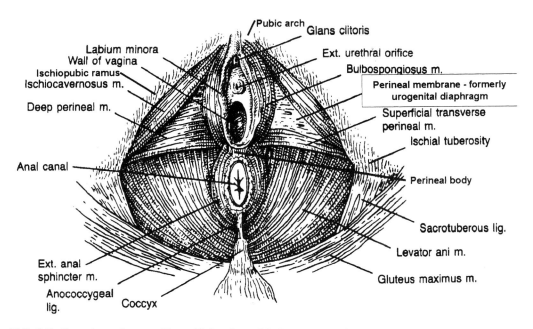

FIG. 2.7. Female perineum. (From Richardson AC, DeLancey JOL. Anatomy of genital support. In: Hurt WG, ed. *The masters' techniques in gynecologic surgery: urogynecologic surgery,* 2nd ed. Philadelphia: Lippincott Williams & Wilkins, 2000:24, with permission.)

necting the endopelvic fascia surrounding the vagina and urethra with the fibromuscular structures that surround the outlet of these viscera (Fig. 2.7).

PERINEAL BODY

The perineal body is that area of the perineum located between the vaginal outlet and anus. It is a three-dimensional pyramidal structure with an orientation in the standing patient such that its base is parallel with the floor. The apex of the perineal body is located at the junction of the lower third and the middle third of the vagina. The height of the perineal body is 3 to 4 cm (Fig. 2.1A). Into the perineal body inserts the bulbocavernosus muscles, the superficial transverse perineal muscles, a portion of levator ani muscles, as well as other fibromuscular structures, most importantly the rectovaginal septum. The rectovaginal septum helps stabilize the perineal body through its upper attachments to the uterosacral ligaments and

then to the sacrum. As a result, there is limited downward mobility of the perineal body in the nulliparous patient.

PELVIC VISCERAL SUPPORT SYSTEM AND AXES OF PELVIC SUPPORT

With the bones, ligaments, and muscles of the female pelvis introduced and briefly discussed, an understanding of vaginal and pelvic organ support continues with a discussion of the visceral or endopelvic fascia and the concept of the three axes of pelvic support in the standing female patient. The bladder, vagina, and rectum are stabilized in the pelvis by the visceral connective tissues, which allow for their independent functions of storage, distention, and evacuation. Three support axes maintain the central position of these pelvic organs (8) (Fig. 2.8). Problems of pelvic support primarily occur in the erect patient whether standing or sitting. The visceral connective tissue provides the physical material of support.

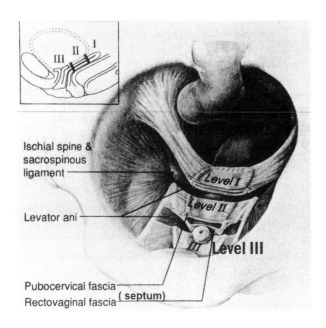

FIG. 2.8. Levels of pelvic support. (From DeLancey JOL. Anatomic aspects of vaginal eversion after hysterectomy. *Am J Obstet Gynecol* 1992;166:1719, with permission.)

The first vaginal support axis (DeLancey level I) (9) is the upper vertical axis, which facilitates an understanding of the cardinal ligament–uterosacral ligament complex. This fascial sheath contains suspensory fibers that coalesce into anatomic leashes. These suspensory leashes serve to pull the top of the vagina, cervix, and lower uterine segment posteriorly toward the sacrum so that the viscera are positioned over the supporting levator plate.

The second support axis (DeLancey level II) is the horizontal axis traveling from the ischial spine to the posterior aspect of the pubic bone. The lateral, or paravaginal, supports of the bladder, upper two thirds of the vagina, and rectum are derived from this axis.

The third vaginal support axis (DeLancey level III) or lower vertical axis is perpendicular to the plane of the levator hiatus and urogenital and anal triangles and defines the vertical orientation of the lower one third of the vagina, urethra, and anal canal.

Upper Vertical Axis: Suspension

The upper vertical axis is oriented vertically from the sacroiliac juncture at the pelvic brim to the ischial spine, running along the anterior border of the greater sciatic foramen. This follows the course and direction of the internal iliac vessels. The cardinal ligament sheath is a broad, fan-shaped collection of visceral collagen fibers that envelope the internal iliac artery and vein in layers of sheets (3). These sheets fuse and form a sheath, which is vertically oriented and follows the uterine artery and vein into the visceral fascial capsule of the cervix, called the pericervical ring (Fig. 2.3).

These fibers also have attachments to the lower uterine segment and upper vagina. Those attachments to the upper vagina form the paracolpium and are seen through the vagina as the lateral fornices. Because of its close association with the internal iliac and uterine vessels, the cardinal ligament sheath is referred to as a vascular leash. Posteriorly and laterally, this cardinal ligament sheath anchors itself firmly to the parietal fascia of the piriformis and obturator internus muscles as well as the parietal fascia on the anterior border of the greater sciatic foramen.

The uterosacral ligament portion of the cardinal ligament sheath is a denser gathering of visceral connective tissue located in the medial and inferior aspects of this sheath. Each uterosacral ligament thickens and narrows as it inserts into the posterior and lateral aspects of the pericervical ring (10,11). The uterosacral ligaments then curve around the rectum horizontally and attach to tough presacral fascia overlying the second, third, and fourth sacral vertebra. Therefore, each uterosacral ligament may be conceptualized as a sacral leash.

The cardinal ligaments and uterosacral ligaments form a complex of visceral supporting tissues to the upper vagina and cervix and, after hysterectomy, to the vaginal cuff. They pull the upper vagina horizontally back toward the sacrum and thus suspend it over the muscular levator plate. Anatomically, the insertion of the cardinal ligaments and uterosacral ligaments to the pericervical ring occurs at the level of the ischial spines. Clinically, detachment of the cardinal ligament–uterosacral ligament complexes (sheaths or leashes) from the pericervical ring occurs at the level of the ischial spines and provides the anatomic rationale for the development of uterine descensus, posthysterectomy vaginal vault prolapse, and enterocele (apical prolapse).

Horizontal Axis: Sidewall Attachment

The horizontal vaginal support axis explains the horizontal orientation of the bladder, the upper two-thirds of the vagina, and the rectum. The two fascial platforms that are responsible for the horizontal orientation of these viscera are the pubocervical fascia and rectovaginal septum (fascia). Both of these structures are flexible, trapezoidal in shape, and parallel to each other with the vagina between them. However, the anatomic origin of each of these structures is different. An understanding of the horizontal axis explains anterior vaginal wall support (prevention of cystoceles) and posterior vaginal wall support (prevention of rectoceles). In the horizontal axis of pelvic support, the pubocervical fascia and rectovaginal septum ultimately attach laterally to

each pelvic sidewall at the arcus tendineus fasciae pelvis or fascial white line.

The pubocervical fascia, or fibromuscular coat of the vaginal wall, is a thickening of the visceral fascial coat of the vagina anteriorly (12). The term pubocervical fascia is a clinical and surgical reference, not a histologic designation. On each side, this fibromuscular coat attaches indirectly to the fascial white line through a short (1 to 2 cm in width) transverse visceral septum called the fascia endopelvina (Fig. 2.3), which travels the distance from the pubic arch to the ischial spine. Recall the nearly horizontal relationship between the posterior aspect of the pubic bone and the ischial spine. The pubocervical fascia is intimately fused with the vaginal epithelium (13) and provides a physical platform upon which the bladder rests.

When intact, the pubocervical fascia and its lateral attachments to the fascial white lines prevent a cystocele, which is prolapse of the anterior vaginal wall. Just as important, the posterior edge of the pubocervical fascia fuses with the pericervical ring and thus connects with the cardinal ligament–uterosacral ligament complexes. Therefore, the integrity of the pubocervical fascia to prevent anterior vaginal wall prolapse (cystocele) includes not only its attachments to the fascial white lines but also its fusion with the pericervical ring. This relationship positions the upper vagina horizontally over the levator plate (Fig. 2.9).

Inferiorly, the pubocervical fascia travels underneath the urethra and inserts onto the perineal membrane near the lower one-third of the urethra (Fig. 2.5). Anterior reflections of the pubocervical fascia around the urethra insert on the underside of the pubic arch to help stabilize the urethra. These anterior reflections are called the pubourethral ligaments by anatomists and provide a role in urinary continence at the midurethral level. In addition, the pubocervical fascia forms a hammock of visceral connective tissue underneath the urethrovesical junction, thus explaining another mechanism of urinary con-

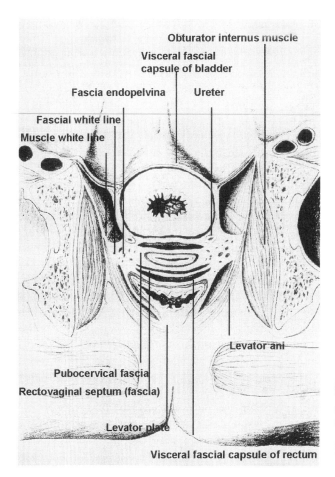

FIG. 2.9. Coronal section through the junction of the upper third and middle third of the vagina demonstrating endopelvic fascia, septa, and spaces. (Adapted from Peham HV, Amreich J. *Operative gynecology,* Vol. 1. Philadelphia: JB Lippincott, 1934: 194, with permission.)

tinence (14). The anterolateral sulci seen in the normal nulliparous patient during vaginal examination are the manifestations of the pubocervical fascia inserting on each fascia endopelvina, which then inserts onto each fascial white line bilaterally.

Again to emphasize, the pubocervical fascia is fused to the visceral fascial ring surrounding the supravaginal portion of the cervix, thus contributing to the pericervical ring of supportive tissue. The pericervical ring is responsible for the continuity of pelvic support from the cardinal ligament–uterosacral ligament complexes of the upper vertical support axis to the horizontal support axis of the pubocervical fascia and rectovaginal septum. The transition of the upper vertical supports to the horizontal

supports occurs at the pericervical ring focus, which is found anatomically at the level of the ischial spines bilaterally. Thus, the upper vertical supports are continuous with the horizontal supports at the level of the ischial spines.

The rectovaginal septum (also known as the rectovaginal fascia) is the horizontal platform of visceral support tissue between the vagina and the rectum (15). This fascia is not a thickened endopelvic fascial coat but is a separate endopelvic fascial platform formed by the fusion of two peritoneal layers that have been modified histologically. In the developing female fetus, the cul-de-sac peritoneum rests on the perineal body. As the fetus develops, these two peritoneal layers fuse and are modified histologically

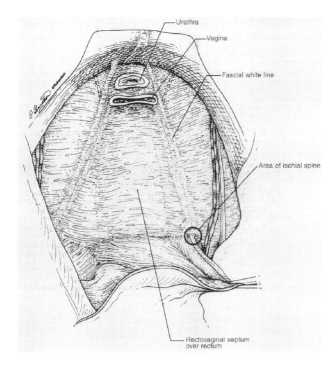

Urethra

Vagina

Fascial white line

Area of ischial spine

Rectovaginal septum over rectum

FIG. 2.10. The rectovaginal septum connects with uterosacral ligaments superiorly, fascia of levators laterally, and perineal body distally. (From Richardson AC. The anatomic defects in rectocele and enterocele. *J Pelvic Surg* 1995;1(4):216, with permission.)

to form a tough, wide fibroelastic sheath. The rectovaginal septum attaches to the apex of the perineal body inferiorly; ultimately to the parietal fascia of the iliococcygeus muscles laterally; and posteriorly to the cul-de-sac peritoneum and both uterosacral ligaments where these latter structures insert into the pericervical ring (Fig. 2.10).

The rectovaginal septum is oriented horizontally in the standing patient and is thus parallel to the pubocervical fascial platform that supports the bladder. It travels between the visceral fascial coats of the vagina and rectum. When intact, the rectovaginal septum clinically prevents the formation of rectoceles or prolapse of the posterior vaginal wall. Also, the intact rectovaginal septum actually suspends the perineal body from the sacrum by its attachments to the uterosacral ligaments. The upper half of the rectovaginal septum is attached laterally to each iliococcygeus fascia by the fascia endopelvina (Fig. 2.9), which inserts onto the fascial white line. As the rectovaginal septum travels to-

ward the perineal body at the midportion of the vagina, it inserts onto the linear thickening of the iliococcygeus fascia, the arcus tendineus fasciae rectovaginalis (6), thus leading into the apex of the perineal body. This attachment is responsible for the posterolateral sulci found in the nulliparous patient in the front half of the vagina.

Lower Vertical Axis: Fusion

The lower vertical support axis is responsible for the vertical orientation of the urethra, lower one-third of the vagina, and anal canal. This axis travels perpendicularly through the levator hiatus and through the perineum, including both urogenital and anal triangles. The levator hiatus is responsible for the vertical orientation of the lower one third of the vagina, the 90-degree rectoanal junction angle (owing to the puborectalis sling) (Fig. 2.1), and the pubocervical fascial hammock at the urethrovesical junction. The deep compartment of the urogenital triangle is the location of the pubourethral ligaments at the midportion of the urethra, just superior to the perineal membrane. The perineal body is also responsible for closure of the vaginal introitus, whereas the anal triangle of the perineum is responsible for the functioning of the anal canal and anus. The lower vertical support axis is formed by the direct attachments and fusion of the visceral fascial capsules around the distal urethra, lower one-third of the vagina (fibers of Luschka), and anal canal to the parietal fascia of the pubococcygeus and puborectalis muscles, in addition to the perineal membrane and perineal body.

CONCLUSIONS

The continuity of the endopelvic fascial network in the pelvis is focused on the pericervical ring at the level of the ischial spines and on the perineal body between the anus and vaginal introitus. The visceral connective tissue of the upper vertical supports (cardinal ligament–uterosacral ligament complexes) merge into the posterior and lateral aspects of the cervix. From the horizontal support axis, the pubocervical fascia inserts into the anterior aspect of the cervix, whereas the rectovaginal septum posteriorly has a relationship to the pericervical ring through its connections with the uterosacral ligaments. The formation of the pericervical ring of visceral fascia around the supravaginal portion of the cervix ensures continuity and interdependency between the endopelvic connective tissue meshwork of the upper vertical support axis and the horizontal support axis. This pericervical ring must be reconstructed after hysterectomy and especially during reconstructive vaginal surgery in order to provide this uninterrupted and continuous support for the vaginal apex as well as the upper anterior and posterior vaginal walls.

The perineal body is the key structure for the support of the urogenital and anal triangles of the perineum. It serves as a support for the structures of the superficial and deep compartments of the urogenital triangle, which contain the supporting structures for the distal urethra and vagina. This fibromuscular structure functions as a converging point for the horizontal supports and the lower vertical supports. The rectovaginal septum merges with the perineal body directly, whereas the pubocervical fascia connects to the perineal membrane of the urogenital triangle, which then connects around the vagina with the perineal body. Integrity of the perineal body helps maintain the competency of the various outlets found in the female perineum. It is a keystone support for the lower pelvic viscera and ensures continuity of support of the horizontal axis with the lower vertical axis.

The female pelvic visceral support system supports all of the pelvic viscera *en bloc,* yet is flexible and versatile enough to allow each organ its own distensibility and its own physiologic function, independent of the other organs and surrounding anatomic structures. The unifying concepts of normal support anatomy must be visualized clearly in order to understand the vaginal examination of the nulliparous patient. The concept of specific, defined breaks in the continuity of the pelvic visceral support system allows the examiner an understanding of how vaginal support defects can evolve. The visualization of these support defects in the surgeon's mind is essential for successful reparative vaginal surgery.

REFERENCES

1. Williams PL, Bannister LH, Berry MM, et al., eds. *Gray's anatomy,* 38th ed. New York: Churchill Livingstone, 1995:88.
2. DeLancey JOL. Standing anatomy of the pelvic floor. *J Pelvic Surg* 1996;2:260–263.
3. Uhlenhuth ER, Day E, Smith R, et al. The visceral endopelvic fascia and the hypogastric sheath. *Surg Gynecol Obstet* 1948;86:9.
4. Retzky SS, Rogers RM, Richardson AC. Anatomy of female pelvic support. In Brubaker LT, Saclarides TJ, eds. *The female pelvic floor: disorders of function and support.* Philadelphia: FA Davis, 1996:3–21.
5. Peham HV, Amreich J. Preface. In: *Operative gynecology,* Vol. 1. Philadelphia: JB Lippincott, 1934:ix.
6. DeLancey JOL. Vaginographic examination of the pelvic floor. *Int Urogynecol J Pelvic Floor Dysfunct* 1994;5:19–24.

7. Leffler KS, Thompson JR, Cundiff GW, et al. Attachment of the rectovaginal septum to the pelvic sidewall. *Am J Obstet Gynecol* 2001;185:41–43.

8. Peham HV, Amreich J. *Operative gynecology,* Vol. 1. Philadelphia: JB Lippincott, 1934:166–242.

9. DeLancey JOL. Anatomic aspects of vaginal eversion after hysterectomy. *Am J Obstet Gynecol* 1992;166: 1717–1728.

10. Buller JL, Thompson JR, Cundiff GW, et al. Uterosacral ligament: description of anatomic relationships to optimize surgical safety. *Obstet Gynecol* 2001;97:873–879.

11. Campbell R. The anatomy and histology of the sacrouterine ligaments. *Am J Obstet Gynecol* 1950;59: 1–12.

12. Weber AM, Walters MD. Anterior vaginal prolapse: review of anatomy and techniques of surgical repair. *Obstet Gynecol* 1997;89:311–318.

13. Farrell SA, Dempsey T, Geldenhuys L. Histologic examination of "fascia" used in colporrhaphy. *Obstet Gynecol* 2001;98:794–798.

14. DeLancey JOL. Structural support of the urethra as it relates to stress urinary incontinence: the hammock hypothesis. *Am J Obstet Gynecol* 1994;170:1713–1723.

15. Uhlenhuth E, Wolfe W, Smith E, et al. The rectogenital septum. *Surg Gynecol Obstet* 1948;86:148.

Ostergard's Urogynecology and Pelvic Floor
Dysfunction, Fifth Edition. edited by A.E. Bent, et al.
Lippincott Williams & Wilkins, Philadelphia © 2003.

3

Epidemiology of Pelvic Organ Prolapse

Steven E. Swift

*Department of Obstetrics and Gynecology, Division of Benign Gynecology, Medical University of
South Carolina, Charleston, South Carolina*

The epidemiology of pelvic organ prolapse is an area that has received much attention in the literature but that remains poorly understood. There are several reasons for this, but prominent among them is the problem with defining pelvic organ prolapse. The American College of Obstetrics and Gynecology technical bulletin defines pelvic organ prolapse as the protrusion of the pelvic organs into or out of the vaginal canal (1). This is a very loose definition and could technically encompass any woman who has the slightest relaxation of the cervix, such that it descends 1 to 2 cm into the vaginal tube with Valsalva, to the woman who has complete vaginal eversion and uterine procidentia. Currently, there is no clear definition to distinguish between normal support and pelvic organ prolapse, and although the extremes of pelvic support are obvious to most practitioners, identifying the more subtle cases can be difficult. Without a clear definition of what represents pelvic organ prolapse, it is difficult to describe its epidemiology.

INCIDENCE OF PELVIC ORGAN SUPPORT DEFECTS

Determining the difference between normal and abnormal pelvic organ prolapse is complicated by a lack of knowledge regarding the distribution of pelvic organ support in the normal female population. Before describing the etiology of pelvic organ prolapse, discussion of the state of our current understanding regarding the distribution of pelvic organ support in the female population will be presented.

Several investigators have recently attempted to document and describe the degree of pelvic organ support in various female populations. One study reported the distribution of pelvic organ support in all women between the ages of 20 and 59 in a small Swedish town (2). They noted that 2% of their population had significant pelvic organ prolapse defined as prolapse that reached the vaginal introitus. However, they did not describe the distribution of pelvic organ support but only commented on its presence or absence using the above definition.

Two other recently published reports have further described the distribution of pelvic organ support in female populations (3,4). These studies employed the pelvic organ prolapse quantification system (POPQ) to define the degree of pelvic organ support in their subjects. The POPQ is a classification system for documenting the degree of pelvic organ support that describes five stages (0 through 4), with stage 0 representing excellent support and stage 4 representing complete vaginal vault inversion or uterine procidentia (5). This classification system has been found to be a reliable and reproducible tool for describing defects in pelvic organ support (6,7). In one report, women between the ages of 45 and 55 years participating in a study on the effects of soybean supplements on menopausal symptoms were recruited, and their pelvic organ support was described (3). The authors reported stage 0 support in 73% of their population, stage 1 support in 23%, and stage 2 support in 4%. No subjects had stage 3 or 4 support defects. A second report involved subjects between the ages of 18 and 86 years presenting for routine annual gynecologic examinations to four outpatient gynecology clinics (4). The degree of support varied with age and demonstrated a bell-curve distribution (Fig. 3.1). These investigators reported 6.4% of their population with stage 0 support, 43.3% with stage 1 support, 47.7% with stage 2 support, and 2.6% with stage 3 support or prolapse. No subjects in this report had stage 4 prolapse. Stage 3 pelvic organ prolapse represents a condition in which the leading edge of the prolapse is greater than 1 cm through or beyond the hymenal remnants. This is prolapse that the patient can see or feel and generally represents symptomatic pelvic organ prolapse. Therefore, in one report, no subjects had clinically significant pelvic organ prolapse, and in the other two reports, at least 2% of the subjects had significant prolapse. It is difficult to reconcile the results of these studies; however, the populations were different in a number of variables other than age, which may explain some of the discrepancy noted.

The drawback to all of these reports is that the populations studied may not necessarily be reflective of the general female population.

Another way of determining the incidence of clinically significant pelvic organ prolapse is to describe the incidence of surgical procedures to correct pelvic organ prolapse in a given population. This was done in two reports: one involved patients attending a family planning clinic and the other described all patients participating in one insurance plan (8,9). They reported an incidence of 2.04 to 2.63 surgical procedures to correct prolapse or genuine stress incontinence (a common symptom of pelvic organ prolapse) per 1,000 woman-years, with an increasing incidence as women age, and a lifetime risk of undergoing surgery for prolapse or incontinence of 5% to 11.1%. The problem with these reports is that women who treated their prolapse with conservative measures were not represented, and not all subjects with stress incontinence have significant pelvic organ prolapse.

In summary, it appears that roughly 2% to 3% of women have significant or pathologic pelvic organ support defects. This represents a fairly common condition with very little information on its causes. The remainder of this

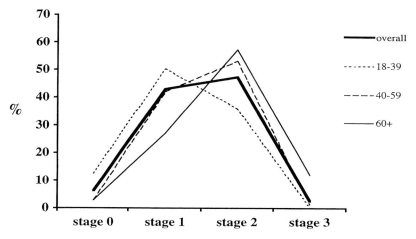

FIG. 3.1. Distribution of pelvic organ support by pelvic organ prolapse quantification system stage in a population of women seeking routine gynecologic health care. ▬▬ , overall curve for the entire population; ------, curve for women aged 18–39 years; – – – – , curve for women aged 40–59 years; ____ , curve for women older than 60 years of age.

chapter is devoted to identifying and discussing the suspected etiologies of pelvic organ prolapse.

ETIOLOGY OF PELVIC ORGAN PROLAPSE

Increasing parity, advancing age, and antecedent surgery to correct pelvic organ support defects are consistently identified as risk factors for the development of pelvic organ prolapse. Several other factors have also been implicated, including vaginal versus abdominal delivery of a term infant, hysterectomy, congenital defects, race, lifestyle, and chronic disease states that increase intraabdominal pressure (e.g., chronic constipation, pulmonary disease, obesity). However, here the literature is not as consistent, and the role that these factors play is still not fully understood.

Childbirth

Vaginal delivery of a term infant has been postulated to be the most significant contributor to the subsequent development of pelvic organ prolapse (2,8–11). It is postulated that as the fetal vertex passes through the vaginal canal, it stretches the levator ani muscles and the pudendal nerve, leading to damage with permanent neuropathy and muscle weakness. This damage is thought to be ultimately responsible for pelvic organ prolapse noted later in life. There is one study that demonstrated an 11-fold increase in pelvic organ prolapse risk in women with greater than four vaginal deliveries as opposed to nulliparous subjects (2). It has also been suggested that larger infants cause greater damage to the pelvic floor at the time of delivery. When this was specifically addressed, it was reported that there is a 10% increase in the risk for developing severe pelvic organ prolapse with each 1-lb increase in the birth weight of a vaginally delivered infant (11).

From the literature, it appears that vaginal delivery causes damage to the pudendal nerve and promotes the development of pelvic organ prolapse. Which patients will eventually develop pelvic organ prolapse, and what other aspects of the delivery process affect the subsequent development of pelvic organ prolapse, remain elusive. There are suggestions that instrumented vaginal deliveries increase the risk and that mediolateral episiotomies lessen the risk. At this time, the data are incomplete; therefore, no recommendations regarding the delivery process can be made. It has also been demonstrated that the pudendal nerve damage caused by vaginal delivery can be avoided by cesarean section (12–14). However, a recent article failed to demonstrate a reduction in the incidence of pelvic floor dysfunction in women delivered by cesarean section (15). Therefore, it remains unclear how and whether we can lessen the risk for developing pelvic organ prolapse by intervening in the delivery process.

Age

Another area in which the literature is in agreement involves the increasing prevalence of pelvic organ prolapse in a population as it ages (2,10,11). This is intuitive to the clinician because there are few patients in their 20s and 30s with significant pelvic organ prolapse. Figure 3.1 demonstrates the distribution of pelvic organ support as women age. The peak or median POPQ stage of support shifts to the right as the population described increases in age. It has been shown that there is a 12% increase in the incidence of severe pelvic organ prolapse with each year of advancing age, or roughly a doubling of the incidence for every decade of life (11). Another study likewise identified age as a statistically significant etiologic risk factor and noted that the incidence of pelvic organ prolapse roughly doubled with every decade of life in women between the ages of 20 and 59 years (10). These studies confirm data on the incidence of surgically managed pelvic organ prolapse from two large studies that showed a 100% increase per decade in the incidence of surgically managed pelvic organ prolapse (2,9).

Menopause

The literature is consistent that the risk for pelvic organ prolapse increases with advancing age, but what roles do menopause and hormone replacement therapy have on pelvic organ prolapse? One study has identified menopausal status as a risk factor, with postmenopausal women being at higher risk for prolapse (10). However, the investigators did not determine which patients were taking hormone replacement therapy and which were not. In another study, menopausal status and hormone replacement therapy were not identified as risk factors for pelvic organ prolapse (11). Therefore, it may be that advancing age is more responsible for the increased risk for pelvic organ prolapse than is menopausal status. Currently, the role of estrogen in the area of pelvic organ prolapse is unclear. However, although it may not prevent the development of prolapse, it probably does not promote its development; therefore, its use in subjects with significant pelvic organ support defects should be viewed as neutral. Whether it can prevent or delay the onset of pelvic organ prolapse remains to be determined.

Previous Surgery to Correct Pelvic Organ Support Defects

Prior surgery may not be a fair addition to the etiologies of pelvic organ prolapse because these subjects have already manifested pelvic organ support defects and have the underlying pathologic processes that lead to this disease. Recurrence rates for surgical correction of pelvic organ prolapse are in the 10% to 30% range (9,16). Therefore, it is not surprising that when subjects with previous surgery to correct prolapse are included in regression analysis and case-control studies, this is consistently identified as a risk factor. When the various risk factors for developing severe (POPQ stage 3 and 4) pelvic organ prolapse were analyzed, it was determined that previous surgery to correct prolapse was the single greatest risk factor for the subsequent development of severe prolapse (11). Therefore,

this appears to be a statement on the inadequacies of our current surgical procedures for correcting significant pelvic organ prolapse. However, it is a strong predictor for women who are at risk for pelvic support defects.

Hysterectomy

The role of hysterectomy as a cause of subsequent development of pelvic organ prolapse is controversial and can stimulate heated exchanges with no current consensus. The overall incidence of severe pelvic organ prolapse following hysterectomy has been estimated to be 2 to 3.6 per 1,000 woman-years (17,18). This is similar to the rates of surgically corrected pelvic organ prolapse and incontinence noted for the general population (2.04 to 2.63 per 1,000 women-years) and would suggest that there is no excess of pelvic organ prolapse in subjects with a prior hysterectomy (8,9). However, when the role of hysterectomy was specifically addressed in a case-control study, it was identified as a significant risk factor for severe pelvic organ prolapse (11). The next question regarding hysterectomy is whether the route of surgery influences the subsequent development of pelvic support defects. There is the general opinion that the incidence of pelvic support defects is greater following a vaginal hysterectomy than after an abdominal hysterectomy (4,17,19). When studied, the rates and degree of prolapse appear similar regardless of the type of antecedent hysterectomy (8,17). Although the route of hysterectomy may not predict subsequent development of pelvic organ prolapse, there is a correlation between subsequent prolapse and the initial indication for the hysterectomy. Pelvic organ prolapse rates as high as 15 per 1,000 woman-years have been noted in patients whose indication for hysterectomy was uterine prolapse (9). This confirms the previously discussed findings of an increased risk for pelvic organ prolapse following surgery to correct pelvic support defects and may explain some of the data suggesting vaginal hysterectomy as a cause of pelvic organ prolapse. More vaginal than abdominal hysterectomies are performed for prolapse.

It is thought that disruption of the attachments of the uterosacral ligament–cardinal ligament complex to the cuff is responsible for post-hysterectomy vaginal vault prolapse. Most authors believe that paying particular attention to reattaching these ligaments to the cuff and obliterating the cul-de-sac can reduce the incidence of prolapse. There are a few uncontrolled reports that the incidence of enterocele following a hysterectomy can be reduced by more than 50% if cul-de-sac obliteration is performed at the time of hysterectomy (18,20). It would seem that if disruption of the attachments of the uterosacral and cardinal ligaments were the main reason for subsequent prolapse, supracervical hysterectomies would provide some degree of protection. In one older study, an individual reported that in his practice, there were 31 cases of eversion of the vagina and cervical stump and only 7 cases of vaginal eversion of the cuff. This was despite the mention that more total abdominal than supracervical hysterectomies were performed in that practice (21). This suggests that preservation of the uterosacral and cardinal ligamentous attachment to the cervix does not prevent subsequent prolapse.

Prolapse after hysterectomy appears to be unrelated to the route of surgery but may be related to the indication, with vaginal vault prolapse occurring most commonly after a hysterectomy for prolapse. Which aspects of a hysterectomy lead to subsequent prolapse are still unknown, but if attention is paid to securing the cardinal and uterosacral ligaments to the cuff and obliterating the cul-de-sac, the incidence may be reduced.

Congenital Defects

One of the biggest issues concerning the etiology of pelvic organ prolapse is determining which patients are at risk. From the previous discussion, it appears that pudendal neuropathy and pelvic floor damage occur with almost all vaginal deliveries, yet severe pelvic organ prolapse occurs in only roughly 2% to 3% of the population. Therefore, do those patients destined to develop prolapse have an underlying congenital defect that prevents recovery of their pelvic support mechanism from the trauma of vaginal delivery, and might this also account for prolapse that is occasionally seen in the nulliparous patient?

One obvious congenital anomaly that could be involved in pelvic support defects is collagen vascular disease. There is evidence that women with pelvic organ prolapse have less total collagen in their pubocervical fascia when compared with controls and that the collagen present is of a weaker type than noted in controls with normal support (22,23). There is also the observation that subjects with pelvic organ prolapse have a greater degree of joint hypermobility, suggesting a collagen defect (24). Therefore, if pelvic organ prolapse is related to collagen defects, women with congenital connective tissue diseases should have a greater incidence of prolapse. However, when women with Ehlers-Danlos syndrome were evaluated, there was no relationship between greater degree of joint mobility and more prominent pelvic organ prolapse (25).

Another congenital defect that is thought to play a role in pelvic organ prolapse is spina bifida. Although this is often cited as a cause of prolapse, particularly in the young nulliparous patient, only a few case reports have described its relationship to prolapse, and most of these were in the newborn (26,27). Torpin reported on a group of adult women with prolapse who had a 28% incidence of spina bifida occulta, compared with a 10% incidence in a control population without prolapse (28). Although the relationship may not be straightforward, in the young nulliparous woman with severe prolapse, an evaluation to identify spina bifida occulta is warranted.

Is there a congenital predilection for pelvic support dysfunction in some subjects that may be responsible for the more severe degrees of pelvic organ prolapse? If so, can these patients be identified and recommendations made for ways to protect their pelvic floor support structures, particularly during childbirth? Or should subjects who present with pelvic organ prolapse be screened for various congenital anomalies? Currently, these questions remain unanswered, and no recommendations regarding screening or prevention can be made.

Racial Differences

One factor that may predict those subjects likely to develop pelvic organ prolapse is their genetic makeup as reflected in their race. There are a few anecdotal reports that certain populations have a higher or lower incidence of pelvic organ prolapse, but these tend to be more opinion than fact (29–31). One study that specifically addressed racial differences showed a similar rate and severity of prolapse between black and white populations (31). In this study, the population examined was selected for the symptom of prolapse, and study results may be more a reflection of the racial makeup of the local population than a statement on the relative incidence of prolapse in a given race. There is also a study examining the difference in anatomy and collagen content of cadaver specimens between white and Asian women (30). There appears to be a greater collagen content in the fascial supports of Asian women than white women. The populations compared and contrasted were not adequately described to determine what other influences may have explained the results. Also, a recent study on the incidence of urinary incontinence (a condition commonly associated with pelvic organ prolapse) in Asian women demonstrated similar rates to those published for predominately white populations (32).

There is anecdotal evidence that white women are at greater risk for developing prolapse than either black or Asian women; however, there is little objective evidence. Although there may be differences in pelvic anatomy between races, how this translates into a risk for pelvic organ prolapse remains speculative.

Lifestyle

It is widely believed that women who participate in high-impact activities, whether at work or play, have more complications with prolapse and associated symptoms than their sedentary counterparts. Heavy lifting at work appears to be related to pelvic organ prolapse. In one study, the number of prolapse surgeries performed on more than 28,000 nursing assistants demonstrated a 60% increase over the general population (33). It was thought that this was secondary to their work-related duties. A similar increase in the risk for undergoing surgery for herniated disk was also noted, validating the selection of this population as one participating in heavy lifting and manual labor.

There are reports on the incidence of urinary incontinence during high-impact activities, particularly sports, with up to 25% of young physically fit women reporting some urinary incontinence while participating in their sport (34). However, when elite athletes are followed over time, the incidence of incontinence developing later in life is similar to that for age-matched controls (35). These reports did not comment on pelvic organ prolapse; hence, how this relates to high-impact sports remains unknown.

Although there does not appear to be an increased risk in athletes for subsequent pelvic floor dysfunction, it does appear that heavy lifting on the job may play a role in its development.

Chronic Disease

Chronic illnesses that result in constant stress and strain on the pelvic floor are often quoted as a significant predisposing condition for pelvic organ prolapse (1,36). Conditions such as chronic obstructive pulmonary disease or chronic cough, chronic constipation, and obesity are the diseases most often implicated, but there are few data in the literature to substantiate this. There is one study that described an association between chronic constipation and pelvic organ prolapse (37). In this study, 61% of subjects with uterovaginal prolapse reported straining with stool as young adults before the onset of the prolapse. In a control group, only 4% reported straining with stool as young women. Also, studies of severely constipated women have demonstrated abnormalities in pudendal nerve function similar to those noted in subjects with uterovaginal prolapse (38).

The relationship between obesity and a common symptom of pelvic support defects, genuine stress incontinence, has been investigated, with the evidence demonstrating that obesity appears to predispose the individual to genuine stress incontinence (39,40). However, the association between obesity and pelvic organ prolapse has not been objectively documented. There is a relationship between cigarette smoking and genuine stress incontinence, with smokers having a 2.5-fold increase in the risk for genuine stress incontinence independent of other factors (41). It was thought that the forceful coughing associated with cigarette smoking was responsible for the increased incidence of stress incontinence in smokers. What effect chronic obstructive pulmonary disease has on stress incontinence or severe pelvic organ prolapse is unknown.

Another disease that is associated with poor wound healing and therefore has been mentioned as a factor in the development of pelvic organ prolapse is diabetes mellitus. It is thought that diabetics may not be able to recover fully from the damage that occurs to the pelvic floor with childbirth and that this puts them at increased risk for pelvic organ prolapse later in life.

One case-control study looked at pulmonary disease, hypertension, diabetes, and obesity as risk factors for severe pelvic organ prolapse (11). These investigators did not find a relationship between these chronic illnesses and prolapse. However, although they had adequate numbers of subjects with diabetes, hypertension, and obesity to identify a relationship, they had very few subjects with pulmonary disease in their population and

may have missed an association between pulmonary disease and prolapse.

Chronic constipation, obesity, and cigarette smoking all appear to be related to the development of pelvic floor dysfunction in the form of stress incontinence; however, what role they play in the development of pelvic organ prolapse has not been defined. Other conditions, such as chronic obstructive pulmonary disease, that result in insults to the pelvic floor also probably play a role in the etiology of this condition but have not been sufficiently investigated.

SUMMARY

The role of childbirth in the development of pelvic floor dysfunction and prolapse remains central. Whether there are congenital conditions that place the individual at risk remains controversial. Are there conditions that can be identified and corrected to reduce the individual's risk for pelvic organ prolapse? These are important considerations that need more investigation before conclusions can be made.

REFERENCES

1. American College of Obstetricians and Gynecologists. *Pelvic organ prolapse.* ACOG Technical Bulletin 214. Washington, DC: ACOG, 1995.
2. Samuelsson EC, Victor FTA, Tibblin G, et al. Signs of genital prolapse in a Swedish population of women 20 to 59 years of age and possible related factors. *Am J Obstet Gynecol* 1999;180:299–305.
3. Bland DR, Earle BB, Vitolins MZ, et al. Use of the pelvic organ prolapse staging system of the International Continence Society, American Urogynecologic Society, and the Society of Gynecologic Surgeons in perimenopausal women. *Am J Obstet Gynecol* 1999; 181:1324–1328.
4. Swift SE. Normative data on the degree of pelvic organ support in women presenting for routine gynecologic healthcare. *Am J Obstet Gynecol* 2000;183:277–285.
5. Bump RC, Mattiasson A, Bo K, et al. The standardization of terminology of female pelvic floor dysfunction. *Am J Obstet Gynecol* 1996;175:10–17.
6. Hall AF, Theofrastous JP, Cundiff GW, et al. Interobserver and intraobserver reliability of the proposed International Continence Society, Society of Gynecologic Surgeons, and American Urogynecologic Society pelvic organ prolapse classification system. *Am J Obstet Gynecol* 1996;175:1467–1471.
7. Kobak WH, Rosenberger K, Walters MD. Interobserver

variation in the assessment of pelvic organ prolapse. *Int Urogynecol J Pelvic Floor Dysfunct* 1996;7:121–124.

8. Mant J, Painter R, Vessey M. Epidemiology of genital prolapse: observations from the Oxford Family Planning Association study. *Br J Obstet Gynaecol* 1997;104: 579–585.

9. Olsen AL, Smith VJ, Bergstrom JO, et al. Epidemiology of surgically managed pelvic organ prolapse and urinary incontinence. *Obstet Gynecol* 1997;89:501–506.

10. Gurel H, Gurel SA. Pelvic relaxation and associated risk factors: the results of logistic regression analysis. *Acta Obstet Gynecol Scand* 1999;78:290–293.

11. Swift SE, Pound T, Dias JK. Case-control study of the etiologic factors in the development of severe pelvic organ prolapse. *Int Urogynecol J Pelvic Floor Dysfunct* 2001;12:187–192.

12. Snooks SJ, Swash M, Henry MM, et al. Risk factors in childbirth causing damage to the pelvic floor innervation. *Int J Colorectal Dis* 1986;1:20–24.

13. Smith ARB, Hosker GL, Warrell DW. The role of partial denervation of the pelvic floor in the aetiology of genital prolapse and stress incontinence of urine: a neurophysiological approach. *Br J Obstet Gynaecol* 1989;96: 24–28.

14. Allen RE, Hosker GL, Smith ARB, et al. Pelvic floor damage and childbirth: a neurophysiological study. *Br J Obstet Gynaecol* 1990;97:770–779.

15. MacLennan AH, Taylor AW, Wilson DH, et al. The prevalence of pelvic floor disorders and their relationship to gender, age and mode of delivery. *Br J Obstet Gynaecol* 2000;107:1460–1470.

16. Benson JT, Lucente V, McClellan E. Vaginal versus abdominal reconstructive surgery for the treatment of pelvic support defects: a prospective, randomized study with long-term outcome evaluation. *Am J Obstet Gynecol* 1996;175:1418–1422.

17. Symmonds RE, Williams TJ, Lee RA, et al. Posthysterectomy enterocele and vaginal vault prolapse. *Am J Obstet Gynecol* 1981;140:852–859.

18. Richter K. Massive eversion of the vagina: pathogenesis, diagnosis and therapy of the "true" prolapse of the vaginal stump. *Clin Obstet Gynecol* 1982;25:897–899.

19. Virtanen HS, Makinen JI. Retrospective analysis of 711 patients operated on for pelvic relaxation in 1983–1989. *Int J Obstet Gynecol* 1993;42:109–115.

20. Waters EG. Vaginal prolapse: technique for prevention and correction at hysterectomy. *Obstet Gynecol* 1956;8: 432–436.

21. Phaneuf LE. Inversion of the vagina and prolapse of the cervix following supracervical hysterectomy and inversion of the vagina following total hysterectomy. *Am J Obstet Gynecol* 1952;64:739–743.

22. Jackson SR, Avery NC, Tarlton JF, et al. Changes in metabolism of collagen in genitourinary prolapse. *Lancet* 1996;347:1658–1661.

23. Makinen J Soderstrom KO, Kiilholma P, et al. Histological changes in the vaginal connective tissue of patients

with and without uterine prolapse. *Arch Gynecol* 1986; 239:17–20.

24. Norton PA, Baker JE, Sharp HC, et al. Genitourinary prolapse: relationship with joint mobility. *Neurourol Urodyn* 1990;9:321–322.

25. McIntosh LJ, Stanitski DF, Mallett VT, et al. Ehlers-Danlos syndrome: relationship between joint hypermobility, urinary incontinence, and pelvic floor prolapse. *Gynecol Obstet Invest* 1996;41:135–139.

26. Ajabor LN, Okojie SE. Genital prolapse in the newborn. *Int Surg* 1976;61:496–497.

27. van Dongen L. The anatomy of genital prolapse. *S Afr Med J* 1981;60:357–359.

28. Torpin R. Prolapse uteri associated with spina bifida and clubfeet in newborn infants. *Am J Obstet Gynecol* 1942;43:892–894.

29. Cox PSV, Webster D. Genital prolapse amongst the Pokot. *East Afr Med J* 1975;52:694–699.

30. Zacharin RF. "A Chinese anatomy": the pelvic supporting tissues of the Chinese and occidental female compared and contrasted. *Aust N Z J Obstet Gynecol* 1977; 17:1–11.

31. Bump RC. Racial comparisons and contrasts in urinary incontinence and pelvic organ prolapse. *Obstet Gynecol* 1993;81:421–425.

32. Brieger GM, Yip SK, Hin LY, et al. The prevalence of urinary dysfunction in Hong Kong Chinese women. *Obstet Gynecol* 1996;88:1041–1044.

33. Jorgensen S, Hein HO, Gyntelberg F. Heavy lifting at work and risk of genital prolapse and herniated disc in assistant nurses. *Occup Med* 1994;44:47–49.

34. Nygaard IE, Thompson FL, Svengalis SL, et al. Urinary incontinence in elite nulliparous athletes. *Obstet Gynecol* 1994;84:183–187.

35. Nygaard IE. Does prolonged high-impact activity contribute to later urinary incontinence? A retrospective cohort study of female Olympians. *Obstet Gynecol* 1997; 90:718–722.

36. DeLancey JOL. Pelvic floor dysfunction: causes and prevention. *Contemp Obstet Gynecol* 1993;Jan:68–80.

37. Spence-Jones C, Kamm MA, Henry MM, et al. Bowel dysfunction: a pathogenic factor in uterovaginal prolapse and urinary stress incontinence. *Br J Obstet Gynaecol* 1994;101:147–152.

38. Snooks SJ, Barnes PRH, Swash M, et al. Damage to the innervation of the pelvic floor musculature in chronic constipation. *Gastroenterology* 1985;89:977–981.

39. Wingate L, Wingate MB, Hassanein R. The relationship between overweight and urinary incontinence in postmenopausal women: a case control study. *Menopause* 1994;1:199–203.

40. Dwyer PL, Lee ET, Hay DM. Obesity and urinary incontinence in women. *Br J Obstet Gynaecol* 1988;95: 91–96.

41. Bump RC, McClish DK. Cigarette smoking and urinary incontinence in women. *Am J Obstet Gynecol* 1992; 167:1213–1218.

Ostergard's Urogynecology and Pelvic Floor Dysfunction, Fifth Edition. edited by A.E. Bent, et al.
Lippincott Williams & Wilkins, Philadelphia © 2003.

4

Pathophysiology

Alfred E. Bent

Department of Gynecology and Obstetrics, Johns Hopkins School of Medicine; and Department of Gynecology, Greater Baltimore Medical Center, Baltimore, Maryland

PELVIC FLOOR

The anatomy of pelvic floor support has been presented in Chapter 2. The clinical examination of pelvic floor defects is presented in Chapter 8. This section is designed to explain the changes in normal anatomy that lead to poor function.

The muscles of the pelvic diaphragm provide poor support when they have been weakened. The descent of the pelvic diaphragm causes further weakening of the pelvic fascial supports. Increases in intraabdominal pressure through coughing, lifting, and straining at stool cause breaks and attenuation of endopelvic fascia. Trauma may cause direct damage to vaginal walls and supports, and lack of estrogen predisposes to an unhealthy vaginal environment. The weaknesses induced affect the anterior vaginal wall with breaks in the fascia (see Fig. 8.6 in Chapter 8). Likewise, rectovaginal fascial defects are present in rectoceles, with breaks notable laterally, centrally, inferiorly, and superiorly. Injury to superior vaginal supports and an intact pubocervical fascia ring lead to uterine descent, vault prolapse, and enterocele (1).

Childbirth

Labor and vaginal delivery are major factors in direct damage to pelvic soft tissues, disruption of endopelvic fascia, and injury to the vaginal walls. Indirect damage occurs as a result of damage to the muscles and nerves of the pelvic floor (2–4). A protective effect of cesarean section before labor has been reported, especially as related to prolonged labor (5). It is thought that nerve damage may result from direct compression of nerves or stretching of nerves. Immediately after delivery, there is frequent evidence of pudendal and perineal nerve injury, although over time, this recovers (6,7). Pelvic floor muscles become denervated after vaginal delivery the same way they do with aging (8). Anal sphincter tears may be occult or overt and impair the function of external and internal components, leading to fecal incontinence (9).

Connective Tissue Disorders

Defective endopelvic connective tissue is projected as a cause of incontinence and prolapse in young, sometime nulliparous women, when there is no other obvious cause. Collagen deficiency has been associated with pelvic organ prolapse (10,11). Estrogen deficiency may also play a role in poor collagen content and weakened tissue support.

Pelvic Neuropathy

Vaginal childbirth, chronic constipation with straining at stool, and descending perineum syndrome with repeated straining for defecation result in progressive stretching and damage to the pudendal nerve. Levator ani muscles may be affected independently of damage to the external anal sphincter.

Congenital Disorders

Conditions of spinal cord and pelvic nerve root pathways, including muscular dystrophy, myelodysplasia, meningomyelocele, bladder exstrophy, and spina bifida, can result in flaccid paralysis of the pelvic floor muscles and pelvic organ prolapse (12).

Postoperative Effects

At the time of hysterectomy, the vaginal vault must be reattached to the suspensory ligaments (uterosacral and cardinal). Additionally, the continuity of the endopelvic fascia must be maintained by suturing anterior pubocervical fascia to posterior rectovaginal fascia over the vaginal vault cuff (1). Ventral fixation may lead to posterior weakness and predispose to enterocele and vault relaxation. Similarly, sacrospinous fixation with posterior fixation of the vagina may lead to cystocele defects (13).

Other Causes

Obesity is thought to contribute to increased intraabdominal pressure transmitted to pelvic organs, affecting the development of pelvic organ prolapse. Additionally, chronic forced and repetitive coughing, which may occur as a result of cigarette smoking, can predispose to prolapse and incontinence (14,15). Work involving heavy lifting or the forces generated by paratrooping can result in markedly increased intraabdominal pressure.

INCONTINENCE

Reversible causes of incontinence may result from systemic or local conditions, and patients can present with symptoms of overactive bladder or stress incontinence (16). Urinary tract infection may be associated with both urgency and urge incontinence as well as with stress incontinence. An inflamed bladder wall causes symptoms of urgency. Some strains of *Escherichia coli* release an α-adrenergic blocking agent that causes relaxation of the urethral smooth muscle, leading to stress incontinence. The effect of inadequate estrogen can cause further tissue irritation and urge symptoms and may also be associated with atrophic mucosal changes in the urethra, leading to poor coaptation and stress incontinence. Numerous medications have varied effects on the bladder by affecting urine production, cognition, and sympathetic and parasympathetic pathways. Medical conditions such as diabetes, congestive heart failure, peripheral edema, and excessive fluid intake may lead to increased urine production or alteration in day–night urinary excretion, leading to rapid bladder filling and symptoms of urgency and urge incontinence. The loss of mobility through disease may compromise timely bladder emptying. Loss of cognition or loss of sensation may lead to uncontrolled voiding.

OVERACTIVE BLADDER (STORAGE DYSFUNCTION)

The bladder normally functions as a reservoir, and then as a conduit for expelling urine from the body. During filling, the bladder should remain relaxed and the urethra contracted. At the appropriate time, the urethra relaxes and the bladder contracts to allow bladder emptying. An overactive bladder is associated with a disruption in various components of this coordinated mechanism, which leads to symptoms of urgency, frequency, nocturia, and urinary urge incontinence (see Chapter 20).

Neurologic

The neural control of the lower urinary tract is an integrated system comprising the local organs (bladder and urethra), sacral micturition area, the spinal cord, and central centers (frontal cortex, pons, and hypothalamus). The cerebral cortex (medial frontal lobes) and basal ganglia suppress micturition. Cortical lesions as occur from tumor, stroke, and cerebrovascular disease may result in loss of awareness or cognition of appropriate voiding situations, loss of sensation of bladder full-

TABLE 4.1. *Suprapontine causes of impaired bladder control*

Frontal lobe disease
Tumors
Encephalitis
Cerebrovascular accident
Head injury
Hydrocephalus
Dementia
Parkinsonism
Idiopathic Parkinson's disease
Multiple system atrophy

TABLE 4.2. *Causes of pontine disease*

Localized plaques of multiple sclerosis
Brain-stem encephalitis
Developmental tumors
Brain-stem glioma

ness, and inappropriate urethral relaxation (17) (Tables 4.1 and 4.2). Parkinson's disease is characterized by low levels of dopamine, which normally suppress bladder overactivity. These patients frequently have bladder overactivity (18).

Sympathetic innervation (T-10 to L-2) of the bladder and urethra may be disrupted from local injury, spinal cord disorders, or dysfunction of the cortical micturition center (19) (Table 4.3). A lesion above the lumbosacral cord level eliminates voluntary control of micturition, leading to bladder overactivity. The detrusor hyperreflexia in humans with spinal cord injury is most likely mediated by C-fiber afferents. Intravesical capsaicin may improve function in these patients (20). Parasympathetic function (S-2 to S-4) is particularly affected through pudendal nerve injury at childbirth, which leads to sensory disorder and impaired pelvic muscle function. Relative cholinergic overactivity may also lead to an overactive bladder (21).

There are also lesions that affect bladder innervation distal to the sacral spinal cord, and these are listed in Table 4.4 (17).

Nonneurogenic

Outflow Obstruction

It has long been determined that bladder outlet obstruction as occurs in prostatic hypertrophy is frequently associated with bladder instability. Removal of the obstruction through transurethral resection of the prostate results in cure of the instability in two thirds of patients (22). A reduction in acetylcholine esterase nerves has been demonstrated in obstructed human bladder muscle (23). Furthermore, pharmacologic studies on muscle specimens from patients with outlet obstruction demonstrated supersensitivity to acetylcholine and reduction in nerve-mediated responses compared with normal bladder (24). It was thought that obstructed detrusor muscle was associated with partial denervation of the muscle, and this led to postjunctional supersensitivity and to an unstable bladder. Either the raised intravesical pressure during voiding or increased tissue pressure of the hypertrophied bladder wall may cause reduced blood flow and denervation of the muscle. The abnormal detrusor muscle may not contract as effectively, which can lead to a combined problem of impaired contractility and bladder overactivity, a process seen in detrusor hyperactivity with impaired contractility (DHIC).

TABLE 4.3. *Causes of spinal cord disease*

Traumatic spinal cord injury
Multiple sclerosis
Transverse myelitis
Tropical spastic paraparesis (human T-cell leukemia virus type 1)
Other infections
Tumors
Arteriovenous malformation

TABLE 4.4. *Subsacral lesions affecting bladder innervation*

Spina bifida
  Myelomeningocele
  Tethered cord
Cauda equina injury
  Trauma
  Central disk prolapse
  Tumors
Small fiber neuropathy
  Diabetes
  Leprosy
  Amyloid
  Inherited autonomic neuropathies

Another theory is a reorganization of the spinal micturition reflex following outlet obstruction. An increased expression of nerve growth factor may be demonstrated in the bladder and sacral autonomic center, leading to facilitation of the spinal reflex and subsequent detrusor overactivity (25).

Aging

As many as 60% of institutionalized elderly patients have detrusor overactivity (26). It is difficult to measure the impact of neurologic cause in this group because there are many age-related neurologic conditions, including subclinical stroke and autonomic neuropathy. Ultrastructural studies reveal dysfunction in electrical couplings between muscle cells. There can be increased myogenic contractions in the overactive bladder, but widespread degeneration of muscle cells and nerve axons cause impaired detrusor contractility. These again are features of DHIC (27–29).

Anatomic

Correction of bladder neck hypermobility has been shown to improve detrusor instability (30). It is conjectured that afferent nerve activity is impaired secondary to poor pelvic support, and this leads to unstable detrusor contractions. There has not been a study on the effectiveness of surgery in pelvic floor prolapse and its effect on detrusor instability.

Hypersensitivity Disorders

Unmyelinated C fibers (capsaicin sensitive) transmit sensations of bladder fullness, urgency, and pain. It is hypothesized that increased afferent activity can induce bladder overactivity in patients with hypersensitivity disorders (31).

Muscular

The detrusor muscle has three intertwined muscle layers, and there are both smooth and striated muscle fibers in the urethra. The detrusor may become weakened through effects of aging, atrophy, overdistention, and impaired innervation, as described earlier. Detrusor contractions are partly related to a rise in intracellular calcium, which occurs through several pathways, including adenosine triphosphate (ATP) phosphorylation, protein kinases, and calcium and potassium channels. Disruption may lead to overactivity or underactivity of the bladder.

Myogenic changes may be the common pathway for the effects of denervation no matter what the etiology. Partial denervation of detrusor muscle may alter properties of smooth muscle, leading to increased excitability and coupling between cells. Activity locally spreads through the bladder wall and eventually produces a coordinated contraction (32).

STRESS INCONTINENCE

Genuine stress incontinence occurs when the urethra and bladder neck (urethrovesical junction) fail to maintain a watertight seal. This implies an abnormality in the components of continence, including the urethral wall (mucosa, vascularity, and smooth muscle), urethral support at the bladder neck (muscular and fascial), periurethral striated muscle, and urethral innervation (see Chapter 1). More simply, stress incontinence may result from damage to urethral support, loss of urethral sphincter function, or both. The disorders of stress incontinence are first discussed as those resulting from anatomic defects and those resulting from defects in the urethral sphincter mechanism. The effects of childbirth are also presented.

Anatomic (Hypermobility) Stress Incontinence

The anatomic defect leading to anatomic stress incontinence is the loss of muscular and fascial supports from the bladder neck and proximal urethra to the arcus tendineus fascia pelvis and pelvic diaphragm (see Chapter 1). With increased intraabdominal pressure, there is mobility and descent of the urethra and bladder neck. Pressure transmission to the urethra is compromised as it moves below the effective intraabdominal pressure range. The hammock of tissue under the urethra may also be poorly supported, and there is no backstop against which the urethra can be compressed. Finally, the periurethral striated muscle may offer little resistance because the efficiency of contraction is compromised by the malposition of the urethra.

The amplitude of intraabdominal pressure affects the demonstration, severity, and social impact of stress incontinence. Some women are essentially continent, but with a full bladder and a forceful event, such as vomiting, spasmodic coughing, or sneezing, they have disturbing urine loss. Forceful intraabdominal pressure is seen with aerobic exercise, especially jumping jacks or trampoline activity, and with obesity, chronic or acute pulmonary conditions, and some occupations. It is not unusual for young, nulliparous patients to have leakage related to physical events (33) such as gymnastics, volleyball, and other sports. Female paratroopers have a similar problem.

Intrinsic Sphincter Deficiency

Intrinsic sphincter deficiency (ISD) is caused by abnormalities of the urethral sphincter mechanism (34). These components include the important layers that make up the urethra (see Fig. 1.2 in Chapter 1) as well as the surrounding muscles and an intact neurologic supply.

The urethral epithelial surface or mucosa has numerous furrows and folds that allow external compression to seal the lumen. The submucosal layer is composed of collagen and elastin that provide substance to the folds and contribute to a sealing effect. A rich submucosal venous plexus also contributes to the closure of the urethral lumen and contributes significantly (one third) to urethral pressure (35). These inner urethral components are estrogen sensitive and probably have an aging component as well because estrogen supplementation does not prevent degenerative changes. Age also includes a factor of reduced muscle strength and loss of elasticity of tissues. Surgery near the urethra, such as aggressive anterior repair, may lead to scarring in the submucosal tissues and altered vascularity. Radiation therapy may cause direct tissue injury or vascular injury. Any factor that interferes with the normal urethral components can reduce resting urethral tone or resistance and increase the compressive forces needed to occlude the urethral lumen.

The urethra has a thick inner longitudinal and a thin outer circular layer of smooth muscle external to the submucosal layers. These layers contribute to resting urethral tone (36).

There are three striated muscle components of the urethra. The striated urogenital sphincter, which surrounds the smooth muscle, is located proximally and contains slow-twitch fibers. There are two extrinsic striated muscles: the urethrovaginal sphincter and the compressor urethrae muscles (37). The periurethral muscles contain both slow- and fast-twitch muscle fibers and are responsible for urethral pressure increases during sudden increase in intraabdominal pressure, as in coughing. The neurologic supply to these muscles can be impaired after childbirth and with aging, with subsequent loss of intraurethral tone and an abnormal response to increased intraabdominal pressure.

The pelvic floor muscles and fascial connective tissues provide a base on which the other components of continence depend. The pubococcygeal muscle contracts involuntarily in conjunction with the periurethral striated muscle during physical stress to close the urethral lumen. The pelvic diaphragm and perineal membrane provide a firm backstop for compression of the urethra. Additionally, another portion of the pubococcygeus muscle can be trained to contract voluntarily and improve compression of the urethra both at rest and during physical stress. These muscles function inadequately if the neurologic supply has been interrupted through aging, childbirth, and other factors. Both muscular and connective tissue components may be disrupted by childbirth, radical surgery, severe coughing, heavy work, and other trauma. The connective tissue in some patients may be inadequate from the start, and this may explain incontinence difficulties in the young, nulliparous patient (38,39).

Stress incontinence may be due to a peripheral neuropathy affecting innervation of pudendal nerve branches to the pelvic floor and striated muscle of the urethra (40). This occurs through childbearing, aging, chronic abdominal straining, and other factors. As stated previously, appropriate muscle activity requires normal nerve supply.

Childbirth Effect

The four mechanisms by which childbirth contributes to urinary incontinence are (a) injury to connective tissue supports by mechanical pressure effects, (b) vascular damage to pelvic structures through compression by the presenting part, (c) damage to pelvic nerves and muscles, and (d) direct injury to the urinary tract (41).

Even in the early 1900s, Delee described childbirth effects on pelvic floor anatomy (42).

Passage of the fetal head through the genital hiatus disconnects the vagina from its fascial anchors, allowing the vagina to slide down and out. The rectum is separated from its fascial and levator ani attachments. The fetal head distends, stretches, and may break levator muscles. The fascia or fibromuscular layer between bladder and vagina (many physicians believe there is no fascial layer here) is stretched, and the bladder connection to the endopelvic fascia can be severed. In addition to these anatomic disruptions, pudendal and perineal nerve damage has been described. This damage occurs distal to the ischial spine in the pudendal canal. Nerve damage results from direct compression by the fetal head and also from longitudinal stretching during perineal descent of the fetus. The changes of denervation of pelvic floor muscles are normal with aging but are increased by childbirth (8). Women with stress incontinence, fecal incontinence, or pelvic organ prolapse have greater denervation of pelvic floor muscles than women without symptoms. The denervated muscles cause inefficient activity of periurethral, anal, and pelvic striated muscles. The overall effects can be lower resting urethral resistance, decreased striated muscle activity with physical stress, increased descent of the urethra and bladder base with physical stress, and lower anal squeeze pressure. The effects of neurologic injury may affect continence or pelvic floor relaxation indirectly through loss of muscle strength or directly through loss of neurologic control. The levator hiatus may widen, increasing pelvic prolapse, and the anal sphincter weakness can cause fecal incontinence.

A number of studies have documented childbirth-related injury to the pudendal nerve and to the perineal branch of the pudendal nerve, which innervates the periurethral striated muscle (17). The normal perineal nerve terminal motor latency is 2.0 milliseconds, and in a group of patients with stress incontinence, the motor latency was 3.9 milliseconds (43). The pudendal nerve is also involved in the process, and studies have shown both delayed conduction to the muscles of the pelvic floor and morphologic evidence of nerve-mediated damage to the levator ani muscles after childbirth (44). Studies after vaginal delivery have shown both increased fiber density indicating denervation and reinnervation to pelvic floor muscles and prolonged pudendal motor terminal latency. Weaker levator ani muscles have been demonstrated in patients with stress incontinence (45). Studies have also shown histologic-histochemical and morphometric abnormalities in the pubococcygeal muscles of incontinent women. There were abnormalities in fiber-type pattern and muscle fiber cross-sectional area. There were also degenerative changes in connective tissue (46). Biochemical analyses of muscle specimens from women with stress incontinence showed imbalance in the biochemistry of glycogen with activation of hydrolytic decomposition (47).

Stress incontinence exists before first pregnancy in a substantial number of patients (5% or more) and confuses the discussion surrounding childbirth as an etiologic event (48).

Women who develop incontinence in middle life may be predestined, and pregnancy rather than delivery may first uncover the defect.

SUMMARY

There is overlap in function relative to anatomic support and the ability of the sphincter to work in an incorrect anatomic position. An abnormal position of the bladder neck can prevent normal pressure transmission during intraabdominal stress. Also, the laxity of pelvic floor musculature and fascia (collagen deficiency) can prevent the compression of the urethra against a normal backstop. The term urethral sphincter incompetence may be appropriately applied to all cases of stress incontinence. There may never be a single defect leading to stress incontinence; most likely, it results from an interaction of the many components described previously. Physicians may continue to refer to the two types of incontinence as anatomic and ISD, relative to treatment approach. The former can be managed by a repositioning operation, whereas the latter requires additional support to a weakened urethral sphincter, with or without support of the bladder neck. ISD can also be managed by periurethral bulking agents in cases in which there is adequate support of the bladder neck, although successes have been reported in cases of bladder neck hypermobility (49). More widespread use of

sling surgery and the development of newer sling techniques, such as tension-free vaginal tape, may lure one into the mindset that one operation fits all. It remains essential to investigate and understand the mechanics of the defects leading to stress incontinence in the individual patient and to apply the most effective therapy based on this knowledge.

REFERENCES

1. Gill EJ, Hurt WG. Pathophysiology of pelvic organ prolapse. *Obstet Gynecol Clin North Am* 1998;25:757–769.
2. Gainey HL. Post-partum observation of pelvic tissue damage. *Am J Obstet Gynecol* 1943;45:457–466.
3. Gainey HL. Postpartum observation of pelvic tissue damage: further studies. *Am J Obstet Gynecol* 1955;70:800–807.
4. Meyer S, Schreyer A, deGrandi P, et al. The effects of birth on urinary continence mechanisms and other pelvic-floor characteristics. *Obstet Gynecol* 1998;92:613–618.
5. Tetzscher T, Sorensen M, Jonsson L. et al. Delivery and pudendal nerve function. *Acta Obstet Gynecol Scand* 1997;76:324–331.
6. Peschers UM, Schaer GN, DeLancey JOL, et al. Levator ani function before and after childbirth. *Br J Obstet Gynaecol* 1997;104:1004–1008.
7. Snooks SJ, Setchell M, Swash M, et al. Injury to innervation of pelvic floor sphincter musculature in childbirth. *Lancet* 1984;2:546–550.
8. Smith ARB, Hosker GL, Warrell DW. The role of partial denervation of the pelvic floor in the aetiology of genitourinary prolapse and stress incontinence of urine. *Br J Obstet Gynaecol* 1989;96:24–28.
9. Nygaard IE, Rao SS, Dawson JD. Anal incontinence after anal sphincter disruption: a 30-year retrospective cohort study. *Obstet Gynecol* 1997;89:896–901.
10. Makinen J, Soderstrom K, Kiilhoma P, et al. Histological change in the vaginal connective tissue of patients with and without uterine prolapse. *Arch Gynecol* 1986;239:17–20.
11. Norton P, Boyd C, Deak S. Abnormal collagen ratios in women with genitourinary prolapse. *Neurourol Urodyn* 1992;11:2–4.
12. DeMola JRL, Carpenter SE. Management of genital prolapse in neonates and young women. *Obstet Gynecol Surv* 1996;51:253–260.
13. Shull BL, Capen CV, Riggs MW, et al. Preoperative and postoperative analysis of site-specific pelvic support defects in 81 women treated with sacrospinous ligament suspension and pelvic reconstruction. *Am J Obstet Gynecol* 1992;166:1764–1771.
14. Bump RC, Sugerman HJ, Fantl JA, et al. Obesity and lower urinary tract function in women: effect of surgically induced weight loss. *Am J Obstet Gynecol* 1992;167:392–399.
15. Bump RC, McClish DK. Cigarette smoking and urinary incontinence in women. *Am J Obstet Gynecol* 1992;167:1213–1218.
16. Robinson D. Pathophysiology of female lower urinary tract dysfunction. *Obstet Gynecol Clin North Am* 1998;25:747–756.

17. DeLancey JOL, Fowler CJ, Keane D, et al. Pathophysiology. In: Abrams A, Khoury S, Wein A, eds. *First international consultation on incontinence.* Plymouth, MA: Health Publication Ltd, 1999:227–294.

18. Yoshimura N, Mizuta E, Kuno S. et al. The dopamine D, receptor agonist SKF 38393 suppresses detrusor hyperreflexia in the monkey with parkinsonism induced by 1-methyl-4-phenyl-1,2,3,6–tetrahydropyridine (MPTP). *Neuropharmacology* 1993;32:315–321.

19. DeGroat WC. A neurologic basis for the overactive bladder. *Urology* 1997;50:36.

20. Geirsson G, Fall M, Sullivan L. Effect of intravesical capsaicin treatment on posttraumatic spinal detrusor hyperreflexia and the bladder cooling reflex. *Neurourol Urodyn* 1994;13:346–347.

21. Andersson KE. Neurotransmitters and neuroreceptors in the lower urinary tract. *Curr Opin Obstet Gynecol* 1996;8:361–365.

22. Abrams PH. Detrusor instability and bladder outlet obstruction. *Neurourol Urodyn* 1985;4:317–328.

23. Gosling JA, Gilpin SA, Dixon J, et al. Decrease in the autonomic innervation of human detrusor muscle in outflow obstruction. *J Urol* 1986;136:501–504.

24. Harrison SCW, Hunnan GR, Farman PAT, et al. Bladder instability and denervation in patients with bladder outflow obstruction. *Br J Urol* 1987;60:519–522.

25. Steers WD, de Groat WC. Effect of bladder outlet obstruction on micturition reflex pathways in the rat. *J Urol* 1988;140:864–871.

26. Resnick NM, Yalla SV, Laurino E. The pathophysiology of urinary incontinence among institutionalized elderly persons. *N Engl J Med* 1989;320:1–7.

27. Elbadawi A, Yalla SV, Resnick NM. Structural basis of geriatric voiding dysfunction. Aging detrusor: normal vs. impaired contractility. *J Urol* 1993;150: 1657–1667.

28. Elbadawi A, Yalla SV, Resnick NM. Structural basis of geriatric voiding dysfunction. III. Detrusor overactivity. *J Urol* 1993;150:1668–1680.

29. Resnick NM, Yalla SV. Detrusor hyperactivity with impaired contractile function: an unrecognized but common cause of incontinence in elderly patients. *JAMA* 1987;257:3076–3081.

30. Sand PK, Bowen LW, Ostergard DR, et al. The effect of retropubic urethropexy on detrusor stability. *Obstet Gynecol* 1988;71:818–822.

31. Maggi CA, Barbanti G, Santiciolo P, et al. Cystometric evidence that capsaicin-sensitive nerves modulate the afferent branch of micturition reflex in humans. *J Urol* 1989;142:150–154.

32. Brading AF. A myogenic basis for the overactive bladder. *Urology* 1997;50[Suppl 6A]:57–73.

33. Nygaard IE, Thompson FL, Svengalis SL, et al. Urinary incontinence in elite nulliparous athletes. *Obstet Gynecol* 1994;84:183–187.

34. Urinary Incontinence Guideline Panel. *Urinary incontinence in adults: clinical practice guideline update.* AHCPR Pub. No. 96-0686. Rockville, MD: Agency for Health Care Policy and Research, Public Health Service, U.S. Department of Health and Human Services, March 1996.

35. Raz S, Caine M, Ziegler M. The vascular component in the production of intraurethral pressure. *J Urol* 1972; 108:93–96.

36. Nordling J. Alpha blockers and urethral pressure in neurological patients. *Urol Int* 1978;33:304–309.

37. DeLancey JOL. Correlative study of paraurethral anatomy. *Obstet Gynecol* 1986;68:91–97.

38. Norton P, Baker J, Sharp H, et al. Genitourinary prolapse and hypermobility in women. *Obstet Gynecol* 1995;85:225–229.

39. Keane DP, Sims TJ, Abrams P, et al. Analysis of collagen status in premenopausal nulliparous women with genuine stress incontinence. *Br J Obstet Gynaecol* 1997;104:994–998.

40. Anderson RS. A neurogenic element to urinary genuine stress incontinence. *Br J Obstet Gynaecol* 1984;91:41–45.

41. Walters MD, Newton ER. Pathophysiology and obstetrics issues of genuine stress incontinence and pelvic floor dysfunction. In: Walters MD, Karram MM eds. *Urogynecology and reconstructive pelvic surgery,* 2nd ed. St. Louis: Mosby, 1999:135–144.

42. Delee JB. The prophylactic forceps operation. *Am J Obstet Gynecol* 1920;1:34.

43. Snooks SJ, Badenoch DF, Tiptaft RC, et al. Perineal nerve damage in genuine stress urinary incontinence. *Br J Urol* 1985;57:422–426.

44. Snooks SJ, Swash M, Henry MM, et al. Risk factors in childbirth causing damage to the pelvic floor innervation. *Int J Colorectal Dis* 1986;1:20–24.

45. Gunnarsson M, Mattiasson A. Circumvaginal surface electromyography in women with urinary incontinence and in healthy volunteers. *Scand J Urol Nephrol Suppl* 1994;157:89–95.

46. Fischer W, Pfister C, Tunn R. Histomorphology of pelvic floor muscles in women with urinary incontinence. *Zentralb Gynakol* 1992;114:189–194.

47. Jozwik M Jr, Lotocki W, Jozwik M. Stress urinary incontinence in women. II. Abnormalities of glycogenolysis in tissues related to the lower urinary tract. *Int Urol Nephrol* 1996;28:485–494.

48. Wolin LH. Stress incontinence in young healthy nulliparous subjects. *J Urol* 1969;101:545–549.

49. Bent AE, Foote J, Siegel S, et al. Collagen implant for treating stress urinary incontinence in women with urethral hypermobility. *J Urol* 2001;166:1354–1357.

Ostergard's Urogynecology and Pelvic Floor Dysfunction, Fifth Edition. edited by A.E. Bent, et al. Lippincott Williams & Wilkins, Philadelphia © 2003.

5

Outcome Assessment

Vik Khullar

Faculty of Medicine, Imperial College School of Medicine; and Department of Obstetrics and Gynecology, St. Mary's Hospital, London, England

Urogynecologic disorders are common, affecting up to 40% of women attending a gynecologic clinic. The problems of urinary incontinence and vaginal prolapse alter the lives of women dramatically such that they can no longer continue their usual daily activities. Unfortunately, despite the severely limiting nature of these problems, women do not seek help for many years. The impact of the disease on a woman's daily life will not relate to the severity of the incontinence. When a woman realizes that she is leaking, she will develop strategies to minimize urinary incontinence, such as restricting fluid intake or voiding frequently. These changes in behavior reduce the severity of the woman's symptoms but lead to a reduction in her quality of life (QoL).

An assessment of urinary symptoms is usually made with a standardized symptom questionnaire. The diagnosis of the underlying cause may require urodynamic testing. Based on these investigations and an assessment of symptom severity, the appropriate treatment can be started. A woman's own views may be distorted by the physician–patient interaction. This problem may be worsened when the outcome of treatment is being assessed.

Symptoms of lower urinary tract dysfunction vary greatly for different women. Standard forms without proper psychometric testing in the assessment of lower urinary tract dysfunction are invalid. This assessment alters according to the patient's physical, psychological, social, domestic, and interpersonal lifestyle. The impact of the disease on the individual are modified by other factors, including age, race, and culture; personal goals and experience; interpersonal relationships; general physical and mental health; and life expectancy. The absence of a structured and standardized patient-completed assessment makes any meaningful quantification of the impact of urinary incontinence on the individual inaccurate. When objective measures of lower urinary tract dysfunction have been compared with the degree of improvement felt by the woman, no relationship has been found. Many authors have found that measurement of urinary frequency and urine loss are only weakly associated with perceived impact of incontinence.

This chapter describes QoL assessment and how it has been applied to women with urinary incontinence. Validated QoL questionnaires have become established in a number of settings, including interventional randomized controlled trials for the assessment of women with urinary incontinence.

There are many definitions of QoL, but there is no agreed definition. Early definitions involved the assessment of health because it was thought that this would be associated with QoL. Unfortunately, although health is associated with socioeconomic factors, economic factors are not closely linked to health to allow it to be used as a surrogate. QoL is not just the absence of ill health. The World Health Organization (WHO) definition

TABLE 5.1. *Aspects (dimensions) of quality of life*

- Social function: meeting people, leisure activities, and social support
- Physical function: activity, exercise, self-containment
- Emotional function: anxiety, depression
- Role performance: work, care of the home, and shopping
- Sleep
- Pain
- Personal function: intimate activity, family relationships
- Disease-specific symptoms

of health is not merely the absence of disease, but complete physical, mental, and social well-being. QoL has many different facets and involves a combination of patient-assessed measures of health, including physical function, social and role function, sense of well-being, burden of symptoms and emotional or mental state.

QoL is usually measured with questionnaires that are self-completed or filled in at interview. Self-completed questionnaires are an inexpensive and practical method of obtaining information on QoL. They do rely on the patient understanding the questions, and the questionnaire must be designed to allow this to happen. The problem with self-completion is that the questionnaire may be interpreted differently in different populations and cultures. Thus, QoL questionnaires should always be pretested in the population in which they are to be used before clinical trial. Although many different questionnaires are now available, each conforms to the same basic structure. The questionnaires consist of a variable number of domains (or sections), usually one to seven, that gather information focused on particular aspects of health and QoL (Table 5.1).

QoL measures have been used in many different patient groups and illnesses. They are useful in assessing outcome measures in clinical trials, particularly when the measures take into account the patient's perception of her overall well-being.

There are two major types of QoL questionnaires: generic and disease specific. Generic questionnaires can be used in different groups of women whatever the disease being studied. They allow the comparison of different groups of women. Disease-specific questionnaires are designed for particular diseases and focus on clinically important areas for that disease. This makes the disease-specific questionnaires more sensitive to change and outcome than generic questionnaires.

DEVELOPING A QUESTIONNAIRE

Irrespective of their type, all questionnaires have been previously validated and their reliability has been tested to ensure their psychometric value for the assessment of QoL. To develop a questionnaire, there are a number of crucial steps (1) (Table 5.2).

Reliability assesses how often the same results are obtained when the tests are repeatedly determined. There are two main areas of reliability. The first is internal reliability, and this estimates how the individual questions in a questionnaire relate to each other and the total score. The Cronbach's alpha measures this, and values greater than 0.7 are acceptable, values greater than 0.8 are good, and values greater than 0.9 are excellent. Test–retest reli-

TABLE 5.2. *Steps to develop a quality-of-life questionnaire*

- Focus groups of patients for disease effects
- Test–retest reliability, reproducibility of questionnaire
- Validity; construct, criterion, and content/face of questionnaire
- Test responsiveness, ideally in interventional study

ability assesses the reproducibility of the questionnaire scores using correlation coefficients, such as Spearman's rho or Pearson's r, or interclass correlation coefficients. There is high reliability when the values are greater than or equal to 0.8.

The validity of a questionnaire assesses whether it measures what is intended. This can be determined in a number of ways and requires evaluation of the questionnaire at different times and usually against different measures of the disease. Validity has three major aspects: content/face, construct, and criterion.

Content/face validity is an assessment of whether the questionnaire makes sense to the patients and the clinical experts using the questionnaire, and whether all the important or relevant domains are included. This is achieved by using literature reviews, interviews with patients, and consultations with other experts in the field. This should be carried out early in the development of a questionnaire. In particular, the questions must make clinical sense and be understandable and unambiguous to the patient. For example, if the questionnaire aims to measure a woman's perspectives of incontinence, it is essential that attention be devoted to understanding how women perceive such symptoms and what words are used to describe them. These aspects are developed through interviews with women, and then the completed draft versions of questionnaires are given to women who have the disease under study. After the questionnaire has been developed and administered, levels of missing data can be used as an indicator of inappropriate questions.

Construct validity assesses the possible relationship between QoL measures and other areas, such as pain, anxiety, and satisfaction with life. The measures are related using the Pearson or Spearman correlation coefficients. There are no absolute values for determining a good correlation, but the better the correlation, the greater the relationship between the questionnaire and underlying disease effects. A common method of testing the construct validity of a questionnaire is to examine its ability to differentiate between patient groups, such as women who attend a community clinic and those who attend a hospital clinic.

Criterion validity describes how well the questionnaire correlates with a gold standard that already exists. The gold standards may be clinical or other validated measures. In many areas, there is no clear gold standard, or there may be debate. For incontinence, there is no clear gold standard against which to measure the criterion validity of questionnaires. Although it is acknowledged that urodynamic studies or pad tests represent the most accurate representation of leakage and thus of a clinical diagnosis of incontinence, these factors are not the only ones that one would want to have reflected by a questionnaire. There should be some relationship between a questionnaire that assesses incontinence and a clinical finding of the condition. Because these questionnaires do assess the woman's perception of incontinence and its impact on their QoL, the diagnosis and the condition may not correlate well. An ideal gold standard is another questionnaire that measures the same QoL areas but does not cover it completely. Thus, comparisons can be made between the two questionnaires.

Reproducibility is an assessment of variability between and within observers (interrater and intrarater reliability). This is important if the questionnaire is completed at interview. The analysis of variance (ANOVA) test is used to determine variance.

Finally, responsiveness is assessed. This is controversial because there is no agreement about the best method of determining whether a questionnaire has the optimum measurement of change. This is best done in a study comparing an intervention and control group.

QUALITY OF LIFE AND URINARY INCONTINENCE

The QoL of incontinent women has been determined in a number of studies, and the design of the studies has been varied. Unfortunately, most studies have not tried to characterize the cause of the urinary incontinence. This is unfortunate because urinary symptoms and urodynamic diagnoses do not correlate well. It has been shown that incontinence does cause embarrassment and reduced self-esteem (2,3). Incontinence also leads to impaired emotional and psychological well-being (4), poorer sexual relationships (5–7), and impairment of social activities and relationships (8–10). Thus, the impacts of urinary incontinence on many aspects of life are undeniable, but the main problem is how best to quantify these impacts and to use the most sensitive method to detect changes in trials of treatments.

GENERIC QUALITY-OF-LIFE QUESTIONNAIRES

Generic questionnaires are designed to measure general aspects of QoL. This means they can be used for different populations and the comparison of different diseases. The generic questionnaires that have been used to assess incontinence include the Sickness Impact Profile (SIP) (11), Nottingham Health Profile (NHP) (12), the Short Form 36 (SF-36) (13), and the Psychosocial Adjustment to Illness Scale (PAIS) (14). The questionnaires have been used extensively to assess the impact of lower urinary tract symptoms and their effects on QoL. Thus, there are extensive comparative and normative data, with manuals that have data stratified for age, sex, and social class. The normative data are obtained from large groups of subjects without medical complaints.

When comparing women with detrusor instability to those with rheumatoid arthritis and to those with no symptoms, the women with detrusor instability had worse QoL values than the other two groups in the domains of vitality, social function, and emotional problems (15).

The generic questionnaires need nonspecific questions and scoring for a variety of diseases. This reduces the sensitivity of the measure for specific diseases such as lower urinary tract dysfunction. Reduced sensitivity for a ques-

tionnaire may prevent it from detecting changes in clinical trials. Disease-specific questionnaires are designed to be sensitive to lower urinary tract dysfunction and changes. A number of questionnaires have been recommended by the Second International Consultation on Incontinence (Table 5.3). It has been recommended that studies use generic and disease-specific questionnaires.

Generic QoL questionnaires have been used to assess urinary incontinence in women. Grimby and colleagues (16) used the NHP for 120 elderly women with urinary incontinence and 313 elderly women without urinary symptoms. Overall, 70% of women replied from the study group. The women with urinary symptoms were divided into the following groups: those with stress incontinence (28%), those with urge incontinence (40%), and those with mixed symptoms (31%) after a clinical history, urinary diary, cough test, and pad test. Urodynamic testing was not carried out. The incontinent women had a significantly higher level of both social isolation and emotional impairment than the control group. Interestingly, there was more emotional disturbance in women suffering urge incontinence and mixed symptoms than in those suffering stress incontinence. Women with urge incontinence also had greater sleep disturbance than the control group. This underlines the unpredictable nature of urge incontinence, which can lead to greater emotional problems, and the probable effects of nocturia.

The SF-36 is a widely used generic questionnaire. Sand and co-workers (17) used the SF-36 questionnaire to assess the efficacy of treatment in women with urodynamic stress incontinence in a randomized, double-blind, placebo-controlled trial com-

TABLE 5.3. *Recommended condition-specific quality-of-life questionnaires*

- King's Health Questionnaire
- Urogenital Distress Inventory
- Incontinence Impact Questionnaire
- Incontinence Quality-of-Life Questionnaire

paring electrical vaginal stimulation with the use of a sham device. Thirty-five women used the active stimulator and 17 the sham device. The objective outcome measures of urinary diary, pad test, and vaginal muscle strength showed a significant benefit of the active device. Subjective measures (urinary symptom questionnaire and visual analogue scale) also showed benefit. No significant difference was seen in the score changes for the SF-36. This nonsignificant result was due to the low power of the study and the lack of sensitivity of the generic questionnaire to detect change.

Generic questionnaires have been used to determine which women will not respond favorably to treatment. Kelleher and associates (18) has used the PAIS questionnaire to assess women with detrusor overactivity before and 6 months after treatment for detrusor instability with anticholinergic therapy. This questionnaire showed that women with the worst pretreatment scores had the worst posttreatment scores. Interestingly, women who had a worse QoL because of stress incontinence were more likely to consider themselves subjectively cured after continence surgery.

DISEASE-SPECIFIC QUALITY-OF-LIFE QUESTIONNAIRES

Many disease-specific questionnaires have been developed in recent years. Many were not properly validated before their publication, and these will not be reviewed. The questionnaires are divided into two types: the first assesses the "bother" of the urinary symptoms on the woman and her life, and the other measures the impact of the urinary symptoms on the woman's QoL. Because these two areas are so closely linked, the two types are complementary.

The Bristol Female Lower Urinary Tract Symptoms questionnaire was designed to be sensitive to changes in women's symptoms (19). This questionnaire quantifies symptoms in severity and frequency, and then determines in a separate group of questions the bother of these symptoms on the woman. It

has been validated but is principally a symptom questionnaire.

The Symptom Impact Index is a three-item questionnaire developed for use with the Symptom Severity Index (a five-item questionnaire) (20). The questionnaire has been validated and has been used as a sensitive method of assessing incontinence after continence surgery. It has the benefit of being short and easy to fill in. The questions are aimed mainly at the symptoms of stress incontinence and hence may not be as helpful in patients with urge incontinence or irritative symptoms.

The Incontinence Impact Questionnaire (IIQ) is again a self-administered questionnaire (21) that has undergone rigorous validation (22). It shows weak but significant correlations with urinary frequency and quantity of urine lost (23,24). A short form of this questionnaire has been developed with seven questions (IIQ-7), and this is more useful for clinical situations.

The King's Health Questionnaire (25) has three parts. The first part has questions on general health and the second on urinary symptoms. The third part has questions on seven domains of QoL, including role; physical, social, and personal domains; and emotional problems, sleep disturbance, and incontinence impact. This questionnaire has been extensively validated and used in clinical trials and is available in several languages, including German, U.S. English, Canadian English, Greek, Spanish, Swiss, Italian, and French versions.

The Incontinence Quality-of-Life Questionnaire (I-QoL) was designed for clinical trials to measure the impact of incontinence in men and women (26). This can be obtained through the Medical Outcomes Trust.

The Urogenital Distress Inventory was developed in the United States to assess which irritative symptoms are troubling (22). The questionnaire enquires about 19 symptoms and has been tested in community-dwelling women with incontinence and in women older than 60 years of age (27). The questionnaire has good levels of validity, responsiveness, and reliability. Using regression analysis, a shorter version of the Urogenital

Distress Inventory was developed, the UDI-6 (28,29). It has been suggested that this questionnaire may be used to predict the urodynamic diagnosis.

Other questionnaires, such as the York Incontinence Perceptions Scale (24), Stress Incontinence Questionnaire (30), and Psychosocial Consequences Questionnaire (31) have not fully completed their psychometric evaluation and thus cannot be recommended for clinical use.

USES OF QUALITY-OF-LIFE QUESTIONNAIRES IN UROGYNECOLOGY

QoL measurements give an extra perspective when used in outcome studies. Their importance is emphasized when objective measures show no changes, for example, when a drug is used to investigate the treatment of the overactive bladder with frequency–volume charts and QoL questionnaires. As a result of the medication and an ability to drink more, the women may still have the same urinary frequency as before. However, because the women are able to drink more, their QoL is improved because of decreased morbidity. QoL measurements also allow clinicians to determine whether there has been a true improvement in a woman's life when the changes in parameters are small but significant or when a treatment improves one symptom while making other symptoms worse.

Many women in the community appear to have urinary symptoms. It is not clear why these women tolerate their symptoms rather than attempting to get treatment. Interestingly, the length of time a woman has her problem, and the time to seeking help, are not related to severity or duration of the incontinence nor the level of the woman's education (32). QoL questionnaires help assess the overall impact of the disease on the individual and would ultimately be useful in determining the true costs of incontinence.

QoL questionnaires are helpful in allowing the assessment of need and the effects of treatment. This allows health improvement to be assessed and compared with other diseases. One method of comparing health improvement with different diseases is the use of quality-adjusted life years (QALY), which combine both QoL and survival (33). This allows a very simplistic method of comparing the effects of different treatments using these two different outcome measures.

Predicting Quality-of-Life Impairment for Incontinent Women

Urinary incontinence has many different effects on the QoL of women. One would expect that severity and duration of symptoms has a major impact on QoL, but interestingly, they do not appear to correlate. However, women with detrusor overactivity and poor QoL do not respond well to treatment (34). It is possible that this may be because the disease is more severe and the treatments are less effective.

Urodynamic diagnosis has a major influence on the QoL impairment of women. Women with detrusor overactivity have been shown to have greater impairment of QoL than women with urodynamic stress incontinence (16,35). The reason these women have a worse QoL is that the incontinence due to detrusor overactivity is unpredictable and more severe, and the woman feels she has less control (23). This appears to be the same for the sexual problems of women suffering from detrusor overactivity (7,36).

Elderly women are sometimes denied surgical treatment for urodynamic stress incontinence because the improvement in QoL is not justified by the morbidity of the surgery. The improvement in QoL in older women is often better than that in younger women (CJ Kelleher, personal communication), even though older women often have more severe urinary symptoms. Elderly women may delay presentation for investigation and treatment (37), although there is no evidence that urinary incontinence causes less bother to elderly women than younger women.

Quality of Life in Patients with Vaginal Prolapse

Vaginal prolapse is a common, distressing, and disabling condition affecting up to 30% of women of all ages attending gynecology outpatient clinics. The incidence of vaginal prolapse increases with advancing age, menopause, and parity and has been thought to be most common in whites, less common in Asian, and uncommon in blacks, although one study has shown no racial differences (38). There are few epidemiologic data about urogenital prolapse, but it has been reported to be the most common reason for hysterectomy in women older than 50 years of age. It has been estimated that more than half a million operations for vaginal prolapse are performed annually in the United States.

The symptom of feeling "something coming down" is almost universally described. Women may describe a lump or a "feeling of pressure" in the vagina, which is worse toward the end of the day, is relieved by lying down, and may be totally asymptomatic in the morning. Urinary symptoms, such as poor stream, hesitancy, straining to void, incomplete emptying, recurrent urinary tract infections, and the need to reduce the bulge digitally to void or defecate may be also present. Management of vaginal prolapse has usually relied on the physician's findings to decide whether or not a woman needs to be treated and whether or not she is cured by that treatment. Nevertheless, interviewing a woman about her vaginal prolapse symptoms may cause embarrassment, and a symptomatic assessment by the physician may be difficult or inaccurate. There appears to be little correlation between symptoms from vaginal prolapse and clinical findings (39). Thus, a valid, reliable, and easily comprehensible questionnaire designed to assess the severity of symptoms of prolapse and their impact on QoL has been developed, the Prolapse Quality-of-Life Questionnaire (40). This questionnaire has been used to assess the impact on prolapse of different surgical procedures (40). Even though women who had either operation felt that the result of their vaginal prolapse repair was adequate, the QoL was significantly better in those women who had a mesh inserted compared with a standard anterior repair. It has also been shown that there is no correlation between prolapse QoL scores and vaginal examination findings supine. There is significant correlation between prolapse QoL scores and vaginal examination if it is performed standing.

Copies of the King's Health Questionnaire and Prolapse Quality-of-Life Questionnaire can be obtained from the author (Urogynaecology Unit, Department of Obstetrics and Gynaecology, Mint Wing, ICSM, St. Mary's Hospital, Norfolk Place, London W21PG, UK; vik.khullar@ic.ac.uk).

CONCLUSIONS

QoL assessment allows a detailed evaluation of the effects of lower urinary tract dysfunction and vaginal prolapse on the individual. This allows the individual to be assessed in her totality rather than assessing simply a change in symptoms. QoL measurements are recognized to be an essential component of the assessment of women in trials of new treatments in urogynecology, and they disclose important areas that should improve our investigation and practice.

REFERENCES

1. Streiner DL, Norma GR. *Health measurement scales, a practical guide to their development and use.* Oxford: Oxford Medical Publications, 1993.
2. Lagro-Janssen AL, Debruyne FM, Van Weel C. Psychological aspects of female urinary incontinence in general practice. *Br J Urol* 1992;70:499–502.
3. Ouslander JG, Hepps K, Raz S, et al. Genitourinary dysfunction in a geriatric outpatient population. *J Am Geriatr Soc* 1986;34:507–514.
4. Herzog AR, Diokno AC, Fultz NH. Urinary incontinence: medical and psychosocial aspects. *Annu Rev Gerontol Geriatr* 1989;9:74–119.
5. Sutherst JR. Sexual dysfunction and urinary incontinence. *Br J Obstet Gynaecol* 1979;86:387–388.
6. Kelleher CJ, Cardozo LD, Khullar V, et al. The impact of urinary incontinence on sexual function. *J Sexual Health* 1993;8:186–191.
7. Hilton P. Urinary incontinence during sexual intercourse: a common, but rarely volunteered, symptom. *Br J Obstet Gynaecol* 1988;95:377–381.

8. Iosif S, Henriksson L, Ulmsten U. The frequency of disorders of the lower urinary tract, urinary incontinence in particular, as evaluated by a questionnaire survey in a gynecological health control population. *Acta Obstet Gynecol Scand* 1981;60:71–76.

9. Breakwell SL, Walker SN. Differences in physical health, social interaction, and personal adjustment between continent and incontinent homebound aged women. *J Commun Health Nursing* 1988;5:19–31.

10. Kutner NG, Schechtman KB, Ory MG, et al. Older adults' perceptions of their health and functioning in relation to sleep disturbance, falling, and urinary incontinence. FICSIT Group. *J Am Geriatr Soc* 1994;42: 757–762.

11. Bergner M, Bobbitt RA, Carter WB, et al. The Sickness Impact Profile: development and final revision of a health status measure. *Med Care* 1981;19:787–805.

12. Hunt SM, McEwen J, McKenna SP. Measuring health status: a new tool for clinicians and epidemiologists. *J R Coll Gen Pract* 1985;35:185–188.

13. Jenkinson C, Coulter A, Wright L. Short form 36 (SF36) health survey questionnaire: normative data for adults of working age. *BMJ* 1993;306:1437–1440.

14. Derogatis LR, Derogatis MF. *The Psychosocial Adjustment to Illness Scale (PAIS and PAIS SR) administration, scoring and procedures manual—II. London:* Clinical Psychometric Research, 1990.

15. Johannesson M, O'Conor RM, Kobelt-Nguyen G, et al. Willingness to pay for reduced incontinence symptoms. *Br J Urol* 1997;80:557–562.

16. Grimby A, Milsom I, Molander U, et al. The influence of urinary incontinence on the quality of life of elderly women. *Age Ageing* 1993;22:82–89.

17. Sand PK, Richardson DA, Staskin DR, et al. Pelvic floor electrical stimulation in the treatment of genuine stress incontinence: a multicenter, placebo-controlled trial. *Am J Obstet Gynecol* 1995;173:72–79.

18. Kelleher CJ, Khullar V, Cardozo LD. Psychoneuroticism and quality of life impairment in healthy incontinent women. *Neurourol Urodyn* 1993;12:393–394.

19. Jackson S, Donovan J, Brookes S, et al. The Bristol Female Lower Urinary Tract Symptoms questionnaire: development and psychometric testing. *Br J Urol* 1996; 77:805–812.

20. Black N, Griffiths J, Pope C. Development of a symptom severity index and a symptom impact index for stress incontinence in women. *Neurourol Urodyn* 1996; 15:630–640.

21. Norton PA, MacDonald LD, Sedgwick PM, et al. Distress and delay associated with urinary incontinence, frequency, and urgency in women. *BMJ* 1988;297: 1187–1189.

22. Shumaker SA, Wyman JF, Uebersax JS, et al. Health-related quality of life measures for women with urinary incontinence: the Incontinence Impact Questionnaire and the Urogenital Distress Inventory. Continence Program in Women (CPW) Research Group. *Qual Life Res* 1994;3:291–306.

23. Wyman JF, Harkins SW, Choi SC, et al. Psychosocial impact of urinary incontinence in women. *Obstet Gynecol* 1987;70:378–381.

24. Lee PS, Reid DW, Saltmarche A, et al. Measuring the psychosocial impact of urinary incontinence: the York Incontinence Perceptions Scale (YIPS). *J Am Geriatr Soc* 1995;43:1275–1278.

25. Kelleher CJ, Cardozo LD, Khullar V, et al. A new questionnaire to assess the quality of life of urinary incontinent women. *Br J Obstet Gynaecol* 1997;104: 1374–1379.

26. Wagner TH, Patrick DL, Bavendam TG, et al. Quality of life of persons with urinary incontinence: development of a new measure. *Urology* 1996;47:67–71.

27. Robinson D, Pearce KF, Preisser JS, et al. Relationship between patient reports of urinary incontinence symptoms and quality of life measures. *Obstet Gynecol* 1998; 91:224–228.

28. Uebersax JS, Wyman JF, Shumaker SA, et al. Short forms to assess life quality and symptom distress for urinary incontinence in women: the Incontinence Impact Questionnaire and the Urogenital Distress Inventory. Continence Program for Women Research Group. *Neurourol Urodyn* 1995;14:131–139.

29. Dugan E, Cohen SJ, Robinson D, et al. The quality of life of older adults with urinary incontinence: determining generic and condition-specific predictors. *Qual Life Res* 1998;7:337–344.

30. Nochajski TH, Burns PA, Pranikoff K, et al. Dimensions of urine loss among older women with genuine stress incontinence. *Neurourol Urodyn* 1993;12:223–233.

31. Seim A, Hermstad R, Hunskaar S. Management in general practice significantly reduced psychosocial consequences of female urinary incontinence. *Qual Life Res* 1997;6:257–264.

32. Burgio KL, Ives DG, Locher JL, et al. Treatment seeking for urinary incontinence in older adults. *J Am Geriatr Soc* 1994;42:208–212.

33. Kobelt G. Economic considerations and outcome measurement in urge incontinence. *Urology* 1997;50: 100–107.

34. Moore KH, Eadie AS, McAlister A, et al. Response to drug treatment of detrusor instability in relation to psychosomatic. *Neurourol Urodyn* 1989;8:412.

35. Hunskaar S, Vinsnes A. The quality of life in women with urinary incontinence as measured by the sickness impact profile [erratum appears in *J Am Geriatr Soc* 1992;40(9):976–977]. *J Am Geriatr Soc* 1991;39: 378–382.

36. Kelleher CJ, Cardozo LD, Khullar V, et al. The impact of urinary incontinence on sexual function. *J Sexual Health* 1993;8:186–191.

37. Fonda D, Resnick NM, Colling J, et al. Outcome measures for research of lower urinary tract dysfunction in frail older people. *Neurourol Urodyn* 1998;17: 273–281.

38. Bump RC. Racial comparisons and contrasts in urinary incontinence and pelvic organ prolapse. *Obstet Gynecol* 1993;81:421–425.

39. Athanasiou S, Hill S, Gleason C, et al. Validation of the ICS proposed pelvic organ prolapse descriptive system. *Neurourol Urodyn* 1995;14:414–415.

40. Digesu GA, Khullar V, Cardozo L, et al. P-QoL: a validated quality of life questionnaire for the symptomatic assessment of women with uterovaginal prolapse. *Int Urogynecol J* 2000;11:S25.

SECTION II

Evaluation

Ostergard's Urogynecology and Pelvic Floor Dysfunction, Fifth Edition. edited by A.E. Bent, et al. Lippincott Williams & Wilkins, Philadelphia © 2003.

6

Differential Diagnosis of Urinary Incontinence

Michael W. Weinberger

Department of Obstetrics and Gynecology, Kaiser Permanente, Southern California; and Deparment of Obstetrics and Gynecology, Division of Urogynecology, Kaiser Permanente– Los Angeles Medical Center, Los Angeles, California

The International Continence Society (ICS) defines urinary incontinence as involuntary urine loss that is severe enough to constitute a social or hygienic problem and that is objectively demonstrable (1). According to this definition, urinary incontinence may be a symptom, sign, or diagnosis. The symptom is the patient's report of urine loss, the sign is objective demonstration of urine loss, and the diagnosis is established with urodynamic testing.

The various causes of incontinence in women are listed in Table 6.1. In clinical practice, many cases ultimately are diagnosed as either genuine stress incontinence (urine leakage caused by urethral hypermobility or impaired sphincter function), detrusor instability (urine loss due to involuntary bladder contractions), or mixed incontinence (a combination of stress and urge incontinence). Nonetheless, urinary incontinence is often multifactorial in etiology. In some instances, incontinence occurs despite normal bladder and urethral function. Such would be the case for women with incontinence due to acute

lower urinary tract infection and for those with functional incontinence, for whom environmental or physical impediments prevent reaching the toilet before leakage occurs. Occasionally, urinary incontinence is the presenting symptom of another medical illness, such as delirium, pneumonia, diabetes mellitus, or congestive heart failure. In this circumstance, the incontinence is classified as transient incontinence and remits when the underlying medical condition is treated. Knowledge of the multiple causes of incontinence facilitates diagnosis and treatment.

GENUINE STRESS INCONTINENCE

The ICS defines genuine stress incontinence as the involuntary loss of urine occurring when, in the absence of a detrusor contraction, the intravesical pressure exceeds intraurethral pressure (1). A major cause of genuine stress incontinence is the loss of anatomic support of the urethra, bladder, and urethrovesical junction. Normally, these structures rest in a "hammock" of supporting tissue comprised of endopelvic fascia and the anterior vaginal wall. The hammock extends across the pelvic floor attaching laterally to the arcus tendineus fascia pelvis (white line) and levator ani muscles (2). There is also direct connection between the pubococcygeus muscle and the suburethral endopelvic fascia that may further limit bladder neck descent during physical stress. When the bladder

TABLE 6.1. *Types of urinary incontinence*

Genuine stress incontinence
Overactive bladder
Mixed incontinence
Overflow incontinence
Bypass of anatomic continence mechanism
Functional incontinence
Transient incontinence

and proximal urethra are well supported, increases in intraabdominal pressure are transmitted equally to both structures, and continence is maintained. This occurs, at least in part, because coughing or straining compresses the anterior urethral wall against the well-supported posterior urethral wall, thereby occluding the lumen. Loss of anatomic support allows displacement of the urethrovesical junction during physically stressful activities. Intraabdominal pressure increases are then fully transmitted to the bladder, but to a lesser extent to the urethra, and urine loss occurs. Historically, the pathophysiology of stress incontinence was believed to be urethral displacement outside the "zone of intraabdominal pressure." There is, however, no anatomic structure through which the urethra passes to exit the abdomen. Based on cadaver dissections, DeLancey hypothesized that the integrity of the suburethral hammock is more important for continence than the location of the urethra relative to the pelvic floor (2).

Genuine stress incontinence also occurs when the urethra, regardless of support, fails to function as an effective sphincter. Various terms have been used to describe this condition, including type III urethra, low-pressure urethra, and intrinsic sphincter deficiency (ISD). ISD may result from congenital weakness secondary to myelomeningocele or epispadias. It may be acquired after trauma, radiation, or a sacral cord lesion. In women, ISD is common after multiple anti-incontinence operations (Table 6.2).

The importance of identifying patients with ISD before surgery is the 33% to 54% failure rate after conventional urethral suspension procedures (3,4). By contrast, suburethral sling operations effectively restore long-term continence in 76% to 96% of these patients (5,6). Periurethral collagen injection cures ISD in 45% of cases and improves incontinence severity in an additional 34% to 55% of patients (7,8).

Many urodynamic and radiographic tests are used to evaluate genuine stress incontinence, but none is considered diagnostic by all investigators. Early research emphasized the importance of the posterior urethrovesical angle (PUVA) in maintaining continence. Using lateral cystourethrography, Jeffcoate and Roberts (9) reported that 80% of patients with stress incontinence had loss of the PUVA. Green (10) used bead chain cystograms to classify patients with stress incontinence based on the support of the urethrovesical junction. Type I incontinence is characterized by loss of the PUVA, and type II by loss of the PUVA with posterior, inferior, and rotational descent of the bladder base and urethra (10). Green advocated treating type I defects with anterior colporrhaphy and type II defects with retropubic bladder neck suspension. Most authorities have abandoned Green's approach.

Blaivas and Olsson (11) recommend video urodynamics to evaluate the urethral sphincter mechanism. They found in women with stress incontinence that the bladder neck is closed at rest but opens with increased intraabdominal pressure. Their modification of Green's classification system includes types 0, I, IIA, and IIB, distinguished by the resting position of the bladder neck relative to the symphysis pubis. The finding that 25% to 50% of continent women have an incompetent bladder neck during straining has led to considerable controversy about the role of the bladder neck in maintaining continence (12,13).

In 1981, McGuire (14) reported that 75% of women who failed previous antiincontinence operations had an open fibrotic urethra at rest. Resting proximal urethral closure pressure in these individuals was less than 20 cm H_2O. McGuire called this condition the type III urethra. Research by Sand and colleagues (4) sup-

TABLE 6.2. *Causes of genuine stress incontinence*

Anatomic
  Inadequate support of urethrovesical junction
Intrinsic sphincter deficiency
  Congenital
    Meningomyelocele
    Epispadias
  Acquired
    Trauma
    Postirradiation
    Spinal cord injury
    Previous anti-incontinence surgery

ported the hypothesis that static low urethral closure pressure was a risk factor for failure of colposuspension procedures. These investigators reported that the failure rate following Burch colposuspension was three times higher in patients who demonstrated low urethral closure pressure preoperatively (maximum urethral closure pressure less than or equal to 20 cm H_2O) than in those having "normal" closure pressures (maximum urethral closure pressure more than 20 cm H_2O): 54% and 18% failure rates, respectively. These reports led to the widespread adoption of subtracted urethral pressure profilometry to evaluate urethral function.

Recently, abdominal leak point pressure has been advocated as a test of urethral sphincteric function (15). Leak point pressure was originally used to determine whether a myelodysplastic child was at risk for vesicoureteral reflux and hydronephrosis. It is measured by inserting a pressure catheter into the bladder and infusing water until leakage occurs around the catheter; intravesical pressure at that time is the leak point pressure. McGuire modified this technique to determine the abdominal leak point pressure (15). Urethral and bladder pressure are recorded as contrast is infused into the bladder under fluoroscopic guidance. After filling the bladder to 150 mL, the patient increases abdominal pressure by straining and coughing. The process is videotaped, and the abdominal pressure at the time of urine leakage is noted. McGuire found that 76% of patients with leakage at low abdominal pressures (5 to 60 cm H_2O) had type III incontinence on video urodynamic testing. In contrast, 90% of patients with leak point pressure greater than 60 cm H_2O had type I or II incontinence. Currently, measurements to determine leak point pressure have not been standardized.

Numerous investigators have attempted to correlate urethral closure pressure and leak point pressure. McGuire and associates (15) found that maximum urethral pressure was unrelated to the "force required to drive urine across the sphincter." In contrast, Sultana (16) and Swift and Ostergard (17) reported statisti-

cally significant, but clinically weak, correlation between maximum urethral closure pressure and Valsalva leak point pressure (correlation coefficients of 0.62 and 0.56, respectively). Because these tests are purported to evaluate the integrity of the urethral sphincter, a high degree of correlation would be expected. The inconsistency among these reports is due, in part, to differences in the technique of measuring leak point pressure. More importantly, the tests probably evaluate different aspects of urethral function: urethral pressure profilometry measures static forces occluding the urethral lumen at rest, whereas leak point pressure reflects the ability of the urethra to resist expulsive forces of abdominal pressure.

Although many clinicians equate ISD with a low-pressure urethra or type III incontinence, the terms are not necessarily interchangeable. Further research into normal urethral function, as well as clinical trials comparing the ability of urethral closure pressure and leak point to predict surgical outcome, will clarify the role of these tests.

OVERACTIVE BLADDER

The International Continence Society defines overactive bladder function as a disorder of the urine storage phase characterized by involuntary detrusor contractions (1). A number of terms have been used in the past to describe this condition, including unstable bladder, detrusor instability, hyperreflexic bladder, detrusor dyssynergia, motor urge incontinence, and uninhibited bladder. Currently, two terms are accepted by the ICS for use in describing overactive bladder function: unstable bladder (or detrusor instability) and detrusor hyperreflexia.

The ICS defines the unstable bladder as one that contracts spontaneously or with provocation during bladder filling while the patient is attempting to inhibit micturition. When the ICS first standardized urodynamic terminology in 1976, the diagnosis of detrusor instability required a rise in bladder pressure of 15 cm H_2O during filling cystometry. A less restrictive definition was adopted in

1988 when it was recognized that contractions measuring less than 15 cm H_2O often cause symptoms of frequency, urgency, and incontinence (18). Currently, an unstable bladder is diagnosed if detrusor contractions occur during provocative cystometry. The contraction may be of any amplitude and need not cause either symptoms or incontinence. A gradual increase in bladder pressure without subsequent decrease reflects a change of compliance rather than detrusor instability.

The term detrusor hyperreflexia is used when bladder overactivity is due to disturbance of nervous control mechanisms. The ICS definition of detrusor hyprerreflexia requires objective evidence of a relevant neurologic disorder. Neurologic disorders commonly associated with detrusor hyperreflexia include stroke, dementia, multiple sclerosis, brain tumor, and Parkinson's disease.

The ICS defines urinary urgency as a strong desire to void accompanied by fear of leakage or fear of pain. Patients with urgency may be divided into two categories: those having motor urgency and those with sensory urgency. Motor urgency is diagnosed in those patients who report having a strong desire to urinate and who have urodynamic findings consistent with an unstable bladder. Sensory urgency refers to a subset of patients who report symptoms of urinary frequency and urgency but lack cystometric evidence of an overactive bladder.

MIXED INCONTINENCE

Detrusor instability and genuine stress incontinence coexist in 4% to 30% of patients (19,20). The degree to which each component contributes to the patient's urinary incontinence varies, but one factor often predominates. Patients with mixed incontinence leak larger volumes of urine and tend to have more incontinent episodes per week than patients with either pure stress incontinence or detrusor instability alone (21).

There is controversy whether coexisting detrusor instability decreases the surgical cure rate of genuine stress incontinence. Stanton and co-workers (22) reported that colposuspension cured stress incontinence in 85% of patients when this was the singular diagnosis but in only 43% of patients with mixed incontinence. Lockhart and colleagues (23) divided patients with mixed incontinence into two groups based on the increase in detrusor pressure during bladder filling. If the pressure increase was less than 25 cm H_2O, the stress incontinence cure rate was 90%; when the pressure increase exceeded 25 cm H_2O, the cure rate was only 50%. Other investigators have reported that detrusor instability does not affect the ability to cure genuine stress incontinence with surgery (19,24). Differing patient selection criteria, definitions of detrusor instability, diagnostic techniques, and outcome analysis may account for the discrepancies.

OVERFLOW INCONTINENCE

The ICS defines overflow incontinence as the involuntary loss of urine associated with overdistention of the bladder (1). In most cases, overdistention is caused by outflow tract obstruction or detrusor underactivity.

Outflow tract obstruction is uncommon in women. Pelvic prolapse, uterine leiomyomas, ovarian neoplasms, acutely retroverted gravid and nongravid uteri, and large vaginal wall mesonephric and paramesonephric cysts are reported as causes of urethral obstruction (25). Bladder neck obstruction is a potential iatrogenic complication of anti-incontinence surgery. The true incidence of this complication is difficult to determine, but voiding dysfunction and urinary retention occur in 2.9% to 25% of women who undergo surgery; varying by procedure, the aggressiveness of bladder neck elevation, and the patient's preoperative voiding mechanism (26).

Detrusor function may be compromised by neurogenic or myogenic factors (Table 6.3). Herniated intervertebral disks, peripheral neuropathy (caused by diabetes mellitus, hypothyroidism, vitamin B_{12} deficiency, or tabes dorsalis), spinal cord injury, and central nervous system lesions may produce

TABLE 6.3. *Causes of overflow incontinence*

Bladder atony
  Neurologic causes
    Autonomic neuropathy
    Peripheral neuropathy
    Central nervous system pathology
  Pharmacologic causes
    Anticholinergic agents
    Calcium-channel blockers
    α-Adrenergic agonists
    β-Adrenergic agonists
  Endocrine disease
    Diabetes mellitus
    Hypothyroidism
Decreased bladder wall compliance
  Radiation fibrosis
  Intrinsic bladder disease
    Interstitial cystitis
    Recurrent urinary tract infection
Outflow tract obstruction
  Pelvic organ prolapse
  Benign and malignant pelvic neoplasms
  Previous anti-incontinence surgery

a hypotonic or an acontractile bladder. Medications that induce overflow incontinence include anticholinergics, calcium-channel blockers, α- and β-adrenergic agonists, and diuretics.

The bladder wall may be damaged by radiation therapy, interstitial cystitis, or recurrent urinary tract infection. Overflow incontinence can develop if bladder fibrosis produces a small-volume, noncompliant, functionally inadequate urine reservoir.

Increased tone of the pelvic floor and urethral sphincter apparatus has been reported as a cause of urinary retention (27). Local factors such as pain, infectious or inflammatory processes, and trauma may cause involuntary, tonic contraction of the pelvic floor muscles and reflex inhibition of detrusor function.

Patients with overflow incontinence commonly complain of unconscious urine loss throughout the day and night. Many experience hesitancy, intermittent flow with diminished stream, having to lean or bend to a certain position, or using suprapubic pressure to empty their bladders. Increased residual urine volumes predispose these individuals to recurrent urinary tract infections. During physical examination, the bladder may be palpable above the pubic symphysis.

Overflow incontinence is always included in the differential diagnosis of urinary incontinence. In practice, overflow incontinence is rarely diagnosed unless one is dealing with a special patient population, such as elderly or neurologically impaired patients. Measurement of postvoid residual urine identifies patients at risk for overflow incontinence.

BYPASS OF ANATOMIC CONTINENCE MECHANISM

An uncommon cause of incontinence is the bypass of the normal continence mechanism (Table 6.4) by nonphysiologic conduits for urine such as epispadias, ectopic ureters, and fistulas (ureterovaginal, vesicovaginal, urethrovaginal, or vesicouterine). These patients usually experience continuous urine loss, and the diagnosis is relatively easy.

In some cases, diagnosis may be more difficult. For example, patients with epispadias may occasionally reach adulthood before an association is made between the incomplete midline fusion of their genitalia, the absence of pubic hair at the center of the mons pubis, and lifelong urinary incontinence. An ectopic ureter can cause incontinence if it empties distal to the urethral sphincter mechanism. One third of ectopic ureters empty at the level of the bladder neck; these women are usually continent. When the ureter opens into the mid or distal urethra (33% of cases), the vagina (25%), or the cervix and uterus (5%), urine loss may be continuous or infrequent.

Patients with urethral diverticula present with dysuria, dyspareunia, and postmicturition dribbling. Urine accumulates within the

TABLE 6.4. *Bypass of anatomic continence mechanism*

Ectopic ureter
Epispadias
Fistula
  Ureterovaginal
  Urethrovaginal
  Vesicouterine
  Vesicovaginal
Urethral diverticulum

diverticulum and empties when the patient stands. Physical findings of a large reducible suburethral mass can suggest the diagnosis, which is confirmed with urethroscopy, urethral pressure profilometry, or radiographic techniques.

FUNCTIONAL INCONTINENCE

Functional incontinence occurs when a patient with an intact lower urinary tract is unable or unwilling to reach the toilet to urinate. Visual impairment, limited manual dexterity, and multiple layers of undergarments or pads may prevent undressing before urine loss occurs. Patients should be encouraged to wear comfortable, loose-fitting clothing that is easy to remove.

Environmental factors may impair the elderly patient's ability to reach the bathroom before incontinence occurs. These factors may include inaccessible facilities, unfamiliar surroundings, inattentive staff, and physical restraints. Correcting environmental factors may restore continence.

EFFECTS OF AGING

The prevalence and type of urinary incontinence vary with the age and health of the population being evaluated. Several investigators have reported that the prevalence of genuine stress incontinence decreases with advancing age, with commensurate increases in detrusor instability and mixed incontinence (28,29). Among ambulatory adult incontinent women, genuine stress incontinence is diagnosed in 50% to 70% of cases. In this population, detrusor instability and mixed incontinence each account for 20% to 40% of cases. Among elderly community-dwelling incontinent women undergoing urodynamic testing, genuine stress incontinence is diagnosed less frequently (36% to 46% of cases); detrusor instability and mixed incontinence are more common, accounting for 27% to 46% and 19% of diagnoses, respectively (30,31). Urodynamic evaluation of incontinent institutionalized el-derly women diagnosed detrusor instability in 61%, genuine stress incontinence in 21%, and mixed incontinence in 4% (32).

The effect of aging on urinary tract function has not been studied longitudinally. Cross-sectional observations suggest that bladder capacity, the ability to postpone voiding, maximum urethral closure pressure, and urinary flow rate decrease with age. Postvoid residual urine volume and the prevalence of uninhibited detrusor contractions are probably increased (33). Even in the absence of congestive heart failure, peripheral venous insufficiency, or renal disease, an age-related decline in glomerular filtration rate causes elderly people to excrete the bulk of their daily-ingested fluid at night. As a result, the healthy 80-year-old may experience one to two episodes of nocturia.

None of these age-related changes cause incontinence, but they reduce the capacity of the lower urinary tract to withstand further insult. Factors outside the urinary tract often precipitate or exacerbate incontinence. Reversal of the precipitating factor will restore continence even if underlying urogynecologic abnormalities are not corrected.

TRANSIENT CAUSES OF INCONTINENCE

Recognizing that physiologic changes in lower urinary tract function make elderly people more susceptible to incontinence, Resnick devised the mnemonic DIAPPERS to categorize the causes of transient incontinence (34) (Table 6.5).

TABLE 6.5. *Transient causes of urinary incontinence*

Delirium
Infection
Atrophic vaginitis
Pharmacologic
Psychological
Endocrine
Restricted mobility
Stool impaction

Delirium

Delirium is a confusional state characterized by acute or subacute onset. Its insidious onset and slow progression distinguish it from dementia. Delirium may result from any drug or medical illness, including pneumonia, deep venous thrombosis, congestive heart failure, or the pain associated with a fracture. These underlying causes may present atypically and, if unrecognized, may be associated with significant morbidity and mortality. Incontinence is a symptom that will abate when the cause of the patient's confusion is identified and treated.

Infection

Increased postvoid residual urine and postmenopausal urogenital atrophy predispose elderly women to develop urinary tract infections. Symptoms of urinary tract infection in elderly patients may differ from those in younger patients. Dysuria is often absent, and incontinence may be the patient's only symptom.

Bacteriuria can cause mucosal irritation leading to unsuppressible detrusor contractions and urge incontinence. Bacterial endotoxins inhibiting α-adrenergic receptors may cause urethral relaxation and stress incontinence (35). Among patients with undiagnosed urinary tract infections at the time of urodynamic evaluation, 30% of those with stress incontinence and 60% of those with detrusor instability became continent after treatment of bacteriuria (36).

Atrophic Urethritis

Postmenopausal estrogen deficiency causes increased genitourinary tract sensitivity and irritative symptoms. Patients may complain of urethral burning, dysuria, dyspareunia, urinary urgency, or urge incontinence. Despite theoretical benefits, clinical studies evaluating the effects of estrogen replacement on urinary incontinence have yielded inconsistent results.

Pharmacologic Causes

Virtually any medication that affects the autonomic nervous system also influences lower urinary tract function. Commonly prescribed antihypertensives, antidepressants, and sedative hypnotics may exacerbate incontinence. Many over-the-counter multicomponent cold medications, decongestants, and antihistamines can affect the lower urinary tract. Incontinent patients should be asked about nonprescription medication use.

Psychological Causes

Incontinence may occasionally be used to gain attention or to manipulate others. Patients may be so profoundly depressed that they do not care about continence.

Endocrine Causes

Diabetes mellitus and hypercalcemia may induce an osmotic diuresis that exacerbates other causes of incontinence.

Restricted Mobility

Arthritis, hip deformity, or gait instability may impair the elderly patient's ability to reach the bathroom. If mobility cannot be improved, a nearby commode may improve the incontinence.

Stool Impaction

Fecal impaction is a common cause of urinary incontinence in bedridden or immobile patients. It should be suspected in the patient who develops fecal oozing and urinary incontinence with a palpable bladder.

SUMMARY

The etiologies of urinary incontinence are many. The pathophysiology may be multifactorial. History alone is inadequate to establish the etiology of incontinence. It is incumbent on the clinician to perform a thorough evaluation of all incontinent patients before any therapy. Many patients benefit from comprehensive urodynamic evaluation before treatment.

REFERENCES

1. Abrams P, Blaivas JG, Stanton SL, et al. The standardization of terminology of lower urinary tract function. *Scand J Urol Nephrol* 1988;114[Suppl]:5–19.
2. DeLancey JOL. Structural support of the urethra as it relates to urinary incontinence: the hammock hypothesis. *Am J Obstet Gynecol* 1994;170:1713–1723.
3. Koonings PP, Bergman A, Ballard CA. Low urethral pressure and stress urinary incontinence in women: risk factor for failed retropubic surgical procedure. *Urology* 1990;36:245–248.
4. Sand PK, Bowen LW, Pangawiban R, et al. The low pressure urethra as a factor in failed retropubic urethropexy. *Obstet Gynecol* 1987;69:399–402.
5. Weinberger MW, Ostergard DR. Long-term clinical and urodynamic evaluation of the polytetrafluoroethylene suburethral sling for treatment of genuine stress incontinence. *Obstet Gynecol* 1995;86:92–96.
6. McGuire EJ, Lytton B. Pubovaginal sling procedure for stress incontinence. *J Urol* 1978;119:82–84.
7. McGuire EJ, Appell RA. Transurethral collagen injection for urinary incontinence. *Urology* 1994;43: 413–415.
8. Herschorn S, Radomski SB, Steele DJ. Early experience with intraurethral collagen injections for urinary incontinence. *J Urol* 1992;148:1797–1800.
9. Jeffcoate TNA, Roberts H. Observations on stress incontinence of urine. *Am J Obstet Gynecol* 1952;64: 712–738.
10. Green TH. Development of a plan for the diagnosis and treatment of urinary stress incontinence. *Am J Obstet Gynecol* 1962;83:632–648.
11. Blaivas JG, Olsson CA. Stress incontinence: classification and surgical approach. *J Urol* 1988;139:727–731.
12. Versi E, Cardozo LD, Studd JWW, et al. Internal urinary sphincter in maintenance of female continence. *BMJ* 1986;292:166–167.
13. Hilton P, Stanton SL. Urethral pressure measurement by microtransducer: the results in symptom-free women and in those with genuine stress incontinence. *Br J Obstet Gynaecol* 1983;90:919–933.
14. McGuire EJ. Urodynamic findings in patients after failure of stress incontinence operations. *Prog Clin Biol Res* 1981;78:351–360.
15. McGuire EJ, Fitzpatrick CC, Wan J, et al. Clinical assessment of urethral sphincter function. *J Urol* 1993; 150:1452–1454.
16. Sultana C. Urethral closure pressure and leak-point pressure in incontinent women. *Obstet Gynecol* 1995; 86:839–842.
17. Swift SE, Ostergard DR. A comparison of stress leak-point pressure and maximal urethral closure pressure in patients with genuine stress incontinence. *Obstet Gynecol* 1995;85:704–708.
18. Coolsaet BLRA, Blok C, van Venrouijj GEFM, et al. Subthreshold detrusor instability. *Neurourol Urodyn* 1985;4:309–311.
19. McGuire EJ, Savastano JA. Stress incontinence and detrusor instability/urge incontinence. *Neurourol Urodyn* 1985;4:313–316.
20. Herzog AR, Fultz NH. Prevalence and incidence of urinary incontinence in community-dwelling populations. *J Am Geriatr Soc* 1990;38:273–281.
21. Fantl JA, Bump RC, McClish DK. Mixed urinary incontinence. *Urology* 1990;36[Suppl]:21–24.
22. Stanton SL, Cardozo L, Williams J, et al. Clinical and urodynamic features of failed incontinence surgery in the female. *Am J Obstet Gynecol* 1978;51:515–520.
23. Lockhart J, Vorstman B, Politano VA. Anti-incontinence surgery in females with detrusor instability. *Neurourol Urodyn* 1984;3:201–207.
24. Bowen LW, Sand PK, Ostergard DR, et al. Unsuccessful Burch urethropexy: a case-controlled urodynamic study. *Am J Obstet Gynecol* 1989;160:452–458.
25. Polsky MS, Agee RE, Berg SR, et al. Acute urinary retention in women: brief discussion and unusual case report. *J Urol* 1973;110:541–543.
26. Bump RC, Cundiff GW. Prevention and management of complications after continence surgery. In: Ostergard DR, Bent AE, eds. *Urogynecology and urodynamics,* 4th ed. Baltimore: Williams & Wilkins, 1996:595–608.
27. Raz S, Smith RB. External sphincter spasticity syndrome in female patients. *J Urol* 1976;115:443–446.
28. Yarnell JWG, Voyle GJ, Richards CJ, et al. The prevalence and severity of urinary incontinence in women. *J Epidemiol Community Health* 1981;35:71–74.
29. Brocklehurst JC, Fry J, Griffith LL, et al. Urinary infection and dysuria in women aged 45–64 years: their relevance to similar findings in the elderly. *Age Ageing* 1972;1:41–47.
30. Ouslander J, Staskin D, Raz S, et al. Clinical versus urodynamic diagnosis in an incontinent geriatric female population. *J Urol* 1987;137:68–71.
31. Bent AE, Richardson DA, Ostergard DR. Diagnosis of lower urinary tract disorders in postmenopausal patients. *Am J Obstet Gynecol* 1983;145:218–222.
32. Resnick NM, Yalla SV, Laurino E. The pathophysiology of urinary incontinence among institutionalized elderly persons. *N Engl J Med* 1989;320:1–7.
33. Resnick NM, Yalla SV. Aging and its effect on the bladder. *Semin Urol* 1987;5:82–86.
34. Resnick NM, Yalla SV. Management of urinary incontinence in the elderly. *N Engl J Med* 1985;313:800–805.
35. Nergardh A, Boreus LO, Holme T. The inhibitory effect of coli-endotoxin on alpha-adrenergic receptor functions in the lower urinary tract: an in vitro study in cats. *Scand J Urol Nephrol* 1977;11:219–224.
36. Bergman A, Bhatia NN. Urodynamics: effect of urinary tract infection on urethral and bladder function. *Obstet Gynecol* 1985;66:366–371.

*Ostergard's Urogynecology and Pelvic Floor
Dysfunction, Fifth Edition.* edited by A.E. Bent, et al.
Lippincott Williams & Wilkins, Philadelphia © 2003.

7

Basic Evaluation of the Incontinent Female Patient

Steven E. Swift* and Alfred E. Bent**

*Department of Obstetrics and Gynecology, Division of Benign Gynecology,
Medical University of South Carolina, Charleston, South Carolina
**Department of Gynecology and Obstetrics, Johns Hopkins School of Medicine;
and Department of Gynecology, Greater Baltimore Medical Center, Baltimore, Maryland

Currently, there is considerable debate over what constitutes the minimal or basics of an evaluation of the incontinent female. Although there are a few published guidelines, no studies to date have determined the effectiveness of these recommendations or their relationship to therapeutic outcomes. Therefore, we are left with conflicting expert opinion regarding which if any testing should be done before initiating therapy for incontinence in the female patient. This can make it difficult if not impossible for the physician to determine what to employ in clinical practice when faced with these patients.

Any basic evaluation of the incontinent female should be able to distinguish reliably among genuine stress incontinence, detrusor instability, and mixed incontinence because these entities are responsible for most cases of female urinary incontinence (Table 7.1). Also, the evaluation should be able to detect those uncommon forms of incontinence that require further specialized evaluation and referral to a specialist. Finally, the evaluation should allow the physician to determine appropriate therapy.

BACKGROUND

The Agency for Health Care Policy and Research (AHCPR) first published consensus guidelines for evaluation and management of urinary incontinence in 1992 (updated in 1996) (1). These guidelines were drawn up by a panel of experts who based their recommendations on a critical review of the literature and on expert opinion. They recommended that a basic evaluation should include the following: a thorough history (including a voiding diary), physical examination, postvoid residual, and urinalysis. The evaluation criteria were subsequently applied retrospectively to a referral-based practice and were found to diagnose roughly 30% of subjects with the complaint of stress urinary incontinence incorrectly or incompletely (2). Remember that these guidelines were developed for a primary care practice but in this study were applied to a tertiary referral population. Therefore, it remains to be determined how effective they are for patients in a primary clinical practice. However, this study did point out some of the shortcomings of the AHCPR guidelines and demonstrated that these recommendations should be constantly tested and updated to reflect changes in our knowledge base.

This chapter focuses on simple testing techniques for evaluating the incontinent female that are available to most practitioners and points out some of the situations that require more specialized testing or referral.

TABLE 7.1. *Findings during the basic evaluation of the incontinent patient that require further evaluation*

Finding	Suggested further evaluation
History	
1. Recurrent UTI*	1. Cystoscopy and possibly IVP versus renal U/S
2. Continuous incontinence/non-episodic	2. R/O fistula
3. Previous failed incontinence surgery*	3. Comprehensive evaluation
4. Painful frequent voids/urge incontinence	4. Cystoscopy and CMG
5. Greater then 4,000 mL voided volume on 24-hr voiding diary	5. Evaluation of diabetes insipidus
6. Neurologic disease suspected of contributing to the patient's symptoms*	6. Referral to a local expert on female urinary incontinence and/or neurologist
Physical exam	
1. Vagina with obvious urine	1. R/O fistula
2. Suburethral tender mass	2. Cystoscopy/radiographic study to R/O diverticula
3. Large pelvic mass	3. Age-appropriate W/U
4. Pelvic organ prolapse extending beyond the hymen (POPQ stages 3 and 4)*	4. Evaluation of severe pelvic organ prolapse
Urodynamics	
1. PVR >100 mL*	1. Referral for evaluation of obstructive voiding or underactive detrusor
2. Persistent microscopic hematuria on dip urinalysis in the absence of infection*	2. Appropriate referral for cystoscopy and upper tract evaluation
3. Small volume bladder on cystometrogram (<300 mL)	3. Cystoscopy with sedation to R/O interstitial cystitis
4. Mixed incontinence on cystometrogram and cough stress test	4. Multichannel urodynamics or other comprehensive evaluation
5. Positive supine empty stress test	5. Multichannel urodynamics or other comprehensive evaluation
Overall impression of results	
1. Confusion regarding the results of testing*	1. Referral to a local expert on female urinary incontinence
2. Patients failing treatment based on your evaluation*	2. Referral to a local expert on female urinary incontinence

*Correspond to Agency for Health Care Policy and Research guidelines for further evaluation after a basic workup of the incontinent female (1).
UTI, urinary tract infection; IVP, intravenous pyelogram; U/S, ultrasound; R/O, rule out; CMG, cystometrogram; POPQ, pelvic organ prolapse quantification system; W/U, workup; PVR, postvoid residual

HISTORY

Patient history should be used for identifying reversible causes of incontinence and determining the impact that incontinence has on the patient's quality of life. However, it has demonstrated a poor ability to differentiate between the various types of incontinence and should not be relied on to make a diagnosis (3–6).

The following statement, as true today as it was in 1972, sums up the role of history in diagnosing the type of urinary incontinence in females: ". . . urinary symptoms in the female can be extremely misleading and do not form a scientific basis for treatment. . . . Without some form of objective investigation, the gynecologist who relies on clinical impression is likely to submit some of his patients to ineffective surgery, and others to needless surgery" (7).

Although history is a poor predictor for the diagnosis, it does play a major role in evaluation and treatment. A comprehensive urogynecologic history should include duration and characteristics of the incontinent episodes, frequency of incontinent episodes, use of protective devices, previous therapy, history of recurrent urinary tract infections, menopausal status, functional status, and other medical conditions and medications. Determining the nature and severity of the patient's incontinence will help direct future therapies with more severe symptoms suggesting more aggressive therapeutic choices and milder symptoms suggesting less invasive interventions. Although this may seem obvious, it can be overlooked in the evaluation process; for example, a patient who has two or three incontinence episodes a year might be offered invasive surgery or placed on daily medication with all the attendant side effects. Therefore, documenting the degree and severity of the problem is important before offering therapy. There are no standardized severity scales to use in documenting the degree of incontinence, and there is no severity measurement value or cutoff for determining when a patient has incontinence and when she is considered continent. Instead, there exists a continuum of patients. Those with symptoms at either extreme represent obvious examples of minimal or severe incontinence for whom the decision to intervene or not is readily apparent. It is the patient with mild to moderate symptoms who represents the greatest challenge in determining the extent of evaluation and treatment. Therefore, documenting the degree of her problem and desire for therapeutic interventions will aid greatly in treatment planning.

Reversible and transient causes of incontinence should also be identified. These are summarized in Chapter 6 with the mnemonic DIAPPERS and can be reviewed in more detail there. One area that deserves special attention is the use of antihypertensive agents, which are commonly prescribed for older females. It has been demonstrated that patients attending hypertension clinics have a relative risk for urinary incontinence of 3.3, with α-adrenergic blockers (i.e., prazosin, terazosin, or doxazosin) being the primary culprits (8). A simple change in medication from an α-adrenergic blocker can often provide significant clinical improvement. Diuretics, although often implicated in incontinence, may aggravate symptoms but have not been shown to have a causal relationship (9).

The history is also useful for identifying potentially modifiable risk factors for incontinence. Cigarette smoking has been shown to increase the incidence of both stress and urge incontinence (10). Constipation is reported almost 10 times more often in incontinent women than in continent controls (11). The history is the starting point for any evaluation of incontinence and usually determines the severity of the problem and the need for further evaluation and intervention.

VOIDING DIARY

The voiding diary is a helpful evaluation tool for documenting and measuring the severity of incontinence. A 1-week record of leak episodes and voiding is highly reliable for demonstrating urinary frequency, nocturia, and number of incontinent episodes; however, it cannot diagnose the type of incontinence (12). A 24-hour record of fluid intake and voided volumes has a weak correlation with frequency of voids and incontinent episodes, but it does measure the fluid intake and voided bladder volumes (13). A fluid intake of greater than 4 L/d mandates consideration of diabetes insipidus, and frequent small voids can point to a diagnosis of interstitial cystitis.

PHYSICAL EXAMINATION

The physical examination should include a general physical examination, pelvic examination, local neurologic testing, cotton swab test, postvoid residual, and cough stress test (1). Some aspects of an overall general physical examination include comment regarding peripheral edema. Significant peripheral edema in conjunction with a 24-hour voiding diary that demonstrates nocturia and nocturnal urge incontinence suggests that the patient is mobilizing fluid in the recumbent position. Mobilizing this fluid before bed may aid in the treatment of her symptoms. The individual with limited mobility requires consideration of this in any treatment plan. Use of bedside commodes and teaching better transfer technique are often all that is necessary to treat her incontinence.

A focused neurologic examination is recommended to screen for neurologic disease but has a low detection rate in the patient with no history of neurologic disease (see Chapter 10). The findings of a thorough physical examination can aid in various aspects of therapy and form the basis of the evaluation of the incontinent female.

Pelvic Examination

A pelvic examination is central to evaluating the incontinent female, and the presence of uncommon forms of incontinence can be suggested from a careful inspection. The presence of a large pool of urine in the vagina should suggest a vesicovaginal, ureterovaginal, or urethrovaginal fistula. On bimanual examination, a large tender mass palpated along the anterior vaginal wall suggests a suburethral diverticulum. In addition, a large pelvic mass may contribute to urinary frequency and urgency as it presses down on the bladder, although it is unlikely to be the cause of the incontinence. If the examination suggests any of these findings, further evaluation should be directed toward making the proper diagnosis.

During the examination, attention should be paid to pelvic organ support. The pelvic organ prolapse quantification system (POPQ) is a standardized system for measuring and reporting changes in vaginal support (14). Other techniques for describing pelvic organ support are covered in Chapters 8 and 9. The assessment of pelvic organ support should be conducted during a Valsalva maneuver or cough, and the degree of movement of the various components of the vagina should be noted. A Sims or disarticulated Graves speculum can be used to retract the posterior vaginal wall, allowing for visualization of the entire anterior vaginal wall during straining. A similar technique is employed to visualize the posterior vaginal wall by retracting the anterior vagina. The cervix and apex or cuff can be either visualized directly with a speculum or palpated during straining to determine the degree of support. There is some controversy regarding whether the patient should be examined in the supine dorsal lithotomy position or standing. In one study, there did not appear to be any difference between examining the subject supine or standing (15).

Q-tip Test

The mobility of the urethrovesical junction (UVJ) should be assessed by Q-tip test or by imaging techniques such as ultrasound or cystography (16). The Q-tip, or cotton swab, test is performed by first cleaning the external urethral meatus with an appropriate antibacterial solution. Next, a sterile Q-tip that has been lubricated with an anesthetic ointment is gently inserted into the urethra until the tip has reached the bladder. Generally, there is a slight decrease in resistance as the tip passes the bladder neck. The Q-tip is then drawn back until a slight resistance is felt, which ensures that the tip is at the UVJ. The resting angle is measured with a simple goniometer, with the reference being parallel to the floor. The subject is then asked to perform the Valsalva maneuver or cough, and the excursion is measured. By Q-tip test, hypermobility is defined as an excursion with straining of more than 30 degrees from the resting angle or more than 30 degrees from the horizontal (17,18) (Fig. 7.1). The Q-tip test has been a mainstay of the basic evaluation since its introduction in 1971 and has demonstrated good interobserver reliability (19–21). It has never demonstrated clinical utility in diagnosing the type of incontinence but can only determine whether there is UVJ hypermobility or good support. It has been suggested that mobility of the UVJ can be assessed by simply visualizing the degree of descent of the anterior vaginal wall with Valsalva. However, when direct visual assessment was compared with the Q-tip test, it was deemed inadequate (22). For a full discussion of ultrasound and cystourethrographic definitions of hypermobility, refer to Chapter 14. If surgery is not being contemplated, the Q-tip test can be omitted from a basic evaluation. Its main role is to determine which subjects would benefit from a surgical elevation of the bladder neck and which subjects already have adequate UVJ support.

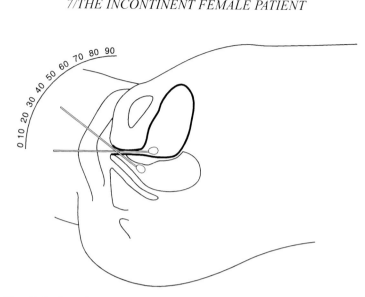

FIG. 7.1. The Q-tip test demonstrating a resting angle of 0 degrees (bladder outlined in *bold line*) and the Q-tip angle with strain of about 40 degrees.

Postvoid Residual

A postvoid residual urine determination (PVR) should be made immediately after spontaneous voiding to rule out overflow incontinence in all patients. It has been suggested that postvoid residual can be estimated on bimanual examination by feeling for an enlarged distended bladder. However, this technique had a 14% sensitivity rate for detecting PVR of greater then 50 mL. A more accurate technique is performed by a simple in-and-out catheterization or ultrasound, if available. Consensus seems to exist that a PVR of less than 50 mL is normal, a PVR of more than 200 mL is abnormal, and any values in between require clinical correlation (1). Abnormal tests should be repeated because the reliability of a single determination is poor (23). There are currently few if any data available to determine what constitutes a clinically significant elevated PVR that results in morbidity (i.e., increased urinary tract infections, overflow incontinence, sensation of bladder pressure or urgency, or reflux with upper tract damage). Therefore, every patient should have a PVR determined, and values of less than 50 mL should reassure the clinician. Values of greater then 50 mL but less than 200

mL should be repeated and correlated clinically. If the patient is asymptomatic with clean urinalysis and no history of urinary tract infections, no therapy is indicated. The patient should be referred for a voiding study to determine whether she has any other pathology (e.g., detrusor–sphincter dyssynergia). If the PVR is greater than 200 mL, the patient should be referred for evaluation by an expert.

Urinalysis

A test to evaluate for an occult bladder infection should be performed. A dipstick urinalysis had poor sensitivity but high specificity and negative predictive values of 97% to 99% in a urogynecology clinic population (24,25). Therefore, a negative dipstick urinalysis reliably predicts the absence of infection. A positive dipstick urinalysis (meaning the presence of heme, leukocytes, or nitrates) mandates a clean-catch or catheterized microscopic urinalysis with culture and sensitivity to determine whether an infection is present. Alternatively, if a microscope is available, a sample of un-spun urine can be inspected for the presence of leukocytes, red blood cells, and bacteria.

There is controversy regarding the need for all patients with incontinence to have a urine culture and sensitivity as part of their initial evaluation. From the previously given data, a good policy would be to screen all patients with either a dipstick or office microscopic urinalysis. In high-risk patients and in subjects undergoing invasive testing, a stronger case can be made to ensure sterile urine by culture and sensitivity.

The physical examination makes up an important part of the basic examination of the incontinent female but does not always lead to the diagnosis. However, empiric conservative treatment can often be initiated after the history and physical examination are completed, with complex testing reserved for treatment failures.

URODYNAMIC TESTING

The diagnosis of urinary incontinence often rests with the urodynamic studies that are performed as part of the evaluation. Although they can be very sophisticated, there are simple means of performing these tests that are readily available to most practitioners in the office setting.

Cystometrogram

Routine office cystometry, which was left out of the AHCPR recommendations, should be considered an essential part of the basic evaluation of the incontinent patient because it plays a central role in the diagnosis of both stress incontinence and detrusor instability. It has demonstrated a limited ability to diagnose detrusor instability, and even sophisticated multichannel studies detect uninhibited detrusor contractions in only 60% of subjects noted to have detrusor instability on ambulatory urodynamics (26). In view of this, the sophistication of the technique employed to perform cystometry may be of limited importance, and simple eyeball cystometry may suffice.

The technique for performing eyeball cystometry uses 500 mL of sterile saline, a Foley catheter, and a 60-mL Foley tip syringe (Fig.

7.2). The urethral meatus is prepped with a cleansing solution. The catheter is placed, and the bladder is emptied. If the subject has just voided, this can be recorded as the PVR. The subject is then asked to stand, if possible. The plunger of the 60-mL Foley tip syringe is removed, and the barrel is attached to the catheter. The barrel is held about 10 to 15 cm above the pubic symphysis. The sterile saline is then poured into the open barrel of the Foley-tipped syringe, filling the bladder in 60-mL increments until the patient states she cannot tolerate more fluid in the bladder. The meniscus of the saline in the syringe barrel is noted throughout the filling process, and if it begins to rise, this should be described as a detrusor contraction. The results of eyeball cystometry were found to be comparable to more sophisticated urodynamics (27).

The other piece of information that a cystometrogram can provide is bladder capacity. Normal bladder capacity is at least 350 to 400 mL. If the bladder volume by cystometry is very small (less than 300 mL), interstitial cystitis should be considered; conversely, if the capacity is more than 350 mL, interstitial cystitis is effectively ruled out (28). Various tech-

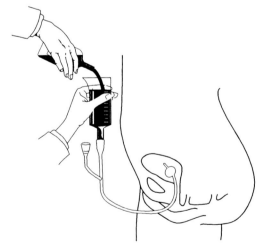

FIG. 7.2. Eyeball cystometry is done in the standing position if possible. The barrel of the Foley tip syringe is held roughly 10 cm above the upper extent of the pubic symphysis.

niques for performing simple cystometry have been described employing the intrauterine pressure channel of a fetal monitor and an old-fashioned manometer (29,30). Regardless of the technique employed, the results of cystometry should always be interpreted with an open mind, remembering that a negative cystometrogram does not rule out the presence of detrusor instability.

Cough Stress Test

A cystometrogram allows for bladder filling so that the cough stress test can be performed with a known bladder volume. The cough stress test involves filling a patient's bladder to at least 300 mL or symptomatic fullness. Then, while standing (or supine if she is unable to stand), the patient coughs while the physician directly visualizes the urethral meatus. If urine is noted to leak from the external urethral meatus, the result is a positive cough stress test. It has been demonstrated that performing a cough stress test before filling the bladder is extremely unreliable and may miss 80% of cases of stress incontinence, but when performed at a bladder volume of 300 mL or symptomatic fullness, this test becomes highly reliable (31–35). A negative cough stress test effectively rules out most cases of stress incontinence (36).

Some patients do not cough forcibly in the laboratory setting, and they may consciously hold in during the test. A positive cough stress test correlates highly with the presence of stress incontinence; however, if uninhibited detrusor contractions are noted during a cystometrogram preceding the cough stress test, the results become suspect (35,36). One other caveat regarding the cough stress test is the supine empty stress test. This refers to subjects who are noted to leak urine from the urethral meatus during a cough or Valsalva maneuver at the time of the pelvic examination. Generally, the patient has voided just before the pelvic examination and is asked to cough or perform the Valsalva maneuver to evaluate her pelvic organ support. If the subject demonstrates urine loss under these circumstances, she has a positive supine empty cough stress test. A positive supine empty stress test has correlated strongly with a severe form of stress incontinence referred to as intrinsic sphincter deficiency (37). This entity is further discussed in Chapter 11. These patients generally respond poorly to conservative therapy and often require referral to a specialist for more extensive testing.

The cystometrogram and cough stress test are not essential to the basic evaluation, particularly if one is contemplating conservative therapy. If more invasive therapy is being considered, however, these tests should be performed as indicated.

SUMMARY

The AHCPR clinical practice guidelines for evaluation and treatment of urinary incontinence in adults took the initial step in defining those components of a basic evaluation that should be required in the testing of all women with urinary incontinence. For empiric conservative therapy, these guidelines should suffice. However, if more invasive treatment is being considered, a simple cystometrogram and a cough stress test should be included. Most of the suggestions presented here reflect those made by the AHCPR in their published guidelines (1).

REFERENCES

1. Fantl JA, Newman DK, Colling J, et al. *Urinary incontinence in adults: acute and chronic management.* Clinical Practice Guideline, No. 2, 1996 Update. Rockville, MD: U.S. Department of Health and Human Services. Public Health Service, Agency for Health Care Policy and Research. AHCPR Publication No. 96-0682, March 1996.
2. Handa VL, Jensen JK, Ostergard DR. Federal guidelines for the management of urinary incontinence in the United States: which patients should undergo urodynamic testing. *Int Urogynecol J Pelvic Floor Dysfunct* 1995;6:198–203.
3. Harvey MA, Versi E. Predictive value of clinical evaluation of stress urinary incontinence: a summary of the published literature. *Int Urogynecol J Pelvic Floor Dysfunct* 2001;12:31–37.
4. Videla FL, Wall LL. Stress incontinence diagnosed without multichannel urodynamic studies. *Obstet Gynecol* 1998;91:965–968.
5. Diokno AC, Wells TJ, Brink CA. Urinary incontinence

in elderly women: urodynamic evaluation. *J Am Geriatr Soc* 1987;35:940–946.

6. Jensen JK, Nielsen FR, Ostergard DR. The role of patient history in the diagnosis of urinary incontinence. *Obstet Gynecol* 1994;83:904–910.

7. Moolgaoker AS, Ardran GM, Smith JC, et al. The diagnosis and management of urinary incontinence in the female. *J Obstet Gynaecol Br Commw* 1972;79:481–497.

8. Marshall HJ, Beevers DG. Alpha-adrenoceptor blocking drugs and female urinary incontinence: prevalence and reversibility. *Br J Clin Pharmacol* 1996;42:507–509.

9. Fantl JA, Wyman JF, Wilson MS, et al. Diuretics and urinary incontinence in community-dwelling women. *Neurourol Urodyn* 1990;9:25–34.

10. Bump RC, McClish DK. Cigarette smoking and urinary incontinence in women. *Am J Obstet Gynecol* 1992; 167:1213–1218.

11. Spence-Jones C, Kamm MA, Henry MM, et al. Bowel dysfunction: a pathogenic factor in uterovaginal prolapse and urinary stress incontinence. *Br J Obstet Gynaecol* 1994;101:147–152.

12. Wyman JF, Choi SC, Harkins SW, et al. The urinary diary in evaluation of incontinent women: a test-retest analysis. *Obstet Gynecol* 1988;71:812–817.

13. Wyman JK, Elswick RK, Wilson MS, et al. Relationship of fluid intake to voluntary micturitions and urinary incontinence in women. *Neurourol Urodyn* 1991; 10:463–473.

14. Bump RC, Mattiasson A, Bo K, et al. The standardization of terminology of female pelvic organ prolapse and pelvic floor dysfunction. *Am J Obstet Gynecol* 1996;175:10–17.

15. Swift SE, Herring MD. Comparison of pelvic organ prolapse in the dorsal lithotomy versus the standing position. *Obstet Gynecol* 1998;91:961–964.

16. Karram MM, Bhatia NN. The Q-tip test: standardization of the technique and its interpretation in women with urinary incontinence. *Obstet Gynecol* 1988;71:807–811.

17. Walter, MD, Shields LE. The diagnostic value of history, physical examination, and the Q-tip cotton swab test in women with urinary incontinence. *Am J Obstet Gynecol* 1988;159:145–149.

18. Fantl JA, Hurt WG, Bump RC. Urethral axis and sphincteric function. *Am J Obstet Gynecol* 1986;155: 554–558.

19. Lobel RW, Sand PK, Gore RM. *The cotton swab test in healthy continent women.* Abstract presented at the 22nd Annual International Urogynecologic Association meeting, Amsterdam, The Netherlands, July 30–August 2, 1997.

20. Thorp JM, Jones LH, Wells E, et al. Assessment of pelvic floor function: a series of simple tests in nulliparous women. *Int Urogynecol J Pelvic Floor Dysfunct* 1996;7:94–97.

21. Crystle CD, Charme LS, Copeland WE. Q-tip test in stress urinary incontinence. *Obstet Gynecol* 1971;38: 313–315.

22. Montella JM, Ewing S, Cater J. Visual assessment of urethrovesical junction mobility. *Int Urogynecol J Pelvic Floor Dysfunct* 1997;8:13–17.

23. Stoller ML, Millard RJ. The accuracy of a catheterized residual volume. *J Urol* 1989;141:15–16.

24. Graham CA, Mallett VT, Ransom SB. *Routine urine culture and sensitivity in the evaluation of incontinent women: a utility and cost effectiveness study.* Abstract presented at the 19th Annual American Urogynecology Society meeting, Washington, DC, November 12–15, 1998.

25. Steele AC, Neff J, Mallipeddi P, et al. *The utility of screening urinalysis in female incontinence and pelvic prolapse.* Abstract presented at 19th Annual American Urogynecology Society meeting, Washington, DC, November 12–15, 1998.

26. van Waalwijk van Doorn ES, Remmers A, Janknegt RA. Extramural ambulatory urodynamic monitoring during natural filling and normal daily activities: evaluation of 100 patients. *J Urol* 1991;146:124–131.

27. Ouslander J, Leach G, Abelson S, et al. Simple versus multichannel cystometry in the evaluation of bladder function in an incontinent geriatric population. *J Urol* 1988;140:1482–1486.

28. Parsons CL. Interstitial cystitis: clinical manifestations and diagnostic criteria in over 200 cases. *Neurourol Urodyn* 1990;9:241–250.

29. Swift SE. The reliability of performing a screening cystometrogram using a fetal monitoring device. *Obstet Gynecol* 1997;89:708–712.

30. Sand PK, Brubaker LT, Novak T. Simple standing incremental cystometry as a screening method for detrusor instability. *Obstet Gynecol* 1991;77:453–457.

31. Kadar N. The value of bladder filling in the clinical detection of urine loss and selection of patients for urodynamic testing. *Br J Obstet Gynaecol* 1988;95:698–704.

32. Swift SE, Ostergard DR. Evaluation of current urodynamic testing methods in the diagnosis of genuine stress incontinence. *Obstet Gynecol* 1995;86:85–91.

33. Scotti RJ, Myers DL. A comparison of the cough stress test and single-channel cystometry with multichannel urodynamic evaluation in genuine stress incontinence. *Obstet Gynecol* 1993;81:430–433.

34. Summitt RL, Stovall TG, Bent AE, et al. Urinary incontinence: correlation of history and brief office evaluation with multichannel urodynamic testing. *Am J Obstet Gynecol* 1992;166:1835–1844.

35. Swift SE, Yoon EA. The test re-test reliability of the cough stress test in women with urinary incontinence. *Obstet Gynecol* 1999;94:99–102.

36. Weidner AC, Myers ER, Visco AG, et al. Which women with stress incontinence require urodynamic evaluation? *Am J Obstet Gynecol* 2001;184:20–27.

37. McClennan MT, Bent AE. Supine empty stress test as a predictor of low Valsalva leak point pressure. *Neurourol Urodyn* 1998;17:121–127.

Ostergard's Urogynecology and Pelvic Floor Dysfunction, Fifth Edition. edited by A.E. Bent, et al. Lippincott Williams & Wilkins, Philadelphia © 2003.

8

Clinical Evaluation of Pelvic Support Defects with Anatomic Correlations

Robert M. Rogers, Jr.* and A. Cullen Richardson**

*Department of Obstetrics and Gynecology, The Reading Hospital and Medical Center, West Reading, Pennsylvania
**(Deceased) Department of Gynecology and Obstetrics, Emory University School of Medicine, Atlanta, Georgia

The continuous and interdependent construction of the pelvic visceral support system is an essential concept when visualizing the underlying anatomic defects that result in clinically evident pelvic support failures. In our current conceptualizations of pelvic support defects, the unseen supporting visceral connective tissues stretch somewhat, but then break to cause pelvic support defects, while allowing the overlying vaginal epithelium and underlying peritoneum to stretch endlessly. These breaks in the integrity of the visceral connective tissue support system have been confirmed by empiric observations. Older methods of reparative vaginal surgery were based on the concept that the visceral supporting connective tissues (endopelvic fascia) stretch to great lengths (attenuation) along with the covering peritoneum and vaginal epithelium. Current procedures for repairing vaginal support defects concentrate on finding these visceral connective tissue breaks, and then reattaching the broken edges, usually with permanent suture. Older techniques repair the perceived attenuated or generally stretched visceral connective tissues by plication and shortening of this visceral fascia, usually with absorbable suture. Problems of female pelvic and vaginal support are currently referred to as pelvic support defects, whereas the former conceptualization talked of pelvic support relaxation. The controversy between those who believe that the visceral support tissues "break" as opposed to "stretching" continues to this day.

This chapter is based on the current observations of breaks and defined, specific disruptions at specific anatomic sites within the integrity of the pelvic visceral support system. The reader must have a three-dimensional, working knowledge of this pelvic support system (see Chapter 2).

The most common problems of pelvic support include uterine prolapse, vaginal vault prolapse, enterocele, high cystocele, high rectocele, urethrocele (urethral hypermobility), low rectocele, gaping introitus, and perineal descent. These are physical findings, not descriptions of anatomic defects. These findings are a visible bulge or prolapse of some portion of the vaginal wall (Fig. 8.1). The quantitative description of the bulges (see Chapter 9) aids in understanding the amount of separation of the broken edges of the support tissues but does not identify the underlying support defects.

Importantly, the reader must always keep in mind that pelvic support defects definitely involve varying contributions of damage to the pelvic floor muscles and their vital innervations. These contributions have yet to

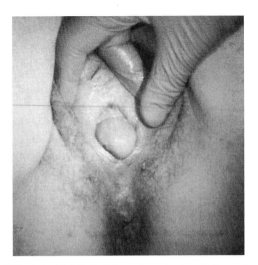

FIG. 8.1. Visible bulging of vaginal wall through introitus.

be studied and fully appreciated. This is a "wild card" in the success of current reparative vaginal procedures. In addition, the quantity and quality of the pelvic support connective tissues themselves are highly variable from patient to patient and are dependent on many constituent factors. Factors that affect the visceral endopelvic support tissues include mechanical, genetic, hormonal, nutritional, and environmental along with the functional state of the surrounding pelvic muscular support and the somatic and visceral innervation of these tissues. Mechanical stresses include childbirth, chronic constipation, repetitive heavy lifting, and high-impact athletic activities. The most common environmental factor is cigarette smoking, which is antiestrogenic and affects connective tissue integrity.

Reparative vaginal surgeons can only repair the breaks in the underlying visceral connective tissue, thereby hopefully restoring the continuous and interdependent function of the visceral support system. The surgeon cannot restore nor strengthen the quality or quantity of the patient's visceral connective tissue, nor can the surgeon restore damaged muscles and nerves. Great

humility on the part of the vaginal surgeon is in order here. The descriptions of pelvic support defects must be based on a full appreciation of the mobility and feel of the healthy tissues in the nonpregnant, normal nulliparous young patient. In addition to the obvious bulges that may be demonstrated in the vagina, the examiner must also appreciate the importance of the appearance of the vaginal epithelium itself and the presence of rugae (Fig. 8.2).

Vaginal rugae are the result of two factors. The first is the irregular surface of the vaginal epithelium owing to variations in its thickness. Second, and more important in diagnosing vaginal support defects, the pleated rugosity of the vaginal epithelium is a result of the intact, underlying visceral connective tissue. Healthy, functional visceral fascia contains contractile smooth muscle and elastin fibers, both of which are physiologically active. These findings are best demonstrated in the well-estrogenized vagina. In the very elderly patient with marked vaginal atrophy, the prominent vaginal rugae are flattened and subtle but are still seen by the careful observer. The appli-

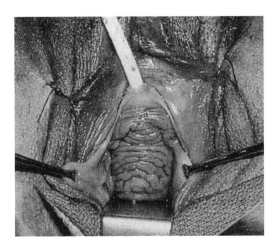

FIG. 8.2. Rugated anterior vaginal wall. (From Baggish MS, Karram MM, *Atlas of pelvic anatomy and gynecologic surgery.* Singapore: WB Saunders, Singapore, 2001:382, with permission.)

cation of a small amount of topical vaginal estrogen restores the prominent vaginal rugae in 1 to 2 weeks.

PELVIC EXAMINATION WHEN VAGINAL SUPPORT DEFECTS ARE NOT PRESENT

Successful diagnostic examination of a patient with pelvic support defects is based on knowledge and experience with the examination of the vaginal support anatomy in the normal nulliparous young woman. The examiner's eyes must focus on specific support locations in the vagina for detailed observations. The examiner's gloved fingers must be trained for fine, discriminative palpation. The following vaginal areas need to be inspected, palpated, and appreciated from the vaginal apex to the vaginal walls to the vaginal introitus and perineum: cervix or vaginal cuff; the four vaginal fornices; vaginal walls—anterior, lateral and posterior; urethrovesical junction and urethra; levator hiatus and lower third of the vagina; and perineal body and rectoanal canal. The examining physician needs a Sims retractor or the lower blade of a Graves speculum, in addition to a gentle instrument to grasp the cervix, such as a single-toothed tenaculum, Babcock clamp, or lightly applied long Allis clamp.

Each area should be evaluated and appreciated with the patient resting and then with the patient straining in a Valsalva maneuver. The appearance and movement of these areas must be appreciated as well as the palpable feel of the thickness, tension, and strength of the underlying visceral fascia. Patients with normal anatomy do not have vaginal bulges nor demonstrate prolapse. Usually, the patient is examined in the dorsolithotomy position. However, examination of the patient in a standing position is also advised to evaluate these vaginal support areas in order to give the examiner more appreciation of the stresses that occur in the patient's normal active position. Prolapse symptoms generally occur when the patient is sitting or standing, not lying down.

Examination of the Vaginal Apex—Normal

With a bivalved speculum carefully placed into the vagina, the examiner can view the cervix. The cervix is stabilized by the attachments of the pericervical ring to the cardinal ligament–uterosacral ligament complexes bilaterally. The cervix is found at the level of the ischial spines and is attached to the hollow of the sacrum by the uterosacral ligaments. These ligaments only allow the cervix to move downward in the long axis of the vagina within the confines of the upper one third of the vagina. With gentle traction on the cervix, the physician can palpate the thick, firm uterosacral ligaments as they attach to the posterolateral aspects of the pericervical ring of visceral fascia. This relationship is better appreciated during a gentle rectal examination during cervical traction. It is also more readily demonstrated during examination under anesthesia.

Because of the vertical and oblique fiber components of each cardinal ligament sheath, the cervix is also positioned slightly anterior to the midpelvic, ischial spine diameter because of the upward pull toward the pelvic brim. The attachments of the cardinal ligaments to the pericervical ring only allow limited lateral motion of the cervix because of the attachment of each cardinal ligament to the sidewall of the pelvis, along the anterior edge of the greater sciatic foramen down to near the ischial spine, and to the iliococcygeus muscle near the ischial spine. Traction on the cervix in the longitudinal axis of the vagina allows the examiner to palpate the cardinal ligaments as they insert laterally onto the pericervical ring.

The cardinal ligaments also attach to the upper portion of the vagina bilaterally to help secure the lateral fornices seen within the vagina. Surgically, this area is the paracolpium. These fornices demonstrate an upward concavity with the patient resting.

With the patient straining down, the examiner can see and feel the limited motion of the cervix and lateral fornices during this maneuver.

The anterior fornix is formed by the fusion of the pubocervical fascia just underneath the anterior vaginal epithelium onto the pericervical ring anteriorly. There should be little excursion of the anterior fornix when the patient bears down. Again, the examiner should palpate this area and get an appreciation for the thickness and continuity of this area.

The posterior fornix is bounded by the uterosacral ligaments inserting into the posterolateral aspects of the pericervical ring and by the rectovaginal fascia traveling underneath the posterior vaginal epithelium and inserting onto the cul-de-sac peritoneum as well as the posterior aspect of the pericervical ring. The examiner must appreciate its normal excursion at times of rest and during Valsalva maneuver. This knowledge assists the surgeon when assessing posterior enteroceles.

Examination of the Vaginal Walls— Normal

The anterior vaginal wall is covered by thickened epithelium with a thickened underlying fibromuscular coat known clinically and surgically as the pubocervical fascia. The transverse rugations in the anterior vaginal wall demonstrate the well-estrogenized vaginal epithelium, but more importantly, they demonstrate the thick, intact, and healthy nature of the underlying pubocervical fascia (Fig. 8.2). The rugosity is the result of smooth muscle contraction and tension of the elastin fibers within the collagen matrix of the visceral fascia. Using a Sims retractor to depress the posterior vaginal wall, the observer should be able to visualize the anterolateral sulci going from the midvagina back toward the ischial spines. Each of these anterolateral sulci represents the attachment of the pubocervical fascia along each pelvic sidewall through the fascia en-

dopelvina to the fascial white line (arcus tendineus fasciae pelvis). The excursion of these areas is important to note with the patient straining in order to appreciate what is normal. The anterior vaginal wall should be inspected and palpated both centrally and laterally and from the pericervical ring to the urethrovesical junction.

The urethrovesical junction is supported by the hammock of pubocervical fascia with attachments to each fascial white line laterally. Gentle traction with a Babcock clamp in the area of the vesical neck demonstrates the limited lateral mobility of the urethra. A Q-tip test (see Chapter 7) demonstrates posterior rotation of the urethrovesical junction in a range of 20 to 25 degrees anteriorly. The examiner's finger along the side of the urethra does not reach the superior pubic ramus because of the attachment of the pubocervical fascia to the fascial white line on each sidewall. With a well-lubricated cervical or urethral dilator gently inserted into the urethra, the examiner can appreciate the thickness of the pubocervical fascia underneath the urethra.

The posterior vaginal wall likewise demonstrates transverse rugations for the same reasons. The vaginal epithelium is well epithelialized, and the underlying posterior visceral vaginal fascia contains smooth muscle and elastin. However, the visceral fascial coat around the posterior vaginal epithelium is generally thinner than the anteriorly placed pubocervical fascia. Between the rectum and vagina is found the fibroelastic sheath of rectovaginal fascia. Rectovaginal examination allows the examiner to appreciate the thickness and the mobility of this fascia.

The examiner should gently palpate each of the lateral sidewalls of the vagina from each ischial spine in a linear fashion to the pubic arch. The examiner should feel a "banjo string," which represents the fascial white line or arcus tendineus fasciae pelvis. On inspection of each lateral vaginal wall at the midvaginal area, the observer sees the separation of the anterolateral sulcus from a posterolateral sulcus, which represents the line of attachment of the rectovaginal fascia to the parietal fascia of the levator ani muscles (arcus tendineus fasciae rectovaginalis). The anterolateral sulcus travels toward the pubic arch, whereas the posterolateral sulcus courses down toward the perineal body.

Examination of the Levator Hiatus—Normal

The examiner should then place two fingers within the opening of the vagina and lower third of the vagina in order to appreciate the size, length, width, and muscle tone of the levator hiatus muscles—namely, the pubococcygeus and puborectalis muscles. The levator hiatus should be appreciated both in the resting state and in the contracted state. The medial edge of the pubococcygeus muscle is found slightly inside the level of the hymenal ring.

Examination of the Perineum—Normal

Rectovaginal examination allows the examiner to appreciate the downward (inferior) movement of the perineal body. The perineal body should feel very thick and broad between the anus and vaginal introitus. As the finger moves through the anal canal toward the rectum, the observer should appreciate the pyramidal shape of the perineal body as the examining fingers palpate the close approximation of the rectum with the mid and upper portions of the vagina. The apex of the perineal body is found at the level of the lower third and middle third of the vagina. Because of the attachment of the rectovaginal fascia to the apex of the perineal body and then to the uterosacral ligaments at the level of the ischial spines, the downward movement of the perineal body should not be more than about 1 cm.

The perineum is normally concave owing to the attachment of the rectovaginal fascia from above. In reality, the perineal body is suspended from the sacrum by the rectovaginal fascia and the uterosacral ligaments.

Examination of the Rectoanal Canal—Normal

Finally, the examiner needs to understand, visualize, and palpate the rectoanal canal. The examiner can palpate the walls of the rectal canal. These walls are the rectovaginal fascia anteriorly, the levator plate posteriorly, and the downward extensions of the uterosacral ligaments by the lateral walls. The muscular levator plate travels from the rectoanal junction toward the lower sacrum and coccyx. The levator plate is formed by the midline fusion of the levator ani muscles just underneath the rectum and is about 4 cm in length. In the standing patient, the levator plate when contracted is almost horizontal to the floor (see Fig. 2.1B in Chapter 2). In the dorsolithotomy position, the levator plate presents in a vertical fashion in impressive strength against the examiner's finger. This is the primary action that is responsible for preventing uterine and vaginal prolapse. The levator plate when contracted is easily palpated during digital rectal examination.

The examiner can then palpate the walls of the anal canal, which are surrounded on three sides by the puborectalis muscle and anteriorly by the perineal body. Again, these areas need to be evaluated with the patient at rest, with the appropriate Valsalva maneuver, as well as with a strong pelvic floor contraction.

Of course, as the physician performs more numbers of pelvic examinations on normal nulliparous patients, increasing his or her experience and powers of observation and palpation, more subtleties and normal variations are appreciated and stored for future reference.

PELVIC EXAMINATION WHEN VAGINAL SUPPORT DEFECTS ARE PRESENT

Visualization of the vaginal bulging with straining, and palpation of the thickness of these tissues with appreciation of the presence or absence of rugae, are important in understanding where the underlying breaks in the visceral endopelvic fascial network have occurred. These visceral support breaks most commonly occur at peripheral attachment sites, and uncommonly occur centrally.

Bulges in the Apex of the Vagina

With the cervix or vaginal cuff descending into the middle third or lower third of the vagina, the examiner needs to search for the uterosacral ligaments and cardinal ligaments. In a cervical and uterine prolapse or vaginal cuff prolapse, the examiner feels a thin line going from the posterolateral aspect of the pericervical ring back toward the ischial spine. This thin line represents the empty peritoneal sleeve, which used to contain the strong, thick uterosacral ligament. The uterosacral ligament usually becomes detached from the pericervical ring at the level of the ischial spines. Therefore, with proper traction and palpation in the examination room or at surgery, the examiner should be able to find good, useful uterosacral ligament cord about 1 to 2 cm medial and posterior to the ischial spine, just beneath the parietal peritoneum in the pelvis. The uterosacral ligament by observation does not break in its midportion, nor does it break away from its attachment to the sacrum. Observations confirm that the uterosacral ligament in prolapse breaks away from the cervix and vaginal cuff from the pericervical ring at the anatomic level of the ischial spines. Because cervical elongation has been observed with uterine prolapse, the examining physician should use a uterine sound to estimate the length of the cervix from the external cervical os to the internal cervical os. All these findings should be recorded. With each aspect of the examination, the physician should evaluate and appreciate the mobility and thickness of the structures as well as the subtle movements of the layers underneath the vaginal epithelium and overlying the pelvic peritoneum.

When the patient bears down during a Valsalva maneuver, the lateral fornices of the vagina bulge down significantly owing to the detachment from the cardinal ligament sheaths. The posterior fornix also significantly bulges down because of the detachment of the rectovaginal fascia from each uterosacral ligament, as described previously. Because of these detachments from the cardinal ligament–uterosacral ligament complexes, the cervix demonstrates wide lateral mobility (Fig. 8.3).

Most vaginal cuff prolapses (Fig. 8.4) include apical enteroceles (prolapse of the vaginal apex), whereby the pubocervical fascia and rectovaginal fascia have physically separated to further disrupt the pericervical ring. The underlying support feels very thin as a result of the stretching of the peritoneum, which is now in direct contact with the vaginal epithelium. These are true hernias with no intervening visceral fascia. The overlying vaginal epithelium is stretched and

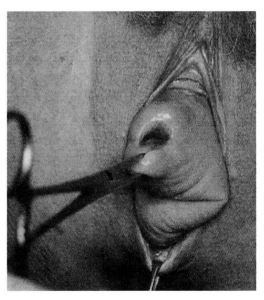

FIG. 8.3. Uterine prolapse with bulging of the posterior and lateral vaginal walls and a loose introitus. (From Baggish MS, Karram MM, *Atlas of pelvic anatomy and gynecologic surgery.* Singapore: WB Saunders, Singapore, 2001:402, with permission.)

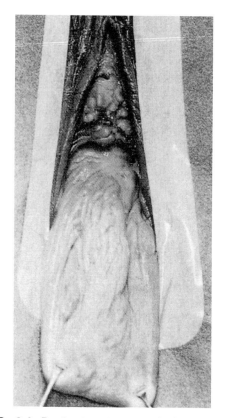

FIG. 8.4. Posthysterectomy vaginal vault prolapse. (From Brubaker L. Diagnostic evaluation of pelvic organ prolapse. In: Benson JT. *Atlas of clinical gynecology: urogynecology and reconstructive pelvic surgery.* Philadelphia: Current Medicine, 1999:5.5, with permission.)

of the pericervical ring and its attachment to each uterosacral ligament at the level of each ischial spine but also must include a reattachment of the pubocervical fascia, as well as the rectovaginal fascia, to each fascial white line laterally.

Bulges in the Anterior Vaginal Wall

A cystocele is a bulging of the anterior vaginal wall down into the vagina beyond its normal limits. The normal limits must be learned from the examination of many nulliparous patients. Generally, an anterior vaginal wall prolapse beyond the midportion of the vagina constitutes a cystocele. However, the word cystocele implies a defect concerning the bladder itself. This is certainly not true. A cystocele represents a defect in the visceral supporting tissues to the pubocervical fascia. The intact pubocervical fascia and its peripheral attachments prevent cystocele and support the bladder. Defects within the pubocervical fascial support system that cause anterior vaginal wall prolapse are found in the following areas: the peripheral attachments of the pubocervical fascia to the fascial white lines; transversely as the pubocervical fascia inserts into the pericervical ring; transversely as the pericervical ring with intact pubocervical fascia inserts onto the uterosacral ligaments; less often centrally underneath the bladder itself; and very rarely, distally, where the urethra detaches from the perineal membrane and from the overlying symphysis pubis (Fig. 8.6).

The detachment of the pubocervical fascia from the lateral attachment edges to the fascial white lines constitutes a paravaginal defect. A paravaginal defect is the partial or complete tearing away of the fascia endopelvina and attached pubocervical fascia from one or both fascial white lines. The paravaginal defect can be caused by the detachment of the pubocervical fascia from the fascial white line, with the fascial white line remaining on the levator ani muscle; or there may be a complete detach-

very smooth without rugae (Fig. 8.5).The examiner should also appreciate that as the disrupted pericervical ring descends down the longitudinal axis of the vagina away from the level of the ischial spines, there must also be a lateral detachment of the pubocervical fascia and the rectovaginal fascia away from the fascial white lines bilaterally. In the patient who has not had reparative vaginal surgery, therefore, cervical and uterine prolapse or vaginal vault prolapse also includes some degree of high cystocele formation and high rectocele formation. Therefore, repair of a cervical or vaginal cuff prolapse not only must address reconstruction

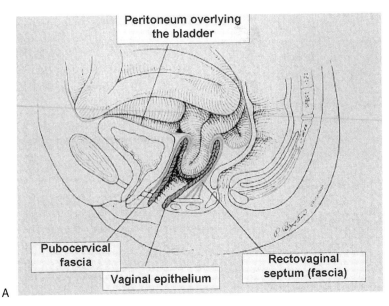

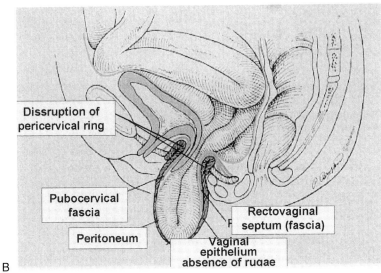

FIG. 8.5. A: Beginning of apical enterocele with some separation of pubocervical and rectovaginal fascia. **B:** Further separation of pubocervical and rectovaginal fascia and descent of vaginal vault with accompanying cystocele and rectocele. (*continued on next page*)

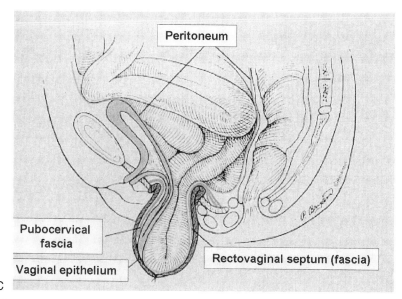

FIG. 8.5. *(Continued)* **C:** The vaginal epithelium is thicker in this diagram of vault prolapse with apical enterocele. (From Richardson AC. The anatomic defects in rectocele and enterocele. *J Pelvic Surg* 1995;1(4):219, with permission.)

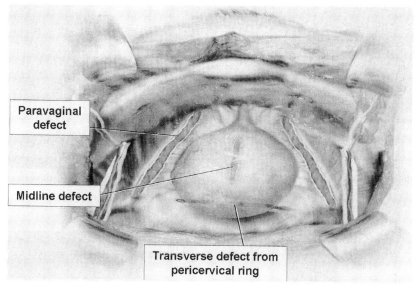

FIG. 8.6. Defects in pubocervical fascial support causing cystocele. (From Baggish MS, Karram MM. *Atlas of pelvic anatomy and gynecologic surgery.* Singapore: WB Saunders, 2001:381, with permission.)

ment of the pubocervical fascia with the attached fascial white line away from the parietal fascia of the levator ani; or there may be a combination of both. With a Sims retractor or the lower blade of a Graves speculum depressing the posterior vaginal wall, a paravaginal defect is diagnosed by observing the significant loss of one or both anterolateral sulci as the patient bears down. Most cystoceles are also accompanied by a bulging down of the vaginal apex and loss of vaginal fornices, as noted in the prior discussion (Fig. 8.7A).

A paravaginal defect is further substantiated by supporting the anterolateral regions of the vagina up against each fascial white line, traveling from the pubic arch back toward the ischial spines. The examiner may use a ring forceps, a Bozeman forceps, or a Baden vaginal defect analyzer. The ends of this instrument also support the vaginal apex against each ischial spine, thus approximating the reattachment of the pericer-

vical ring to each uterosacral ligament at that level. With such instrument support, straining by the patient does not demonstrate the cystocele bulge (Fig. 8.7B). Therefore, proper surgical repair must include a bilateral paravaginal defect repair accompanied by the reconstruction of the pericervical ring and the attachment of this pericervical ring to each uterosacral ligament at the level of the ischial spines.

The transverse tear, which is also accompanied by some degree of a paravaginal defect, can either be caused by a transverse tearing of the pubocervical fascia away from the anterior margin of the pericervical ring (Fig. 8.6) or by a transverse tearing away of the pericervical ring with intact pubocervical fascia from each uterosacral ligament. In the first case, a straining patient causes a distinct bulging out of the anterior vaginal fornix and a loss of thickness and strength in the underlying visceral fascia in this area. In the second case, a detachment

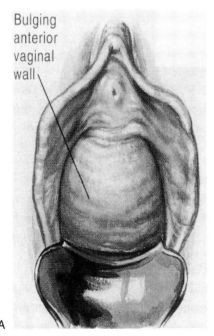 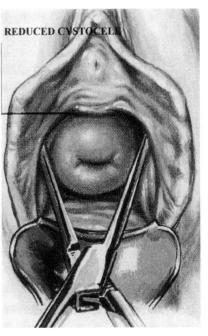

A   B

FIG. 8.7. A: Bulging anterior vaginal wall defect. **B:** Paravaginal defect cystocele reduced with ring forceps placed laterally to elevate the pubocervical fascial detachment toward the white line. (From Retzky SS, Rogers RM. *Urinary incontinence in women.* Summit, NJ: Clinical Symposia Ciba-Geigy Corp, 1995;47(3):22, adapted from Plate 11. Copyright © 1995. ICON Learning Systems, LLC, a subsidiary of MediMedia USA Inc. Reprinted with permission from ICON Learning Systems, LLC, illustrated by John A. Craig, M.D. All rights reserved.)

of each uterosacral ligament to the pericervical ring results in a significant cervical descensus or vaginal vault descensus, with no thickness of uterosacral ligaments being palpated near the pericervical ring.

With a complete paravaginal defect of one side, the examiner's fingers can readily ascend the pelvic sidewall to the bony arcuate line of the ilium. With a paravaginal defect, excellent rugae in the well-estrogenized vagina are still present. In the transverse defect where there is a bulging out of the anterior fornix, the bulge normally has very poor rugations owing to the loss of the underlying pubocervical fascia. The surgically useful pubocervical fascia is found immediately beneath the well rugated vaginal epithelium.

An anterior enterocele (prolapse of the upper anterior wall) develops after hysterectomy when the posterior attachments of the pubocervical fascia are torn from the uterosacral ligaments (Fig. 8.8). The peritoneum of the anterior fornix herniates through this visceral fascial break to push directly against the vaginal epithelium in this area to cause the bulge. When seen, this is usually associated with a posthysterectomy patient who has had a retrop-

ubic colposuspension or sacrospinous ligament colpopexy without full surgical attention to the reconstruction of the pericervical ring.

Again, the point must be emphasized that a cystocele not only includes partial or complete paravaginal defects but in many cases also includes detachment and disruption of the pericervical ring from the uterosacral ligaments as described. The network of visceral supporting fascia within the female pelvis is continuous and interdependent from the pelvic brim to the level of the ischial spines, along the muscular pelvic sidewalls, to the pubic symphysis and perineum. Although the current gynecologic surgical literature speaks of isolated, site-specific defects, in reality in the unoperated patient, the support defects are rarely isolated to one specific support area.

The general rule of vaginal support anatomy is that support defects are not due to one visceral fascial break in one specific area but are caused by two or more fascial breaks in the same support area as well in two or more other vaginal support areas. These are important guidelines in patients who have vaginal support defects but who have not had prior reparative vaginal surgery. Obviously, in

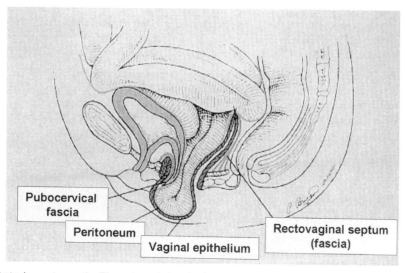

FIG. 8.8. Anterior enterocele. There is a defect in the pubocervical fascia of the anterior vaginal wall with just vaginal epithelium covering the peritoneum lining the enterocele defect. Compare rectovaginal septum with Fig. 8.5B and C. (From Richardson AC. The anatomic defects in rectocele and enterocele. *J Pelvic Surg* 1995;1(4):218, with permission.)

patients who have had prior reparative vaginal surgery, certain breaks in certain areas may have been successfully repaired, and another break in another area may have been missed or not properly repaired, thus causing a single distinct defect in these patients.

Central breaks or central defects (Fig. 8.6) in the pubocervical fascia are surprisingly uncommon and result in a midvaginal bulge when the lateral sulci and apex of the vagina are supported by an instrument such as ring forceps, a Baden vaginal analyzer, or Bozeman forceps. Most of these central breaks occur around the bladder neck or urethrovesical junc-

tion. The examiner may put a dilator in the urethra and feel for the thinness between the vaginal epithelium and urethra. The vesical neck is hypermobile in all directions. Central defects are most easily repaired by a traditional anterior colporrhaphy with an incision centrally through the anterior vaginal wall, followed by a search for the broken pubocervical fascial edges. Closing this defect requires reapproximation of these edges with a series of interrupted permanent sutures.

When performing an anterior colporrhaphy within the confines of the true vesicovaginal space, the operator must recognize that the

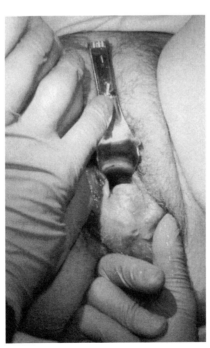

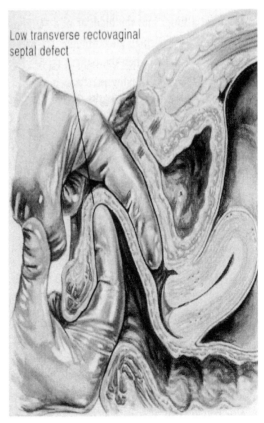

Low transverse rectovaginal septal defect

A   B

FIG. 8.9. A: Low rectocele defect demonstrated by rectal examination with retraction of the anterior vaginal wall in order to view the full length of the posterior vagina. **B:** Demonstration of examination for low defect type rectocele. (From Retzky SS, Rogers RM. *Urinary incontinence in women.* Summit, NJ: Clinical Symposia Ciba-Geigy Corp, 1995;47(3):23, adapted from Plate 12. Copyright © 1995. ICON Learning Systems, LLC, a subsidiary of MediMedia USA Inc. Reprinted with permission from ICON Learning Systems, LLC, illustrated by John A. Craig, M.D. All rights reserved.)

pubocervical fascia is the thick fibromuscular connective tissue remaining on the vaginal flaps. This fascia can be mobilized by sharp dissection using forceps and sharp scissors or knife. The thin visceral fascia surrounding the bladder is not pubocervical fascia. Therefore, plication of the bladder fascia does not successfully repair a cystocele. Reconstruction of the integrity of the pubocervical fascia in the midline and to each fascial white line laterally, back toward the ischial spine, and then attachment of the posterior edge of the pubocervical fascia to each uterosacral ligament repairs a cystocele (anterior vaginal wall prolapse).

A distal defect results from the distal urethra detaching from the perineal membrane and thus from the overlying symphysis. These defects are very rare. Such defects demonstrate telescoping of the urethra straight outward with straining. There is little downward motion. Correction of this defect is usually accomplished by a urethral sling procedure.

Bulges in the Posterior Vaginal Wall

A bulge in the posterior vaginal wall, commonly known as a rectocele, indicates a break or breaks in the integrity of the rectovaginal septum, also known as the rectovaginal fascia. During a rectovaginal examination, an appreciation of the normal feel and attachments of the rectovaginal fascia allows the examiner to appreciate some of the breaks and defects in the rectovaginal fascial support system. The breaks of the rectovaginal fascia most commonly are away from the perineal body and away from the lateral attachments to the pubococcygeus muscles of the levator hiatus, along the arcus tendineus fasciae rectovaginalis. These defects are manifested as a low rectocele or, more clinically, as a low posterior vaginal wall prolapse (Fig. 8.9).

In the upper one third of the vagina, the peritoneum covers the surface of the rectovaginal fascia, whereas in the middle third of the vagina, the rectovaginal fascia is in contact with and loosely attached just underneath the posterior vaginal wall. A rectocele is a tearing of the rectovaginal fascia that allows the rectal

muscularis to push upward against the vaginal epithelium with no intervening visceral fascia. In a high rectocele (prolapse of the upper posterior wall), the break in the rectovaginal fascia allows the peritoneum to be pushed into contact with the vaginal epithelium of the upper third of the vagina with no intervening visceral fascia. The vaginal epithelium is smooth without rugae because there is no intervening visceral fascia (Fig. 8.10).

High rectoceles are associated with posterior and apical enteroceles (Fig. 8.11). These are manifested by a bulging down or prolapse

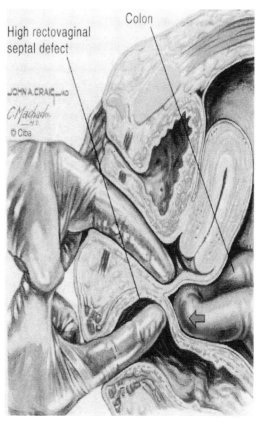

FIG. 8.10. Demonstration of high rectocele defect. (From Retzky SS, Rogers RM. *Urinary incontinence in women.* Summit, NJ: Clinical Symposia Ciba-Geigy Corp, 1995;47(3):23, adapted from Plate 12. Copyright © 1995. ICON Learning Systems, LLC, a subsidiary of MediMedia USA Inc. Reprinted with permission from ICON Learning Systems, LLC, illustrated by John A. Craig, M.D. All rights reserved.)

of the cul-de-sac and posterolateral walls of the vagina toward the middle third of the vagina or lower. The high rectocele is a result of the separation of the rectovaginal fascia from each uterosacral ligament and from its posterior insertion onto the pericervical ring. In addition, the rectovaginal fascia has torn away from the fascial white lines, usually in conjunction with a high cystocele where the pubocervical fascia has also torn away from the fascial white lines near the ischial spines.

Therefore, vaginal repair of a high rectocele with accompanying enterocele requires opening the vaginal epithelium posteriorly, finding the rectovaginal fascia, and then reattaching the fascia to each uterosacral ligament

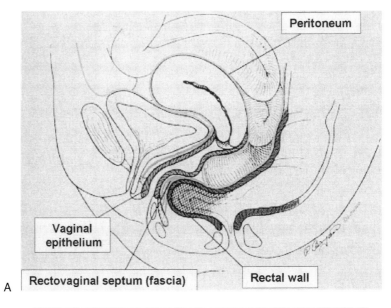

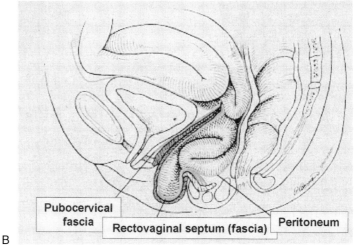

FIG. 8.11. Posterior enteroceles. **A:** The uterus is preserved, but there is a defect in the low rectovaginal fascia. **B:** The uterus has been removed and there is good fusion of pubocervical and rectovaginal fascia at the apex of the vagina, but there is a low defect in the rectovaginal fascia leading to both rectocele and enterocele. (From Richardson AC. The anatomic defects in rectocele and enterocele. *J Pelvic Surg* 1995;1(4):219, with permission.)

and to the reconstructed pericervical ring as well as laterally to the levator ani muscles at the level of the fascial white lines. This latter procedure has previously been described as an iliococcygeus colpopexy. Sometimes, the underlying defects that cause the bulging rectocele cannot be confidently diagnosed preoperatively in the examination room and require careful surgical dissection in order to find the underlying rectovaginal fascia. The rectovaginal fascia is found just beneath the posterior vaginal epithelium in front of the perirectal fat in the rectovaginal space.

The Gaping Vaginal Introitus and Levator Hiatus

The examiner should also palpate, examine, and describe the levator hiatus and compare it with the normal levator hiatus. In addition, the examiner should evaluate the position, strength, thickness, and contractility of the pubococcygeus and puborectalis muscles. Also, the examiner should do a rectal

examination and assess the strength and position of the levator plate. If the levator plate is inclined downward, this increases the shearing stress on any intact visceral pelvic support structures, especially the cardinal ligament–uterosacral ligament complexes (Figs. 8.3 and 8.12).

Perineal Bulges and Rectoanal Canal Disruption

Normally, the perineum is concave because the intact perineal body is attached to the sacrum by the uterosacral ligaments and rectovaginal fascia. Any significant break along this continuity results in an outward bulging of the perineal body as well as its descent far below its normal position. In addition, when a straight edge is placed between the two ischial tuberosities, the anus should lie along that line but pulled 1 to 2 cm above it or superiorly toward the promontory of the sacrum. The anus is fused with the perineal body. Therefore, any descent of the perineal body, as de-

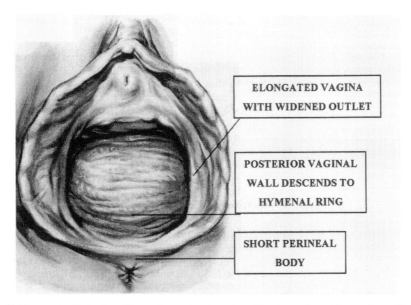

FIG. 8.12. Wide vaginal introitus. There is minimal perineal body and a wide vagina with poor muscle support. (From Retzky SS, Rogers RM. *Urinary incontinence in women.* Summit, NJ: Clinical Symposia Ciba-Geigy Corp, 1995;47(3):20, adapted from Plate 10. Copyright © 1995. ICON Learning Systems, LLC, a subsidiary of MediMedia USA Inc. Reprinted with permission from ICON Learning Systems, LLC, illustrated by John A. Craig, M.D. All rights reserved.)

scribed previously, allows the anus to descend and be deflected outward and down toward the coccyx. This results in abnormal angulation of the anal canal as indicated by a Q-tip placed in the canal. During a rectal examination, palpation of the lateral attachments, the posterior attachment, the uterosacral liga-

ments, and lower attachments to the perineal body can be felt. Again, comparison must be made in the normal nulliparous patient.

In a perineal rectocele, the rectal muscularis is in direct contact with the perineal skin, with no intervening fascia (Fig. 8.13). The underlying defect is a complete disruption of the in-

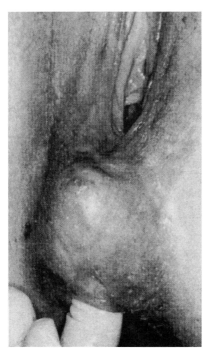

A

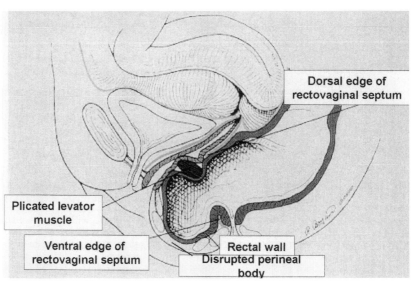

B

FIG. 8.13. Perineal rectocele. **A:** Defect demonstrated by digital rectal examination. **B:** The break in the rectovaginal fascia brings rectal wall in contact with perineal skin. (From Richardson AC. The anatomic defects in rectocele and enterocele. *J Pelvic Surg* 1995;1(4):218, with permission.)

Dorsal edge of rectovaginal septum

Plicated levator muscle

Ventral edge of rectovaginal septum

Rectal wall
Disrupted perineal body

tegrity of the perineal body itself. Obviously, there has been a complete disruption of the fibrous connective tissue as well as the superficial transverse perinei muscles, the bulbocavernosus muscles in the midline, and the contributing levator ani muscles. Physically, there is a wide area of skin between the vaginal opening and the anus. Bimanual examination of the perineum reveals the presence of only skin and rectal muscularis. With a Valsalva maneuver, the perineum demonstrates a significant bulge. The skin is stretched and smooth. Anal examination reveals a loss of the normal funneling of the anus and a marked widening above the anal sphincter in the rectum. Careful reconstruction of the perineal body in a symmetric and defined manner is the procedure of choice, followed by attachment to the rectovaginal septum at its apex.

AFTERTHOUGHT

The role of the reparative vaginal surgeon is to find and repair the breaks in the integrity of the visceral fascial supporting system in the female patient. All observations concerning the various bulges in and around the vagina need to be assessed and recorded for each individual patient. All defects need to be identified and addressed. Importantly, the operative gynecologist must anatomically visualize the various breaks in the visceral support system that explain the observed areas of vaginal prolapse. Then, and only then, can the gynecologic surgeon plan appropriate procedures to correct these underlying support defects for the purposes of restoring normal

axes, normal anatomy, and hopefully, normal function to the vagina and its support structures as well as the bladder and urethra and the rectum and anal canal. Occasionally, the surgeon plans a procedure that creates an anatomic abnormality to compensate for each of the defects. Restoration of normal anatomy during the first surgery has the best chance for the restoration of normal function. However, because of damaged somatic nerves and muscles, a compensatory defect sometimes must be created surgically. The surgeon must understand the anatomic alterations resulting from each reparative procedure *and* how these alterations affect the continuity and function of the visceral pelvic support system.

It is advised to repeat a structured and focused examination of the patient in the operating room after the patient is asleep, immediately before the proposed surgery. This examination sometimes reveals findings that were not noted previously in the office. After the proposed pelvic reparative surgeries have been completed, the surgeon must reexamine the patient in order to ensure that all the fascial defects have been properly repaired. If not, further surgery is required to complete the defect repair procedures. Unrecognized or unrepaired endopelvic fascial defects are not magically healed as the patient is moved from the operating table onto the stretcher and during her trip to the recovery room. These unrepaired defects eventually result in renewed symptoms and repeat reparative vaginal procedures. The best course is to identify and repair all pelvic support defects during the first surgery.

Ostergard's Urogynecology and Pelvic Floor Dysfunction, Fifth Edition. edited by A.E. Bent, et al. Lippincott Williams & Wilkins, Philadelphia © 2003.

9

Standardization of the Description of Pelvic Organ Prolapse

Kimberly W. Coates and Bob L. Shull

Department of Obstetrics and Gynecology, Texas A&M University College of Medicine/Health Science Center; and Department of Obstetrics and Gynecology, Scott & White Clinic, Temple, Texas

Lack of a standardized system for objective and quantifiable description of pelvic organ prolapse has historically been a significant problem in gynecology. Gynecologists had been unable to document physical findings objectively and follow them longitudinally and to compare preoperative and postoperative pelvic support in series reported by different investigators. These handicaps adversely affected the advancement of knowledge of the natural history of pelvic organ prolapse and refinement of surgical techniques for treatment of pelvic organ prolapse. A standardized system that allows reproducible and reliable descriptions of pelvic organ support was believed to be imperative. Although multiple systems were proposed, it was not until 1996 that a system, commonly referred to as the pelvic organ prolapse quantification system (POPQ), was published and approved by the International Continence Society (ICS), American Urogynecologic Society (AUGS), and the Society of Gynecologic Surgeons (SGS) (1).

HISTORY

Dr. Norman Miller, one of the early American gynecologic surgeons to note the importance of observing end results of surgical therapy, reported a creative system for quantifying the size of cystoceles (2). "Enormous" was used to describe a cystocele the size of an "average orange," "large" for the size of a "lemon," "moderate" for the size of a "hen's egg," and "small" for the size of a "bantam's egg or plum." Although he aspired to quantify the amount of prolapse observed, his system was fraught with limitations because descriptions such as these are subjective and vary greatly between observers. The use of multiple classification methods for pelvic organ prolapse led some investigators to become frustrated about the lack of a standardized description for grading prolapse. In 1961, Friedman and Little (3) concisely summarized the state of disarray: "Specious and misleading discrepancies exist with reference to classification of the extent of descent of the uterus in disorders involving fascial relaxation."

In 1980, Dr. C. T. Beecham (4) proposed a grading system "in the interests of standardization" that included three degrees of severity to describe "rectocele," "cystocele," "uterine prolapse" or "vaginal apex prolapse," and "enterocele." His classification system strictly prohibited straining by the patient or the examiner's use of traction on pelvic structures. Digital depression of the perineum was an integral part of this method. Each site of prolapse was graded by degree, from first to third, based on visual inspection. When the site of evaluation was seen with depression of the perineum, a first-degree grade of severity was assigned to that site. For example, when the perineum was depressed and the cervix was visible, first-degree uterine prolapse was diagnosed. For second- and third-degree prolapse, the examiner would note progressively more descent of the prolapsing site with the patient at rest. Specific definitions were assigned for each site of prolapse. A major fallacy of this classification is the requirement that the patient is not allowed to strain during the examination. Consider how much could be learned from auscultation of the lungs if the patient was asked *not* to breathe. We know patients must be examined with a maximum increase in intraabdominal pressure to reproduce prolapse findings at their worst. All recently proposed grading systems recommend the use of straining efforts or standing to elicit the maximum amount of prolapse.

In 1996, Brubaker and Norton (5) reviewed a sample of 157 manuscripts published in the English language from 1966 to 1990 and found the state of affairs described by Little and Friedman had not improved in the subsequent three decades (Tables 9.1 and 9.2). While pelvic reconstructive surgeons saddled themselves with the lack of any precise classification system, oncologists developed clinical and surgical staging systems and infertility

TABLE 9.1. *Overall category of disorder*

Category	No %
Prolapse	53 (34%)
Genital prolapse	37 (24%)
Pelvic relaxation	14 (9%)
Procidentia	4 (3%)
Other	
Descensus	
Descent	
Eversion	
Genital relaxation	
Genital tract prolapse	
Genitourinary prolapse	
Pelvic floor defect	
Pelvic floor dysfunction	
Pelvic floor lesion	
Pelvic prolapse	
Perineal hernia	
Perineal relaxation	
Urogenital prolapse	
Uterovaginal prolapse	
Vaginal inversion	
Vaginal prolapse	

From Brubaker L, Norton P. Current clinical nomenclature for description of pelvic organ prolapse. *J Pelvic Surg* 1996;2:257–259, with permission.

TABLE 9.2. *Grading systems used in 157 prolapse papers*

Grading system	N
Mild/moderate/severe	19
Grade 0–3/1–3	12
Grade 0–4/1–4	8
Incomplete/complete	3
Alternative grading system	37
No grading system	78

From Brubaker L, Norton P. Current clinical nomenclature for description of pelvic organ prolapse. *J Pelvic Surg* 1996;2:257–259, with permission.

surgeons introduced staging for endometriosis. Now all scientific reports regarding outcome of cancer therapy can be understood by gynecologists worldwide, results from different treatment modalities can be critically compared, and patients can be given information about treatment options and prognosis for cure. Pelvic reconstructive surgeons and their patients, on the other hand, have not been able to enjoy these advantages.

THE HALFWAY SYSTEM

From the late 1960s to the 1990s, Drs. Baden and Walker (6) developed and refined a site-specific classification for pelvic organ prolapse that addresses all potential sites of support loss. Initially published in 1968 and known as the vaginal profile, their original classification was perceived to be too difficult for general use. After review of their original classification by a committee of the American College of Obstetricians and Gynecologists, Baden and Walker created a simplified version known as the halfway system (Table 9.3).

For almost two decades, we have used the halfway system for describing pelvic organ prolapse. Consequently, we have been able to follow patients longitudinally to determine changes in pelvic support and to document long-term responses to surgical intervention. This site-specific analysis of pelvic organ prolapse has led to significant refinement in our diagnostic skills and to modifications in surgical techniques (7–10). Although this system provides a means to quantify the amount of prolapse at six vaginal sites, it provides

TABLE 9.3. *Halfway system for grading relaxations*

Urethrocele, cystocele, uterine prolapse, culdocele, or rectocele: patient strains firmly. Grade descent of desired sites. Grade posterior urethral descent, lowest part other sites.
   Grade 0: normal position *for each* respective site
   Grade 1: descent *halfway* to the hymen
   Grade 2: descent to the hymen
   Grade 3: descent *halfway past* the hymen
   Grade 4: maximum possible descent for each site
Anterior perineal laceration: grade with patient holding
   Grade 0: normal; superficial epithelial laceration
   Grade 1: laceration *halfway* to the anal sphincter
   Grade 2: laceration to the anal sphincter
   Grade 3: laceration involves anal sphincter
   Grade 4: laceration involves rectal mucosa

When choosing between two grades, use the greater grade (i.e., if there is a question as to grade 2 or 3 cystocele, use cystocele, grade 3). Grade still in doubt? Regrade with patient standing. Grade worst site, worst segment, or vaginal canal PRN. Grades are interchanged with mild to severe and degrees methods.

From Baden W, Walker T. Surgical repair of vaginal defects. Philadelphia: JB Lippincott, 1992:14, with permission.

only an estimate and not an exact measurement of descent of the prolapsing structure proximal or distal to the hymen (11).

STANDARDIZATION OF TERMINOLOGY

In September 1993, a subcommittee of the ICS met in Rome to draft a system to enable accurate quantitative description of pelvic support findings (1). The subcommittee completed a final draft of their recommendations that was distributed to members of the ICS, the AUGS, and the SGS in late 1994 and early 1995. This quantification system, the POPQ system, was formally adopted by the ICS in October 1995, the AUGS in January 1996, and the SGS in March 1996 (1). This standardized system was published in the *American Journal of Obstetrics and Gynecology* in July 1996 (1). The system is an adaptation of Baden and Walker's site-specific system that requires measuring eight sites to create a tandem vaginal profile before assigning site-specific ordinal stages.

Keys to this classification scheme are specifically defined points of measurement and use of a defined anatomic landmark as a fixed point of reference. The hymen is the fixed point by which measurements of six vaginal points are referenced. The report discourages the use of imprecise terms, such as introitus (1). Points of measurement

within the vaginal canal are defined for the anterior and posterior vaginal wall and vaginal apex. Anteriorly, the two points of reference include a point 3 cm proximal to the external urethral meatus and a point that represents the most distal or dependent portion of the anterior vaginal wall (Fig. 9.1).

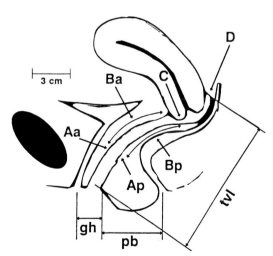

FIG. 9.1. Six sites (points *Aa, Ba, C, D, Bp,* and *Ap*), genital hiatus (*gh*), perineal body (*pb*), and total vaginal length (*tvl*) used for pelvic organ support quantitation. (From Bump RC, Mattiasson A, Bø K, et al. The standardization of terminology of female pelvic organ prolapse and pelvic floor dysfunction. *Am J Obstet Gynecol* 1996;175:10–17, with permission.)

Posteriorly, the points of reference are similar by use of a midline posterior point 3 cm proximal to the hymen and a point representing the most distal or dependent position of the posterior vaginal wall (Fig. 9.1). The vaginal apex is defined by two points: the most distal edge of the cervix or vaginal cuff scar and the location of the posterior fornix or pouch of Douglas (Fig. 9.1). This last point is omitted in patients who have no cervix. Measurements of the genital hiatus, perineal body, and the total vaginal length are also included in this classification scheme (Fig. 9.1). A grid or line diagram may be used to describe normal support as well as support defects of the vaginal cuff and anterior and posterior vaginal walls (Fig. 9.2 and 9.3).

All measurements are made in centimeters and expressed as above (proximal) or below (distal) the hymen and designated negative or positive, respectively. The numbers may then be listed as a simple line of numbers (tandem profile) or as a three-by-three grid (Table 9.4).

In addition, the report establishes an ordinal staging system to be used after the quantitative description is completed (Table 9.5). The committee acknowledges the arbitrary nature of such a staging system but

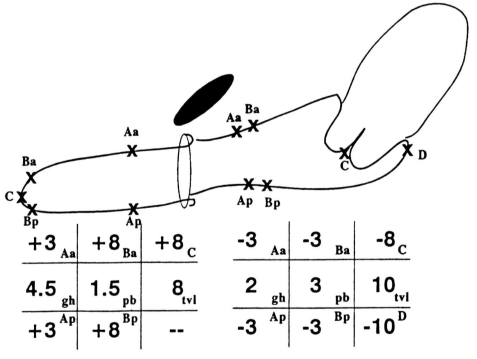

A   B

FIG. 9.2. A: Grid and line diagram of complete eversion of vagina. Most distal point of anterior wall (point *Ba*), vaginal cuff scar (point *C*), and most distal point of the posterior wall (point *Bp*) are all at same position (+8), and points *Aa* and *Ap* are maximally distal (both at +3). Because total vaginal length equals maximum protrusion, this is stage IV prolapse. **B:** Normal support. Points *Aa* and *Ba* and points *Ap* and *Bp* are all −3 because there is no anterior or posterior wall descent. Lowest point of the cervix is 8 cm above hymen (−8) and posterior fornix is 2 cm above this (−10). Vaginal length is 10 cm, and genital hiatus and perineal body measure 2 and 3 cm, respectively. This represents stage 0 support. (From Bump RC, Mattiasson A, Bø K, et al. The standardization of terminology of female pelvic organ prolapse and pelvic floor dysfunction. *Am J Obstet Gynecol* 1996;175:10–17, with permission.)

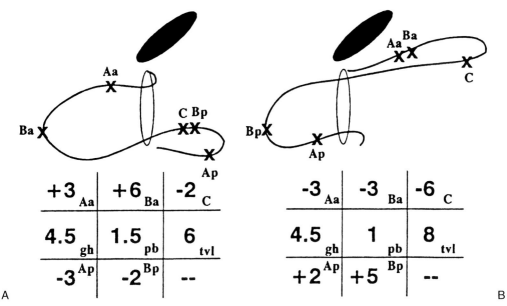

FIG. 9.3. A: Grid and line diagram of predominant anterior support defect. Leading point of prolapse is upper anterior vaginal wall, point *Ba* (+6). There is significant elongation of bulging anterior wall. Point *Aa* is maximally distal (+3), and vaginal cuff scar is 2 cm above hymen (*C* = −2). Cuff scar has undergone 4 cm of descent because it would be at −6 (total vaginal length) if it were perfectly supported. In this example, total vaginal length is not maximum depth of vagina with elongated anterior vaginal wall maximally reduced but rather depth of vagina at cuff, with point *C* reduced to its normal full extent, as specified in text. This represents state III *Ba* prolapse. **B:** Predominant posterior support defect. Leading point of prolapse is upper posterior vaginal wall, point *Bp* (+5). Point *Ap* is 2 cm distal to hymen (+2), and vaginal cuff scar is 6 cm above hymen (−6). Cuff has undergone only 2 cm of descent distal to hymen (+2), and vaginal cuff scar is 6 cm above hymen (−6). Cuff has undergone only 2 cm of descent because it would be at −8 (total vaginal length) if it were perfectly supported. This represents stage III *Bp* prolapse. (From Bump RC, Mattiasson A, Bø K, et al. The standardization of terminology of female pelvic organ prolapse and pelvic floor dysfunction. *Am J Obstet Gynecol* 1996;175:10–17, with permission.)

TABLE 9.4. *A three-by-three grid for recording the quantitative description of pelvic organ prolapse*

Point Aa	Point Ba	Point C
Anterior wall	Anterior wall	Cervix or cuff
Genital hiatus	Perineal body	Total vaginal length
Point Ap	Point Bp	Point D
Posterior wall	Posterior wall	Posterior fornix

From Bump RC, Mattiasson A, Bø K, et al. The standardization of terminology of female pelvic organ prolapse and pelvic floor dysfunction. *Am J Obstet Gynecol* 1996;175:10–17, with permission.

TABLE 9.5. *International continence society pelvic organ prolapse ordinal staging system*

Stage 0	Points Aa, Ap, Ba, and Bp are all at −3 cm and either point C or D is at no more than −(X − 2) cm
Stage I	The criteria for stage 0 are not met and the leading edge of prolapse is less than −1 cm
Stage II	Leading edge of prolapse is at least −1 cm but no more than +1 cm
Stage III	Leading edge of prolapse is greater than +1 cm but less than +(X − 2) cm
Stage IV	Leading edge of prolapse is at least +(X − 2) cm

X, total vaginal length in centimeters in stages 0, III, and IV. Stages I through IV can be subgrouped according to which portion of the lower reproductive tract is the leading edge of the prolapse using the following qualifiers: a, anterior vaginal wall; p, posterior vaginal wall; C, vaginal cuff; Cx, cervix; and Aa, Ba, Ap, Bp, and D for the defined points of measurement (e.g., IV-Cx, II-a, or III-Bp).

From Bump RC, Mattiasson A, Bø K, et al. The standardization of terminology of female pelvic organ prolapse and pelvic floor dysfunction. *Am J Obstet Gynecol* 1996;175:10–17, with permission.

concludes that it is necessary. Staging allows for description and comparison of populations of patients, correlation of symptoms with severity of prolapse, and assessment of treatment outcomes.

Observation and description of the maximum amount of pelvic organ prolapse are critical and must be consistent with the amount of prolapse experienced by the patient. It is suggested that the maximum prolapse observed be confirmed by the following: by observation that the protrusion of the vaginal wall becomes "tight" when the patient strains; by observation that traction on the prolapse produces no further descent; by the patient's confirmation that the size of prolapse observed is consistent with the most extensive prolapse she has experienced; or by examination of the standing and straining patient and observing that the extent of prolapse is consistent with the other positions used (1). We have found it useful to ask the patient to use a handheld mirror to observe and confirm the maximal extent of prolapse during the examination. It has been reported that the degree of prolapse observed varies by patient position, with an increase in prolapse with the patient in a sitting "45% upright" position in a birthing chair as compared with the patient in a dorsal lithotomy position (12–14). This difference did not seem to be related to other patient characteristics, including age, race, parity, weight, or the prolapse stage or genital hiatus measurement in the lithotomy position (14). POPQ measurements have also been compared by Swift and Herring in the standing and dorsal lithotomy positions (15). A high degree of correlation of measurements in the two positions was found, and it has been postulated that this was related to differences in pelvic tilt produced by standing and dorsal lithotomy positions as compared with a sitting position (15). As with the McRoberts maneuver, maximum hip flexion is likely to occur in the birthing chair, which results in opening of the pelvic outlet (14,15).

The subcommittee report also addresses the use of ancillary techniques for describing pelvic organ prolapse (1). These ancillary techniques may be used to characterize further the observed prolapse; however, careful description by investigators of the technique and the methods used is essential. Ancillary techniques may include digital rectal and vaginal examination, cotton swab testing for mobility of the urethral axis, and endoscopic or imaging studies.

The subcommittee report addresses the presence of functional symptoms related to the presence of pelvic organ prolapse. Although the functional deficits are not well established, there is a great need to characterize the occurrence of these symptoms with prolapse. The report acknowledges four functional symptom groups including urinary, bowel, sexual, and other local symptoms. They rpecommend that investigators attempt to standardize and validate symptom scales when possible. Specifically, investigators should ask precisely the same questions before and after the treatment has been implemented.

The subcommittee's efforts in creating this classification scheme and incorporating objective criteria for the description of pelvic organ prolapse were a first step toward establishing a standard, reliable, and validated description of pelvic anatomy and function. They acknowledged the need for studies designed to evaluate and validate the descriptions and definitions they propose. In 1996, Hall and associates evaluated the interobserver and intraobserver reliability of the POPQ system (13). The reproducibility of the nine site-specific measurements and the summary stage and substage were evaluated. There was substantial and highly significant correlation between measurements for both interobserver and intraobserver examinations (13). Although it took new POPQ examiners an average of 1.7 minutes longer than experienced POPQ examiners to complete the examination, the reliability did not vary between the groups (13).

Recently, concern has been expressed that the POPQ system may be complicated, confusing, and difficult to learn (16,17). An informal questionnaire was distributed to a select group of the ICS, and only 20% of the respondents were using the system, with the most commonly reported reason being that the POPQ was "too difficult to learn and teach" (17). Subsequently, alternative classification methods are being explored. The International Federation of Gynecologists and Obstetricians (FIGO) has expressed interest in developing a system that allows for description of common physical examination findings in women with pelvic organ prolapse, demonstrates good reproducibility, and can be easily learned by health care providers worldwide (17). The Standardization of Terminology Committee of the International Urogynecology Association is preparing an opinion regarding the current classification systems and anticipates publication of the system for worldwide adoption.

Despite reported concerns regarding the complexity of the POPQ system, Steele and colleagues reported that the POPQ system could be effectively taught to obstetric and gynecology residents and medical students (18). Likewise, we have found that it can be readily taught to interested medical students, residents, and practicing gynecologists. It has become a useful clinical and research tool to allow for the longitudinal study of patient populations and evaluation of nonsurgical and surgical treatment outcomes.

REFERENCES

1. Bump R, Bø K, Brubaker L, et al. The International Continence Society Committee on Standardization of Terminology, Subcommittee on Pelvic Organ Prolapse and Pelvic Floor Dysfunction. The standardization of terminology of female pelvic organ prolapse and pelvic floor dysfunction. *Am J Obstet Gynecol* 1996;175:10–17.
2. Miller NF. End-results from correction of cystocele by the simple fascia pleating method. *Surg Gynecol Obstet* 1928;46:403–410.
3. Friedman EA, Little WA. The conflict in nomenclature for descensus uteri. *Am J Obstet Gynecol* 1961;81:817–820.
4. Beecham CT. Classification of vaginal relaxation. *Am J Obstet Gynecol* 1980;136:957–958.
5. Brubaker L, Norton P. Current clinical nomenclature for description of pelvic organ prolapse. *J Pelvic Surg* 1996;2:257–259.
6. Baden W, Walker T. *Surgical repair of vaginal defects.* Philadelphia, PA: JB Lippincott, 1992.
7. Shull BL, Baden WF. Paravaginal defect repair for urinary incontinence: a six year experience. *Am J Obstet Gynecol* 1989;160:1432–1440.
8. Shull BL, Capen CV, Riggs M, et al. Pre- and postoperative analysis of site-specific pelvic support defects in 81 women treated by sacrospinous ligament suspension and pelvic reconstruction. *Am J Obstet Gynecol* 1992;166:1764–1768.
9. Shull BL, Capen CV, Riggs M, et al. Bilateral attachment of the vaginal cuff to iliococcygeus fascia: an effective method of cuff suspension. *Am J Obstet Gynecol* 1993;168:1669–1677.
10. Shull BL, Benn SJ, Kuehl TJ. Surgical management of prolapse of the anterior vaginal segment: an analysis of support defects, operative morbidity, and anatomic outcome. *Am J Obstet Gynecol* 1994;171:1429–1439.
11. Coates KW, Galan HL, Shull BL, et al. The squirrel monkey: an animal model of pelvic relaxation. *Am J Obstet Gynecol* 1995;172:588–593.
12. Montella JM, Cater JR. Comparison of measurement obtained in supine and sitting position in the evaluation of pelvic organ prolapse. *Int Urogynecol J* 1995;6:304 [abst].
13. Hall AF, Theofrastous JP, Cundiff GW, et al. Interobserver and intraobserver reliability of the proposed International Continence Society, Society of Gynecologic Surgeons, and American Urogynecologic Society pelvic organ prolapse classification system. *Am J Obstet Gynecol* 1996;175:1467–1471.
14. Barber MD, Lambers AR, Visco AG, et al. Effect of patient position on clinical evaluation of pelvic organ prolapse. *Obstet Gynecol* 2000;96:18–22.
15. Swift SE, Herring M. Comparison of pelvic organ prolapse in the dorsal lithotomy compared with the standing position. *Obstet Gynecol* 1998;91:961–964.
16. Scotti RJ, Flora R, Greston WM, et al. Characterizing and reporting pelvic floor defects: the revised New York classification system. *Int Urogynecol J* 2000;11:48–60.
17. Swift S, Freeman R, Petri E, et al. Proposal for a worldwide, user-friendly classification system for pelvic organ prolapse (abstract). 26th annual meeting of the International Urogynecologic Association, Melbourne, Australia, December 5–7, 2001.
18. Steele A, Mallipeddi P, Welgoss J, et al. Teaching the pelvic organ prolapse quantitation system. *Am J Obstet Gynecol* 1998;179:1458–1464.

Ostergard's Urogynecology and Pelvic Floor Dysfunction, Fifth Edition. edited by A.E. Bent, et al.
Lippincott Williams & Wilkins, Philadelphia © 2003.

10

Screening Neurologic Examination with Clinical Correlations in the Evaluation of the Incontinent Patient

Lawrence R. Lind* and Narender N. Bhatia**

*Department of Obstetrics and Gynecology, Division of Urogynecology, North Shore–Long Island Jewish Health System, New York University School of Medicine, Manhasset, NY
**Department of Obstetrics and Gynecology, UCLA School of Medicine; and Division of Urogynecology, Harbor/UCLA Medical Center, Los Angeles, California

A comprehensive neurologic examination is an integral part of the history and physical examination of female patients with lower urinary tract symptoms. Electrophysiologic studies demonstrate an increasing role of neurologic evaluation of patients with voiding dysfunction (1–6). The urogynecologist must understand the neurophysiology of normal voiding, be familiar with the physical findings that may suggest a neurologic explanation for voiding dysfunction, and know which urodynamic and electrophysiologic tests are required as they relate to neurologic causes of voiding dysfunction (see Chapter 13). This chapter describes the details of the neurologically oriented physical examination, followed by a clinical overview of the most common neurologic disorders that have urologic sequelae. Guidelines are provided for selecting patients who require formal neurologic consultation or advanced electrophysiologic testing.

NEUROLOGIC EVALUATION

When evaluating patients with voiding disorders, a neurologic history and examination should be an integral part of the general physical examination. To perform an effective general screening neurologic examination, a basic understanding of neuroanatomy is necessary. The localization of a lesion to the cerebrum, brain stem, cerebellum, spinal cord, or peripheral nervous system is accomplished by systematic examination of the cranial nerves, neck, and trunk; motor, reflex, and sensory function of the lower extremities; and sphincteric and autonomic nervous system functions, gait, and station. Each component of the neurologic examination is presented with emphasis on the clinical correlations between findings on the neurologic examination and concomitant voiding abnormalities.

HISTORY

The neurologic examination always begins with a detailed yet focused history. Attention is necessary not only to the presented facts but also to the speech and manner of patient responses to questions. The mode of onset, evolution, and course of each symptom are of paramount importance. It is tempting to shorten the time spent on history taking when the patient is a poor historian. The presence of poor speech or disorganized thoughts may be the first clue to a central nervous system lesion that is related to the urologic complaints. The elicited history should include sequentially the same categories to be explored in the neurologic examination: mental status, strength and sensory changes of the upper and lower extremities, and gait and station.

GENERAL SCREENING NEUROLOGIC EXAMINATION

Mental Status

Mental status testing is performed by determining accuracy in the following areas: recent and past memory; orientation to date, place, and person; calculations; comprehension of simple directions; and reading and writing abilities. The Mini Mental Status Examination is available as a structured, well-tested tool for brief assessment of a patient's mental status (7). Disorders associated with mental status aberrations that may also produce urologic abnormalities include senile and presenile dementia, Parkinson's disease, brain tumors, and normal pressure hydrocephalus. Patients with these disorders may present with either detrusor instability (when the frontal lobe is primarily affected) or overflow incontinence (when the paracentral gyrus is primarily affected).

It is important to define the severity of any mental deficit because the patient's cognitive and physical abilities will affect treatment options. Further information regarding cerebral injuries, neurologic evaluation, and urinary function are detailed in the clinical correlations section.

Cranial Nerves

A detailed review of each cranial nerve is beyond the scope of this chapter. Most of the nerves can be evaluated in a series of maneuvers that takes less than 1 minute. A reasonably thorough examination includes assessment of smell; eye movements; fundoscopic examination; facial symmetry; use of eye, facial, and tongue muscles; jaw strength; head movement; and shoulder shrug.

Muscle Strength

Skeletal muscles should be inspected for muscle atrophy and fasciculations, spasticity, rigidity, and strength. Muscle strength is assessed by having the patient either resist movement or actively move against resistance. Strength is graded on a scale of 0 to 5: 0, no movement; 1, trace of contraction; 2, ac-

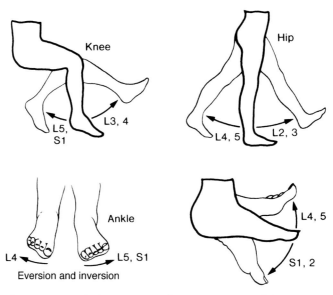

FIG. 10.1. Testing of motor strength. Lower extremity movements and the corresponding spinal cord segments are indicated.

tive movement when gravity eliminated; 3, active movement against gravity only; 4, active movement against resistance but less than normal; and 5, normal strength.

The maneuvers required to test sacral spinal cord integrity focus on the lower extremities. The basic maneuvers are extension and flexion of the hip, knee, and ankle and inversion or eversion of the foot (Fig. 10.1).

Deep Tendon Reflexes

Evaluation of the deep tendon reflexes provides information regarding segmental and suprasegmental spinal cord function. For urologic patients, the essential reflexes include the jaw jerk and the biceps, triceps, knee, ankle, and plantar responses. Any asymmetry of the reflexes may closely reflect the nature of bladder dysfunction. In supranuclear lesions, there is hyperreflexia of the deep tendon reflexes. This is often associated with uninhibited detrusor contractions as demonstrated by cystometry.

An upper motor neuron lesion may also be detected with the plantar toe reflex. The plantar toe reflex is elicited by stroking the handle of a reflex hammer along the lateral aspect of the foot, from the heel to the ball of the foot, and then curving it medially. A normal response produces plantar flexion of the toes. An abnormal (Babinski) response produces fanning of the toes and dorsiflexion of the big toe and indicates interruption of the corticospinal tracts, an upper motor neuron lesion.

Although the absence of a patellar reflex is always abnormal, the ankle reflex diminishes with age; its absence in elderly patients, therefore, may be of no clinical significance (8). In patients with cauda equina lesions or with peripheral neuropathy (lower motor neurons), the deep tendon reflexes may be diminished or absent. Clinically, patients demonstrate detrusor areflexia or varying degrees of decreased bladder contractility. The presence of peripheral nerve impairment, autonomic neuropathy, or spinal cord disease below T-12 may be suggested by absent or diminished reflexes and clinically correlated with symptoms of urinary retention or voiding difficulties.

Sensory Function

Accurate assessment of sensory function is challenging because of the subjective nature of the response and the need for patient cooperation. Despite these limitations, the examiner can usually determine whether the patient can perceive a stimulus and whether the response is symmetric. The spinal pathways of importance are the lateral spinothalamic tract (pain and temperature), the posterior columns (position, vibration, and light touch), and the anterior spinothalamic tract (crude touch). Only the distal extremities need to be evaluated for position sense and vibration; however, both proximal and distal extremities should be evaluated for pain, touch, and temperature.

A dermatome is an area of skin innervated by a sensory nerve from a single nerve root. Dermatome charts (Fig. 10.2) are useful when a deficit is noted on examination. Dermatomes overlap, and levels can vary considerably.

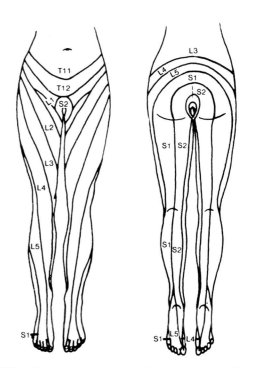

FIG. 10.2. An exemplary dermatome map for use with sensory testing.

Sacral Cord Integrity

Spinal cord segments S-2 to S-4 contain important neurons involved with micturition. In short, autonomic parasympathetic detrusor muscle fibers arise from the intermediolateral cell column of the spinal cord at levels S-2 and S-3, with minor contributions from S-1. The principal action of these fibers, traveling as the pelvic nerve, is contraction of the detrusor muscle. Sympathetic motor neurons, traveling with the hypogastric nerve, regulate bladder storage. α-Adrenergic stimulation primarily affects the proximal urethra, causing constriction. β-Adrenergic stimulation has minor detrusor effect causing relaxation, whereas the predominant regulator of detrusor activity is the parasympathetic system as described previously.

In addition to the autonomic innervation, the periurethral striated muscle is also innervated by the pudendal nerve, originating in the S-2 to S-4 segments. Stimulation of this nerve causes contraction of the distal periurethral striated muscle.

The external voluntary anal sphincter is representative of the pelvic floor striated musculature. Anal sphincter testing involves a determination of resistance to the entry of the examining finger and the ability of the patient to contract the anal sphincter voluntarily. A full bladder or rectal ampulla may interfere with anal sphincter reflex activity but will not change muscle tone. The presence of a voluntary contraction of the anal sphincter suggests integrity of the pelvic floor innervation, both segmental and suprasacral. Preservation of tone in the absence of a voluntary contraction indicates a suprasacral lesion; diminished tone implies a sacral or peripheral nerve abnormality.

Reflexes, including the anal sphincter, clitoral-anal reflex, and cough reflexes, can produce contraction of the pelvic floor. Stroking the skin lateral to the anus elicits the anal reflex. Contraction of the anus should be observed. When the contraction is not visible, often a contraction can be palpated with an examining finger (Fig. 10.3). The clitoral-anal reflex involves contraction of the bulbocavernosus, ischiocavernosus, and anal sphincter in response to tapping or squeezing of the clitoris (Fig. 10.3). Pulling on a suprapubic or intraurethral Foley catheter or touching the urethral or vesical mucosa also stimulates this reflex. Because the external anal sphincter and pelvic floor muscles have similar neurologic innervation, the anal sphincter usually responds concomi-

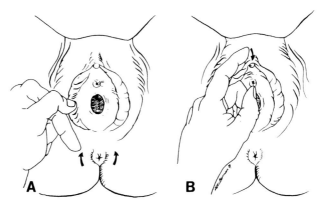

FIG. 10.3. Tests of sacral cord integrity. **A:** The anal reflex. The skin lateral to the anus is stroked. Contraction of the anus is observed or palpated with an examining finger. **B:** The clitoral-anal reflex. Contraction of the bulbocavernosus and ischiocavernosus muscles is observed in response to tapping or squeezing the clitoris.

tantly in the reflex tests described. Integrity of these reflexes indicates functional normality of the fifth lumbar to the fifth sacral segments.

The cough reflex involves the same spinal cord efferents and also the volitional innervation of the abdominal muscles (T-6 to L-1). Both coughing and deep inspiration cause a contraction of the periurethral striated sphincter (Fig. 10.4). Unfortunately, these reflexes can be difficult to evaluate clinically because of the rapidity of response. The ability to detect the responses of all three reflexes can be improved by placing a pressure-sensitive catheter in either the urethra or the anal sphincter and recording pressure changes. In about 10% of normal adults, the reflex response may not be strong enough to be appreciated on physical examination (9). In these patients, electromyogram (EMG) and latency studies may be helpful in distin-

guishing diminished responses from absence of reflex activity (10).

Cerebellum

The cerebellum has four major functions in the control of micturition: maintenance of the tone of the periurethral striated muscle and the pelvic floor, suppression of the detrusor reflex by modulation of the brain-stem detrusor centers, coordination of bladder contraction with urethral relaxation, and regulation of the strength of detrusor and periurethral muscle contractions. Truncal ataxia and the ataxic gait characteristic of midline cerebellar dysfunction are frequently observed in patients with multiple sclerosis. Additional cerebellar testing consists of evaluation of finger–nose and heel–shin coordination and examination of the patient's gait, including tandem gait.

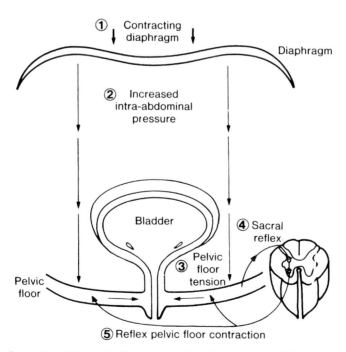

FIG. 10.4. Tests of sacral cord integrity. The cough reflex. Contraction of the diaphragm during cough generates increased abdominal pressure that places tension on the pelvic floor. Tension on the pelvic floor initiates a sacral reflex, resulting in contraction of the pelvic floor and periurethral striated muscles.

Cerebellar disease characteristically produces spontaneous high-amplitude detrusor reflex contractions as observed during cystometry. Poor hand coordination in these patients can impede the use of intermittent self-catheterization.

NEUROLOGIC DISORDERS AND CLINICAL SEQUELAE: CLINICAL CORRELATIONS

Diseases at or above the Brain Stem

Cerebrovascular Disease

Disorders affecting the cerebrum include dementia, atrophy, cerebral vascular accident, tumor, trauma, and hydrocephalus. Neurologic examination may reveal abnormal mental status, speech impairment, and asymmetry in strength and reflexes. At the time of the acute episode, urinary retention may occur. After a variable recovery period, the most common expression of lower urinary tract dysfunction is detrusor hyperreflexia because there is release of the detrusor reflex response from voluntary control. Sensation is variable but usually intact; thus, the patient complains of urgency. When sensation is intact and the cerebral insult has not affected the patient's awareness of the problem, voluntary contraction of the urethral sphincter mechanism may maintain continence. This compensation makes the difference between urgency and urgency with incontinence. Smooth and striated muscle activity is usually synergic. Urodynamic findings suggesting detrusor–sphincter dyssynergia may truly represent appropriate sphincter activity in a patient who is attempting not to soil herself, a syndrome named pseudodyssynergia (11,12).

A stroke or cerebrovascular accident is a common, often devastating occurrence. Because the site of brain injury can vary, the consequences on urinary function can vary. By far, the most common urologic sequela of a stroke or cerebrovascular accident is detrusor hyperreflexia. Although some patients regain normal urinary function, permanent bladder overactivity with clinical incontinence is an unfortunate possibility.

Brain Tumor

Voiding dysfunction secondary to a solid mass is dependent on the localized region involved. The most frequent area that affects voiding function is the frontal lobe, with resultant detrusor hyperreflexia. Mass lesions in this area often result in decreased awareness of all voiding events; therefore, the patient has no thoughts concerning voluntary suppression of the reflex and may not care to wait for a socially acceptable time before soiling herself. This type of cognitive deficit is commonly elicited on the Mini Mental Status Examination. When the cerebral insult is in the midline affecting the paracentral gyrus, volitional control of urethral sphincteric relaxation is lost, resulting in urinary retention.

Parkinson's Disease

Parkinson's disease is characterized by a relative dopamine deficiency with a predominance of cholinergic activity in the corpus striatum. Neurologic findings include bradykinesia, tremor, and skeletal rigidity. Voiding dysfunction occurs in 25% to 75% of patients and is usually characterized by urgency, frequency, nocturia, and urge incontinence (12). Urodynamically, detrusor hyperreflexia is the most common finding. In one study of 70 patients with urinary symptoms and Parkinson's disease, 47 (67%) had detrusor hyperreflexia, 11 (16%) had hyporeflexia or areflexia, 6 (9%) had hyperreflexia with impaired contractile function, 2 had detrusor–sphincter dyssynergia, and 4 had normal function (13). The only urodynamic parameter that correlated with disease severity was postvoid residual urine volume. Smooth and striated muscle activity is synergic, but it is less clear whether these patients retain striated sphincter control (14).

Shy-Drager Syndrome

Shy-Drager syndrome is a rare degenerative disorder affecting the cerebellum, brain stem, peripheral autonomic ganglia, and thoracolumbar preganglionic sympathetic neurons (14). Patients present parkinsonian symptoms, orthostatic hypotension, and anhydrosis. Voiding dysfunction varies but most often includes detrusor hyperreflexia and an open bladder neck at rest with denervation of the striated sphincter.

Cranial Nerve Abnormalities

Cranial nerve deficits in combination with urinary dysfunction suggest a brainstem lesion or a generalized neurologic disorder. A history of optic neuritis, the detection of pallor of the optic discs, or the presence of nystagmus may suggest the diagnosis of multiple sclerosis. Although the brain stem may not be directly responsible for the urinary symptoms, the finding of cranial nerve dysfunction promotes the search for similar plaques elsewhere in the nervous system. Because the lesions of multiple sclerosis may be in the upper spinal cord, lower spinal cord, or both locations, urinary derangements may include detrusor instability, detrusor areflexia, or a combination of detrusor overactivity with incomplete emptying.

Diseases Affecting the Spinal Cord

Spinal cord injury may be the result of trauma, vascular disease, arteriovenous malformation, myelopathy, arachnoiditis, or myelitis. The spinal level of the insult dictates the motor and urologic sequelae of spinal cord injury. It is important to recognize that the vertebral level does not correspond to the neural cord level. The sacral spinal cord begins about the level of T-12 to L-1. The spinal cord terminates in the cauda equina at about the level of the second lumbar vertebra.

Suprasacral Injury

Bladder contractility and reflex bladder contractions require an intact conus medullaris (sacral spinal cord segments) and its afferent and efferent connections. Complete lesions above this level but below the level of sympathetic outflow usually result in detrusor hyperreflexia, absent sensation below the level of the lesion, smooth sphincter synergia, and striated sphincter dyssynergia (12). If the insult is above the spinal column level of T-6 (spinal cord level T-7 to T-8), there may also be dyssynergia of the smooth muscle sphincter.

General neurologic and urologic findings vary depending on the amount of time that has passed before the physical evaluation. Immediately after a major spinal injury, spinal shock occurs. There is a global decrease in nerve excitability below the level of the lesion. There are decreased or absent somatic reflexes and flaccid muscle paralysis below the level of the injury (15,16). The exception to this rule is that the peripheral somatic reflexes (anal and bulbocavernosus reflexes) may never disappear. If they do, they may return in hours or minutes (16). Autonomic activity is depressed, resulting in an acontractile and areflexic bladder. The smooth component of the sphincter usually is intact, and EMG recordings can usually be obtained from the striated sphincter (17). Continence is usually preserved secondary to the sphincter tone, and urinary retention is the usual clinical problem requiring intermittent or continuous catheterization.

After an injury, if the distal spinal cord is intact but isolated from the upper cord, detrusor contractility will eventually return, causing involuntary voiding, usually with incomplete emptying secondary to weak involuntary detrusor contractions. Bladder reflex activity should parallel return of lower extremity reflex activity. In these patients, preserving low-pressure bladder storage is a priority. After a period of spinal shock, the longstanding dysfunction that follows a complete lesion above the sacral spinal cord includes detrusor hyper-reflexia, smooth sphincter synergia (unless the lesion is above T-6), and striated sphincter dyssynergia (12). Neurologic examination demonstrates skeletal muscle spasticity below the level of the insult, hyperreflexic deep tendon reflexes, extensor plantar (Babinski) reflexes, and decreased sensation. Bladder emptying is usually incomplete as a result of striated sphincter dyssynergia.

For some upper spinal lesions, reflex activity of the spinal cord does not follow the areflexic stage, and the bladder remains hypotonic. In these patients, referral for electrophysiologic testing is indicated. Abnormalities in evoked potential from the perineal region may be demonstrated.

The pontine-mesencephalic formation is responsible for coordinating bladder and striated sphincter activity. Any lesion between this center and the sacral spinal cord may interfere with this coordination, resulting in true detrusor–sphincter dyssynergia. Although management of the incontinence is often of great concern to the patient, clinical priority lies with protecting the upper urinary tracts from the sequelae of high intravesical pressure. Cystometry is essential to determine the bladder pressure before detrusor contractions occur and the bladder capacity at a safe intravesical pressure and to detect the pressure at which leakage occurs. To avoid upper tract injury, bladder pressures at vesical volumes obtained during the intermittent catheterization schedule must be less than 40 cm H_2O. Alternatively, the pressure at which the bladder involuntarily empties must be below 40 cm H_2O.

Lesions above T-6

Many of the findings with lesions above T-6 are the same as those below T-6 but above the sacral cord. As mentioned previously, there may be smooth muscle sphincter dyssynergia in addition to the dysfunctions described earlier for lower lesions. Autonomic dysreflexia is a syndrome of exaggerated sympathetic activity below the level of the spinal lesion (15,16,18). It occurs most often in patients with cervical spine injuries but can occur with any lesion above T-6. The syndrome includes hypertension, headache, profuse sweating, and reflex bradycardia. The stimulus for this response usually comes from the rectum or bladder. Hemodynamic effects of the syndrome can be managed acutely with parenteral ganglionic α-adrenergic blockade or parenteral chlorpromazine (Thorazine). Stimuli that initiate this reflex must be identified on an individual case basis. Catheter management protocols often must be altered to decrease bladder overactivity that is often the stimulus for acute exacerbations. Alternatively, surgical measures may be required to decrease outlet resistance so that leakage occurs at lower bladder volumes and pressures.

Lesions of the Sacral Spinal Cord

After sacral spinal injury and spinal shock, there is depression of the deep tendon reflexes, varying degrees of flaccid paralysis, and absent sensation below the level of the lesion. This is in contrast to upper spinal lesions in which hyperreflexia and muscle spasticity are the rule. Detrusor areflexia is the most common urologic result. The smooth sphincter is competent but fails to relax. The striated sphincter retains some tone (diminished EMG activity) but is usually no longer under voluntary control. The classic urologic findings include a reasonable bladder capacity with high compliance. However, depending on the obstructive abilities of the nonrelaxing sphincter, decreased compliance is also a possible clinical outcome. When bladder pressure becomes greater than urethral pressure, leakage occurs. If this leak point is high enough, the upper tracts are affected.

Multiple Sclerosis

Multiple sclerosis is one of the most common neurologic causes of voiding dysfunction (19). The pathophysiology involves impaired nerve conduction secondary to focal neural demyelination. Neurologic abnormalities are subject to exacerbation and remission over time. Symptoms are dependent on the extent and locations of the demyelinating plaques. Cranial nerve findings are common, but all levels of the spinal cord are vulnerable.

Voiding abnormalities are common because the process commonly involves the posterior and lateral columns of the spinal cord, which are of import for bladder and outlet function. Fifty to 80% of patients with this disease have voiding complaints, and in 10%, a voiding complaint is part of the initial symptom complex. Patients may present with acute urinary retention, but detrusor hyperreflexia is the most common abnormality. In addition, 30% to 65% of patients with detrusor hyperreflexia secondary to multiple sclerosis also have striated sphincter dyssynergia (18–20). Bladder areflexia may occur but is less common. Voiding function in the presence of detrusor–sphincter dyssynergia is variable, and physician priority lies with protecting the upper tracts from the potential consequences of elevated bladder pressures. Patients are often treated with high-dose anticholinergics with or without a requirement for self-catheterization.

Diseases of the Peripheral Nervous System

Diabetes Mellitus

Diabetes is the most common cause of peripheral and autonomic neuropathies. The pathophysiology involves segmental demyelination and impaired nerve conduction secondary to metabolic abnormalities of the Schwann cell (19,20). Physical examination may reveal decreased sensation in the lower extremities secondary to vascular and nerve compromise. Urinary symptoms are insidious in onset as bladder sensation gradually diminishes. Typically, with impaired sensation, voiding intervals increase and may progress to only once or twice daily with no real sensation or urgency. Stretch of the detrusor muscle and neural impairment eventually result in decreased contractility. Recruitment of abdominal muscles or use of mechanical ma-

neuvers is common to initiate and maintain a weak stream of urine. Urodynamic testing demonstrates decreased sensation to bladder filling, large bladder capacity, poor contractility, prolonged voiding time with low peak flows, and high residual volumes. Early diagnosis and institution of timed voiding with periodic evaluation of residual volumes is the best treatment. Tabes dorsalis and pernicious anemia may result in similar sensory neurogenic voiding abnormalities (15).

Herpes

Invasion of the sacral spinal ganglia with the herpesvirus results in typical vesicular skin eruptions, reflecting the affected dermatomes. There are urologic sequelae related to herpes zoster. One review noted that 26% of patients with herpes zoster had urologic complaints, including retention, incontinence, dysuria, and frequency (21). Another article reported symptoms of retention in seven patients with both herpes zoster and herpes simplex viruses. Six patients had skin eruptions on the saddle area (S-2 to S-4 dermatome), and one had a skin lesion at the L-4 to L-5 dermatome. All seven patients had detrusor areflexia without bladder sensation. Clean intermittent self-catheterization was used, with recovery in 4 to 6 weeks (22).

Spinal Disk Disease

Patients with spinal disc disease usually present with low back pain radiating down the back of the thigh (15). When spinal root compression in the L4-5 or L5-S1 disk interspace causes voiding dysfunction, the most common urodynamic finding is detrusor hyperreflexia. The striated sphincter may be normal or show signs of decreased function. The status of the striated sphincter will dictate whether the patient experiences incontinence secondary to involuntary detrusor contractions or retention or straining secondary to the failure of relaxation of the striated sphincter. Laminectomy may not restore bladder function. It is thus important to identify the problem preoperatively to separate disk protrusion from the surgical intervention as the causative agent.

Radical Pelvic Surgery

Voiding dysfunction after surgery is most common after abdominoperineal resection and radical hysterectomy (12). The frequency varies, with reports of up to 60% of patients having voiding difficulties and 15% to 20% experiencing permanent dysfunction (18). Neurologic examination in these patients may be normal. Urinary retention with varying degrees of sensory awareness is usually the first abnormal urologic finding. In the long term, there is absent or diminished bladder contractility with distal obstruction secondary to preserved striated sphincter tone that is no longer under voluntary control. Decreased compliance is common. Depending on the degree of distal obstruction, the patient may manifest both storage and emptying dysfunction. Urodynamic studies are essential in such complex patients. Risks to the upper urinary tracts depend on the filling leak point. Therapy is directed to establish low-pressure storage and periodic emptying.

NEUROLOGIC CONSULTATION AND ELECTROPHYSIOLOGIC TESTING

In certain patients, urinary bladder dysfunction could be the initial manifestation of an underlying neurologic disease. On the other hand, many patients with multiple urinary symptoms have no symptoms or signs suggestive of overt neurologic disease. In these patients, detailed electrophysiologic and urodynamic testing of the lower urinary tract may suggest neuropathy as the underlying cause of the symptoms. In patients with known neurologic disease and associated bladder symptoms, the urodynamic and related testing assists to define the nature, location, and extent of end-organ involvement. The questions of when and to whom to refer are often difficult. Any patient with a neurologic deficit and voiding complaints should

undergo multichannel urodynamics, including uroflowmetry, cystometry, and pressure-voiding studies. Patients with established neurologic diagnoses whose urinary complaints, physical examination, and urodynamics are in agreement regarding the mechanism of the voiding disorder do not require advanced electrophysiologic testing. However, if a treatment plan fails or when history, physical examination, and urodynamics do not lead to a clear etiology of the voiding dysfunction, electrophysiologic testing is indicated by a qualified specialist. This may be a neurologist, urologist, or urogynecologist, depending on specialized training. In addition, patients presenting with incontinence or pelvic organ prolapse despite having no risk factors may also be good candidates for electrophysiologic testing. In this scenario, evoked responses may localize an atypical explanation for the voiding dysfunction such as a paraspinal mass. In this case, imaging studies can be selected more specifically, and perhaps inappropriate surgical intervention may be avoided for the elective problem of incontinence.

Similar reasoning applies to patients with intrinsic sphincter deficiency. In the absence of established risk factors [age more than 50 years, previous incontinence surgery, radiation, known neurologic impairment (23)], patients with urodynamic evidence of intrinsic sphincter deficiency may also benefit from electrophysiologic testing. The association of intrinsic sphincter deficiency with myelomeningocele is well established (24,25), and thus in the absence of historical or examination evidence to explain the sphincteric incompetence, electrophysiologic testing to investigate spinal cord integrity is indicated. The specific tests available and their applications are discussed in Chapter 13.

There should be a low threshold for referral to a neurologist. Although the mechanism of correcting a voiding dysfunction may be clear after history, physical examination, and urodynamics, the presence of any underlying neurologic disorder necessitates ongoing care by a neurologist. Any patient with a new neurologic finding or a change in character of existing deficits requires neurologic consultation.

CONCLUSIONS

A variety of diseases cause urethral and bladder disturbances with associated neurologic signs and symptoms. Although the urologic neuroanatomy is complex, some patterns of neurologic deficits and their urologic manifestations are well established. Familiarity with these patterns, combined with appropriate neurologic history and physical examination, is essential for evaluation of women with lower urinary complaints. Gynecologists and urologists need to be familiar with the clinical correlations between general neurologic findings and urologic dysfunction to treat and triage patients with lower urinary tract complaints.

REFERENCES

1. Kiff ES, Swash M. Slowed conduction in the pudendal nerves in idiopathic (neurogenic) fecal incontinence. *Br J Surg* 1984;71:614–616.
2. Bradley WE, Timm GW, Rockswold GL, et al. Detrusor and urethral electromyelography. *J Urol* 1975;114: 69–71.
3. Swash M, Henrey MM, Snooks SJ. Unifying concept of pelvic floor disorders and incontinence. *J R Soc Med* 1985;78:906–911.
4. Benson JT, ed. *Female pelvic floor disorders: investigation and management.* New York: Norton Medical Books, 1992:142–166.
5. Benson JT. Neurophysiologic control of lower urinary tract. *Obstet Gynecol Clin North Am* 1989;16:733–740.
6. Benson JT, McClellen E. The effect of vaginal dissection on the pudendal nerve. *Obstet Gynecol* 1993;82: 387–389.
7. Folstein MF, Robins LM, Helzer JE. The mini mental state examination. *Arch Gem Psychiatr* 1983;40:812–816.
8. DeJong RN. *The neurologic examination.* Hagerstown: Harper & Rowe, 1995:439–440.
9. Bruskewitz R. Female incontinence: signs and symptoms. In: Raz S, ed. *Female urology.* Philadelphia: WB Saunders, 1983:45–50.
10. Ortiz OC, Bertitti AC, Nunez JD. Female pelvic floor responses. *Int J Urogynecol* 1994;5:278–282.
11. Wein AJ, Barrett DM. Etiologic possibilities for increased pelvic floor electromyography activity during bladder filling. *J Urol* 1982;127:949–952.
12. Barrett DM, Wein AJ. Voiding dysfunction: diagnosis, classification, and management. In: Gillenwater JY, Grayhack JT, Howards SS, et al., eds. *Adult and pediatric urology,* 2nd ed. St. Louis: Mosby Year Book, 1991:1001–1099.
13. Ariki I, Kitahara M, Oida T, et al. Voiding dysfunction and Parkinson's disease: urodynamic abnormalities and urinary symptoms. *J Urol* 2000;164:1640–1643.
14. Blaivas JG. Non traumatic neurogenic voiding dysfunction in the adult. I. Physiology and approach to therapy. *AUA Update Series* 1985;4, lesson 11.
15. Hald T, Bradley WE. *The urinary bladder-neurology and dynamics.* Baltimore: Williams and Wilkins, 1982: 160–165.
16. Thomas DG. Spinal cord injury. In: Mundy AR, Stephenson TP, Wein AJ, eds. *Urodynamics: principles, practice, and application.* Edinburgh, Great Britain: Churchill Livingstone, 1984:260–272.
17. Awad S, Bryniak SR, Downie JN, et al. Urethral pressure profile during spinal shock stage in man: a preliminary report. *J Urol* 1777;117:91–94.
18. McGuire EJ. Clinical evaluation and treatment of neurogenic vesical dysfunction. In: Libertino J, ed. *International perspectives in urology.* Baltimore: Williams & Wilkins, 1984:303–312.
19. Blaivas JG. Non traumatic neurogenic voiding dysfunction in the adult. II. Multiple sclerosis and diabetes mellitus. *AUA Update Series* 1985;4, lesson 12.
20. Mundy AR, Blaivas JG. Non-traumatic neurologic disorders. In: Mundy AR, Stephenson TP, Wein AJ, eds. *Urodynamics: principles, practice and application.* New York: Churchill Livingstone, 1984:278–287.
21. Broseta E, Osca JM, Morera J, et al. Urologic manifestations of herpes zoster. *Eur Urol* 1993;24(2):244–247.
22. Yamanishi T, Yasuda K, Sakakibara R, et al. Urinary retention due to herpes virus infections. *Neurourol Urodyn* 1998;17:613–619.
23. Horbach NS, Ostergard DR. Predicting intrinsic sphincter deficiency in women with stress incontinence. *Obstet Gynecol* 1994;84:188–192.
24. McGuire EJ, Woodside JR, Borden TA, et al. Prognostic value of urodynamic testing in myelodysplastic children. *J Urol* 1980;126:205–208.
25. Wan J, McGuire EJ, Bloom DA, et al. Stress leak point pressure: a diagnostic tool for incontinent children. *J Urol* 1993;150:700–702.

Ostergard's Urogynecology and Pelvic Floor Dysfunction, Fifth Edition. edited by A.E. Bent, et al. Lippincott Williams & Wilkins, Philadelphia © 2003.

11

Urodynamic Testing

James Paul Theofrastous* and Steven E. Swift**

*Department of Obstetrics and Gynecology, University of North Carolina Chapel Hill School of Medicine, Chapel Hill, North Carolina; and Department of Urogynecology and Reconstructive Pelvic Surgery, Mountain Area Health Education Center, Regional OB.GYN Specialists, Asheville, North Carolina
**Department of Obstetrics and Gynecology, Medical University of South Carolina, Division of Benign Gynecology, Charleston, South Carolina

"The bladder is an unreliable witness."
Richard Turner-Warwick

INDICATIONS FOR URODYNAMIC STUDIES

The goal of urodynamic testing is to illuminate the most appropriate therapy to improve the quality of life of a woman who is suffering from urinary dysfunction. Urodynamic testing provides practical clinical information and may be used to delineate the pathophysiology of urinary dysfunction and the mechanism of action of continence surgery. Like any diagnostic test, clinical urodynamic testing should only be performed if the results will alter management. If a woman's incontinence does not improve with a trial of empiric therapy, it is reasonable to proceed with urodynamic testing to determine a specific diagnosis and treatment options. A vast array of urodynamic tests exists, but most can be categorized as evaluating either bladder storage, urethral resistance, or voiding function. The choice of test technique depends on the clinical situation, available resources, and clinician's training. A healthy young parous female with urethral hypermobility and pure stress incontinence symptoms that have not responded to pelvic floor muscle exercises is very unlikely to have detrusor instability or voiding dysfunction, and simple office urodynamic testing (see Chapter 7) is appropriate for her preoperative evaluation. For populations of women in whom the prevalence of abnormal detrusor function is higher, multichannel testing may be more accurate and cost-effective (1).

Unfortunately, the symptoms of urinary dysfunction are often nonspecific. There is a wide overlap of clinical symptoms and findings in women with genuine stress incontinence and detrusor instability. In a study of 90 women with urinary incontinence who underwent urodynamic evaluation, 71% of those diagnosed with detrusor instability complained of stress incontinence with coughing or sneezing, and 24% of women who were diagnosed with genuine stress incontinence had the symptom of urge incontinence (2). Other studies have reported that the symptom of pure stress incontinence is only 78% sensitive and 84% specific for the diagnosis of genuine stress incontinence (3), and even incorporating a thorough symptom-specific questionnaire and pelvic examination yields a correct diagnosis in only 81% of women (4). These studies demonstrate that clinical symptoms and basic findings on pelvic examination are not accurate enough to rely on for determining invasive and expensive therapy.

Women seen in most general practices are usually less complicated than those who are seen by specialists in referral services (5) and may not require complex testing. The U.S. Agency for Health Care Policy and Research (AHCPR) published guidelines in 1992 (6) that were updated in 1996 (7) for determining the appropriate level of preoperative evaluation for patients with urinary incontinence. These recommendations were developed by a multidisciplinary review of published data by clinicians, researchers, and biostatisticians. Although referral-based practices may have a minority of patients who meet these criteria (8), many women who present to a general practitioner are likely to fall within these parameters. A clinical decision tree for selecting women who may benefit from more complex urodynamic testing based on the AHCPR guidelines is presented in Fig. 11.1.

Some authors have questioned the need for urodynamic testing before continence surgery with the pragmatic criticism that it would not alter their decision to perform urethropexy. These urodynamic critics argue that surgery may improve or cure detrusor instability so that the documentation of a specific diagnosis is moot. A study of women after pubovaginal sling urethropexy suggested that 67% of preoperative detrusor instability resolved and that only severe detrusor instability increased the chance of failure, and the authors com-

mented that the urodynamic testing itself does not resolve detrusor instability (9). Many more studies have noted that the presence of detrusor instability is a significant risk factor for failure after continence surgery (10–13). One study of 86 women who underwent Burch urethropexy noted a markedly decreased success rate of only 30% in women with mixed incontinence (14). In addition to confirming the presence of genuine stress incontinence, which would justify surgery, the decision to identify preoperative detrusor instability through urodynamic testing seems reasonable if for no other reason than to enable realistic counseling of a woman before subjecting her to invasive surgery.

COMPLEX CYSTOMETRY

Cystometry is the evaluation of bladder filling and is usually performed to determine whether abnormal detrusor activity is present during filling. Complex cystometry refers to the use of devices to measure pressures within the bladder and intraabdominal cavity during filling. Galen conceived of the bladder as a reservoir for urine that was evacuated by abdominal wall contraction overcoming urethral resistance (15). This passive role of the bladder dominated medicine for nearly two millennia. In the mid-19th century, physiologists began to investigate bladder function in human cadavers and live animals and postulated a connection between bladder and neurologic function (16,17). The first *in vivo* measurement of vesical pressure was made in desperation after being foiled by rectal peristalsis during an attempt to measure abdominal pressure (18). In 1882, Mosso and Pellacani discovered the role of detrusor activity in normal voiding (19). Retrograde filling of the bladder with concomitant recording of intravesical pressure was performed in 1884, but the significance of periodic increases in detrusor pressure was not appreciated (20). The concept of unsuppressible bladder contractions leading to incontinence was recognized

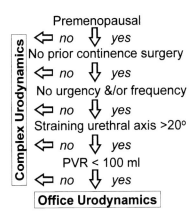

FIG. 11.1. Triage for the performance of complex urodynamics in women complaining of incontinence.

through studying urge incontinence and frequency in German soldiers stationed in trenches during the First World War (21).

Given the slow rate of antegrade bladder filling through diuresis, a cystometrogram is usually performed by filling the bladder retrograde through a urethral catheter that simultaneously records pressure within the bladder. Although a purist in physics may debate the use of the term pressure rather than force as measured by a catheter with a single recording transducer in a fluid filled cavity, pressure is used by consensus. Given that any increases in abdominal pressure will be transmitted to the bladder, a second vaginal or rectal catheter is often used in order to reflect any increases in abdominal pressure. True detrusor pressure is calculated by subtracting abdominal pressure from vesical pressure. The ability to monitor abdominal pressure reduces the chance of a false-positive test result of detrusor instability.

In 1988, an international group of clinicians and researchers outlined several recommendations regarding urodynamic-testing terminology in an attempt to facilitate the meaningfulness of test results from different clinicians (22). Much of the following terminology stems from that report. These details may affect the interpretation of test results and should be specified.

Terminology

Patient Position. Bladder filling may be performed with the patient semierect, standing, or sitting. A supine test may not reveal detrusor instability. No woman is relaxed and comfortable in lithotomy in an examination room surrounded by intimidating instrumentation and machinery. A semierect position in a fully adjustable mechanical chair may minimize discomfort while facilitating examination and providing a reasonable approximation of a woman's anatomy during her daily activities (Fig. 11.2). Most standard examination tables can be adjusted to provide a more upright position by raising the top of the table and using a pillow.

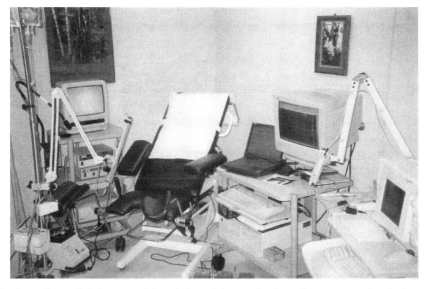

FIG. 11.2. A urodynamic laboratory. From left to right: urethral profilometry mechanical arm with infusion pump; urethrocystoscopy video cart; adjustable examination chair, multichannel urodynamic computer; electromyography computer.

Filling Medium. Various media for bladder filling include sterile fluids, such as water, saline, or radiologic contrast. Room- or body-temperature fluids should be used because cold fluid may precipitate detrusor activity in normal patients. Earlier studies used gas filling, such as carbon dioxide, which is still occasionally used, and air, which was abandoned because of instances of embolism. The use of fluid for filling has the advantage of allowing the performance of a stress test.

Filling Rate. The bladder is usually filled continuously but may also be filled incrementally or by diuresis with ambulatory monitoring. There is some evidence that high rates of filling may result in a false-negative cystometrogram results because of suppression of detrusor activity (23). The rate of filling is usually characterized using the following terms:

• *Slow* or *physiologic*—less than 10 mL/min
• *Medium*—10 to 100 mL/min
• *Fast* or *rapid*—more than 100 mL/min

Catheter Size and Type. A cystometry catheter has a port for filling and a channel for recording pressure. Most catheters are between 3 and 12 French (0.95 to 3.82 mm) in diameter. The transducers for recording pressure are either mounted externally or integrated into the end of the catheter with a recording membrane (microtip or fiberoptic transducers) or within a balloon containing fluid (Fig. 11.3). The choice of a catheter system depends on individual preference, patient volume, availability of skilled personnel to maintain reusable catheters, and resources. Reusable microtip catheters may be used repetitively for hundreds of studies without performance deterioration but generally cost $1,000 to $2,000. Disposable microtip, fiberoptic, or water transducer catheters are in the $40 to $80 range, and some manufacturers offer multiple-use disposable catheters. Catheters should be able to record pressure up 300 cm H_2O. The catheter is zeroed to atmospheric pressure before placing it in the bladder. External transducers are placed level with the symphysis pubis before calibration to atmospheric pressure.

An important part of cystometry is to assess the patient's level of urgency and comfort during filling. Although the subjective nature of bladder sensation limits reproducibility (24), it is useful to identify patients with excessive or absent sensation during filling. Marked urgency at low volumes (less than

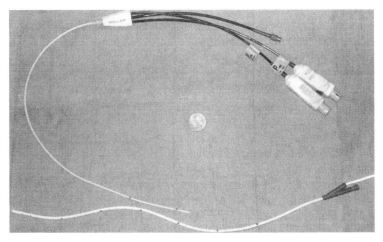

FIG. 11.3. Urodynamic catheters. *Top:* Two-channel microtip catheter with vesical and urethral pressure transducers; *bottom:* disposable single-channel fiberoptic catheter.

150 mL) may be seen with severe detrusor instability or interstitial cystitis, and a woman with neurogenic bladder may have no sensation of fullness at any volume. The following descriptive terms are commonly reported during cystometry:

First sensation: when a sense of fullness first appears. This is highly subjective, is frequently related to the presence of urethral catheters, and is most often noted when the patient is first asked to report it.

First desire to void: when the patient would usually pass urine at the next convenient opportunity but could delay voiding if necessary (commonly between 100 and 300 mL).

Strong desire to void: the persistent desire to void without the fear of imminent leakage. (commonly between 300 and 500 mL).

Urgency: the persistent desire to void with the fear of imminent leakage.

Pain: this is abnormal during filling, and the nature and location of the pain should be noted.

Maximum cystometric capacity (MCC): the volume at which the patient feels she can no longer delay voiding (commonly between 300 and 500 mL). In the absence of a strong sensation to void, the MCC is the volume at which the clinician discontinues filling. Overdistending the bladder may result in a false-positive stress test result.

Units of measure: pressure measurements are reported in centimeters of water (cm H_2O).

Detrusor instability: involuntary detrusor contractions of any magnitude during filling while the patient is attempting to inhibit voiding. Detrusor contractions are most often spontaneous but may be provoked by such triggers as coughing, changing posture, or heel bouncing. Detrusor instability may be phasic with discrete contractions, or progressive with a steady increase in detrusor pressure throughout filling. In the past, specific thresholds for significant contractions have been proposed (5 to 15 mm Hg), but current recommendations consider any amplitude contraction as significant.

Detrusor hyperreflexia: detrusor overactivity due to neurologic pathology, such as spinal cord lesions or cerebrovascular accident.

Vesical compliance: the increase in detrusor pressure during filling. Compliance is calculated by dividing the bladder volume by the increase in detrusor pressure and is expressed in milliliters per centimeter of water (mL/cm H_2O). Although early urodynamic literature generally noted biphasic or triphasic increases in vesical pressure in normal subjects (25,26), this is rarely seen in neurologically intact women and may reflect artifact due to the use of boric acid or carbon dioxide in most early investigations. In most neurologically intact women, the detrusor pressure increases less than 5 cm H_2O during filling to capacity. In a recent study of 270 women referred for evaluation of incontinence, 48% had no change in detrusor pressure with filling to capacity, and 75% had a compliance of greater than 130 mL/cm H_2O (27). This study also reported that women who had compliance of less than 40 mL/cm H_2O were 16 times more likely to have detrusor instability and suggested that patients with urge incontinence whose symptoms are not reproduced in the laboratory may have reduced compliance secondary to a variant of detrusor instability. Women with extremely reduced vesical compliance may be at increased risk for renal damage due to vesicoureteral reflux following outlet obstruction such as an aggressive urethropexy.

Choice of Test Technique

For women with a low prevalence of abnormal detrusor function, office urodynamics are usually adequate to make a diagnosis of genuine stress incontinence. The term simple urodynamics is somewhat of an oxymoron but is appropriate when taken in the context of the more complicated technology that exists. In appropriately selected patients, simple, or "eyeball," cystometry (see Chapter 7) can exclude the diagnosis of detrusor instability and confirm the diagnosis of genuine stress incontinence with a reasonable degree of accuracy (28,29). In populations in whom the index of suspicion for detrusor instability is higher, more sensitive testing is indicated. In contrast to simple urodynamic testing, complex testing involves the use of one or more catheters that have the ability to record pressure changes. Complex testing may also attempt to quantitate the amount of pressure required to cause leakage in women with genuine stress incontinence. The frequency response of a transducer used for cystometry should be at least 4 Hz in order to be able to record alterations in detrusor pressure accurately (30).

Single-channel Cystometry

In settings of limited clinical resources, single-channel cystometry may be more readily available than more complicated multichannel devices. In single-channel cystometry, a single catheter is used to fill the bladder and to record intravesical pressure. Single-channel devices include urodynamic monitors with urethral catheters and fetal monitors with intrauterine pressure catheters. A single-channel urodynamic tracing of a woman with genuine stress incontinence is shown in Fig. 11.4. The disadvantage of using a single channel to monitor vesical pressure is the inability to differentiate between increases in abdominal and bladder pressure, but an experienced observer may be able to differentiate between the two. Although some authors have noted a reduced sensitivity in populations with a high prevalence of detrusor instability (31,32), two randomized crossover studies have demonstrated high sensitivity and specificity for single-channel compared with multichannel cystometry (33,34).

Multichannel Cystometry

In multichannel cystometry, a second catheter records abdominal pressure during bladder filling and provocative testing, and a

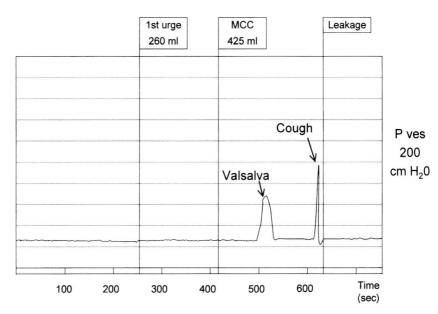

FIG. 11.4. Single-channel cystometrogram of a 42-year-old multiparous woman with symptoms of stress incontinence and urethral hypermobility. She notes the first sensation to void at 260 mL, and the infusion is stopped when she reports fullness at 425 mL (maximum cystometric capacity). Her detrusor remains stable with no increase in pressure during filling. She has no leakage with Valsalva maneuver but demonstrates genuine stress incontinence with coughing.

third pressure recording channel may be used in the transurethral catheter to record the urethral sphincter responses. With increasing consumer and practitioner awareness of the impact of urinary incontinence and treatment options, many commercial multichannel urodynamic systems have been developed and are increasingly available and less expensive. Systems range from mobile two-channel systems that can be mounted on an intravenous pole to computer-integrated systems with six or more channels, urethral profilometry, electromyography, or fluoroscopy. By recording simultaneous pressures within the bladder and abdomen, increases in detrusor pressure can be discriminated from increases in abdominal pressure. Intraabdominal pressure is recorded indirectly by placement of a catheter within the vagina or rectum. Vaginal, rectal, and intravesical pressures have been shown to have a high correlation during abdominal straining (35,36). Placement of the abdominal pressure catheter within the vagina rather than the rectum is more comfortable and avoids the problem of peristalsis. It may be difficult to keep a catheter in place within the vagina in women with severe vaginal vault prolapse, and intrarectal placement may be necessary. In subtracted cystometry, the system automatically subtracts abdominal pressure (P_{abd}) from intravesical pressure (P_{ves}) to yield a recording of detrusor pressure (P_{det}) as a separate channel. A multichannel cystometrogram of a woman with detrusor instability is depicted in Fig. 11.5. Figure 11.6 demonstrates the cystometrogram of a woman with detrusor instability who demonstrates leakage with coughing secondary to detrusor instability. This arrangement of catheters is also often used to evaluate voiding function. Although some

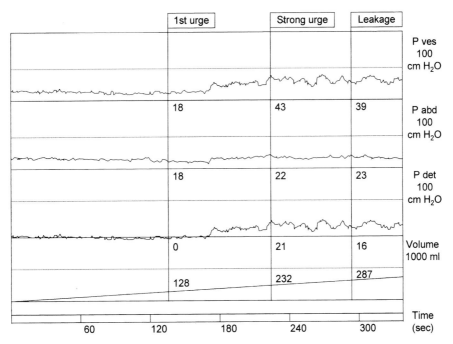

FIG. 11.5. Cystometrogram of a 58-year-old nulliparous woman with mixed symptoms of incontinence demonstrating phasic detrusor instability and normal bladder capacity. True detrusor pressure (P_{det}) is calculated by subtracting abdominal pressure (P_{abd}) from raw vesical or bladder pressure (P_{ves}). She subsequently demonstrated stress incontinence without detrusor activity and was diagnosed with mixed incontinence. The scale on the right lists the range and units for the measurements; the *dotted line* is at the halfway point.

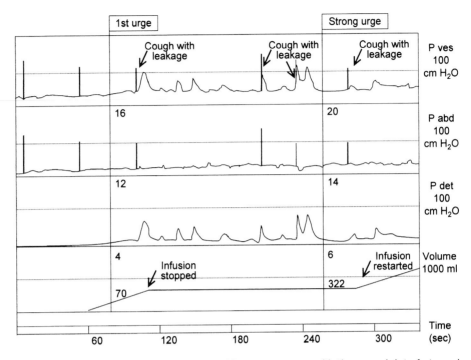

FIG. 11.6. Cystometrogram of a 70-year-old multiparous woman with the complaint of stress incontinence. She develops urgency at a volume of 70 mL and demonstrates leakage due to detrusor instability after several coughs as well as spontaneous detrusor contractions. She had no leakage without triggered detrusor spasms.

practitioners place needles within the striated urethral musculature routinely during filling cystometry, the yield in neurologically intact women is low and does not merit the added discomfort (37). In women in whom detrusor–sphincter dyssynergia is suspected, simultaneous electromyography of the urethral musculature may reveal inappropriate urethral activity during attempts at voiding and is indicative of central nervous system pathology, such as cerebrovascular accident (38), spinal cord injury (39), or multiple sclerosis (40) (Chapter 10).

Performance of Urodynamic Testing

Each clinician develops a testing protocol based on his or her opinion of the relative utility of various components of urodynamic testing in general and specific clinical situations. Urodynamic testing is inherently stressful for the patient because it includes intimidating equipment and an uncomfortable and embarrassing examination. It is important to guide a patient through testing in a compassionate and respectful manner, explaining each procedure. The number of times the urethra is instrumented should be minimized in order to reduce discomfort and the risk for infection. An efficient protocol for performing complex urodynamics is listed in Table 11.1. A busy clinician can usually accomplish a complete

TABLE 11.1. *Suggested efficient protocol for performing complex urodynamics*

1. Postvoid residual
2. Pelvic support evaluation
3. Cystometrogram
4. Urethral profilometry
5. Stress test
6. Provocative maneuvers
7. Urethrocystoscopy
8. Uroflowmetry

study in 20 to 30 minutes, whereas a research academician may add several ancillary test components and require significantly more time. After assessing pelvic support and urethral mobility, the bladder is filled while asking the patient to report urgency and the desire to void and observing detrusor and abdominal activity. It is vital to monitor the patient's symptoms closely and continuously during bladder filling. While abrupt changes in abdominal pressure are generally reflected by concomitant alterations in vesical pressure, small progressive variations in abdominal pressure may not be mirrored in vesical pressure. It is not uncommon for abdominal pressure to decrease gradually without an apparent decrease in vesical pressure during filling as the patient relaxes. Because the detrusor pressure is calculated by subtracting abdominal pressure from vesical pressure, a decrease in abdominal pressure may be displayed as an artificial increase in apparent detrusor pressure. Similarly, if abdominal pressure increases during filling without an increase in vesical pressure, the calculated detrusor channel will display artifact with a decreased or even negative pressure tracing.

Ambulatory Cystometry

Given the artificial atmosphere of the urodynamic laboratory, some authors have proposed that ambulatory urodynamic cystometry may provide a more natural and accurate method to evaluate daily bladder function. Ambulatory urodynamic testing involves placement of a small (3 or 4 French) single transducer catheter in the bladder, which the patient wears home and retains for several hours. A device records periodic alterations in bladder pressure over several hours. Proponents of ambulatory cystometry have noted that higher rates of bladder filling may suppress detrusor activity. In one study of 17 healthy continent volunteers (11 men, 6 women), investigators noted detrusor instability in no subjects at a filling rate of 100 mL/min but demonstrated uninhibited detrusor contractions in 17% of those who were

filled at a rate of 50 mL/min and in 38% of the subjects on ambulatory monitoring (23). A comparison of office and ambulatory cystometry noted that ambulatory monitoring provided a diagnosis of urge incontinence in 27 of 32 subjects who had normal office testing (41). Another study of 72 women with irritative symptoms and a negative cystometrogram with filling to capacity at 50 mL/min noted detrusor instability in all patients with a diuresis cystometrogram obtained by administering intramuscular furosemide and oral fluid bolus (42). Several other reports have noted extremely high rates of some degree of "abnormal" detrusor activity during ambulatory testing (43–45). At a practical level, these findings are not surprising given that some level of detrusor activity with bladder fullness is common and likely to be a normal signal for the individual to find a socially acceptable place to void. Major limitations of ambulatory monitoring include nonstandardized techniques and the fact that it is expensive and labor intensive (46). At a fundamental level, it is unclear where the demarcation between normal and abnormal detrusor activity during daily activities exists.

Reproducibility of Cystometry

Given the multiple variables involved in performing cystometry, it is not surprising that very few intraobserver or interobserver reproducibility studies have been performed. Furthermore, the natural history of detrusor instability relative to variations in symptoms and findings over time in a given subject is unknown. One study using cystometry in 30 women demonstrated resolution of detrusor overactivity in 10% and less severe contractions in 18% without therapy over 2 to 4 weeks (47). Another study of 42 patients with irritative symptoms (32 women and 10 men) questioned the validity of the International Continence Society recommendation to perform cystometry "while the patient is attempting to inhibit micturition." The authors noted that conscious inhibition of urgency during filling decreased the detection of involuntary detrusor contractions in 17% of patients compared with repeat testing without inhibition (48). This is most likely related to the ability to suppress detrusor activity when the urge to void arises (49). Some investigators have queried whether fluctuating hormone levels during the menstrual cycle may affect cystometry, but this does not appear to be so (50).

The ability of the urethra to maintain competence and prevent the leakage of urine during physical activity with increases in vesical pressure is termed urethral resistance. The role of urethral resistance in maintaining continence was recognized by the gynecologist Victor Bonney, who performed retrograde urethral profilometry in 1923 (51). Urethral resistance is multifactorial and represents a complex interaction between neuromuscular, connective tissue, vascular, and anatomic components. The striated musculature of the urethra is thickest in the middle of the urethra (52) and is thought to contribute one third of resting urethral tone, with the remaining two thirds evenly split between smooth muscle and vascular tone (53,54). The measurement of pressure within the urethra is referred to as urethral pressure profilometry. Urethral profilometry may be performed at rest or during

provocative maneuvers. Although early investigators used gas infusion, a comparative study of carbon dioxide and water noted a marked increase in discomfort and technical distortions with carbon dioxide (55). Most practitioners use sterile fluid for urethral profilometry. The frequency response of a transducer used to measure rapid increases in pressure such as coughing should be at least 15 Hz (30).

The following terms are related to urethral profilometry:

Passive urethral profilometry: measurements are obtained at rest.

Dynamic urethral profilometry: measurements are obtained during physical activity, such as coughing, straining, or pelvic floor muscle contraction.

Urethral closure pressure: the difference between urethral and vesical pressure.

Maximum urethral closure pressure (MUCP): the greatest increase in urethral closure pressure noted during catheter withdrawal (usually, 30 to 100 cm H_2O) (Fig. 11.7)

Functional urethral length (FUL): the distance over which urethral pressure exceeds bladder pressure during catheter withdrawal (usually, 2.5 to 3.5 cm).

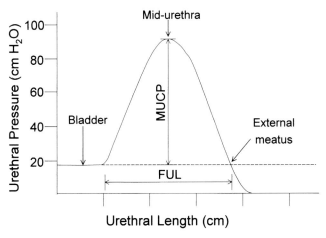

FIG. 11.7. Passive urethral pressure profile. As the catheter is withdrawn through the urethrovesical junction, urethral pressure rises to a maximum urethral closure pressure *(MUCP)* and then drops off and reaches zero as it exits the urethra. Functional urethral length *(FUL)* is defined as the length along which urethral pressure exceeds bladder pressure.

Passive Urethral Profilometry

The urethral pressure profile is obtained by withdrawing a catheter with the pressure transducer starting in the bladder until the transducer is beyond the external meatus. The urethral closure pressure is defined as the difference between urethral pressure and vesical pressure (Fig. 11.7). The closure pressure is initially zero with the transducer in the bladder, it then increases to a MUCP in the midurethra, and it then falls to negative values as the catheter exits the urethra. A single- or double-transducer catheter may be used. A catheter with two transducers has one transducer at the tip and a second transducer 5 to 6 cm from the tip so that the distal transducer will remain in the bladder until the proximal transducer exits the urethra. As the urethral catheter is withdrawn at a fixed rate (usually, 0.2 to 1 mm/s), the proximal transducer will record the increase in urethral pressure while the distal transducer records vesical pressure. The urethral closure pressure area may also be measured by calculating the area under the closure pressure curve, but this appears to add little information and can be tedious. With a mechanical arm to withdraw the urethral catheter at a fixed rate, the FUL may be measured. Most multichannel urodynamic systems display urethral closure pressure as a separate channel (P_{ucp}), and many software packages automatically calculate FUL and MUCP. Urethral profilometry is usually performed at several bladder volumes, including maximum bladder fillings. Given that pressure transducers record pressure from one direction and may be affected by urethral kinking, along with the finding that urethral closure pressure appears to have an asymmetric radial distribution (56), most clinicians orient the transducers laterally (03:00).

Both FUL and MUCP have been shown to decrease slightly with bladder filling and assuming an upright position (57). Although no longitudinal studies exist, both MUCP and FUL have been shown to diminish with age in a cross-sectional study (58). Premenopausal and postmenopausal women demonstrate small fluctuations in urethral closure pressure at a frequency of 0.0015 to 0.035 Hz owing to respiratory and vascular pulsations (59). It is important to note vesical pressure increases during profilometry in women with detrusor instability because any increase in vesical pressure will result in an artificial reduction in closure pressure as the urethral sphincter reflexively relaxes in response to the detrusor contraction.

Although measures of urethral resistance may be useful in understanding the pathophysiology and natural history of incontinence and therapeutic interventions, both FUL and urethral closure pressure have limited clinical utility in any given patient. Both FUL and urethral closure pressure have a wide overlap in symptomatic and asymptomatic women, and the correlation between profilometry values and clinical severity is poor (60). Although both measures appear to have reasonable intraobserver reproducibility, the multitude of techniques and equipment in use precludes any viable comparison of values from different clinicians. Few comparative studies exist, but two studies have noted up to 33% lower MUCPs with fiberoptic than with microtip transducer catheters (61,62).

Dynamic Urethral Profilometry: Pressure Transmission Ratio

Throughout the early to mid-20th century, many urologic and gynecologic surgeons recognized that successful surgical procedures for the treatment of genuine stress incontinence stabilized the urethrovesical junction during physical stress. Despite the explosive proliferation of continence procedures, investigation into the pathophysiology of incontinence and the efficacy of continence procedures was limited to radiographic studies that demonstrated gross anatomic alterations but provided scant physiologic information. With the development of small catheters with sensitive pressure transducers, it became possible to evaluate the relationship of vesical and urethral pressures at rest and during physical stress. The evaluation of alterations in urethral pressures during physical stress is referred to as dynamic profilometry. Dynamic profilometry may be performed during straining, coughing, or contraction of the pelvic floor musculature.

Continence during physical stress requires that urethral pressure exceeds vesical pressure. Bonney noted that urethral pressure increased during coughing and that this increase was blunted in incontinent women with anterior vaginal wall prolapse, but disparaged his methods as "too crude to dogmatize upon" (51). Few improvements in technology were made until the development of sensitive catheter transducers, and in 1961, Enhörning performed seminal research into the relative alterations in urethral and vesical pressures during physical stress and demonstrated that women with genuine stress incontinence had impaired transmission of increases in abdominal pressure to the urethra (63). This was confirmed by Beck and Maughan (1964) (64) and by Toews (1967) (65), who concluded, "if increased intra-abdominal pressure were transmitted equally to bladder and urethra, stress incontinence could never occur even in patients with very low maximal urethral pressure."

The use of a catheter with two pressure transducers allows the urodynamacist to record the changes in vesical and urethral pressures simultaneously during physical stress. In women with normal urethral support, abdominal pressure is transmitted to the urethra to maintain continence (Fig. 11.8). In women with incontinence due to loss of urethral support, transmission of abdominal pressure to the urethra is less efficient (Fig. 11.9). The ratio of the increases in urethral to vesical pressures is expressed as a percentage and is referred to as the pressure transmission ratio (PTR). Most modern urodynamic software can calculate the PTR automatically if the program is able to identify the onset and peak of a cough accurately. Many software programs do this poorly, and the clinician may need to input markers for coughs manually.

PTRs are usually recorded in each quadrant or third of the urethra, and a mean PTR may be calculated. Hilton and Stanton characterized the deficiency in urethral pressure transmission during physical stress as an all-or-none phenomenon. They noted that continent women generally have higher PTRs in the proximal three fourths of the urethra (usually greater than 95%) compared with women with genuine stress incontinence (55% to 83%), and that both groups had diminished transmission in the distal quarter of the urethra (66). Bump and associates reported that a PTR of greater than 90% in the proximal half of the urethra was 97% sensitive and 56% specific for the diagnosis of genuine stress incontinence, with a positive predictive value of 53% and a negative predictive value of 97% (67). Bø and colleagues performed urethral profilometry on 14 young nulliparous women, half of whom reported stress inconti-

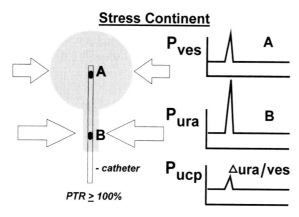

FIG. 11.8. Pressure transmission with normal support. A catheter records pressure simultaneously from within the bladder (A) and urethra (B). The arrows represent force during physical stress. The urethrovesical junction is intraabdominal, enabling abdominal pressure (P_{ves}) to be transmitted efficiently to the urethra (P_{ura}) and to maintain urethral closure pressure (P_{ucp}) and continence. The urethral pressure transmission ratio (PTR) is greater than 100%.

Stress Incontinent

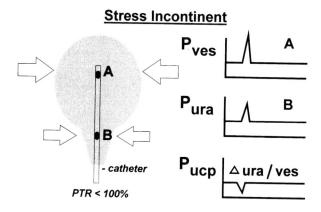

FIG. 11.9. Urethral pressure transmission with urethral hypermobility. A catheter records pressure simultaneously from within the bladder *(A)* and urethra *(B)*. The *arrows* represent force during physical stress. With descent of the urethrovesical junction, abdominal force (P_{ves}) can no longer reach the urethra (P_{ura}) efficiently, and urethral closure pressure drops (P_{ucp}), resulting in stress incontinence. The urethral pressure transmission ratio *(PTR)* is less than 100%.

nence, and noted that all the women with symptoms and only one seventh of the women without symptoms had PTRs of less than 100% (68).

The reproducibility of PTRs with varying cough intensity has been questioned. A study of 16 women noted increased PTRs with cough intensity (69). A study of 36 women with genuine stress incontinence noted marked variations in PTRs with cough pressures of less than 90 cm H_2O (70). A study of 242 women without severe (stage III or IV) pelvic organ prolapse demonstrated that PTRs have reasonable quantitative and qualitative reproducibility that is unaffected by cough strength (Kappa = 0.71 for mean PTR) (71). The major limitation of PTRs is wide overlap in continent and incontinent women. This poor specificity precludes the diagnostic use of PTRs, but PTRs may be used to describe populations in research settings.

Another type of dynamic urethral profilometry is to withdraw the urethral catheter during contraction of the pelvic floor musculature to create a Kegel urethral pressure profile (KUPP). The KUPP has been shown to result in a reproducible increase in MUCP (72), which correlates with increases in vaginal pressure (73), and may be used as a tool to gauge the ability to perform an adequate pelvic floor muscle contraction (increase in MUCP of 20% or more) (74). There is evidence that women with the ability to contract their pelvic floor muscles adequately at

baseline based on increases in urethral closure pressure may be less likely to achieve marked improvement in their level of continence with pelvic floor muscle exercise therapy than women with poor baseline contractility (75).

Urethral Profilometry after Continence Surgery

The measurement of PTRs before and after continence surgery has provided invaluable information on the mechanism of action of efficacy and complications of continence surgery. Hilton and Stanton performed urethral profilometry before and 3 months after Burch retropubic urethropexy and noted that successful surgery generally yielded increases in PTRs with urethral stabilization despite no increase in MUCP (76). Bump and colleagues determined that continence surgery failures demonstrated diminished PTRs (less than 90%) compared with women with successful surgery who had ideal urethral PTRs (close to 100%) (77). Women with postoperative *de novo* detrusor instability had excessively elevated urethral PTRs (greater than 110%), which were not seen in women with primary detrusor instability. Subsequent research has noted that successful continence surgery in women with genuine stress incontinence depends on reaching a balance between providing adequate urethral support to increase dynamic urethral pressure transmission without overcorrecting and creating excessive obstruction and creating excessive obstruction and voiding dysfunction (78).

Reproducibility of Urethral Profilometry

As with cystometry, the absence of standardization of test techniques has been a barrier to studies of reproducibility between investigators, and very few intraobserver studies have been performed. One study of 10 healthy asymptomatic fertile women demonstrated reasonable reproducibility of FUL and MUCP at a 2-year interval (79), and no significant variations have been noted during the menstrual cycle (80,81).

Urodynamic Stress Test Measurements: Leak Point Pressures

The performance of a stress test to document the presence of gross leakage during straining or coughing is the same during complex urodynamic testing as it would be during simpler testing. Some authors have advocated complicated methods of determining leakage by such techniques as measuring urethral conductivity (82), but most clinicians observe leakage by direct observation. Several techniques have been advanced to measure the exact threshold of pressure that is required to overcome urethral resistance and result in

genuine stress incontinence. With a catheter-recording bladder or abdominal pressure, clinicians may measure the increase in pressure that is required to result in leakage during a provocative maneuver such as Valsalva or coughing. This value is referred to as the leak point pressure. Because clinicians with different backgrounds are using leak point pressures in a variety of clinical situations, the variables involved in obtaining the measure are not standardized. Test variables that may effect the value of a leak point pressure include patient position, vesical volume, the placement and diameter of the urethral catheter, the provocative maneuver used, filling medium density, and whether direct visualization or fluoroscopy are used to detect leakage. Terminology for the tests is also controversial with various authors using the terms Valsalva leak point pressure, abdominal leak point pressure, and stress leak point pressure synonymously.

A leak point pressure is measured by filling the bladder to a desired volume and then asking the patient to strain or cough while noting the onset of leakage. Although some clinicians report the total abdominal or vesical pressure at leakage, most define the leak point pressure as the increase in pressure associated with the onset of leakage (Fig. 11.10). Given the myriad of variables that

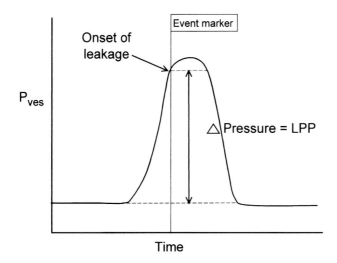

FIG. 11.10. Measurement of Valsalva leak point pressure. A catheter records pressure within the bladder (P_{ves}). Vesical pressure increases with straining, and the Valsalva leak point pressure is defined as the change in vesical pressure at which the onset of leakage is observed.

may affect leakage, the most reasonable utility of leak point is to document the presence of genuine stress incontinence.

Interest in leak point pressures began in 1981 when McGuire and co-workers examined detrusor leak point pressures in myelodysplastic children to assess their risk for upper tract damage due to bladder hyperreflexia and ureteral reflux (83). Valsalva leak point pressures were then used to evaluate women with genuine stress incontinence treated with urethral collagen bulking injections (84,85) and subsequently gained widespread clinical use in the urologic and gynecologic communities. Most women with genuine stress incontinence realize that they are more likely to experience leakage at lower levels of activity as their bladder becomes more full. Studies in which repetitive Valsalva leak point pressures were measured serially at increasing vesical volumes have demonstrated that Valsalva leak point pressures were more likely to be positive. There is decreased magnitude of leak point pressures with increasing vesical volume (86,87). In addition, some women with higher urethral resistance may not leak at all with Valsalva and may demonstrate leakage only with the higher pressures generated during a cough (88). Although various authors have advanced critical values for leak point pressures to diagnose conditions such as intrinsic urethral sphincteric deficiency (see later), no data exist to support the use of any leak point pressure value as a clinical tool for determining prognosis for response to a specific therapy.

Reproducibility of Leak Point Pressures

Although Valsalva leak point pressures have been shown to have reasonable reproducibility at a given vesical volume, the diameter of the catheter and whether it is placed in the bladder or the vagina affect both Valsalva and cough leak point pressures (86,89). Cough leak point pressures are generally higher than Valsalva leak point pressures (86,89), most likely because of augmentation of urethral resistance from pelvic floor mus-

cle activation with coughing (90). Women with worse clinical measures of incontinence and low urethral closure pressure tend to have lower Valsalva leak point pressures (88). Many authors have noted a poor correlation between urethral profilometry measures and leak point pressures (85,88). The correlation between fluoroscopic and direct visualization leak point pressures is unknown.

INTRINSIC URETHRAL SPHINCTERIC DEFICIENCY

Considerable interest has developed in using urodynamic testing to identify women who, due to their genuine stress incontinence, are at higher risk for failure after continence surgery. Although most women experience genuine stress incontinence as a result of mechanical disruption of urethrovesical junction support, some women may have impairment of the ability of the urethra to maintain closure as a component of their incontinence. This condition of impaired urethral resistance is called intrinsic sphincter deficiency (ISD).

Background

The term intrinsic sphincter deficiency was first coined in 1992 by a panel formed by the Agency for Health Care Policy and Research (AHCPR) (6). In this document, ISD was defined as a cause of genuine stress urinary incontinence in which "the urethral sphincter is unable to coapt and generate enough resistance to retain urine in the bladder, especially during stress maneuvers. In women, intrinsic sphincter deficiency is commonly associated with multiple anti-incontinence procedures. Patients with intrinsic sphincter deficiency often leak continuously or with minimal exertion."

Other terms used to describe ISD reflect the varied background of investigators into this area and include low urethral pressure, type III incontinence, sphincteric incompetence, sphincteric incontinence, impaired urethral resistance, incompetent bladder neck, and urethral incontinence.

The definition of ISD as set down by the AHCPR mentions some testing procedures that can suggest the diagnosis but does not establish a set of specific or objective criteria that can be used to make the diagnosis. As with all other aspects of urodynamic testing, clinicians have described different criteria for establishing a diagnosis of ISD from within their niche of test techniques, with sparse comparative or prospective data. The following is a description of several modalities that have been examined in the investigation of ISD.

Clinical Symptoms

Women with ISD are thought to have more severe leakage. McGuire and colleagues noted that 81% of patients with grade 3 incontinence, defined as incontinence without regard to effort, position, or activity, had ISD (85). Other studies have found no clinically significant relationships between incontinence severity and urethral closure or Valsalva leak point pressures (90,91). This is no doubt because women manage their incontinence problems with many individual variations in terms of hygiene, fluid intake, voiding frequency, and physical activity.

Historical Risk Factors

Many surgeons have attempted to identify women who may be at risk for ISD based on a woman's demographic and historical information. In 1940, Kennedy observed that urethral sphincter tone decreased with age (92), and age has been consistently identified in several contemporary observational studies as a risk factor for ISD. Neither parity nor hormonal status appears to be a discrete risk factor for ISD (91,93–95). There is compelling evidence for an association between previous failed continence surgery and intrinsic sphincter deficiency, but whether intrinsic sphincter deficiency precedes or results from surgery is unclear. Any process that damages the neuromuscular components of the urethra would be expected to contribute to ISD. McGuire was the first to note that patients who failed continence surgery frequently had impaired urethral resistance and often had undergone prior continence surgery (97). There is some evidence that surgery, particularly vaginal periurethral dissection, may result in functional damage to the urethra owing to fibrosis and pudendal nerve damage (98). Most surgical series, however, demonstrate little change or a slight increase in MUCP after continence surgery (99,100).

ISD has been observed in patients with lumbosacral spinal dysraphism (101) and spinal cord injuries (102). McGuire and Wagner noted that interruption of the sacral nerve roots S-2 to S-4 to control detrusor hyperreflexia in paraplegics did not alter urethral pressures but that high spinal anesthesia (involving the thoracic cord) did result in complete loss of resting urethral pressure (103). This suggests that a significant part of urethral sphincter function is maintained by the sympathetic nervous system in the thoracic and sacral cord segments and that simple disruption of the sacral cord segments alone does not uniformly result in ISD. Other conditions that have been associated with ISD include pelvic irradiation (104,105) and radical pelvic surgery (106,107). It is likely that ISD represents the end result of a combination of insults to some or all of the fibroelastic and neuromuscular components of the urethral sphincter.

Urodynamic Testing for Diagnosing Intrinsic Sphincter Deficiency

Urethral Axis

Early investigators noted that most women with genuine stress incontinence had loss of urethral and bladder support on radiographic imaging, which was described by Green as type I and type II incontinence in 1962 (108). Genuine stress incontinence in the absence of urethral hypermobility is by definition due to ISD. The absence of urethral hypermobility has been reported to decrease the success rate of continence procedures that are designed to stabilize the urethrovesical junction during physical stress. Bergman and colleagues reported a

50% failure rate in 15 women with a straining axis of less than 30 degrees who underwent either Pereyra needle or Burch urethropexy (109). Summit and associates noted that a straining axis of less than 30 degrees reduced the success of an abdominal wall sling from 93% (27 of 29) to 20% (one fifth) of women with low urethral closure pressure (110).

Although controversy exists as to the ideal method of measuring urethral mobility (111), the most simple and extant technique is to measure deflection of a cotton swab placed at the urethrovesical junction from the horizontal axis during straining (112). A straining axis of less than 20 (113) or 30 (110) degrees from the horizontal is considered to constitute urethral hypermobility. Other techniques described include posterior rotation and descent on lateral fluoroscopic imaging and ultrasound measurement of urethrovesical descent more than 10 mm (114) indicating hypermobility.

Urethral Profilometry

In his early work in urethral profilometry, Bonney was surprised to identify an incontinent woman with profoundly impaired urethral resistance in whom almost no retrograde pressure was required to overcome her urethra (51). In 1976, McGuire and associates described a "fixed posterior urethra" in a small group of women who had failed continence surgery and noted that most had very low urethral pressure (less than 10 cm H_2O) (115). They first coined the term type III incontinence in 1981 to define a group of women who had low closure pressure (less than 20 cm H_2O) in the proximal 1.5 cm of the urethra with or without urethral hypermobility (98,115,116). Sand and co-workers subsequently reported that MUCP of 20 cm H_2O or less decreased the success rate after Burch urethropexy from 82% to 46% at 3 months (93). Using a technique that defies ready categorization but provides a crude measure of urethral resistance, a recent study noted a high correlation between being able to withdraw a pediatric 8-French Foley catheter with an inflated bulb through the urethra and low urethral closure pressure (117). The use of crit-

ical MUCP values to diagnose ISD is hampered by marked variations in techniques used to obtain test results. A comparison of microtip and fiberoptic catheters noted a 30% discrepancy in the diagnosis of low urethral pressure (62).

Urethroscopy

Urethrocystoscopy is not a mandatory component of the evaluation of low risk women with incontinence, but in experienced hands, it may provide valuable information. Urethrocystoscopy can provide an immediate assessment of the ability of the urethra to maintain coaptation at the bladder neck. With normal urethral coaptation, the urethral mucosal surfaces are pliable and come into apposition as a cystoscope is withdrawn through the urethrovesical junction. Women with genuine stress incontinence and urethral hypermobility demonstrate funneling or descent of the urethrovesical junction during straining. A woman with ISD may demonstrate the so-called drainpipe urethra in which the bladder neck is open and patulous at rest and remains fixed or demonstrates minimal funneling during straining (Fig. 11.11). The examiner must

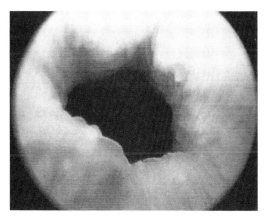

FIG. 11.11. Urethrocystoscopy of a woman with intrinsic sphincter deficiency. This patient has had two prior continence procedures and demonstrates the drainpipe urethra with a straining urethral axis of 5 degrees. The urethrovesical junction is patulous and open at rest and remains fixed during straining.

be careful not to get the end of the scope too close to the urethrovesical junction during this assessment because this can keep the mucosa from coapting, making a normal bladder neck appear patulous.

The association of endoscopic ISD with other measures of urethral resistance is uncertain. In the only comparative study performed, 80% of women with an endoscopic description of ISD had an MUCP of greater than 20 cm H_2O (118). The reproducibility of endoscopic evidence of ISD is unknown, but intraobserver and interobserver reproducibility of the appearance of the bladder neck at the time of continence surgery has been shown to be poor (119). The finding of an open bladder neck on fluoroscopy has also been proposed as a marker for ISD. The diagnostic value of the finding of an open bladder neck on radiographic imaging has been devalued because an open bladder neck during coughing was noted in 20% to 50% of continent women by ultrasound (120) and fluoroscopy (121,122).

Leak Point Pressure

The stress leak point pressure is an attractive concept to determine a woman's continence threshold during her daily activities. Unfortunately, the lack of standard criteria for performing stress leak point pressures severely limits the usefulness of specific test values. The confusion of variations in urodynamic testing is well illustrated in the area of leak points and ISD. McGuire and colleagues reported that 75% of women with type III incontinence have radiographic Valsalva leak point pressures less than or equal to 60 cm H_2O (85), and this cutoff was widely adopted as a criterion for ISD for instituting treatments such as collagen bulking injections. Medicare recently revised the criteria for periurethral bulking to an abdominal leak point pressure of less than 100 cm H_2O with a vesical volume of at least 150 mL (123). Patient position, fluid type, provocative maneuver, method of documenting leakage, and upper limit of bladder distention are not specified.

The correlation between urethral closure and leak point pressures is poor. It appears that lowering the threshold to define ISD based on a low leak point pressure will increase the accuracy of identifying women with low urethral closure pressure. A stress leak point of 60 cm H_2O or less has been reported to be 90% sensitive and 64% specific for diagnosing low-pressure urethra (124). Decreasing the leak point cutoff to 45 cm H_2O resulted in a sensitivity of 80% but increased the specificity to 90%. Other authors have suggested increased accuracy in identifying women with low urethral pressure by using a Valsalva leak point pressure of less than 50 cm H_2O (113). In a study that demonstrated the decrease in Valsalva leak point pressures with increasing volume, all women with low urethral pressure had leakage with Valsalva at 300 mL, but the positive predictive value of leakage at that volume was only 57% (87).

Empty Stress Test

An empty stress test is performed by having a woman perform a stress test soon after emptying her bladder. In a woman with a normal postvoid residual (less than 100 mL), leakage at such a low vesical volume suggests that she may have profound impairment of urethral resistance. In a study of 124 women with a positive empty supine stress test within 20 minutes after voiding, Lobel and Sand reported a sensitivity of 70%, with 66% positive and 90% negative predictive values for the presence of low urethral pressure (125). Most of the patients in that study had urethral hypermobility. Another study of the empty stress test reported a sensitivity of 79% with 40% positive and 90% negative predictive values for low Valsalva leak point pressure, which was defined as 60 cm H_2O or less at a vesical volume of 150 mL (126). If a woman demonstrates a positive stress test soon after voiding, the clinician's index of suspicion for ISD should increase.

Combined Criteria

A single standardized and reproducible diagnostic criteria list for ISD would be convenient, but it does not exist. Some authors have noted an increase in accuracy of identifying ISD by using a composite of urethral profilometry and cystoscopy (118). Others proposed using a composite of urethral axis (less than 20 degrees), profilometry (MUCP less than 20 cm H_2O), and leak point pressure (less than 50 cm H_2O), but noted that although half the subjects fell below at least one cutoff value, only 10% fell below all three (113). The clinical implications of a diagnosis of ISD based on multiple criteria are unknown. A list of criteria proposed to diagnose ISD is given in Table 11.2.

Intrinsic Sphincteric Deficiency: Summary

The goal of identifying women with ISD is to identify those at risk for failure following continence surgery. Because of the spectra of combinations of impairment in urethral support and resistance that may be present in any given woman with urinary incontinence, ISD most likely represents a multifaceted condition rather than a specific diagnosis. No single diagnostic test exists to define ISD, and a combination of clinical incontinence severity and assessment of urethral support and urethral resistance should be used to characterize and follow patients. It is the task of responsible investigators to validate specific continence procedures prospectively for the various subcategories of ISD rather than making overly general conclusions based on limited data.

URODYNAMIC TESTING IN WOMEN WITH SEVERE PELVIC ORGAN PROLAPSE

One of the feared complications of prolapse surgery is to correct vaginal prolapse only to unveil an incontinence problem that was concealed by severe prolapse (127). The term occult genuine stress incontinence is used for a woman who is clinically stress continent but who exhibits stress incontinence when her prolapse is reduced. This phenomenon would not be expected to occur in milder stages of prolapse (stage I or II). Obstruction of the urethra may be due to kinking from anterior or apical prolapse or to direct compression from large

TABLE 11.2. *Diagnostic techniques described for defining intrinsic sphincter deficiency*

Condition	Diagnostic technique	Diagnostic criteria
Lack of urethral hypermobility	Cotton swab test Perineal ultrasound	Straining axis < 20–30 degrees Urethrovesical junction descent < 10 mm
	Urethrocystoscopy	Urethrovesical junction patulous and fixed during straining
Low-pressure urethra	Urethral pressure profile (multichannel urodynamics)	Maximal urethral closure pressure ≤ 20 cm H_2O
Low leak point pressure	Stress leak point pressure (multichannel urodynamics or video cystourethrography)	Gross or fluoroscopically visualized urine loss during Valsalva maneuver at a vesical pressure of less than 45–100 cm H_2O
Type III incontinence	Video cystourethrography (multichannel urodynamics with simultaneous fluoroscopy)	Urethral closure pressure of less than 20 cm H_2O in the proximal 1.5 cm of the urethra. Urethra open at rest

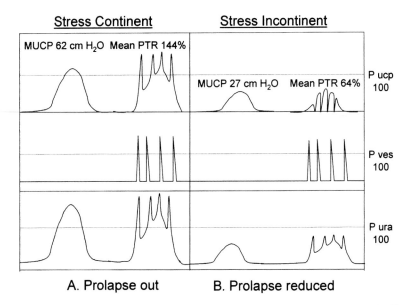

FIG. 11.12. Occult genuine stress incontinence in a patient with severe prolapse. **A:** The patient is continent owing to urethral kinking and compression, and urethral pressure transmission *(PTR)* is exaggerated throughout the urethra. **B:** With barrier reduction of the prolapse, the patient demonstrates stress incontinence with a reduction in urethral pressure transmission and a marked reduction in maximum urethral closure pressure *(MUCP)*.

posterior wall prolapse conditions. A barrier stress test is used to evaluate for occult incontinence and involves reducing the prolapse and then performing a stress test. A barrier urethral pressure profile may be performed to evaluate alterations in MUCP and dynamic urethral profilometry (Fig. 11.12). The technique used for reduction of prolapse during urodynamic testing is not standardized and may affect the demonstration of occult incontinence or low urethral pressure (128). Prolapse may be reduced using a straight retractor, such as the posterior blade of a speculum; using a Sims-type retractor; or placing a diaphragm or pessary. A study of 11 continent women with severe uterovaginal prolapse revealed mechanical obstruction of the urethra with extremely elevated dynamic urethral PTRs (166% to 257%), which were diminished (78% to 101%), along with the MUCP (75 to 45 cm H_2O) with barrier reduction of their prolapse (129). Rosenzwieg and coworkers studied 22 clinically continent women with severe pelvic organ prolapse and discov-

ered 9 women (41%) with occult stress incontinence and 9 with detrusor instability, 5 (56%) of who had irritative urinary tract symptoms (frequency, urgency, or nocturia) (130).

In summary, there are no definitive data for selecting which clinically continent patients with severe prolapse require urodynamic testing before reconstructive pelvic surgery. Urodynamic testing may be moot in the active young woman who will undergo an abdominal vault suspension with urethropexy or the frail elderly woman who will undergo colpocleisis without urethropexy regardless of the results of a barrier stress test. As with any procedure, the surgeon must tailor treatment to the individual patient's risk for morbidity, lifestyle, and expectations.

URODYNAMICS AND URINARY TRACT INFECTION

It is important to assess for cystitis by culture or urine analysis before performing urodynamic testing to avoid infectious morbidity and an erroneous diagnosis. Women with detrusor instability may have increased rates of bacteriuria (131), and instrumentation during urodynamic testing may precipitate cystitis. Furthermore, symptoms of cystitis may mimic detrusor instability. In one study of women with significant bacteriuria (greater than 10^5 organisms/mL), half of the women diagnosed with an unstable bladder had a normal cystometrogram 2 weeks after antibiotic treatment of urinary tract infection (132).

Guidelines for the use of antibiotic prophylaxis at the time of urodynamic testing are nebulous. Although a significant proportion of elderly women with irritative urinary symptoms may have bacteriuria (133), both case-control (134) and randomized prospective placebo-controlled studies (135,136) have shown low rates of cystitis following testing and no benefit with a short course of antibiotic treatment. Based on this information, the routine use of antibiotic prophylaxis following urodynamic testing does not appear to be justified.

THE NEGATIVE URODYNAMIC STUDY

Up to 10% of urodynamic tests may be nondiagnostic (137). A normal urodynamic study in a woman with symptoms poses a diagnostic and therapeutic conundrum. Blaivas refers to a false-negative urodynamic study result as type 0 incontinence (138). Given the subjective nature of lower urinary tract complaints and the artificial environment of the urodynamic laboratory, it is not incomprehensible to have a nondiagnostic urodynamic test. Urodynamic testing in a tense and apprehensive patient is unlikely to provide an accurate reflection of a woman's symptoms during her daily activities. Increased anxiety is likely to result in increased pelvic floor and urethral musculature tone that may affect the patient's level of comfort during filling and instrumentation. Patient anxiety with increased pelvic floor muscle tone may suppress abnormal detrusor activity (49), interfere with the stress test (139), and impair voiding ("stage-fright"

retention). Women with chronic pelvic pain may also present urinary tract symptoms that may or may not be associated with urinary tract disorders, such as interstitial cystitis (140).

A normal or negative test result is frustrating for a patient who is expecting relief for complaints severe enough to subject herself to uncomfortable and expensive testing. A lack of a diagnosis is also frustrating for the clinician whose training favors providing a patient with treatment. Management of negative urodynamic testing may involve reassuring a patient of the absence of a troublesome diagnosis or the need for invasive surgery. It may also be appropriate to institute empiric behavioral or medical therapy regardless of the urodynamic test results. For women with irritative symptoms and a normal cystometrogram, it may be appropriate to institute pelvic floor muscle exercises with bladder training and possible anticholinergic medication with appropriate follow-up. Elderly women may experience irritative symptoms due to atrophic urogenital changes and may benefit from local estrogen therapy. A woman with symptoms of stress incontinence with a negative standing stress test at maximum capacity may have genuine stress incontinence under extreme circumstances in her daily activities but is unlikely to benefit from a urethropexy. In this patient, pelvic floor muscle exercises and bladder training may be the most appropriate options.

URODYNAMIC TESTING: SUMMARY

The ideal urodynamic test will identify women with a specific diagnosis in a reproducible and cost-effective fashion. Clinical urodynamic testing should aid in the selection of specific treatments and identify women who are at increased risk for complications or failure. Although the vast arrays of urodynamic armamentaria each have thoughtful and passionate proponents who have helped our understanding of the pathophysiology of lower urinary tract dysfunction and therapeutic interventions, very few of these tests have been validated clinically. The wide variability in test specifications and the absence of prospective data limit the utility of many published observations. Clinicians should interpret any suggestions that "critical" urodynamic test values, such as closure or leak point pressures, may decrease the efficacy of specific continence procedures with healthy skepticism. As with any clinical test, the clinician must interpret urodynamic test results within the perspective of a patient's complaints and in light of their clinical experience. The challenge for urodynamic investigators is to establish the reproducibility and clinical validity of urodynamic tests rather than to propagate more nonstandardized tests of uncertain utility.

REFERENCES

1. Weber AM, Walters MD. Cost-effectiveness of urodynamic testing before surgery for women with pelvic organ prolapse and stress urinary incontinence. *Am J Obstet Gynecol* 2000;183:1338–1347.
2. Summit RL Jr, Stovall TG, Bent AE, et al. Urinary incontinence: correlation of history and brief office evaluation with multichannel urodynamic testing. *Am J Obstet Gynecol* 1992;166:1835–1844.
3. Lagro-Janssen AL, Debruyne FM, van Weel C. Value of the patient's case history in diagnosing urinary incontinence in general practice. *Br J Urol* 1991;67:569–572.
4. Versi E, Cardozo L, Anand D, et al. Symptoms analysis for the diagnosis of genuine stress incontinence. *Br J Obstet Gynaecol* 1991;98:815–819.
5. Haylen BT, Sutherst JR, Frazer MI. Is the investigation of most stress incontinence really necessary? *Br J Urol* 1989;64:147–149.
6. Urinary Incontinence Guideline Panel. *Urinary incontinence in adults.* Clinical Practice Guideline. AHCPR Pub. No. 92-0038. Rockville, MD: Agency for Health Care Policy and Research, Public Health Service, U.S. Dept Health and Human Services, March 1992.
7. Fantl JA, Newman DK, Colling J, et al. *Managing acute and chronic urinary incontinence.* Clinical Practice Guideline. No. 2 1996 Update. Rockville, MD: U.S. Dept Health and Human Services, Public Health Service, Agency for Health Care Policy and Research, AHCPR Pub. No. 96-0686, March 1996.
8. Widner AC, Myers ER, Visco AG, et al. Which women with stress incontinence require urodynamic evaluation? *Am J Obstet Gynecol* 2001;184:20–27.
9. McGuire EJ, Lytton B, Kohorn EI, et al. The value of urodynamic testing in stress urinary incontinence. *J Urol* 1980;124:256–258.
10. Arnold EP, Webster JR, Loose H, et al. Urodynamics of female incontinence: factors influencing the results of surgery. *Am J Obstet Gynecol* 1973;117:805–813.
11. Stanton SL, Cardozo L, Williams JE, et al. Clinical

and urodynamic features of failed continence surgery in the female. *Obstet Gynecol* 1978;51:515–520.
12. Beck RP, Arnusch D, King C. Results in treating 210 patients with detrusor overactivity incontinence of urine. *Am J Obstet Gynecol* 1976;125:593–596.
13. Colombo M, Zanetta G, Vitobello D, et al. The Burch colposuspension for women with and without detrusor overactivity. *Br J Obstet Gynaecol* 1996;103:255–260.
14. Sand PK, Bowen LW, Ostergard DR, et al. The effect of retropubic urethropexy on detrusor instability. *Obstet Gynecol* 1988;71:818–822.
15. Galen C. *On the natural faculties* [translated by AJ Brock]. Cambridge, MA: Harvard University Press, 1988.
16. Heidenhain R, Colberg A. Versuche uber Tonus des Blasenschliessmuskels. *Mullers Arch f Anat Physiol* 1858:437–462.
17. Rosenplanter H. Heitrage zur Frage des Sphinktertonus. *Petersb Med Ztschr* 1867;1:16–32.
18. Scatz F. Beitrage zur Physiologischen Geburtskunde. *Arch Gynakol* 1872;4:195–202.
19. Mosso A, Pellacani P. Sur la fonctionsde la vessie. *Ital Arch de Biolog* 1882;1:97–127.
20. Guyon F. De la sensibilite de la vessie au contract et la distention dans l'etat physiologique et pathologique. *Ann Mal de Organes Genito-urinaire* 1884:61–74.
21. Schwartz O. Versuch einer Analyse der Miktions anomalien nach Erkeltungen. *Wein klin Wchnschr* 1915;28:1057–1062.
22. Abrams P, Blaivas JG, Stanton SL, et al. The standardisation of terminology of lower urinary tract function. *Scand J Urol Nephrol Suppl* 1988;114:5–19.
23. Robertson AS, Griffiths CJ, Ramsden PD, et al. Bladder function in healthy volunteers: ambulatory monitoring and conventional urodynamic studies. *Br J Urol* 1994;73:242–249.
24. Wyndaele JJ. Are sensations perceived during bladder filling reproducible during cystometry? *Urol Int* 1992; 48:299–301.
25. Watkins KH. The clinical value of bladder pressure estimations. *Br J Urol* 1934;6:104–118.
26. Simeone FA, Lampson RS. A cystometric study of the function of the urinary bladder. *Ann Surg* 1937;106:413–422.
27. Harris RL, Cundiff GW, Theofrastous JP, et al. Bladder compliance in neurologically intact women. *Neurourol Urodyn* 1996;15:483–488.
28. Scotti RJ, Myers DL. A comparison of the cough stress test and single-channel cystometry with multichannel urodynamic evaluation in genuine stress incontinence. *Obstet Gynecol* 1993;81:430–433.
29. Wall LL, Wiskind AK, Taylor PA. Simple bladder filling with a cough stress test compared with subtracted cystometry for the diagnosis of urinary incontinence. *Am J Obstet Gynecol* 1994;171:1472–1479.
30. Bump RC. The urodynamic laboratory. *Obstet Gynecol Clin North Am* 1989;16:795–816.
31. Ouslander J, Leach G, Abelson S, et al. Simple versus multichannel cystometry in the evaluation of bladder function in an incontinent geriatric population. *J Urol* 1988;140:1482–1486.
32. Bergman A, Nguyen H, Koonings PP, et al. Use of fetal cardiotocographic monitor in the evaluation of urinary incontinence. *Isr J Med Sci* 1988;24:291–294.
33. Sutherst JR, Brown MC. Comparison of single and

multichannel cystometry in diagnosing bladder instability. *Br Med J (Clin Res Ed)* 1984;288:1720–1722.

34. Swift SE. The reliability of performing a screening cystometrogram using a fetal monitoring device for the detection of detrusor instability. *Obstet Gynecol* 1997;89:708–712.

35. Richardson DA. Use of vaginal pressure measurements in urodynamic testing. *Obstet Gynecol* 1985;66: 581–584.

36. Al-Taher H, Sutherst JR, Richmond DH, et al. Vaginal pressure as an index of intra-abdominal pressure during urodynamic evaluation. *Br J Urol* 1987;59: 529–532.

37. Blaivas JG, Labib KL, Bauer SB, et al. A new approach to electromyography of the external urethral sphincter. *J Urol* 1978;117:773–777.

38. Khorsandi M, Ginsberg PC, Harkaway RC. Reassessing the role of urodynamics after cerebrovascular accident: males versus females. *Urol Int* 1998;61:142–146.

39. Weld KJ, Dmochowski RR. Association of injury and bladder behavior in patients with post-traumatic spinal cord injury. *Urology* 2000;55:490–494.

40. Barbalias GA, Nikiforidis G, Liatsikos EN. Vesico urethral dysfunction associated with multiple sclerosis: clinical and urodynamic perspectives. *J Urol* 1998; 160:106–111.

41. Remmers A, Janknegt RA. Extramural ambulatory urodynamic monitoring during natural filling and normal activities: evaluation of 100 patients. *J Urol* 1991; 146:124–131.

42. Van Venrooj GEPM, Boon TA. Extensive urodynamic investigation: interaction among diuresis, detrusor instability, urethral relaxation, incontinence, and complications in women with a history of urge incontinence. *J Urol* 1994;152:1535–1538.

43. Bhatia NN, Bradley WE, Halderman S. Urodynamics: continuous monitoring. *J Urol* 1982;128:963–968.

44. Van Waalwijk, Van Doorn ESC, Remmers A, Janknegt RA. Conventional and extramural ambulatory urodynamic testing of the lower urinary tract in female volunteers. *J Urol* 1992;147:1319–1326.

45. Davis G, McClure G, Sherman R, et al. Ambulatory urodynamics of female soldiers. *Milit Med* 1998;163: 808–812.

46. Brown K, Hilton P. Ambulatory monitoring. *Int Urogynecol J* 1997;8:369–376.

47. Homma Y, Kondo Y, Takahashi S, et al. Reproducibility of cystometry in overactive detrusor. *Eur Urol* 2000;38:681–685.

48. Blaivas JG, Groutz A, Verhaaren M. Does the method of cystometry affect the incidence of involuntary detrusor contractions? A prospective randomized urodynamic study. *Neurourol Urodyn* 2001;20:141–145.

49. Romanzi LJ, Groutz A, Heritz DM, et al. Involuntary detrusor contractions: correlation of urodynamic data to clinical categories. *Neurourol Urodyn* 2001;20:249–257.

50. Shimonovitz S, Monga AK, Stanton SL. Does the menstrual cycle influence cystometry? *Int Urogynecol J* 1997;8:213–216.

51. Bonney V. On diurnal incontinence of urine in women. *J Obstet Gynaecol Br Emp* 1923;30:358–365.

52. Gosling JA, Dixon JS, Critchley HOD, et al. A comparative study of the human external sphincter and periurethral levator ani muscles. *Br J Urol* 1981;53: 35–41.

53. Rud T, Andersson KE, Asmussen M, et al. Factors maintaining intra-urethral pressure in women. *Invest Urol* 1980;17:343–347.

54. Bump RC, Friedman CI, Copeland WE Jr. Non-neuromuscular determinants of intraluminal urethral pressure in the female baboon: relative importance of vascular and nonvascular factors. *J Urol* 1988;139:162–164.

55. Shawer M, Brown M, Sutherst JR. Comparative examination of female urethral pressure profiles measured by CO_2 and H_2O infusion techniques. *Br J Urol* 1983; 55:326–331.

56. Haeusler G, Tempfer C, Heinzl H, et al. Value of urethral pressure profilometry in the female incontinent patient: a prospective trial with an 8-channel urethral catheter. *Urology* 1998;52:1113–1117.

57. Bhatia NN, Ostergard DR. Urodynamics in women with stress–urinary incontinence. *Obstet Gynecol* 1982;60:552–9.

58. Rud T. Urethral pressure profile in continent women from childhood to old age. *Acta Obstet Gynecol Scand* 1980;59:331–335.

59. Sorenson S, Waechter PB, Constantinou CE, et al. Urethral pressure and pressure variations in healthy fertile and postmenopausal women with reference to the female sex hormones. *J Urol* 1991;146:1434–1440.

60. Theofrastous JP, Bump RC, Elser DM, et al. Correlation of Valsalva leak point pressures and urethral pressure profilometry variables with measures of incontinence severity in women with pure genuine stress incontinence. *Am J Obstet Gynecol* 1995;173:407–414.

61. Elser DM, London W, Fantl JA, et al. A comparison of urethral profilometry using microtip and fiberoptic catheters. *Int Urogynecol J Pelvic Floor Dysfunct* 1999;10:371–374.

62. Culligan PJ, Goldberg RP, Blackhurst DW, et al. Comparison of microtransducer and fiberoptic catheters for urodynamic studies. *Obstet Gynecol* 2001;98:253–257.

63. Enhörning G. Simultaneous recording of the intravesical and intraurethral pressure. *Acta Chir Scand Suppl* 1961;276:1–68.

64. Beck RP, Maughan GB. Simultaneous intraurethral and intravesical pressure studies in normal women and those with stress incontinence. *Am J Obstet Gynecol* 1964;89:746–753.

65. Toews HA. Intraurethral and intravesical pressures in normal and stress-incontinent women. *Obstet Gynecol* 1967;29:613–624.

66. Hilton P, Stanton SL. Urethral pressure measurement by microtransducer: the results in symptom-free women and those with genuine stress incontinence. *Br J Obstet Gynecol* 1983;90:919–933.

67. Bump RC, Copeland WE, Hurt WG, et al. Dynamic urethral pressure/profilometry pressure transmission ratio determinations in stress-incontinent and stress-continent subjects. *Am J Obstet Gynecol* 1988;159:749–755.

68. Bø K, Stein R, Kulseng-Hanssen S, et al. Clinical and urodynamic assessment of nulliparous young women with and without stress incontinence symptoms: a case-control study. *Obstet Gynecol* 1994;84:1028–1032.

69. Richardson DA. Reproducibility of pressure transmission ratios in stress incontinent women. *Neurourol Urodyn* 1993;12:123–130.

70. Swift SE, Rust PF, Ostergard DR. Intrasubject variability of the pressure-transmission ratio in patients

with genuine stress incontinence. *Int Urogynecol J Pelvic Floor Dysfunct* 1996;7:312–316.

71. Cundiff GW, Harris RL, Theofrastous JP, et al. Pressure transmission ratio reproducibility in stress continent and stress incontinent women. *Neurourol Urodyn* 1997;16:161–166.

72. Loenen NTVM, Vierhout ME. Augmentation of urethral pressure profile by voluntary pelvic floor contraction. *Int Urogynecol J* 1997;8:284–287.

73. Theofrastous JP, Wyman JF, Bump RC, et al., and the Continence Program for Women Research Group. The relationship between urethral and vaginal pressures during pelvic muscle contraction. *Neurourol Urodyn* 1997;16:553–558.

74. Bump RC, Hurt WG, Fantl JA, et al. Assessment of Kegel pelvic muscle exercise performance after brief verbal instruction. *Am J Obstet Gynecol* 1991;165:322–327.

75. Theofrastous JP, Wyman JF, Bump RC, et al., and the Continence Program for Women Research Group. The effects of pelvic floor muscle training on strength and predictors of response in the treatment of urinary incontinence. *Neurourol Urodyn* 2002;21:(in press).

76. Hilton P, Stanton SL. A clinical and urodynamic assessment of the Burch colposuspension for genuine stress incontinence. *Br J Obstet Gynaecol* 1983;90:934–939.

77. Bump RC, Fantl JA, Hurt WG. Dynamic urethral pressure profilometry pressure transmission ratio determinations after continence surgery: understanding the mechanism of success, failure, and complications. *Obstet Gynecol* 1988;72:870–874.

78. Bump RC, Hurt WG, Elser DM, et al. Understanding lower urinary tract function soon after bladder neck surgery. Continence Program for Women Research Group. *Neurourol Urodyn* 1999;18:629–637.

79. Sørensen S, Gregersen, Sørensen SM. Long-term reproducibility of urodynamic investigations in healthy fertile females. *Scand J Urol Nephrol Suppl* 1988;114:35–41.

80. Sørensen S, Knudsen UB, Kirkeky HJ, et al. Urodynamic investigations in healthy fertile females during the menstrual cycle. *Scand J Urol Nephrol Suppl* 1988;114:28–34.

81. Van Geelen JM, Doesburg WH, Thomas CMG, et al. Urodynamic studies in the normal menstrual cycle: the relationship between hormonal changes during the menstrual cycle and the pressure profile. *Am J Obstet Gynecol* 1918;141:384–392.

82. Creighton SM, Plevnik S, Stanton SL. Distal urethral electrical conductance (DUEC)—a preliminary assessment of its role as a quick screening test for incontinent women. *Br J Obstet Gynaecol* 1991;98:69–72.

83. McGuire EJ, Woodside JR, Borden TA, et al. Prognostic value of urodynamic testing in myelodysplastic patients. *J Urol* 1981;126:205–209.

84. McGuire EJ, Wang SC, Appell R, et al. Treatment of urethral incontinence by collagen injection: one year followup. *J Urol* 1990;143:224A.

85. McGuire EJ, Fitzpatrick CC, Wan J, et al. Clinical assessment of urethral sphincteric function. *J Urol* 1993;150:1452–1454.

86. Miklos JR, Sze EHM, Karram MM. A critical appraisal of the methods of measuring leak-point pressures in women with stress incontinence. *Obstet Gynecol* 1995;86:349–352.

87. Theofrastous JP, Cundiff GW, Harris RL, et al. The effect of vesical volume on Valsalva leak point pressures in women with genuine stress urinary incontinence. *Obstet Gynecol* 1996;87:711–714.

88. Theofrastous JP, Bump RC, Elser DM, et al. Correlation of Valsalva leak point pressures and urethral pressure profilometry variables with measures of incontinence severity in women with pure genuine stress incontinence. *Am J Obstet Gynecol* 1995;173:407–414.

89. Bump RC, Elser DM, Theofrastous JP, et al. Valsalva leak point pressures in women with genuine stress incontinence: reproducibility, effect of catheter caliber, and correlations with other measures of urethral resistance. *Am J Obstet Gynecol* 1995;173:551–557.

90. Shafik A. Straining urethral reflex: description of a reflex and its clinical significance. *Acta Anat* 1991;140:104–107.

91. Horbach NS, Ostergard DR. Predicting intrinsic urethral sphincter dysfunction in women with stress urinary incontinence. *Obstet Gynecol* 1994;84:188–192.

92. Kennedy WT. Urinary incontinence relieved by restoration and maintenance of the normal position of the urethra. *Am J Obstet Gynecol* 1941;41:16–28.

93. Sand PK, Bowen LW, Panganiban R, et al. The low pressure urethra as a factor in failed retropubic urethropexy. *Obstet Gynecol* 1987;68:399–402.

94. Hilton P, Stanton SL. Urethral pressure measurement by microtransducer: results in symptom-free women and in those with genuine stress incontinence. *Br J Obstet Gynaecol* 1983;90:919–933.

95. Summitt RL, Sipes DR, Bent AE, et al. Evaluation of pressure transmission ratios in women with genuine stress incontinence and low urethral pressure: a comparative study. *Obstet Gynecol* 1994;83:984–988.

96. Meschia M, Bruschi F, Barbancini P, et al. Recurrent incontinence after retropubic surgery. *J Gynecol Surg* 1993;9:25–28.

97. McGuire EJ. Urodynamic findings in patients after failure of stress incontinence operations. *Prog Clin Biol Res* 1981;78:351–360.

98. Benson JT, McClellan E. The effect of vaginal dissection on the pudendal nerve. *Obstet Gynecol* 1993;82:387–389.

99. Bergman A, Ballard CA, Koonings PP. Comparison of three surgical procedures for genuine stress incontinence: prospective randomized study. *Am J Obstet Gynecol* 1989;160:1102–1106.

100. Herbertsson G, Iosif CS. Surgical results and urodynamic studies 10 years after retropubic colpourethrocystopexy. *Acta Obstet Gynecol Scand* 1993;72:298–301.

101. Barbalias GA, Blavis JG. Neurologic implications of the pathologically open bladder neck. *J Urol* 1983;129:780–782.

102. Nordling J, Meyhoff HH, Olesen KP. Cysto-urethrographic appearance of the bladder and posterior urethra in neuromuscular disorders of the lower urinary tract. *Scand J Urol Nephrol* 1982;16:115–124.

103. McGuire EJ, Wagner FC. The effects of sacral denervation on bladder and urethral function. *Surg Obstet Gynecol* 1977;164:343–346.

104. Zoubek J, McGuire EJ, Noll F, et al. The late occurrence of urinary tract damage in patients successfully treated by radiotherapy for cervical carcinoma. *J Urol* 1989;141:1347–1349.

105. Parkin DE, Davis JA, Symonds RP. Urodynamic findings following radiotherapy for cervical carcinoma. *Br J Urol* 1988;61:213–217.

106. Scotti RJ, Bergman A, Bhatia NN, et al. Urodynamic changes in urethrovesical function after radical hysterectomy. *Obstet Gynecol* 1986;68:111–120.

107. Sasaki H, Yoshida T, Noda K, et al. Urethral pressure profiles following radical hysterectomy. *Obstet Gynecol* 1982;59:101–104.

108. Green TH. Development of a plan for the diagnosis and treatment of urinary stress incontinence. *Am J Obstet Gynecol* 1962;83:632–648.

109. Bergman A, Koonings PP, Ballard CA. Negative Q-tip test as a risk factor for failed incontinence surgery in women. *J Reprod Med* 1989;34:193–197.

110. Summitt RL, Bent AE, Ostergard DR, et al. Stress incontinence and low urethral closure pressure: correlation of preoperative urethral hypermobility with successful suburethral sling procedures. *J Reprod Med* 1990;9:877–880.

111. Caputo RM, Benson JT. The Q-tip test and urethrovesical junction mobility. *Obstet Gynecol* 1993; 82:892–896.

112. Karram MM, Bhatia NN. The Q-tip test: standardization of the technique and its interpretation. *Obstet Gynecol* 1988;71:807–811.

113. Bump RC, Coates KW, Cundiff GW, et al. Diagnosing intrinsic sphincteric deficiency: comparing urethral closure pressure, urethral axis, and Valsalva leak point pressures. *Am J Obstet Gynecol* 1997;177:303–310.

114. Bergman A, Vermesh M, Ballard CA, et al. Role of ultrasound in urinary incontinence evaluation. *Urology* 1989;33:443–444.

115. McGuire EJ, Lytton B, Pepe V, et al. Stress urinary incontinence. *Obstet Gynecol* 1976;47:255–264.

116. McGuire EJ, Woodside JR. Diagnostic advantages of fluoroscopic monitoring during urodynamic evaluation. *J Urol* 1981;125:830–834.

117. Arya LA, Myers DL, Jackson ND. Office screening test for intrinsic urethral sphincter deficiency: pediatric Foley test. *Obstet Gynecol* 2001;97:885–889.

118. Cundiff GW, Bent AE. The contribution of urethrocystoscopy to evaluation of lower urinary tract dysfunction in women. *Int Urogynecol J Pelvic Floor Dysfunct* 1996;7:307–311.

119. Bump RC, Hurt WG, Elser DM, et al. Reliability of intra-operative anatomic, endoscopic, and urodynamic measurements and their correlation with post-operative pressure transmissions in women undergoing bladder neck suspension surgery. *Neurourol Urodyn* 1995;14:490–491.

120. Chapple CR, Helm CW, Blease S, et al. Asymptomatic bladder neck incompetence in nulliparous females. *Br J Urol* 1989;64:357–359.

121. Versi E. The significance of an open bladder neck in women. *Br J Urol* 1991;68:42–43.

122. Versi E, Cardozo LD, Studd JW. Distal urethral compensatory mechanisms in women with an incompetent bladder neck who remain continent, and the effect of menopause. *Neurourol Urodyn* 1990;9:579–582.

123. Medicare Coverage Advisory Committee. Part 65–69: mechanical/hydraulic incontinence control devices. *DMERC Supplier Manual.* Nashville, TN: Cigna Health Care Medicare Adminisration, 2002.

124. Swift SE, Ostergard DR. A comparison of stress-leak-point pressure and maximal urethral closure pressure in patients with genuine stress incontinence. *Obstet Gynecol* 1995;85:704–708.

125. Lobel RW, Sand PK. The empty supine stress test as a predictor of intrinsic urethral sphincter dysfunction. *Obstet Gynecol* 1996;88:128–132.

126. McLennan MT, Bent AE. Supine empty stress test as a predictor of low Valsalva leak point pressure. *Neurourol Urodyn* 1998;17:121–127.

127. Symmonds RE, Jordan LT. Iatrogenic stress incontinence of urine. *Am J Obstet Gynecol* 1960;82:1231–1237.

128. Veronikis DK, Nichols DH, Wakamatsu MM. The incidence of low-pressure urethra as a function of prolapse-reducing technique in patients with massive pelvic organ prolapse (maximum descent at all vaginal points) *Am J Obstet Gynecol* 1997;177:1305–1314.

129. Bump RC, Fantl JA, Hurt WG. The mechanism of urinary continence in women with severe uterovaginal prolapse: results of barrier studies. *Obstet Gynecol* 1988;72:291–295.

130. Rosenzweig BA, Pushkin S, Blumenfeld D, et al. Prevalence of abnormal urodynamic test result in continent women with severe genitourinary prolapse. *Obstet Gynecol* 1992;79:539–542.

131. Moore KH, Simons A, Mukerjee C, et al. The relative incidence of detrusor instability and bacterial cystitis detected on the urodynamic-test day. *Br J Urol* 2000; 85:786–792.

132. Bhatia NN, Bergman A. Cystometry: an unstable bladder and urinary tract infection. *Br J Urol* 1986;58: 134–137.

133. Bergman A, McCarthy TA. Antibiotic prophylaxis after instrumentation for urodynamic testing. *Br J Urol* 1983;55:568–569.

134. Coptcoat MJ, Reed C, Cumming J, et al. Is antibiotic prophylaxis necessary for routine urodynamic investigations? A controlled study in 100 patients. *Br J Urol* 1988;61:302–303.

135. Baker KR, Drutz HP, Barnes MD. Effectiveness of antibiotic prophylaxis in preventing bacteriuria after multichannel urodynamic investigations: a blind, randomized study in 124 female patients. *Am J Obstet Gynecol* 1991;165:679–681.

136. Cundiff GW, McLennan MT, Bent AE. Randomized trial of antibiotic prophylaxis for combined urodynamics and cystourethroscopy. *Obstet Gynecol* 1999;93: 749–752.

137. Katz GP, Blaivas JG. A diagnostic dilemma: when urodynamic findings differ from the clinical impression. *J Urol* 1983;129:1170–1174.

138. Blaivas JG, Olsson CA. Stress incontinence: classification and surgical approach. *J Urol* 1988;139: 727–731.

139. Miller JM, Perucchini D, Carchidi LT, et al. Pelvic floor muscle contraction during a cough and decreased vesical neck mobility. *Obstet Gynecol* 2001;97: 255–260.

140. Parsons CL, Bullen M, Kahn BS, et al. Gynecologic presentation of interstitial cystitis as detected by intravesical potassium sensitivity. *Obstet Gynecol* 2001; 98:127–132.

Ostergard's Urogynecology and Pelvic Floor Dysfunction, Fifth Edition. edited by A.E. Bent, et al. Lippincott Williams & Wilkins, Philadelphia © 2003.

12

Cystourethroscopy

Geoffrey W. Cundiff* and Alfred E. Bent**

*Department of Gynecology and Obstetrics, Johns Hopkins School of Medicine; and Department of Obstetrics and Gynecology, Johns Hopkins Bayview Medical Center, Baltimore, Maryland
**Department of Gynecology and Obstetrics, Johns Hopkins School of Medicine; and Department of Gynecology, Greater Baltimore Medical Center, Baltimore, Maryland

Cystourethroscopy provides a noninvasive method of visually evaluating the lower urinary tract. It has broad applications in urogynecology and general gynecology (1). The ability to recognize normal and pathologic findings is mastered with practice and diligence after acquiring a basic understanding of the equipment.

HISTORICAL PERSPECTIVE

Although many credit Kelly with developing the female cystoscope, endoscopy of the female bladder preceded his report by half a century. Bozzini (2) described an endoscopic technique for evaluating the female bladder in the early 19th century. His invention consisted of a stand that supported different-sized hollow funnels, a candle for illumination, and a reflector to direct the light into the funnel when it was placed into the urethra. Visibility with this device was limited both by poor illumination and by the tendency of the operator to be burned if the stand was tilted for a better view. Desmormeaux (3) introduced a more practical endoscope in 1853 that used different-sized angulated tubes. The tubes increased the surface area of the bladder that could be inspected, and use of an alcohol lamp improved illumination. By 1877, Grünfeld's (4) modification of the endoscope still used a hollow tube but added an obliquely placed glass lens at the vesical end. His endoscope was vastly improved by the adaptation of an electric light source reflected by mirrors. Even with this improvement, visualization was poor without bladder distention, and endoscopy was considered an adjunct to the established method of urethral dilation followed by bimanual palpation. Nitze (5) developed a compound lens system that increased the field of vision and used an incandescent light source to provide illumination, but this cystoscope was considered too complicated for all but the specialist.

Kelly's contribution was in overcoming the deficiencies of both Grünfeld's and Nitze's instruments and techniques. The Kelly cystoscope was a hollow tube, without glass, that used an obturator for placement (6). The knee–chest position allowed air to distend the bladder. A head mirror was used to reflect an electric light into the bladder for illumination (Fig. 12.1). The technique was simple yet provided an excellent view.

Modern endoscopy started with the development of the Hopkins fiberoptic telescope in 1954 (7). The use of glass fibers in place of an air chamber dramatically improved light transmission and resolution and also provided a wider viewing angle. The viewing angle could also be changed, which improved the extent of visualization and facilitated more invasive procedures. Later modifications of the Hopkins system incorporated a series of glass rods with optically finished ends separated by intervening spaces.

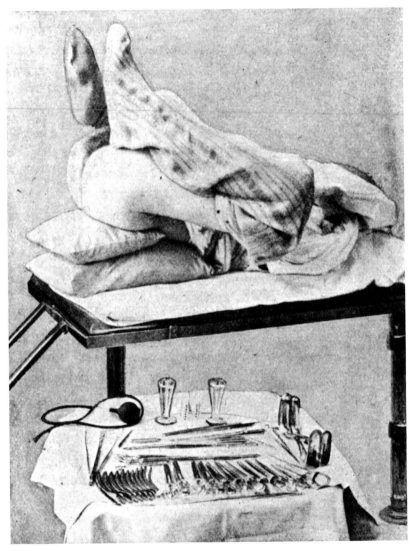

FIG. 12.1. Cystoscopy as described by Kelly used a supine position with the hips elevated. The instruments used by Kelly are arranged in the foreground. (From Kelly HA. The direct examination of the female bladder with elevated pelvis: the catheterization of the ureters under direct inspection, with and without elevation of the pelvis. *Am J Obstet Dis Wom Child* 1894;25:7, with permission.)

The improved view of the bladder provided by the Hopkins cystoscope compromised the view of the urethra. The angled telescope is not effective for evaluating the urethral mucosa because most cystoscopic sheaths have a terminal fenestra for use with a catheter deflector mechanism. This design allows the irrigant to escape during its distal location in the urethra. Robertson (8) addressed the compromised view of the urethra by applying fiberoptic technology to a shorter straight-on telescope, later known as the urethroscope.

The most recent development in cystoscopy is the flexible cystoscope. The flexible fiberoptic lens system permits an instrument that bends, thereby increasing the field of view. Comparisons continue regarding resolution and comfort between rigid and flexible instruments (9,10).

EQUIPMENT

Urethroscopy

The urethroscope is composed of a telescope and sheath. The telescope has a 0-degree (straight-ahead) viewing angle, which provides a circumferential view of the urethral lumen as the distending medium forces the urethra open. The sheath has a port for infusion of media as well as a valve to initiate flow of media or allow bladder emptying. Sheath sizes are 15 and 24 French. The instrument is also useful for vaginoscopy (Fig. 12.2).

Rigid Cystoscopy

The rigid cystoscope is composed of a telescope, bridge, and sheath (Fig. 12.3). Each component serves a different function and is available with various options to facilitate this role.

The telescope transmits light to the bladder cavity and an image to the viewer. Several viewing angles are available, including 0- (straight), 12- (minimal angle for collagen injection), 25- or 30- (forward-oblique), 70- (lateral), and 120-degree (retro view) angles. The angled telescopes have a field marker that assists the viewer with orientation. It is visible as a blackened notch at the outside of the visual field and opposite the angle of deflection.

The 30-degree lens provides the best view of the bladder base and posterior wall, whereas the 70-degree lens permits inspection of the anterolateral walls. The retro view of the 120-degree lens is not usually necessary for cystoscopy of the female bladder but can be useful for evaluating the urethral opening into the bladder. For many applications, a single telescope is not preferable. For diagnosis, the 30-degree telescope is usually sufficient, although the 70-degree telescope may be required in the presence of fixation of the bladder neck [urethrovesical junction (UVJ)]. The 70-degree telescope is preferable when performing operative cystoscopy at the time surgery for stress incontinence.

The cystoscope sheath provides a vehicle for introducing the telescope and distending media into the bladder. It is available in var-

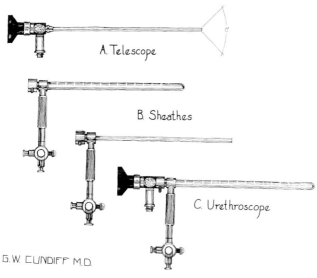

FIG. 12.2. Components of a rigid urethroscope. **A:** Telescope, 0-degree. **B:** sheaths, 15- and 24-French. **C:** Assembled urethroscope.

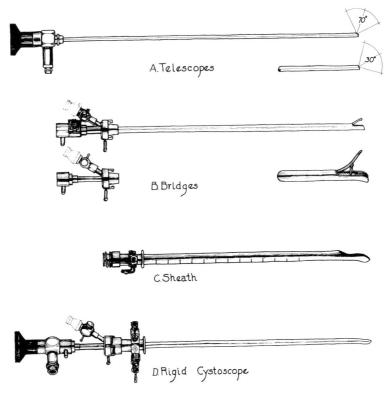

FIG. 12.3. Components of a rigid cystoscope. **A:** Telescopes. The 70-degree lateral angled-view telescope *(above)* and the 30-degree forward-oblique telescope *(below)*. **B:** Bridges. Single-port bridge *(below)* and dual-port bridge with an Albarrán deflecting mechanism *(above)*. The position of the deflecting mechanism within the fenestra of the operating sheath is shown. **C:** Sheath, 22-French operating. **D:** Assembled cystoscope with a diagnostic 17-French sheath.

ious calibers from 15 to 28 French. The telescope partly fills the lumen of the sheath, leaving room for an irrigation-working channel. The smallest-diameter sheath is useful for diagnostic purposes, whereas larger-caliber sheaths allow instruments to be placed in the working channel. The proximal end of the sheath has two irrigating ports: one for introduction of the distending medium and the other for removal. The distal end of the cystoscope sheath is fenestrated to permit the use of instrumentation in the angled field of view. It is also beveled, opposite the fenestrae, to increase comfort on introduction into the urethra. Larger-di-

ameter sheaths may require an obturator for placement.

The bridge serves as the connector between telescope and sheath and forms a watertight seal with both. It may have one or two ports for introduction of instruments into the working channel. The Albarrán bridge is a variation of the bridge that has a deflector mechanism at the end of an inner sheath. When placed in the cystoscopic sheath, the deflector mechanism is located at the distal end of the inner sheath within the fenestra of the outer sheath. At this location, the elevation of the deflector mechanism assists the manipulation of instruments within the field of view.

Flexible Cystoscopy

The flexible cystoscope combines the optical systems and irrigation-working channel in a single unit. The optical system consists of a single image-bearing fiberoptic bundle and two light-bearing fiberoptic bundles. The fibers of these bundles are coated parallel coherent optical fibers that transmit light even when bent. This permits incorporation of a distal-tip deflecting mechanism that will deflect the tip 290 degrees in a single plane. A lever at the eyepiece controls the deflection. The optical fibers are fitted to a lens system that magnifies and focuses the image. A focusing knob is located just distal to the eyepiece. The irrigation-working port enters the instrument at the eyepiece opposite the deflecting mechanism. The coated tip is 15 to 18 French in diameter and 6 to 7 cm in length, with the working unit constituting half the length.

The image may appear somewhat granular, but technology is rapidly closing the gap with the image produced by rigid instrumentation. The flow rate of the working channel is slower than that of rigid instruments, and this may be further curtailed by passage of instruments down the channel. Use of the instrument channel may also limit some of the movement at the tip of the deflector mechanism. Flexible instrumentation is more comfortable, especially for male patients. The short length of the female urethra and ease of passing the rigid cystoscope may offset perceived advantages of flexible instrumentation in the female patient.

Light Sources and Video Monitors

A high-intensity (xenon) light source is recommended for use in video monitoring and photography. The light cable must be checked periodically for transmission properties. Video monitoring eliminates awkward positioning of the operator and improves teaching abilities. It may also help to distract the patient, while allowing her to see important findings.

Distending Media

Water or saline is generally used as a distending medium. Carbon dioxide may be preferred for diagnosing a hard-to-see urethral diverticulum, but otherwise it may cause more discomfort with filling of the bladder, and volumes achieved with liquid more accurately reflect physiologic volumes. The fluid is instilled by gravity through a standard intravenous infusion set, with the bag height about 100 cm above the patient's symphysis to provide adequate flow.

Instrumentation

A wide range of instrumentation is available for use through the cystoscope sheath. The most commonly used in female patients are grasping forceps with either rat-tooth or alligator jaws, biopsy forceps, and scissors. They are available in flexible or rigid styles and come in varying diameters (1). A monopolar ball electrode is useful for electrocautery during operative cystoscopy.

CYSTOURETHROSCOPY TECHNIQUES: DIAGNOSIS

Diagnostic cystourethroscopy in women is easily performed as an office procedure and is well tolerated without anesthesia in most cases. Male patients benefit from topical anesthesia, and it is also useful in the female patient who has any apprehension regarding pain (11). Most indications for endoscopy warrant evaluation of both the bladder and urethra (Table 12.1).

TABLE 12.1. *Indications for cystourethroscopy in female patients*

Hematuria
Chronic irritative voiding symptoms
Obstructive voiding
Recurrent urinary tract infections
Suspected fistula, diverticulum, or foreign body
Suspected interstitial cystitis
Incontinence evaluation
Assessment of ureteral function
Staging for cervical cancer

Urethroscopy

The urethroscope is placed into the urethra with the fluid infusion flowing in order to distend the urethra and facilitate both the view and the passage of the instrument to the bladder. The 24-French sheath allows adequate visualization, although it may be too large in 10% to 15% of patients. Comfort is essential, and the 15-French sheath should be used in these latter patients. The view is not as good with the smaller sheath as with the larger sheath, but it is adequate. The urethra could be dilated to allow passage of the larger sheath, and in this case, topical anesthesia should be used for patient comfort. Topical anesthetic or dilation irritates the urethral mucosa, giving a false impression of inflammation, which should be taken into account if used.

The urethral mucosa is viewed as the instrument is passed slowly to the bladder neck and into the bladder. This causes a small amount of burning-type discomfort. The trigone and ureters may be observed by angling the telescope toward the bladder base and, in some cases, by elevating the trigone with a vaginal finger.

The UVJ is observed during the following commands: "hold your urine," "squeeze your rectum," "strain down like having a bowel movement," and "cough." The hold and squeeze commands are performed with the urethroscope withdrawn enough to allow the UVJ to close two thirds of the way. Movement can then be observed as the UVJ closes during the maneuver. The strain and cough commands are performed with the urethroscope withdrawn enough to allow the UVJ to close two thirds of the way. In this manner, opening of the UVJ can be observed. After modest bladder filling, the vaginal finger compresses and massages the urethra over the end of the urethroscope as the instrument is withdrawn. This allows observation for urethral glands, exudate, fistula, and diverticular openings. The patient has somewhat more discomfort during digital compression of the urethra and should be forewarned concerning the 3 to 5 seconds of discomfort.

Cystoscopy

Cystoscopy is generally performed using a 70-degree telescope with 17-French sheath and with some topical anesthetic on the sheath to facilitate movement in and out of the urethra. The cystoscope is placed into the urethral meatus with the bevel directed posteriorly and is advanced directly into the bladder, aiming at the patient's umbilicus. An obturator is not necessary with a small sheath such as 17 French, but the fluid flow during insertion facilitates passage. A volume of 250 mL or greater is desirable for bladder inspection unless the patient has discomfort before this volume, and a slow trickle is maintained if needed for optimum view. The air bubble is identified at the bladder dome, and this serves as a landmark for the rest of the examination. The examination begins at the bladder dome, making full sweeps with the instrument at each hour of an imaginary clock, going from 12 to 4 o'clock, then 11 to 8 o'clock, and then observing the posterior bladder from 5 to 7 o'clock. Orientation is maintained by placing the field marker directly opposite the area of the bladder to be inspected. The bladder base may require digital vaginal elevation for complete assessment. The bladder volume can be assessed at the end of the inspection by filling the bladder to patient fullness and then measuring the amount of fluid by emptying the bladder through the sheath, or by measuring the volume voided by the patient after the procedure.

Antimicrobial Prophylaxis

A concern after cystourethroscopy is the prevention of infection, which may occur in 5% of cases. A number of these patients already have infection at the time of the examination, even with a recent negative urine culture. Prophylaxis is practiced by many, but recent reports cite no difference in infection rates between patients treated with placebo and nitrofurantoin (12,13). If prophylaxis is used, only a 1- or 2-day course is suggested, and a urinary analgesic (e.g., phenazopyridine) may also be administered for one or two doses.

Patients may experience dysuria, urgency, frequency, and hematuria for several hours after the examination, but most have minimal postprocedure discomfort.

OPERATIVE CYSTOSCOPY

Urogynecologists may do a few minor office procedures, such as biopsy of mucosal lesions, removal of small foreign bodies, and cutting and removal of suture material. These procedures require a larger cystoscope sheath (22 French) and may be associated with discomfort. Anesthesia may be induced by instillation of 50 mL of a 4% lidocaine solution for 5 minutes. A bladder pillar block may augment the anesthesia, and this is performed by injecting 5 mL of 1% lidocaine solution at each bladder pillar. After placement of a bivalve speculum, the bladder pillars are located at 2 and 10 o'clock with respect to the cervix. If the uterus is absent, a Sims speculum is used to expose the anterior vaginal wall, and the pillars are just superior and lateral to the UVJ (14).

The best view for operative procedures is immediately in front of the telescope. With the cystoscope in the bladder, the operative instrument is introduced into the operative port and advanced until it is visible just at the end of the cystoscope. Gross movements are made with the cystoscope as the instrument is brought into apposition with the lesion. Minor adjustments are made by moving the instrument within the cystoscope sheath. Bleeding is self-limited in most cases, although a ball electrode can be used if needed.

INTRAOPERATIVE CYSTOSCOPY

Cystoscopy is an important adjuvant to surgery of the female genitourinary system. It is commonly used to judge coaptation during periurethral collagen injections, to facilitate safe placement of suprapubic catheters, and to evaluate the ureters and bladder mucosa for inadvertent damage. The approach to assessment of the integrity of bladder mucosa after pelvic surgery is similar to the approach described for diagnostic cystoscopy. A thorough survey of the bladder is made, with special attention to the portions of the bladder potentially jeopardized by the specific procedure. Inspection of the anterolateral aspects of the mucosa is important after a bladder suspension procedure, whereas inspection of the trigone is especially important after a difficult vaginal hysterectomy or dissection of an anterior enterocele sac from the bladder. An assessment of ureteral integrity is warranted after any retropubic suspension or culdoplasty, but especially after suspected injury to the ureter. Visualization of efflux of solution from the ureteral orifice is adequate to demonstrate patency, and this is facilitated by injection of 2.5 to 5 mL of indigo carmine dye intravenously 5 minutes before cystoscopy. The absence of efflux is an indication for passage of ureteral catheters to evaluate potential obstruction.

Ureteral Catheterization

Catheterization of the ureteral orifices has been practiced since cystoscopes were first introduced. In gynecology, the primary indications for ureteral catheterization are to evaluate potential ureteral obstruction and to place ureteral markers. Ureteral markers may be useful in radical pelvic surgery and in cases with abnormal pelvic anatomy.

Ureteral catheters are available in various sizes, with a number of specialized tips. Although available from 3 to 12 French, the most useful are 4 to 7 French. The most commonly used catheters are the general-purpose and whistle-tip catheters. Specialized tips include spiral filiform for negotiating strictures and curves and the acorn tip for retrograde studies. Catheters are fabricated from plastic or Dacron and are generally radiopaque. They have graduated centimeter markings for judging depth of insertion.

Once the ureteral orifice is located, the ureteral catheter is advanced into the field of view just outside the fenestrated portion of the cystoscope, with the catheter tip orientated in the axis of the ureteral lumen. The tip is threaded into the first part of the ureteral lumen by advancing the entire cystoscope.

Once the tip passes the ureteral orifice, the catheter is gently threaded along the ureter until resistance is met at the renal pelvis, which is about 25 cm. This is done by grasping the catheter manually proximal to its entry point into the operative channel of the sheath or bridge and gently pushing the catheter into the ureter. The deflecting mechanism of the Albarrán bridge may facilitate the procedure.

Difficulty in passing the catheter may be due to an anatomic variation such as a stenotic orifice, mucosal fold, or ureteral tortuosity. A stenotic orifice is suspected in the presence of immediate resistance to the catheter tip, and a smaller catheter is selected. A mucosal fold may be managed by repositioning the patient, bladder, or cystoscope. Placing the patient in the Trendelenburg position helps to alter the position of the intramural ureter, as does further filling or emptying of the bladder. A filiform-tip catheter is also valuable for negotiating strictures and tortuosities.

If the catheter is to be left in place, it should be secured to a transurethral catheter and connected to a drainage device. Gentle technique is required to prevent hematuria and ureteral spasm.

Suprapubic Teloscopy

Transurethral cystoscopy is applicable during a vaginal surgical approach. Suprapubic teloscopy provides a method to perform cystoscopy from an abdominal approach (15). This may also be accomplished during laparoscopic surgery by passing the telescope through a suprapubic catheter introducer sheath (16).

Suprapubic teloscopy is an extraperitoneal technique that begins with closure of the anterior peritoneum to prevent vesicoperitoneal fistulas and contamination of the peritoneal cavity with spilled urine. Indigo carmine is administered intravenously. The bladder is filled to 400 mL through a transurethral triple-lumen Foley catheter placed at the beginning of the case. A 1- to 2-cm pursestring suture is placed into the bladder muscularis at the bladder dome using a 2-0 or 3-0 absorbable suture. Stay sutures may be placed on either side of the pursestring to facilitate introduction of the tele-

scope. A stab incision is made in the center of the pursestring, the 30- or 70-degree telescope without sheath is inserted into the bladder, and the pursestring is tightened to stabilize the telescope while allowing movement. Orientation is achieved by identifying the Foley bulb and then looking under the bulb to see the trigone. If suprapubic catheterization is planned, the catheter can be placed through the same stab incision as the telescope is removed.

Percutaneous suprapubic teloscopy may be performed during laparoscopic cases by placing a plastic suprapubic catheter introducer through the abdomen under direct vision into the laparoscopic field. The bladder is filled retrograde as in the open technique described previously, and the laparoscopic distention is reduced while the trocar is directed into the bladder. The telescope can fit tightly through an 8-French catheter introducer to allow bladder inspection. The bladder entry site may be sutured or a suprapubic catheter left using an 8-French pediatric Foley catheter.

CYSTOURETHROSCOPIC FINDINGS

Normal Urethra

The normal urethra has a lush, pink epithelium (Fig. 12.4; see Color Plate 1 following page 204), and periurethral gland openings may be seen posteriorly along the length of the urethra. There is often a central posterior ridge called the urethral crest, and there may

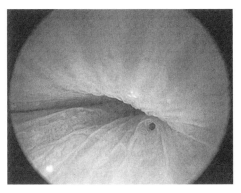

FIG. 12.4. Normal urethra. There is pink, lush epithelium in folds. (See Color Plate 1 following page 204.)

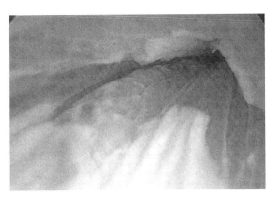

FIG. 12.5. Urethral crest and squamous epithelium of normal urethra. The urethral crest runs posteriorly as a longitudinal ridge, and over it is white epithelium. (See Color Plate 2 following page 204.)

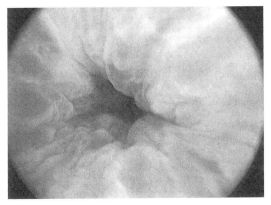

FIG. 12.6. Acute urethritis. The urethra is reddened along its length. (See Color Plate 3 following page 204.)

be white epithelium, especially in the posterior wall of the urethra (Fig. 12.5; see Color Plate 2 following page 204). The UVJ is slightly irregular but rounded in shape. It should normally close with hold maneuvers and with stress maneuvers.

Abnormal Urethroscopic Findings

Acute urethritis is usually caused by infection, trauma, or irritation (Fig. 12.6; see Color Plate 3 following page 204). Findings include inflamed, reddened urethral mucosa, bleeding areas, superficial ulceration, and exudate on the mucosal surface. Polyps and fronds may be present at the UVJ, but their significance is uncertain (Fig. 12.7; see Color Plate 4 following page 204). Palpation over the end of the urethroscope may reveal exudate from urethral glands or may facilitate identification of exudate or pus from a urethral diverticulum. A fistula is an opening usually in the posterior aspect of the urethra, and urine or irrigating fluid may be seen escaping into the vagina (Fig. 12.8; see Color Plate 5 following page 204). A frozen or scarred, functionless urethra may appear pale, may be fixed in an open position, and will have no response to hold or strain maneuvers (Fig. 12.9; See Color Plate 6 following page 204).

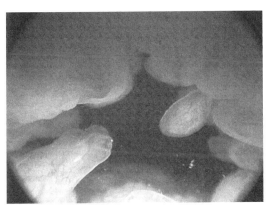

FIG. 12.7. Polyps and fronds at the urethrovesical junction. (See Color Plate 4 following page 204.)

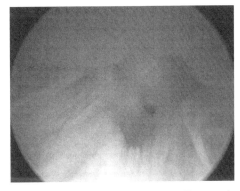

FIG. 12.8. Urethrovaginal fistula. The urethral canal is in the upper right of the photograph, and the opening from the urethra to the vagina is clearly seen as a small opening in the center of the picture. (See Color Plate 5 following page 204.)

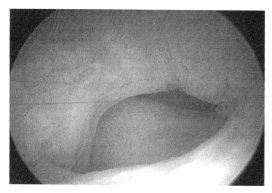

FIG. 12.9. Functionless urethra. The urethra is very short and remains passively open, with the urethroscope barely inside the meatus. The epithelium is smooth, and there is no movement with hold or strain maneuvers. (See Color Plate 6 following page 204.)

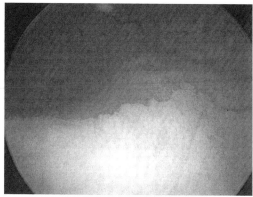

FIG. 12.11. Metaplasia of trigone. The white membrane covers much of the trigone leading up to the ureters. Biopsy reveals squamous metaplasia. (See Color Plate 8 following page 204.)

Normal Bladder

The bladder has a smooth surface with pale pink to glistening white hue. The translucent mucosa affords easy visualization of the branched submucosal vasculature. Infusion of fluid is always accompanied by an air bubble, which marks the dome of the bladder (Fig. 12.10; see Color Plate 7 following page 204). The trigone appears more reddened and granular and may have a thickened white mem-

brane with a villous contour (Fig. 12.11; see Color Plate 8 following page 204). Histologic evaluation of this layer reveals squamous metaplasia, and it is usually referred to simply as metaplasia.

The trigone is triangular, with the inferior apex directed toward the UVJ and the ureteral orifices forming the superior apices (Fig. 12.12; see Color Plate 9 following page 204). As the cystoscope is advanced past the UVJ, the trigone is apparent at the bottom of the field. The interureteric ridge is a visible eleva-

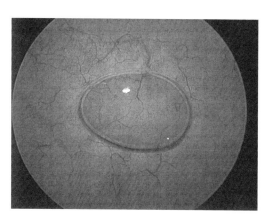

FIG. 12.10. Normal bladder. The air bubble is at the dome of the bladder and serves as a reference marker. The epithelium of the bladder wall is smooth and pale pink and has fine vasculature. (See Color Plate 7 following page 204.)

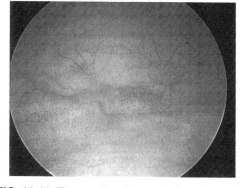

FIG. 12.12. Trigone. The trigone is formed by the urethrovesical junction inferiorly and the ureteral orifices superiorly. The trigone is frequently reddened and granular. (See Color Plate 9 following page 204.)

tion that forms the superior boundary of the trigone and runs between the ureteral orifices. The intramural portion of the ureters can often be seen as they course from the lateral aspect of the bladder toward the trigone. There is marked variation in the ureteral orifices, but they are usually circular or slitlike and located on the apex of a small mound. With urine efflux, the ureter opens, and the mound retracts in the direction of the intramural ureter.

The distended bladder is roughly spherical, but numerous folds of mucosa are evident in the empty or partially filled bladder. The uterus and cervix can be seen indenting the posterior wall of the bladder. Bowel peristalsis may be seen through the bladder wall.

Abnormal Cystoscopic Findings

Bladder pathology either is located in the mucosa or is structural. Mucosal lesions are either inflammatory or neoplastic, although the two may coexist. Cystitis refers to inflammation of the bladder, and generally cystoscopy should be avoided until the infection is treated. Cystitis may be manifested as pink or peach-colored macules or papules. As severity intensifies, the mucosa becomes edematous and hypervascular (Fig. 12.13; see Color Plate 10 following page 204). In hemorrhagic cystitis, there may be individual or con-

fluent mucosal hemorrhages, and the patient complains of hematuria. The hemorrhagic cystitis that follows bladder infusion with toxins such as cyclophosphamide is characterized by diffuse mucosal hemorrhages. In radiation cystitis, areas of hemorrhage are surrounded by pale mucosa, which may be fibrotic or hypovascular. An indwelling catheter produces an inflammatory reaction of the mucosa in contact with the catheter. There may be associated pseudopapillary edema and submucosal hemorrhages and vesical fibrosis.

Interstitial cystitis is suspected in patients with severe frequency, urgency, and suprapubic pain before voiding. The examination is usually performed under anesthesia. The pathognomonic lesions appear after filling and then refilling of the bladder to capacity. Glomerulations are petechial hemorrhages or small red dots and are visible in mild cases. Larger hemorrhagic areas may be seen, and severe areas have linear hemorrhages. Petechiae may be seen in normal patients on the posterior bladder wall and trigone. Patients with interstitial cystitis have at least 10 to 20 glomerulations per field of vision throughout the bladder.

Cystitis cystica consists of clear mucosal cysts, which are usually found on the bladder base and are often found in multiples (Fig. 12.14; see Color Plate 11 following page 204). The cysts are formed by single layers of

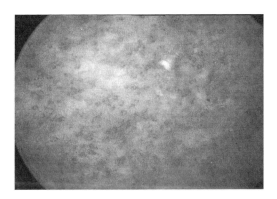

FIG. 12.13. Acute cystitis. The bladder mucosa is reddened and edematous, making it difficult to see clearly. There is often active bleeding further compromising the view. (See Color Plate 10 following page 204.)

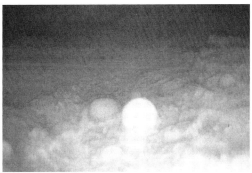

FIG. 12.14. Cystitis cystica. The 1- to 2-mm cysts at the bladder base are smooth-walled and are clear or sometimes pigmented. (See Color Plate 11 following page 204.)

subepithelial transitional cells, which degenerate with central liquefaction. Cystitis glandularis has an appearance similar to cystitis cystica, but the cysts are not clear and have a less uniform contour. There may be associated inflammation. The association of cystitis glandularis with adenovillous carcinoma of the bladder has led to the belief that cystitis glandularis may be a precursor of adenocarcinoma (17).

Bladder cancer is less common in women than in men, but it still may occur, especially after the fifth decade. Transitional cell carcinoma is the most common type, followed by adenocarcinoma and squamous cell carcinoma. Cystoscopic appearance is variable but usually reveals a raised lesion with a villous feathery or papillary appearance (Fig. 12.15; see Color Plate 12 following page 204). Superficial transitional cell carcinoma may be multicentric or may have associated carcinoma *in situ.* Carcinoma *in situ* may be inconspicuous, mimicking the macules or plaques of cystitis.

Trabeculations are smooth ridges, which become evident with distention of the bladder to volumes approaching maximum cystometric capacity. They appear as interlaced cords of different diameters with intervening sacculations (Fig. 12.16; see Color Plate 13 following page 204). They represent hypertrophied detrusor musculature associated with detrusor instability and functional or anatomic ob-

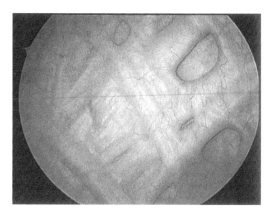

FIG. 12.16. Trabeculation. The muscle bundles appear as prominent ridges with intervening pockets or cellules. (See Color Plate 13 following page 204.)

struction. A bladder diverticulum can occur when high intravesical pressure produces an enlargement of the intervening sacculations. The thick muscular band that creates the neck varies in diameter and gives way to an outpouching of bladder mucosa. The interior of the diverticulum has been reported as the site of neoplasms in a small number of cases.

Fistulas may also be encountered at cystoscopy (Fig. 12.17; see Color Plate 14 fol-

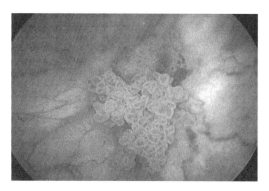

FIG. 12.15. Bladder cancer. The pedunculated papillary lesion is a transitional cell carcinoma. (See Color Plate 12 following page 204.)

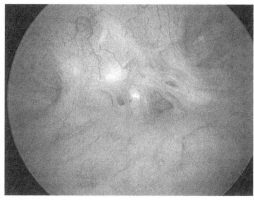

FIG. 12.17. Vesicovaginal fistula. The openings in the bladder with a posthysterectomy fistula occur superior to the trigone in the posterior aspect of the bladder, and there are two distinct holes to the vagina in this picture. (See Color Plate 14 following page 204.)

lowing page 204). Posthysterectomy fistulas are usually located in the bladder base superior to the interureteric ridge, corresponding to the level of the vaginal cuff. The fistula openings range in size from small to several centimeters in diameter. In the immediate postoperative state, the surrounding mucosa is edematous and hyperemic, whereas in later stages, the mucosa has a typical smooth appearance (see Chapter 27). In contrast, vesicoenteric fistulas uniformly have a surrounding inflammatory reaction, often with bulbous edema, and the fistula tract is not discernible in two thirds of cases (18).

Bladder calculi may result from urinary stasis or the presence of a foreign body, or an inflammatory exudate may coalesce and serve as a nidus for stone formation. Stones have extremely variable cystoscopic appearance in terms of color, size, and shape but generally have an irregular surface (19). Foreign bodies and stones are usually accompanied by varying degrees of general or localized inflammatory reaction. A permanent suture may be a nidus for a stone, or may remain in its original state.

Auxiliary ureteral orifices indicate renal collecting abnormalities. When present, they often enter the vesical wall slightly superior to the trigone in near proximity to the other ureteral orifice. In a duplicated collecting system, the upper pole kidney drains into the more distal ureteral opening. A ureterocele is caused by laxity of the distal ureteral lumen with herniation into the vesical cavity during efflux.

SUMMARY

Cystoscopes have evolved into high-resolution instruments that permit excellent visualization of the lower urinary tract. The instrumentation is available with many modifications that increase the applications of the technique. Cystourethroscopy is valuable for diagnosing anatomic lesions of the lower urinary tract that are commonly overlooked by other diagnostic modalities. Cystoscopy is also valuable to assess ureteral function and

vesical integrity during pelvic surgery. The simplicity of the techniques and the breadth of applications make it invaluable to the pelvic surgeon.

REFERENCES

1. Cundiff GW, Bent AE. *Endoscopic diagnosis of the female urinary tract.* London: WB Saunders, 1999.
2. Bozzini P. Lichteiter, eine erfindung zur anschung innerer theile, und krukheiten nebst abbildung. *J Pract Arzeykunde* 1805;24:107.
3. Desmormeaux AJ. *Transactions of the Societé Chirurgie, Paris.* Gazette des Hop, 1865.
4. Grünfeld I. *Der harnröhrenspiegel (das endoscop), seine diagnostische und therapeutische anwendung.* Vienna: Deutsch Chirurgie, 1881.
5. Nitze M. Eine neue balbachtungs-und untersuchunigsmethods fur harnrohre, harnbiase and rectum. *Wien Med Wochenschr* 1879;24:649.
6. Kelly HA. The direct examination of the female bladder with elevated pelvis: the catheterization of the ureters under direct inspection, with and without elevation of the pelvis. *Am J Obstet Dis Wom Child* 1894;25:1–19.
7. Hopkins HH, Kopany NS. A flexible fiberscope, using static scanning. *Nature* 1954;179:39–41.
8. Robertson JR. Air cystoscopy. *Obstet Gynecol* 1968;32:328–330.
9. Clayman RV, Reddy P, Lange PH. Flexible fiber-optic and rigid-rod lens endoscopy of the lower urinary tract; a prospective controlled comparison. *J Urol* 1984;131:715–716.
10. Yoshimura R, Wada S, Kishimoto T. Why the flexible cystoscope has not yet been widely introduced? A questionnaire to Japanese urologists. *Int J Urol* 1999;6:549–559.
11. Choong S, Whitfield HN, Meganathan V, et al. A prospective, randomized, double blind study comparing lignocaine gel and plain lubricating gel in relieving pain during flexible cystoscopy. *Br J Urol* 1997;80:69–71.
12. Cundiff GW, McLennan MT, Bent AE. Randomized trial of antibiotic prophylaxis for combined urodynamics and cystourethroscopy. *Obstet Gynecol* 1999;93:749–752.
13. Kraklau DM, Wolf JS Jr. Review of antibiotic prophylaxis recommendations for office-based urologic procedures. *Tech Urol* 1999;5:123–128.
14. Ostergard DR. Bladder pillar block anesthesia for urethral dilatation in women. *Am J Obstet Gynecol* 1980;136:187–188.
15. Timmons MC, Addison WA. Suprapubic teloscopy: extraperitoneal intraoperative technique to demonstrate ureteral patency. *Obstet Gynecol* 1990;75:137–139.
16. Miklos JR, Kholi N, Sze EH, et al. Percutaneous suprapubic teloscopy: a minimally invasive cystoscopic technique. *Obstet Gynecol* 1997;89:476–478.
17. Edwards PD, Hurm RA, Jaeesehke WH. Conversion of cystitis glandularis to adenocarcinoma. *J Urol* 1972;108:568–570.
18. Farringer JL, Hrabovsky E, Marsh J, et al. Vesicocolic fistula. *South Med J* 1974;67:1043–1046.
19. Schwartz BF, Stoller ML. The vesical calculus. *Urol Clin North Am* 2000;27:333–346.

Ostergard's Urogynecology and Pelvic Floor Dysfunction, Fifth Edition. edited by A.E. Bent, et al.
Lippincott Williams & Wilkins, Philadelphia © 2003.

13

Clinical Neurophysiologic Techniques in Urinary and Fecal Incontinence

J. Thomas Benson

Department of Obstetrics and Gynecology, Indiana University; and Department of Female Pelvic Medicine and Reconstructive Surgery, Methodist Hospital, Indianapolis, Indiana

Urinary and fecal storage and elimination processes are complex and involve the entire nervous system. Reflex interactions occur at local, spinal, and supraspinal levels for quasi-automatic activity, and cortical levels of activity add the dimension of conscious control.

The basic unit of the nervous system is the nerve cell. The nerve cell is intended to last the lifetime of the organism, in contrast to other cells, such as the red blood cell, which lasts only for months. The nerve cell is dynamic—constantly reorganizing, restructuring, and regrowing to retain function. It is composed of a nerve cell body and a process (axon) that may be 5,000 times as long as the nerve cell body. The chief function of the nerve cell is to transmit signals, referred to as action potentials, to an effector (e.g., muscle) or to another neuronal structure. The transmission within the nerve cell process is ionic (electrical), using protein channels in the axon membrane that allow passage of sodium, potassium, and chloride ions. This process is "all or none," whereas at the neuroeffector site or synapse, the transmission is chemical and graded, depending on neurotransmitters acting on receptors. Many of the chemical agents acting as neurotransmitters and the microtubules and neurofilaments used for axonal restructuring are synthesized in the nerve cell (Nissl) body, which is a very highly differentiated secretory cell with prominent nucleolus and rough endoplasmic reticulum. The axon lacks ribosomes and endoplasmic reticulum and cannot synthesize essential constituents. Therefore, a process of axonal transport from nerve cell body throughout the axon, acting both anterograde and retrograde, is vital for the nerve cell's function and survival. Any process that interferes with axonal transport will stop the ability of the axon to transmit action potentials.

The axon is surrounded by endoneurium (Fig. 13.1), which is largely composed of myelin, secreted by Schwann cells in peripheral nerves and by oligodendrocytes within the spinal cord and brain. Evolutionary development has led to myelin sheaths around axons with periodic interruptions of the myelin at nodes of Ranvier, where sodium channels are numerous. This allows increased rates of conduction without requiring massive size of nerves—so-called saltatory conduction. Nerve sizes are dependent, then, on the degree of myelination, and nerve function is related to size, with action potential transmission faster in larger nerves (Table 13.1). A collection of various sized axons surrounded by perineurium, a firm protective structure composed of alternating layers of epithelial cells and basement membranes, constitutes a nerve fascicle. Blood vessels supplying the axons traverse the perineurium at angles, subject to obstruction with nerve stretching. Groups of fascicles are surrounded by loose connective tissue, the epineurium, and constitute the nerve proper.

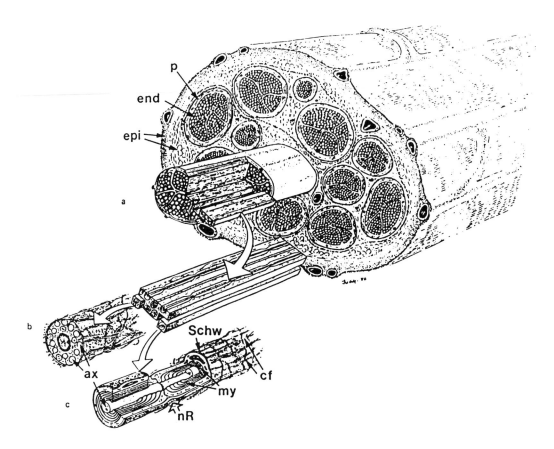

FIG. 13.1. Microanatomy of a peripheral nerve trunk and its components. **A:** Fascicles surrounded by a multilaminated perineurium (*p*) are embedded in a loose connective tissue, the epineurium (*epi*). **B,C:** The outer layers of the epineurium are condensed into a sheath and illustrate the appearance of unmyelinated and myelinated fibers, respectively. Sch, Schwann cell; my, myelin sheath; ax, axon; nR, node of Ranvier. (From Lundburg G. *Nerve injury and repair*. New York: Churchill Livingstone, 1988.)

The nervous system is divided into the central nervous system, composed of spinal cord and brain, and the peripheral nervous system, composed of cranial and spinal nerves connecting the central system to the periphery. Peripheral nerves are formed by dorsal (sensory) and ventral (motor) nerve roots joining together near their exiting site of the vertebral column (Fig. 13.2).

The sacral peripheral nerves supplying the pelvis have features that are clinically significant, making them particularly vulnerable: the cauda equina, the pelvic plexus, and the pu-

dendal nerves. The cauda equina is formed by descent of lumbosacral nerve roots from their origin in the spinal cord to their respective vertebral column exits. Such descent is caused by the spinal cord growing disproportionately to the vertebral column so that in the adult, the cord ends at about the first lumbar vertebra (Fig. 13.3). The roots of the cauda equina do not have the firm protection of the perineurium and are subject to traumatic disease. After the roots meet at the sacral exit foramina, they split into posterior rami, innervating episacral cartilaginous and ligamen-

TABLE 13.1. *Classification of nerve fibers*

Sensory and motor fibers	Sensory fibers	Largest fiber diameter	Fastest conduction velocity (m/s)	General comments
A-α	Ia	22	120	Motor: the large alpha motoneurons of lamina IX, innervating extrafusal muscle fibers Sensory: the primary afferents of muscle spindles
A-α	Ib	22	120	Sensory: Golgi tendon organs, touch and pressure receptors
A-β	II	13	70	Motor: the motoneurons innervating both extrafusal and intrafusal (muscle spindle) muscle fibers Sensory: the secondary afferents of muscle spindles, touch and pressure receptors, and pacinian corpuscles (vibratory sensors)
A-γ		8	40	Motor: the small gamma motoneurons of lamina IX, innervating intrafusal fibers (muscle spindles)
A-δ	III	5	15	Sensory: small, lightly myelinated fibers; touch, pressure, pain, and temperature
B		3	14	Motor: small, lightly myelinated preganglionic autonomic fibers
C	IV	1	2	Motor: all postganglionic autonomic fibers (all are unmyelinated) Sensory: unmyelinated pain and temperature fibers

THE PERIPHERAL NERVOUS SYSTEM

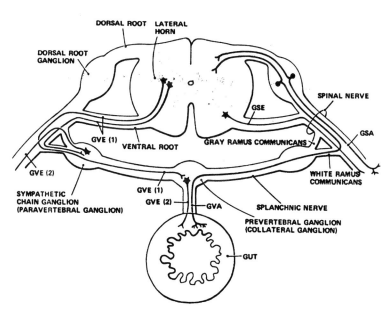

FIG. 13.2. Functional components of a spinal nerve. General somatic afferent (GSA), general visceral afferent (GVA), and general somatic efferent (GSE) fibers and their origin are illustrated on the right and are arbitrarily separated, for clarity, from the general visceral efferent fibers and cells (GVE) (1) and (GVE) (2) on the left. The autonomic (GVE) structures diagrammed here belong to the sympathetic division. (From Gilman S, Gilman SW, eds. *Manter and Gatz's essentials of clinical neuroanatomy and neurophysiology.* Philadelphia: FA Davis, 1992.)

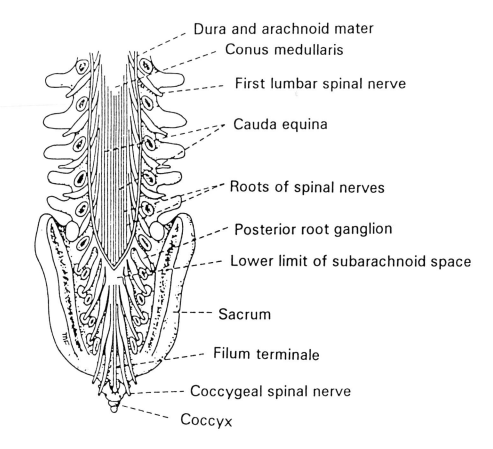

Dura and arachnoid mater
Conus medullaris
First lumbar spinal nerve
Cauda equina
Roots of spinal nerves
Posterior root ganglion
Lower limit of subarachnoid space
Sacrum
Filum terminale
Coccygeal spinal nerve
Coccyx

FIG. 13.3. The cauda equina.

tous structures, and anterior rami. The anterior rami course around and through overlying muscle, forming the lowermost components of the lumbosacral plexus. Branches of the lumbosacral plexus meet with small visceral nerves and form the pelvic plexus. The pelvic plexus overlies and invests in the pelvic muscular floor, thus supplying pelvic floor muscles from a superior aspect, and surrounds and supplies the pelvic viscera. The pelvic plexus is subject to trauma from obstetric delivery or pelvic surgery.

The pudendal nerve is formed in the lower division of the lumbosacral plexus. It leaves the pelvis through the greater sciatic foramen, wraps around the ischial spine, and is firmly invested in obturator fascia (Alcock's canal). It then courses back into the pelvis through the lesser sciatic foramen to provide muscular innervation to the pelvic floor from an inferior aspect. The area of fascial investment of the nerve locks it in place, subjecting it to stretch injury when the pelvic floor descends.

Therapies of neuronal dysfunctions are developing rapidly. Electrical stimulation therapies have provided frequently dramatic improvement in urge incontinence, urgency-frequency syndromes, and nonobstructive retention. As knowledge of protein channels, neurotransmitters, and receptors increases, there is development of new classes of pharmaceutical therapies. With increased availability of therapeutic intervention, diagnosis and localization of pathophysiologic processes is assuming greater importance.

Much of the information necessary for diagnosis may be obtained by careful history and physical examination. When necessary, this information may be supplemented by other measurements of activity, including urodynamics, dynamic cystoproctography, anal manometry, and electrodiagnostic techniques, which are explained in this chapter.

The physiologic processes regarding pelvic organ function involve the central and peripheral nervous system with complex reflex activities, as explained in Chapter 3. Somatic and autonomic motor, somatic, and visceral sensory nerves are all involved.

SOMATIC MOTOR

Somatic motor nerves supply skeletal muscle. Their nerve cell body is in the anterior gray matter of the spinal cord, and a single axon from each cell goes to the effector organ (muscle). Most skeletal muscles are supplied by a large motor axon from an alpha motor neuron cell that goes to extrafascial muscle fibers and a smaller axon from a "gamma" motor neuron cell that goes to intrafascial muscle fibers (spindles) (Fig. 13.4). Using sensory axons, the spindles act in a somatic muscle reflex to control the muscle activity and balance antagonistic muscle action. The somatic motor supply to the urethral and anal sphincter skeletal muscle, however, is different. There are no spindles in the urethral sphincter and relatively few in the anal sphincter; thus, the segmental skeletal reflex system is supplemented by other reflex activities. The sphincters, unlike muscles with abundant spindles, have no antagonist muscle

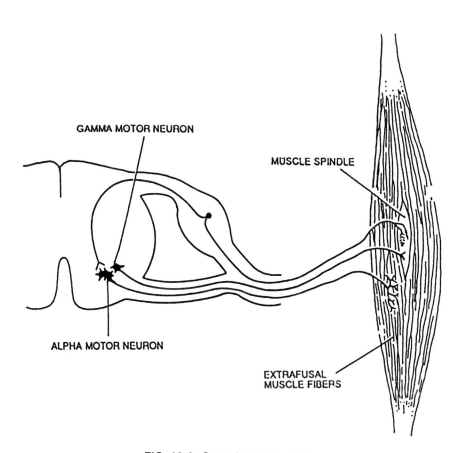

FIG. 13.4. Somatic muscle reflex.

to limit "stretch." They have profuse connective tissue, and length–tension curves are steeper (i.e., the muscle is stiffer), perhaps because of the lack of antagonist.

The group of cell bodies in the spinal cord that give rise to the motor axons supplying the sphincters are collectively called Onuf's nucleus. They are somewhat smaller than alpha anterior horn cells. Unlike other motor neurons, these sacral motor neurons have reciprocal inhibitory interactions with sacral parasympathetic neurons and receive input not only from somatic upper motor neuron pathways but also from the hypothalamus and other autonomic regions. They are also frequently less involved in disease processes affecting other anterior horn cells (e.g., amyotrophic lateral sclerosis or polio).

The sacral somatic motor activity of the pudendal nerve and somatic nerves through the pelvic plexus uses acetylcholine as the chief neurotransmitter, acting through nicotinic receptors, as do most of the body's skeletal muscles. However, there is increasing evidence of striated sphincter muscle having neuromuscular transmission by chemical processes usually seen only with smooth muscle. Both norepinephrine and serotonin mechanisms, usually present with sympathetic activity, are active with the pudendal motor neurons. α_1-Adrenergic receptor antagonists reduce striated urethral sphincter tone, acting through inhibition of sacral pudendal motor neurons, which have noradrenergic nerve terminals and α-adrenergic receptors (1). 5-Hydroxytryptomine (5-HT) (serotonin) systems are also active at the pudendal motor neurons, with evidence that the 5-HT receptor agonists facilitate pudendal reflexes (2). Hence, the sacral motor neurons have distinct properties, unlike other somatic motor neurons.

Somatic Motor Nerve Pathology

Nerve damage may occur at any point from the anterior horn cell to the root (radiculopathy), plexus (plexopathy), peripheral nerve (neuropathy), neuromuscular junction, or muscle fibers.

Anterior horn cell diseases typically do not involve Onuf's nucleus, reflecting the unique properties of these neurons.

Lumbosacral radiculopathies commonly involve bladder and bowel dysfunction. In fact, bladder and bowel involvement is a clinical marker to separate radiculopathy from anterior horn cell disease. The S-2 to S-4 nerve roots going to the pelvis originate in the small terminal portion of the spinal cord (conus medullaris) and constitute the central portion of the cauda equina. Conus medullaris lesions may be produced by ankylosing spondylitis, ependymomas, lipomas, dermoid cysts, transverse myelitis, arteriovenous malformations, and congenital meningomyelocele with cord tethering. They are a fairly common complication of abdominal aortic aneurysm surgery secondary to prolonged aortic clamping.

Cauda equina lesions are very common. Central disk protrusion can affect the bladder and bowel nerve roots, and many clinicians consider bladder and bowel involvement to be a chief indication for surgical treatment of disk protrusion. Cauda equina lesions are seen with congenital caudal aplasia (from diabetic mothers) and congenital and acquired spinal stenosis (pseudoclaudication syndrome). Ankylosing spondylitis, schwannomas, primary and metastatic malignancies, lymphomas, meningiomas, neurofibromas, chordomas, acquired immunodeficiency syndrome, and cytomegalovirus infection are other causes of cauda equina disease. Damage may also occur with distal aortic occlusive disease. Cauda equina lesions secondary to arachnoiditis are seen in episodic fashion, suggesting contamination of epidural agents. Arachnoiditis is also seen with injections of alcohol or phenol or with very high dosages of intrathecal penicillin therapy. Diabetic lumbosacral radiculopathies most commonly involve the L-3 to L-4 roots and are bilateral in half of all cases. These may occur without evidence of diabetic peripheral neuropathy. Radiculopathy should be considered before investigating visceral pathology in diabetic patients with chronic truncal pain. Patients with hereditary motor sensory neuropathies (type I) have increased vulnerability of the cauda equina.

Lumbosacral plexus lesions are most commonly associated with malignancies (cervical, rectal, lymphoma), radiation damage, or hematomas. Electromyography (EMG) is useful in distinguishing plexopathy due to radiation from plexopathy due to recurrence of malignancy, because myokymia (see Needle Electromyography) may be seen with radiation damage.

Mononeuropathies occur frequently in pelvic nerves secondary to injury that may be mechanical, thermal, electrical, radiation, vascular, granulomatous, or from primary or metastatic neoplastic lesions. The leading cause of pelvic mononeuropathy is the mechanical effect (compression and stretching) of labor and delivery. Mechanical compressive nerve damage of permanent nature has been shown to occur with 80 mm Hg pressure for 8 hours. Because second-stage labor forces normally reach maximums of 240 mm Hg pressure (3), it is not surprising to see nerve lesions. Stretch has been shown to cause nerve demyelination if the nerve is stretched 15% of its length (4). The pudendal nerve is stretched 15%, with only 1.35 cm descent of pelvic floor during labor. Thus, pudendal stretch injury is also not surprising.

Pelvic nerve damage that is diffuse and bilaterally symmetric suggests polyneuropathy. Diabetes and alcoholism are likely the leading causes, but polyneuropathies may result from toxicity, metabolic deficiency, immune disorders, and hereditary diseases (Table 13.2). Generally, motor, sensory, and autonomic functions all are affected to some degree. Neuromuscular junction disorders (e.g., myasthenia gravis or myasthenic syn-

TABLE 13.2. *Motor and sensory polyneuropathy*

Acquired immunodeficiency syndrome (AIDS)
Acromegaly
Acute inflammatory polyradiculoneuropathy (Guillain-Barré syndrome)
Angiofollicular lymph node hyperplasia
Arsenic polyneuropathy
Carcinoma
Chronic inflammatory polyradiculoneuropathy
Cryoglobulinemia
Diphtheria
Glue-sniffer's neuropathy
Hereditary neuropathy
Hypothyroidism
Leprosy
Lyme disease
Lymphoma
Monoclonal gammopathy
Motor neuron disease
Multiple demyelinating neuropathy with consistent conduction block
Osteosclerotic myeloma
Pharmaceuticals
  Amiodarone
  Perhexiline
  Suramin
  Lead
  Dapsone
  Didanosine
  Paclitaxel (Taxol)
  Vincristine
Porphyria
Spinal muscular atrophy
Systemic lupus erythematosus
Ulcerative colitis
Waldenström's macroglobulinemia

drome) typically have minor effects on sphincters.

Upper motor neuron lesions may have a profound effect on motor nerves to sphincters as well as on motor neurons to the bladder and bowel. Upper motor neuron control of lower motor neuron skeletal muscle activity is both stimulatory and inhibitory, with the latter predominating. With loss of upper motor neuron control, there is exaggeration of skeletal muscle activity, reflected in increased reflexes. Urodynamically, increased skeletal activity with loss of coordination on visceral activity is typically seen with lesions below the integration center in the pons and is typified by contractions occurring in the sphincter skeletal muscles simultaneously with involuntary vesical contraction (detrusor–sphincter dyssynergia). Cerebral lesions lead to loss of voluntary relaxation of sphincter skeletal activity; hence, a common symptom is hesitancy.

SOMATIC SENSORY

Sensory nerves have their nerve cell bodies outside the spinal cord proper, in the dorsal root ganglion. Embryologically, the dorsal root ganglion neurons, like autonomic ganglion neurons and adrenal medullaris cells, arise from the neural crest, whereas the spinal cord and cell bodies located within it arise from a separate location, the basal plate of the neural groove. This partly explains certain disease processes and growth factors with an affinity for secretory and autonomic nerves.

The sensory nerve cell body gives rise to a single process that splits into a distal component going to the peripheral nerve and a proximal component entering and ascending in the spinal cord.

Peripheral nerves, when injured, have a capacity for repair, whereas nerves within the central nervous system have much less. Hence, the distal process of a sensory nerve may regenerate after injury, but if the proximal branch of the secretory nerve is damaged, it is capable of regeneration up to its junction with the central nervous system only.

Somatic Sensory Nerve Pathology

Sensory effects are possible with involvement of the central nervous system conducting the impulses to the cerebral cortex, involvement of proximal axon of the sensory ganglion such as with radiculopathy, involvement of the nerve cell (neuronopathy), or involvement of the distal axon by plexopathy or neuropathy. Hence, all of the conditions affecting somatic motor axons beyond the central nervous system may also affect somatic sensory. Certain processes, however, have predilection for predominantly sensory neuronal and axonal involvement (Table 13.3). Of particular gynecologic interest is paraneoplastic sensory involvement associated with ovarian cancer. If sensory nerve and cerebellar disease are present in patients demonstrating anti-Purkinje cell antibodies, 80% have ovarian cancer (5).

TABLE 13.3. *Sensory neuronopathy or neuropathy*

Acquired immunodeficiency syndrome (AIDS)
Amyloidosis
B_{12} deficiency
Biliary cirrhosis
Crohn's disease
Drugs
   Cisplatin
   Vincristine
   Aromatic hydrocarbons
   Isoniazid
   Hydralazine
   Nitrofurantoin
   Metronidazole
   Misonidazole
   Pyridoxine toxicity
   Thalidomide toxicity
   Paclitaxel (Taxol)
   Didanosine
   Zalcitabine
Fabry's disease
Friedreich's ataxia
Hereditary sensory neuropathy
Leprosy
Paraneoplastic
Porphyria
Reef fish poisoning
Spinocerebellar degeneration
Tangier's disease
Vasculitic neuropathy
Vitamin E deficiency

The type of sensory involvement relates to the nerve fibers affected. By physical size principles alone, larger fibers are more affected than smaller fibers with focal peripheral nerve damage. Friedrich's ataxia, vitamin B_{12} deficiency, and occasionally subacute sensory neuropathies tend to produce large fiber loss, whereas predominantly small fiber loss is seen in hereditary sensory neuropathy (type I), diabetes, leprosy, amyloidosis, Tangier's disease, Fabry's disease, and congenital insensitivity to pain.

AUTONOMIC OR VISCERAL MOTOR

The autonomic or visceral motor nervous system controls bladder and anorectal smooth muscle activity. It exerts influences that are more continuous and generalized than the somatic system. The continuous tonic activity of visceral motor efferents is due to spontaneous discharge of reticular pacemaker neurons in the brain stem. The visceral motor system, unlike the somatic, is a two-neuron pathway with at least one synapse in the autonomic ganglia. It is separated morphologically and functionally into sympathetic and parasympathetic divisions. The preganglionic autonomic neurons occupy the visceral motor column of the cord (intermediolateral cell column), with sympathetic neurons from T-1 to L-3 segments of the spinal cord and pelvic parasympathetic neurons from S-2 to S-4 segments. These neurons originate from the basal plate of the neural groove and use acetylcholine as principal neurotransmitters. They also synthesize nitric oxide, and some release enkephalin or neurotensin. Their axons leave the cord as small myelinated fibers and synapse with autonomic ganglion neurons.

The autonomic ganglion neurons affect transmission of preganglionic inputs into postganglionic neurons and use acetylcholine with fast excitation (nicotinic receptors), slower excitation (muscarinic receptors), and late slow response mediated by neuropeptides (e.g., substance P). The postganglionic axons are unmyelinated and release acetylcholine (parasympathetic) or norepinephrine (sympathetic) and neuropeptides and adenosine triphosphate (purine) cotransmitters. Sympathetic postganglionic receptors are α- and β-adrenergic receptors. Postganglionic parasympathetic receptors are chiefly muscarinic.

Unlike skeletal muscle, smooth muscle cells have properties of automatism, adaptation, and intramural conduction. Automatism is the ability to sustain rhythmic contractions in the absence of innervation; adaptation is the ability to modify rhythmicity and contractility in response to mechanical factors (e.g., distention); and intramural conduction is the ability to transmit electrical inputs between syncytial fibers, usually by gap junctions. Whereas the main consequence of denervation in skeletal muscle is paralysis and atrophy, the main consequence of autonomic denervation is denervation supersensitivity, involving upregulation of postjunctional receptors. An excellent example of this is detrusor instability occurring as a consequence of postganglionic parasympathetic denervation.

There are basic functional differences in sympathetic and parasympathetic activity. The sympathetic responds to stress, is more diffuse, and its effects have longer duration. The parasympathetic locally controls organs, and its effects are of shorter duration. Most organs have dual sympathetic and parasympathetic control, but the latter predominates in the lower urinary and gastrointestinal tracts.

Pelvic preganglionic sympathetic axons from L-1 to L-3 exit through ventral roots and pass by white rami communicants (white because they are myelinated) of the corresponding spinal nerve to reach the paravertebral chain. At this level, some run rostrally and caudally. Other synapse and postganglionic axons return to peripheral nerves through gray (unmyelinated) rami communicants and travel with the nerves, such as the pudendal and pelvic somatic nerves. Other sympathetic preganglionic neurons constitute the prevertebral sympathetic system.

These neurons pass through the paravertebral chain without synapsing to follow prevertebral vessels. These lumbar splanchnic nerves synapse on inferior mesenteric (presacral) ganglia that provide postganglionic input to hypogastric and pelvic plexuses to innervate pelvic and perineal organs and glands.

Preganglionic parasympathetic fibers arise from S-2 to S-4 spinal cord segments, exit through ventral roots, and join the pelvic plexus by direct branches (nervi erigentes) to synapse at the ganglia. The ganglia are located within the visceral walls, and postganglionic fibers are very short.

Colorectal Effects

The smooth muscle of the gut has intrinsic (myogenic) and neuronal control. The intrinsic gut myogenic activity is coordinated with excitatory and inhibitory motor neurons for peristalsis control and with secretomotor neurons for gastrointestinal exocrine secretion. Generally, sympathetic activity, centered chiefly at the L-3 and L-4 cord levels, acts to reduce gut mechanosensitivity, except at the internal anal sphincter, where noradrenergic activity increases contractility.

The parasympathetic axons act throughout the gut to increase contractility (doing so through the vagus nerve for most of the gastrointestinal tract, with S-2 to S-4 parasympathetic supply going to the descending colon and rectum). At the internal anal sphincter, however, parasympathetic activity promotes relaxation.

Bladder Effects

Sympathetic outflow to the bladder acts on α-adrenergic receptors to contract the outlet (especially in males, presumably to protect against retrograde ejaculation) and relax the detrusor, acting on β-adrenergic receptors. Parasympathetic effects act to contract the detrusor. Sympathetic loss may lead to decreased proximal urethral smooth muscle tone and speculatively may have some association with loss of detrusor relaxation. Parasympathetic effects are much more pronounced, with loss of them leading to loss of effective detrusor contraction (areflexia); hence, cystometric studies are of value. Coordination of bladder visceral efferent and somatic activity is chiefly a function occurring in the pons. Central nervous system lesions above the pons, then, are characterized by coordinated loss of control (uninhibited detrusor contractions), whereas those below the pons have detrusor–sphincter dyssynergia.

Autonomic or Visceral Motor Nerve Pathology

There are generalized autonomic syndromes also involving bladder and bowel dysfunction. The most common neurologic cause of detrusor areflexia is diabetes. Syndromes of pure cholinergic dysfunction exist and are characterized by bladder atony, Adie's pupil, alacrima, constipation, dry mouth, hyperpyrexia, cardiovagal failure, and impotency. Etiologies include Lambert-Eaton syndrome (myasthenia syndrome, frequently associated with malignancies) and neuromuscular junction toxicity from organic phosphates in insecticides or botulinum toxin in improperly canned food. In acute inflammatory demyelinating polyradiculoneuropathy (Guillain-Barré syndrome), urinary retention early in the course of the disease is an early predictor of severity because more than 80% of these patients require ventilatory assistance later (6). Acute intermittent porphyria is an autosomal dominant disease that generally presents in the third or fourth decade with premenstrual abdominal pain, constipation, voiding dysfunction, quadriparesis, and bathing-trunk dyschezia. Generalized sympathetic disorders tend to be length dependent and are characterized by postural hypotension and overactivity early with cold sweaty feet and loss of activity later with red, swollen, anhidrotic distal extremities. Disease processes primarily affecting autonomic nerves are listed in Table 13.4.

TABLE 13.4. *Predominantly autonomic*

Acute inflammatory demyelinating
  polyradiculoneuropathy
Amyloid
Diabetes
Pandysautonomia
Paraneoplastin
Perhexiline
Porphyria
Riley-Day syndrome
Shy-Drager syndrome
Thallium
Vincristine

VISCERAL SENSORY

Volume and tension receptors distributed throughout the bladder muscle wall are carried chiefly by the pelvic nerve to the sacral cord; bladder base pain receptors are in the submucosa and are carried by hypogastric nerve pathways to the L-1 to L-3 portion of the cord. Proximal urethral sensations are carried by both visceral afferent pathways, and sphincter muscle proprioception is also carried by pudendal pathways.

Enteric afferents are in submucosal plexus and mesenteric plexus. Splanchnic nerves carry enteric afferent input to the prevertebral ganglia that act to integrate local reflexes with the organs. The chief afferent neurotransmitters are vasointestinal polypeptide and acetylcholine with neurotensin (facilitating) and enkephalin (inhibiting) cotransmitters. The afferents course through the dorsal roots, directly through the sacral pelvic splanchnics or indirectly through white rami communicants to lumbar levels, to the nerve cell body. The nerve cell body, just as for somatic afferents, is located in the dorsal root ganglion.

The pelvic visceral afferents are A-delta and C fibers. Sensations of filling, fullness, desire to micturate, urgency, and pain can be elicited at different degrees of bladder filling. Anorectally, the ability to distinguish gas, liquid, and solid exists in addition. Most painful sensations are carried in the pelvic and not the hypogastric nerve, and frequency and urgency can be relieved by selective neurectomy of S-3 (7). The sensation that micturition is immi-

nent arises from the bladder neck. Sensory endings are often perivascular. Parasympathetic efferents can excite bladder afferent receptors similarly to the way somatic gamma efferents excite muscle spindle afferents. Spinal transmission of pelvic organ sensation is found in dorsal columns (1-degree afferents, touch, pressure), lateral columns (temperature, fullness, desire to micturate, sexual sensations), and ventral columns (pain, touch).

Visceral Sensory Pathology

Knowledge regarding bladder visceral afferents has expanded greatly, allowing new understanding of bladder dysfunction by appreciating the importance of development of C-fiber afferentation and overactive bladder conditions secondary to such development. The suggestions for such a neurologic basis for the overactive bladder are that damage to central inhibitory pathways or sensitization of peripheral afferent terminals in the bladder can, by neural plasticity, produce or unmask primitive spinal voiding reflexes that trigger bladder overactivity. In other words, pathologic processes either in the nervous system (e.g., spinal cord injury) or in the lower urinary tract (e.g., inflammation or obstruction) lead to a similar type of neuronal rearrangement, nature's attempt at compensating, which produces bladder instability.

Normal supraspinal voiding reflexes are triggered by lightly myelinated A-delta afferent nerve fibers. The primitive spinal–bladder reflexes associated with bladder overactivity are triggered by C-fiber afferent (slowly conducting, unmyelinated pain and temperature) neurons. The C fibers are deactivated by the C-fiber afferent neurotoxin capsaicin. Studying the effect of capsaicin on the micturition reflex in cats revealed that C-fiber afferents are not involved in initiating reflex micturition in normal cats but play an essential role in triggering automatic micturition in chronic spinal cord–injured cats (8).

The phenotypic changes in capsaicin-sensitive, unmyelinated C-fiber bladder afferent neurons (neural plasticity) produced by spinal cord injury and by urethral obstruction are similar. The phenotypic changes include somal hypertrophy (up to 50%) and increased excitability due to changes in the Na^+ and K^+ ion channels (9).

The C fibers are responsible for inducing bladder hyperreflexia by initiating spinal reflexes. An immunocytochemical method to stain fos protein encoded by *c-fos* gene in neurons involved in a stimulated reflex pathway was used to study bladder afferent effects in the spinal cord in spinal cord–injured rats (10,11). Bladder distention in these rats produced increased numbers and an altered distribution of fos-immunoreactive (fos-IR) cells after the spinal injury. The pattern and number of the fos-IR cells were similar to those obtained after noxious irritation of the bladder (stimulation of pain and temperature C fibers by intravesical instillation of acetic acid) in control animals. Pretreatment with capsaicin significantly reduced the number of fos-IR cells, indicating that the capsaicin-sensitive C-fiber afferents mediate the spinal reflex.

Rats with cyclophosphamide-induced cystitis demonstrated similar distributions of fos-IR cells in the cord that, again, were reduced with pretreatment with capsaicin (12).

Thus, local inflammatory bladder processes induce C-afferent spinal reflex pathways.

Urethral obstruction also is associated with enhancement of spinal micturition reflexes and neuronal hypertrophy (13). Interestingly and importantly, the neuronal (and bladder) hypertrophy is avoided if urinary diversion is performed after the spinal transection, suggesting that factors released in the hypertrophied bladder are responsible for the neural changes.

Thus, bladder instability, which clinically is associated with spinal cord injury, inflammatory lower urinary tract disorders, and urethral obstruction, has a common pathophysiologic event characterized by development of C-fiber afferent neural hypertrophy and increased spinal reflexes. These changes may be set into motion by primary spinal cord activity leading to neurogenically mediated bladder changes when associated with spinal cord injury (14). In association with urethral obstruction, these changes are now known to be influenced by neural–target organ interactions induced by neurotrophic signals originating in the bladder.

The neurotrophic signals are produced by nerve growth factor (NGF) that is known to be produced by parenchymal cells in the bladder. Hypertrophy of the bladder after urethral obstruction has a temporal correlation between NGF content, neuronal hypertrophy, bladder weight, and voiding frequency. Autoimmunity to NGF abolished the hypertrophy of the bladder neurons, reduced sacral afferent labeling, eliminated enhancement of spinal micturition reflex, and prevented the urinary frequency that accompanies obstruction (15).

Capsaicin and its ultra potent analogue resinifera toxin, specific C-fiber neurotoxins, are now undergoing intravesical clinical trials for treatment of overactive bladder (16). Additionally, sacral neural stimulation therapy has been shown capable of reversing C-fiber afferentation (17).

DIAGNOSIS OF SOMATIC MOTOR DYSFUNCTION

Somatic motor nerve loss as it reflects bladder or bowel function is related to skeletal muscle activity at the urethra or the anal canal. Rectal examination reveals a loss of squeeze, but resting tone may be relatively normal because it is constituted chiefly (80%) by smooth muscle. Augmenting the physical examination is anal manometry, which can quantitate the squeeze pressure, and dynamic cystoproctography, which can demonstrate loss of puborectalis contraction effect on the anorectal angle. The typical history with pure somatic motor loss is inability to squeeze to prevent passage of flatus or liquid bowel content and inability to squeeze to relocate solid content back into the rectal reservoir.

As for the bladder, loss of somatic motor activity in the urethra leads to symptoms of stress incontinence, and on urodynamics, typical diagnostic features of genuine stress urinary incontinence (vesical pressure exceeding urethral pressure during increased abdominal pressure in the absence of a detrusor contraction) may be seen. On physical examination, pelvic floor muscular weakness may be evident. Reflexes are helpful clinically for localization of lesions. Conus medullaris lesions have more symmetric bilateral loss of clitoral–anal reflex with S2- to S-4 dermatomal sensory changes. Cauda equina lesions may demonstrate varying symmetry in sensory dermatome testing and clitoral–anal reflex and may have absent knee (L-3 to L-4) reflexes and hyperactive Achilles (S-1) reflexes with higher lesions or loss of Achilles reflex with lower lesions.

Electrodiagnostic Features of S-2 to S-4 Somatic Motor Loss

The surface EMG (see Electromyography) reflects total muscle fiber activity and as such gives information of total functioning mass when carefully standardized (Fig. 13.5).

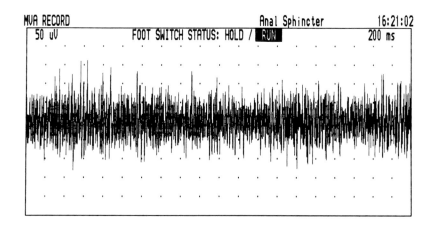

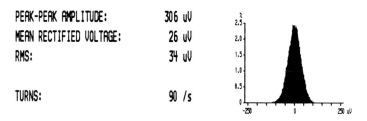

FIG. 13.5. Maximum voluntary activity (MVA) with amplitude histogram of anal sphincter with squeeze. Peak–peak amplitude, amplitude from highest to lowest displayed point on trace; mean rectified voltage, mean amplitude of rectified waveform; RMS, root mean square value of recorded trace; turns, calculated number of peaks exceeding 100 μV normalized to equivalent time base of 1 second. Machine parameters: 200-ms time base, 50-μV gain, 10-kHz and 20-Hz high- and low-cut filters, respectively.

Pudendal and perineal compound muscle action potentials (see Pudendal Nerve Motor Conduction) have reduced amplitude and prolonged distal latencies, reflecting the degree of axonal loss and demyelination, respectively. The changes are bilaterally symmetric with conus lesions, have variable bilaterality with cauda equina lesions, and are unilateral with peripheral mononeuropathies. Sensory conduction studies are normal with radiculopathies, even with clinical sensory loss, because the disease process is proximal to the dorsal root ganglion; hence, the distal axon (the one being tested) is not affected (see Diagnosis of Somatic Sensory Dysfunction). In plexus or peripheral neuropathy, sensory studies are abnormal. Sphincter needle examination (see Needle Electromyography) acutely (0 to 7 days) shows reduced recruitment; at 7 to 15 days, insertional activity will increase, and fibrillation begins to appear. After months, motor unit potential morphology reflects reinnervation by developing increased phases, duration, and amplitude. Those changes are related to the severity and duration of the neuropathic process and hence are helpful adjuncts to determine prognosis.

Sacral Reflex Studies

Clitoral–anal, urethral–anal, and bladder–anal reflex studies are abnormal with conus, cauda equina, or peripheral (pudendal) motor lesions, the abnormality being limited to the affected sides in unilateral radicular or peripheral nerve lesions. Pelvic plexus lesions may be suggested by abnormal urethral–anal and bladder–anal reflexes and normal clitoral–anal reflex.

Supportive evidence for somatic motor involvement with lumbosacral radiculopathy, plexopathy, or peripheral neuropathy is gained by performing lower extremity conduction studies (e.g., peroneal and tibial motor nerve conduction studies and sacral and peroneal sensory nerve conduction

studies) and needle examination of lower extremity and lumbosacral paraspinal muscles. In fact, such studies are necessary to allow correct interpretation of the pelvic nerve studies.

Diagnosis of upper motor neuron lesions can be assisted electrodiagnostically by studying recruitment with needle EMG. Another important sign of upper motor neuron disorder on sacral reflex studies is loss of volitional abolition of the clitoral–anal and urethral–anal reflexes during voiding.

DIAGNOSIS OF SOMATIC SENSORY DYSFUNCTION

Somatic sensory loss to the urethra or anal canal results in the patient not recognizing passage of urine through the urethra or passage of material through the anal canal. The many physiologic reflexes dependent on such somatic sensation are abnormal. The resulting clinical incontinence is difficult to treat, and surgery has disappointing results.

Physical examination may show sensory deficits in S-2, S-3, and S-4 dermatome testing; such loss is not seen with pelvic plexus sensory neuropathy.

Adjuncts to diagnosis include anal manometry, wherein the patient does not perceive filling of the anal canal balloon. Normally, rectal distention leads to internal anal sphincter relaxation by an intrinsic gut reflex, the rectal anal inhibitory reflex. This reflex is an intrinsic enteric reflex, tends to be preserved with most sensory neuropathies, and lost principally with myenteric plexus loss, as in Hirschsprung's disease. However, when somatic sensation is lost, there is a failure of the external anal sphincter to contract to replace content to the rectum for storage, and incontinence occurs without sensation. This can be demonstrated on anal manometry with concomitant surface and sphincter EMG. Likewise, when urine passes into the urethra (without attempt to void), reflex periurethral skeletal muscle activity occurs unless blocked centrally (as during urination). This reflex may be lost with somatic sensory loss.

Electrodiagnostic Adjuncts to Diagnosis of Somatic Sensory Loss

Clitoral–anal reflex testing includes determining the level of sensory perception of pudendal afferents paraclitorally (see Clitoral–Anal Reflex). With complete sensory loss, the reflex is absent. Current perception threshold for different sensory nerve fiber types may also be performed.

If small fiber sensory afferents are affected, urethral–anal reflex may have elevated sensory threshold (see Urethral–Anal Reflex). If the visceral sensory pathway is still intact, the reflex will not be absent. With pure sensory loss, sphincter motor activity is preserved, and with surface or needle sphincter EMG, conscious regulation (e.g., suppressing activity by trying to void) remains intact without evidence of denervation, but reflex activity depending on the somatic sensory loop is absent. In conditions with clinical sensory loss, abnormalities of sensory nerve action potentials are present if the process is at the dorsal root ganglion or distal. In radiculopathy, the sensory nerve function distal to the dorsal root ganglion cell body is preserved. Sacral reflexes may be completely normal in patients with complete loss of sensation if the lesion is above the conus medullaris. A generalized process will be suggested by abnormalities in other sensory studies (e.g., sural and superficial peroneal) or upper limb nerve conduction studies.

Somatosensory evoked potentials (see Cortical Evoked Potentials) are useful in demonstrating and localizing disease process. If pelvic reflexes and the peripheral component of pudendal or posterior tibial evoked potential studies are normal with loss or delay in cervical or cerebral potentials, the disease process may be localized to the spinal cord or supraspinal areas.

DIAGNOSIS OF VISCERAL MOTOR DYSFUNCTION

Most nerve conduction and EMG studies evaluate large nerve fiber activity and hence may not be sensitive to small nerve fiber autonomic dysfunction. When the autonomic process is generalized, quantitative testing is available. Distal small fiber neuropathy is frequently not associated with electrodiagnostic abnormalities but is associated with distal sudomotor abnormalities of either quantitative sudomotor axon reflex (QSART) (see Autonomic Tests) or the thermoregulatory sweat test in more than 80% of cases (18).

Various tests of systemic vasoconstrictor (sympathetic) and cardiovagal (parasympathetic) function are available and helpful in generalized autonomic dysfunction.

The best available test of sacral parasympathetic function remains the cystometric study, and ambulatory cystometrics will improve the poor sensitivity of this test.

DIAGNOSIS OF VISCERAL SENSORY DYSFUNCTION

History of Loss of Sensation with Anorectal or Urinary Tract Filling or Passage

Cystometric testing of the urinary tract may reveal delay of first sensation of filling or of maximum capacity. This is frequently associated with overflow incontinence. On anal manometry, loss of sensation with rectal balloon filling is noted until exaggerated levels may be seen. Megacolon or bladder may be seen on visual studies. Sacral reflexes and delay of sensation (increased threshold) with electrical stimuli may be seen when the proximal urethra or the bladder is stimulated in the urethral–anal and bladder–anal reflex tests. Evoked potentials from the proximal urethra can trace the sensory afferent pathway completely to the cortex.

Visceral afferent dysfunction may be part of a generalized picture of autonomic or peripheral neuropathy, and ancillary testing of the peripheral nerves and autonomic nerves may be helpful.

ELECTRODIAGNOSTIC TESTS

A preliminary report of the World Health Organization committee (19) on pelvic clinical neurophysiology gives an overview of current status of electrodiagnostic testing:

> Although clinical neurophysiology is practiced in every neurology department, uroneurophysiological tests do not seem to be widely available even in university hospitals. They require some special expertise, but particularly additional clinical background knowledge which neurophysiology experts usually do not possess. . . . As in 'general' neurophysiology (in other body areas), patients with malformations, traumatic, compressive, infiltrative or degenerative lesions of the sacral nervous system would be considered candidates for appropriate testing to help with diagnosis and prognosis (and documentation), but always within a framework of the neurourological/uroneurological clinical evaluation. Results from clinical exam and neurophysiological testing should ideally be combined to support a diagnosis of a particular nervous system lesion in an individual patient. All data taken together may be declared compatible with a particular dysfunction, or may be judged insufficient to explain a particular dysfunction (incontinence). All these conclusions are, however, extrapolated from expert opinion, based on experience with patients with known neurological (axonal or demyelinative) lesions, and are not based on controlled studies. . . .

Testing may prove useful in particular subgroups of incontinent patients in whom particular invasive treatment procedures (which rely on well-preserved neuromuscular structures which should be appropriately ascertained and identified) are contemplated, such as implanted therapeutic electrical stimulation.

Electromyography

EMG is the recording of electrical potentials generated by the depolarization of muscle fibers. In most skeletal muscles of the body, the muscle can be voluntarily relaxed to the point of absent electrical activity, but the sphincters are only electrically quiet during voiding.

Surface electrodes are of great value in pelvic function studies, recording skeletal muscle activity over a relatively large area. They are used to monitor voluntary muscle contraction during kinesiologic studies, such as with urodynamics or anal manometry. Surface electrodes are generally square or round metal plates made of platinum or silver and come in different sizes, most commonly 1×1 cm. Reduction of resistance between skin and electrode generally requires cleansing with alcohol and scraping the surface corneum and using electrode conductive cream. Surface electrodes are also used to record evoked compound nerve or muscle action potentials or to stimulate peripheral nerves. They are also used as reference or ground electrodes.

Surface electrodes may be applied to a Foley catheter to record or stimulate from the bladder base or proximal urethra. Various types of surface electrodes on anal plugs or vaginal sponges exist. Reproducibility and standardization requires use of specific types of electrodes, and electrode type and size are important to include when establishing laboratory values. Quantification of surface EMG activity

TABLE 13.5. *Sphincter maximum voluntary activity in 12 subjects aged 35–65 years*[a]

	Peak–peak (µV)	Mean voltage	Rectified	Root mean squared
EAS rest	96 ± 47 (41–191)	5 ± 4 (1–11)		8 ± 4 (3–17)
EAS squeeze	341 ± 165 (125–620)	25 ± 13 (9–40)		35 ± 17 (12–64)
Urethra rest	26 ± 10 (15–50)	2 ± 1 (1–3)		2 ± 1 (1–4)
Urethra squeeze	70 ± 40 (25–166)	6 ± 3 (1–13)		8 ± 5 (2–18)
Urethra rest (needle electromyogram)		9 ± 3 (6–4)		14 ± 4 (10–22)

[a]Values are means ± SD with ranges in parentheses.
EAS, external anal sphincter.

in the proximal urethra and anal canal in normal subjects is given in Table 13.5. This has been helpful in diagnosing patients with intrinsic sphincter deficiency (those patients who respond poorly to standard urethropexy therapy and may require sling or other management) because they typically have loss of urethral skeletal muscle activity. The needle urethral quantification has been found to be predictive of patient response to Burch urethropexy (20).

Needle Electromyography

Placing a needle in a muscle has certain advantages over surface EMG recording. The source of the electrical activity is more certain, and more sensitive testing is possible. Needle EMG can give information concerning denervation, reinnervation, upper and lower motor neuron function, and activity and time course of neurologic disease. There are various types of needles, for example, monopolar, concentric, bipolar, macro, and single fiber, which vary in recording surface, pickup areas, and expense. Most studies today are done with concentric needles because data obtained tend to be more reliable with the fixed electrode and newer disposable needles are arguably as comfortable and inexpensive as monopolar needles. Features studied with needle EMG include insertional activity, spontaneous activity, recruitment, and motor unit potential characteristics.

Insertional activity is the electrical activity created by movement of the needle through muscle fibers. Normally, this activity lasts less than 500 ms. Activity is increased in early denervation states and decreased in conditions of muscle degeneration and replacement with fatty or collagenous tissue.

Spontaneous activity occurs involuntarily. In most skeletal muscles at rest, there is absence of electrical activity except for spontaneous activity. Sphincter needle EMG studies are preceded by local application (for 20 minutes) of lidocaine 2.5% and prilocaine 2.5% cream. The constant firing of activity in the sphincter makes spontaneous activity assessment more difficult but still possible with experience. Spontaneous activity can be normal or abnormal. Normal spontaneous activity is activity at the end plate of the muscle (area of nerve innervation) and is due to muscle fibers firing because the nerve terminal to that fiber is irritated. Abnormal spontaneous activity is composed of fibrillations, fasciculations, myotonia, myokymia, neuromyotonia, and complex repetitive discharges. There are distinctive patterns for each and fairly distinct associations of pathophysiologic states with each. An example is a form of complex repetitive discharge (pseudomyotonia) seen in the urethral skeletal muscle in many cases of urinary retention.

The motor unit action potentials observed with activation of the muscle follow sequential patterns of increasing the rate of firing and acquiring additional motor units when the force of contraction is increased. The type of recruitment can be measured with needle EMG and follows generally distinctive patterns in normal, neurogenic, or myogenic disease states.

The motor unit action potentials reflect the electrophysiologic view of the motor unit, which is defined as anterior horn cell, its axon, and all the muscle fibers innervated by that given axon. In disease states characterized by denervation, active reinnervation occurs, if possible, by adjacent axons sending spouts to reinnervate the denervated muscle fibers. This leads to different morphology of the existing motor unit that is reflected in the motor unit action potential viewed by the exploring needle. Quantifiable features of the motor unit action potential include rise time (time for potential to go from extreme location positive or negative to the opposite, indicates proximity of the needle to the source of the electrical activity), amplitude, duration, and number of phases (Fig. 13.6).

The conversion of analogue to digital needle examination data and the availability of low-cost fast microcomputers are leading to the development of automated techniques of evaluating motor unit action potentials. These techniques have the possible benefits of examining later acquired potentials (those present with increased muscle force); reducing examiner bias; and improving accuracy, reliability, and result comparisons. Automatic de-

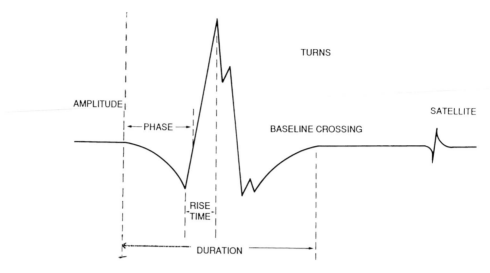

FIG. 13.6. Motor unit action potential.

composition EMG is one such method developed by Dorfman and colleagues (21). Using this methodology, we found the data on sphincter studies in volunteer subjects as presented in Table 13.6. These techniques are as yet problematic, but the potential for development of objective testing with much more uniform application is great.

Needle EMG shows some abnormality virtually anytime there is an organic component of neuromuscular disorder that is significant enough to be symptomatic. Besides urethral and anal sphincters, other pelvic floor muscles (e.g., puborectalis and pubococcygeus) may be examined. Because nerve supply to the puborectalis and external anal sphincter varies, we found it clinically helpful to select the healthiest portion of the anal sphincter closure mechanism to use in sphincter repair.

Previously performed needle EMG mapping of the external anal sphincter has now been replaced by anal ultrasound, but in many situations, it remains more accurate in defining location of skeletal muscle.

Nerve Conduction Studies

Nerve conduction studies can test the integrity of a nerve, the integrity of the muscle supplied by the nerve, and the integrity of the neuromuscular junction. Neuropathies may be categorized as focal or diffuse, root, plexus, nerve, branch, or neuromuscular junction. Time course (e.g., acute, subacute, or chronic) can be depicted, and fiber-type involvement (e.g., sensory, motor, or autonomic) can be suggested. Lower extremity nerve conduction studies are performed in conjunction with

TABLE 13.6. *Automatic decomposition electromyelography of sphincter muscles in asymptomatic female subjects aged 33–45 years (n = 10)*

	Urethral			Anal		
	Rest	Squeeze	Cough	Rest	Squeeze	Cough
Duration (ms)	5.6 ± 3.1	6.7 ± 3.9	4.8 ± 1.3	4.0 ± 1.7	4.7 ± 1.0	4.6 ± 1.5
Amplitude (ms)	58 ± 24	55 ± 16	54 ± 15	39 ± 19	49 ± 7	58 ± 16
Firing rate (Hz)	12.7 ± 10.5	11.1 ± 3.9	14.8 ± 7.5	27.1 ± 12.1	28.9 ± 12.1	19.2 ± 13.8

pelvic floor studies because statuses of the cauda equina, lumbosacral plexus, and generalized neuropathy (which is typically length dependent) are all in part measurable with such studies. Furthermore, interpretation of the pelvic nerve studies must be in the context of the given patient's general neuronal status. Hence, peroneal motor and sensory studies, tibial motor studies, and sural sensory studies are useful as screens when evaluating pelvic neuronal status with pudendal studies.

Pudendal Nerve Motor Conduction

The pudendal nerve can be stimulated at the level of the ischial spine. Such stimulation may be performed with probes or with electrodes attached to the examiner's fingertip. The latter is preferred because the ischial spine may be located more comfortably and reliably if the examiner has the feedback from the finger. The St. Mark's disposable electrode (Fig. 13.7) provides an excellent vehicle for fingertip stimulation of the pudendal nerve. The response to the pudendal nerve stimulation is recorded by 9-mm silver chloride electrodes placed 1 cm lateral (G1) and 1 cm posterior (G2) to the anal opening when testing the inferior hemorrhoidal branch of the pudendal nerve or by electrodes on the Foley catheter when recording the perineal (urethral) branch of the pudendal nerve. The resulting waveform obtained is a compound muscle action potential (CMAP), and measurable quantities include latency, amplitude area, and waveform (Fig. 13.8). The latency

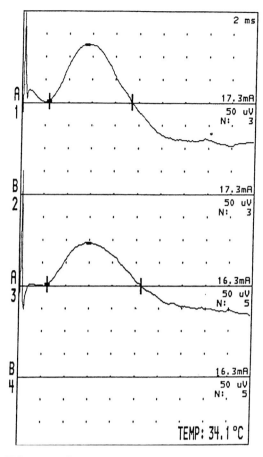

FIG. 13.8. Compound muscle action potentials with pudendal nerve stimulation (pudendal nerve terminal motor latency study). **A1**: Right pudendal stimulation and right anal recording. **A3**: Left pudendal stimulation and left anal recording. Machine parameters: 2-ms time base, 50-μV gain, 0.05-ms pulse duration, 1-Hz repetition rate, 10-kHz and 10-Hz high- and low-cut filters, respectively.

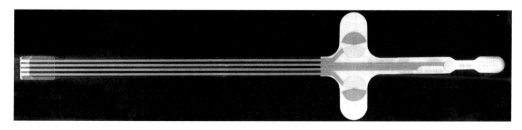

FIG. 13.7. St. Mark's pudendal electrode.

reflects the time involved for nerve conduction from the ischial spine to the muscle, the transmission across the neuromuscular junction, and the resulting muscle fiber contractions, summating to form the CMAP. The latency is somewhat prolonged with loss of large fast conducting axons but even more influenced by processes of demyelination. The latency itself correlates little with strength and hence with clinical muscle force. The amplitude reflects maximal stimulation, wherein the amount of stimulation of the nerve is increased to the level where no further increases in amplitudes of the CMAP is obtainable. The amplitude is related to the total axonal content of the nerve and hence has more relationship clinically with resulting muscle strength. Most processes involving nerve damage have both demyelination and axonal loss, so that latency and amplitude have considerable but not invariable direct relationship.

Most pudendal nerve conduction studies in the literature have used latency as the principal determinant, whereas amplitude is more meaningful. The problem has been one of reproducibility. The standard St. Mark's pudendal technique involves stimulating the nerve at the ischial spine intrarectally, and the pickup electrodes at the base of the examiner's finger records the activity of the external anal sphincter. Interobserver latency determinations have been consistent, but amplitude observations have been variable (Table 13.7). This is apparently because of variations in location of the recording electrode relative to the external anal sphincter, depending on the examiner's finger size. With standard positioning of the recording electrodes on paraanal skin, much more consistency in amplitude has been gained, allowing this valuable parameter to be useful clinically. Amplitudes of the perineal branch CMAP have been shown to be predictive of outcome with sacral neuromodulation therapy in patients with urge incontinence and urgency-frequency syndromes (22).

Another great advantage of this technique modification is that the nerve can now be stimulated vaginally instead of rectally, a comfortable alternative for most women. The pudendal conduction study has other limitations. Conduction blocks cannot be determined because of the inability to stimulate the nerve above and below a possible lesion. Sacral root stimulation can be accomplished, but it is difficult to know in any given patient whether total pudendal root supply has been adequately stimulated. Obtaining proximal motor nerve values by F waves (recording rebound motor axon potentials occurring by impulse traveling to the anterior horn cell and returning to the muscle being recorded) is difficult technically because the short section of nerve under study prevents recording of the rebound event.

Another limitation of pudendal nerve studies is failure, in many studies, to use age-matched control values. Pudendal motor

TABLE 13.7. *Comparison of pudendal motor nerve conduction methodologies in 12 female subjects aged 34–46 years*

	Standard—St. Mark's[a]	Modified methodology[b]
Latency (ms)		
Mean ± SD	2.1 ± 0.3	2.2 ± 0.4
Range	1.5–2.7	1.6–2.9
Interrater variability (%)	4	1
Amplitude (μV)		
Mean ± SD	432 ± 160	99 ± 44
Range	190–760	34–182
Interrater variability (%)	34	1

[a]Stimulation site, ischial spine via rectal approach. Recording, electrodes at base of examiner's finger.

[b]Stimulation site, ischial spine via vaginal approach. Recording, paraanal surface electrodes.

TABLE 13.8. *Normative data for pudendal motor nerve conduction studies*

	Pudendal motor terminal latency (ms)	Perineal motor terminal latency (ms)
Subjects (n = 20) nulliparous, ages 16–30 yr (mean, 23)	2.0 ± 0.3 (1.4–2.4)	2.3 ± 0.3 (1.7–2.9)
Subjects (n = 13) nulliparous, ages 35–65 yr (mean, 46)	2.3 ± 0.4 (1.5–3.5)	2.4 ± 0.4 (1.7–3.8)
Amplitude (μV)	92 ± 51 (34–182)	155 ± 127 (21–466)
Subjects (n = 28), parous, ages 35–66 yr (mean, 43)	2.3 ± 0.4 (1.8–3.3)	2.6 ± 0.4 (2.0–3.1)
Amplitude (μV)		52 ± 27 (26–99)

terminal latencies have age-related normal values, apart from the effects of parity (Table 13.8).

Despite these limitations, pudendal nerve conduction studies provide an important and helpful determinant that, when used in conjunction with other parameters, can be very helpful in increasing understanding of pelvic neuropathy.

Obtaining sensory nerve conduction studies on the pudendal nerve has been technically very difficult.

Current perception threshold studies represent another modality of sensory testing. This test is performed by applying surface electrodes and delivering stimuli at 2 kHz, 250 Hz, and 5 Hz. The relative amount of constant current allowing perception of the stimuli is determined. Normal data have been collected for stimulation of the pelvic floor (Table 13.9).

Sacral Reflexes

Sacral reflexes are reflex contractions of striated muscle structures of the pelvic floor, occurring in response to stimulation of the perineum or other pelvic visceral sites. The three used most commonly in our laboratory are the clitoral–anal, urethral–anal, and bladder–anal reflexes.

Clitoral–Anal Reflex

This reflex may be obtained clinically by touching the clitoral region with a cotton swab and observing contraction in the external anal sphincter. About 10% of neurologically normal females do not have the reflex clinically, although it is present with electrodiagnostic testing, a method first suggested by Rushworth in 1967 (23). The reflex tests the afferent and efferent pudendal nerve pathways and hence the roots of the cauda equina and the conus medullaris. The reflex has two components, the first occurring at a 30- to 50-ms latency and the second at 60- to 70-ms latency. Hence, the response is polysynaptic, with the second component representing suprasacral reflexes. In some normal subjects, a paired stimulus may be required, with the test stimulus applied 5 ms after the conditioning stimulus. The response is recorded by the anal electrodes as described

TABLE 13.9. *Perineal current perception thresholds in 15 subjects aged 23–57 years*

Sensory nerve fiber type	Stimulus frequency	Right paraclitoral[a]	Left paraclitoral[a]	Right paraanal[a]	Left paraanal[a]
Aβ	2 kHz	1.62 ± 0.38 (1.08–2.33)	1.75 ± 0.34 (1.13–2.23)	1.42 ± 0.44 (0.53–2.08)	1.13 ± 0.36 (0.58–1.88)
Aδ	250 Hz	0.34 ± 0.19 (0.08–0.63)	0.41 ± 0.23 (0.13–0.98)	0.40 ± 0.18 (0.08–0.58)	0.40 ± 0.20 (0.03–0.78)
C	5 Hz	0.19 ± 0.15 (0.03–0.58)	0.20 ± 0.13 (0.05–0.48)	0.25 ± 0.17 (0.07–0.58)	0.29 ± 0.28 (0.03–0.93)

[a]Values are means ± SD with ranges in parentheses.

for pudendal nerve terminal motor latency study (see Pudendal Nerve Motor Conduction) and may selectively be recorded on the left and right sides. Stimulation likewise may be done on either the left or right side of the clitoris. Single responses are recorded and compared because averaging works poorly owing to slight variability in response latency. Localized lesions may be indicated as being either afferent or efferent and right or left (Fig. 13.9). This reflex is suppressed during voiding. Failure of such suppression has been found to be highly sensitive in detecting spinal cord lesions above the sacral level (24).

The intensity of stimulation used for the response is 3 to 4 times the intensity at perception threshold, which is generally less than 9 mA of constant current stimulation.

Urethral–Anal Reflex

Using a catheter-mounted ring electrode for stimulation, a reflex response may be obtained at the right and left external anal sphincter with repeated single epochs of stimulation as with the clitoral–anal reflex response. This technique was termed urethral EMG by Bradley (25). This reflex has a long latency of 60 to 90 ms because the very proximal urethral response is carried

by small myelinated or unmyelinated pelvic and hypogastric nerves and the pathway is multisynaptic. The sensory threshold for this reflex is generally less than 13 mA, and the reflex usually requires a stimulus intensity three times the sensory threshold. The reflex is suppressed during voiding, and this is useful as a test of upper motor neuron function. Disease processes involving the proximal urethral afferent nerves or the pelvic plexus may have abnormal urethral–anal reflex activity, and this test has been found to be a sensitive electrodiagnostic test for patients with voiding dysfunction after radical pelvic surgery (Table 13.10). It has also been found to be predictive of outcome with sacral neuromodulation therapy (22).

Bladder–Anal Reflex

The stimulus is with the catheter-mounted ring electrode used for the urethral–anal reflex, now repositioned with bladder emptying and Foley bulb emptying performed to allow contact of the ring electrodes with the bladder wall. Contact is ensured by temporarily connecting the lead to the ring electrodes to the preamplifier and checking resistance. Resistance below 10 kΩ indicates satisfactory contact. The test is then per-

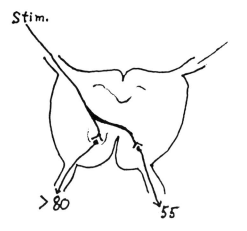
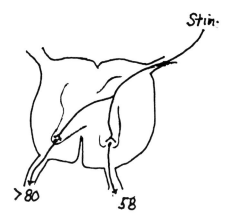

FIG. 13.9. Surface electrodes (instead of concentric needle).

TABLE 13.10. *Electrodiagnostic test results in patients with voiding dysfunction after radical hysterectomy*

	Age (yr)	PNTML (ms)		PeNTML (ms)		Urethral anal reflex (ms)		Urethral sensory threshold (ms)	Clitoral anal reflex (ms)		Lt clitoral anal reflex		Rt clitoral anal reflex	
		Rt	Lt	Rt	Lt	Rt	Lt		Rt	Lt	Rt	Lt	Rt	Lt
Pt 1	39	2.1	2.4	NR*	NR*	NR*	NR*	>100 mA*	40	40	40	40	50	60
Pt 2	50	2.2	NR*	NR*	NR*	226*	NR*	>100 mA*	93	NR*	93	NR*	56	NR*
Pt 3	52	2.3	2.6	3.6*	3.6*	63	78	9.4	55	72	55	72	48	69
Pt 4	32	3.0*	3.3*	2.8	3.4*	NR*	NR*	>100 mA*	81*	66*	81*	66*		
Pt 5	40	3.1*	2.7	2.7	NR*	NR*	NR*	8.6	61*	67*	61*	67*		

PNTML, pudendal nerve terminal motor latency; PeNTML, perineal nerve terminal motor latency; Rt, right; Lt, left; Pt, patient; NR, no response; *, abnormal.

formed just as the urethral–anal reflex test, with similar latency values. Abnormalities in this reflex when the other two reflexes are normal represent isolated bladder afferent disorder. Abnormalities in both the bladder–anal reflex and the urethral–anal reflex with normal clitoral–anal reflex suggest pelvic plexus pathology.

Cortical Evoked Potentials

Any type of synchronizable stimulus reaching the cortex can be studied electrophysiologically. With electrodes at the scalp or over the spinal columns, potentials representing the algebraic summation of electrical activity that is time-locked to a select stimulus delivered through a predetermined sensory pathway are recorded. The evoked potentials are very small and can only be separated from random electrical noise in the body by the computer process of averaging. Hundreds or even thousands of stimuli must be averaged for the specific time-locked response to be recorded. The evoked potentials have early cortical peaks (40 ms or less) produced from large-diameter afferent sensory impulses traveling rostrally through ipsilateral spinal dorsal columns, synapsing at cervicomedullary and ventroposterolateral thalamic nuclei, and activating contralateral primary somatosensory cortex organized in accordance with the classic homunculus. Later responses (more than 70 ms) embody smaller-diameter nerve fibers ascending through anterolateral columns. The lower extremity and the pudendal and bladder afferents activate medial regions of the contralateral hemisphere; hence, recording electrodes are best placed in the midline with an electrode at the nasion (Fz site) and one just posterior to the scalp vertex (Cz1). The ground may be placed over the chin or elsewhere between stimulus and response. Recording is done over the spinal column with one electrode over L-1 vertebra and the second over the iliac crest or alternatively over L-5 vertebra. This arrangement produces a response at the area

where the impulses reach the spinal cord and represents the peripheral component of the evoked potential test. The central component, then, is represented in the impulse transmission from the cord to the cortex.

Pudendal Nerve Somatosensory Evoked Potential

The stimulus may be applied to right or left clitoral region with the anode lateral and cathode adjacent to the clitoris. Three times the sensory threshold current is applied and must be at a comfortable level. The patient must be totally relaxed with eyes closed. Resistance at recording electrodes must be below 3 kΩ; hence, careful skin preparation is necessary. The pudendal nerve afferents at this region are cutaneous sensory only, and achieving reproducible responses over the spinal cord is not usually possible in women, but cortical responses are reliably obtainable. If the pudendal nerve is stimulated at the ischial spine, where muscle afferents are also present, more reproducible spinal column potentials are recordable. The latency to the cortex generally occurs with the first positive-peak deflection between 35 and 43 ms, a value similar to the somatosensory evoked potential when stimulating the posterior tibial nerve at the ankle (Fig. 13.10). In view of the much longer distance traveled by impulses with ankle stimulation, the similar cortical latencies are theorized to represent somewhat slower cord conduction of pudendal afferents relative to tibial nerve afferents.

Proximal Urethral Evoked Potentials

Stimulating through a ring electrode on a Foley catheter (see Pudendal Nerve Motor Conduction) can produce recordable potentials over the scalp, using the same electrode placement as with pudendal somatosensory evoked potentials. The latency is longer (about 50 ms to the first positive peak), suggesting that only visceral afferents are stimulated by this method. The responses are very

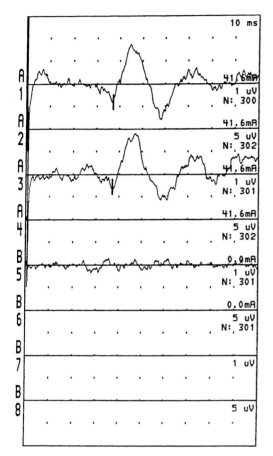

problems causing conduction delay, whereas amplitude variations can reflect loss of axonal content. Careful analysis is required, and a study should never be considered abnormal without knowing the state of the peripheral nervous system. Hence, evoked potential studies may suggest peripheral neuropathy, demyelinating disease, radiculopathies, cortical disorders, or other myelopathies (cord disorders) presenting with visceral or sphincter dysfunction.

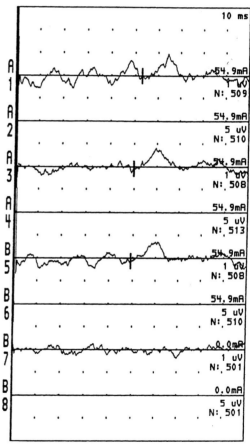

FIG. 13.10. A1: Cortical evoked potential from left pudendal (clitoral branch) stimulation with marker at 37 ms. **A3**: Response replicated. **B5**: Control series without stimulation. Machine parameters: 10-ms time base, 1-μV gain, 0.1-ms pulse duration, 2.5-Hz repetition rate, 1.5-kHz and 3-Hz high- and low-cut filters, respectively.

small (Fig. 13.11), and absence of response may be of uncertain clinical significance because such absence may well be technical. However, obtaining a response with normal latency is valuable in excluding a subpontine neurogenic bladder disorder (26).

Interpretation of Evoked Potential Studies

Comparing absolute and interpeak latencies to standardized data or to uninvolved contralateral study can be used to localize

FIG. 13.11. A1: Cortical evoked potential from bladder base stimulation with marker at 53 ms. **A3**: Response replicated with marker at 50 ms. **B5**: Response replicated with marker at 49 ms. **B7**: Control series without stimulation. Machine parameters: 10-ms time base, 1-μV gain, 0.1-ms pulse duration, 2.5-Hz repetition rate, 1.5-kHz and 3-Hz high and low cut filters, respectively.

Autonomic Tests

Most electrophysiologic testing evaluates larger fiber nerve activity. Tests selective for the small myelinated or unmyelinated autonomic nerves include QSART, sympathetic skin response, orthostatic blood pressure (BP) and heart rate (HR) responses to tilt, HR response to deep breathing, and beat-to-beat BP responses to Valsalva maneuver, tilt, and deep breathing.

QSART

Acetylcholine is iontophoresed into skin, and the impulse travels antidromically to a branch point and then orthodromically to release acetylcholine from the nerve terminal. At the terminal, neuroglandular transmission and binding to muscarinic receptor on eccrine sweat glands evokes a sweat response that ceases secondary to acetylcholinesterase activity in subcutaneous tissue. The recordable response has latency of 1 to 2 minutes, returning to baseline in 5 minutes, and sites are standardized (foot, proximal and distal leg, and forearm). Excessive or persistent response is often seen in painful neuropathies and florid reflex sympathetic dystrophy (27). Absent response indicates failure of postganglionic sympathetic sudomotor axon and is length dependent, so that distal anhidrosis is commonly seen in peripheral neuropathies. A reflex with anhidrosis present and with core temperature rise suggests preganglionic lesions occurring anywhere along the sympathetic efferent neuraxis.

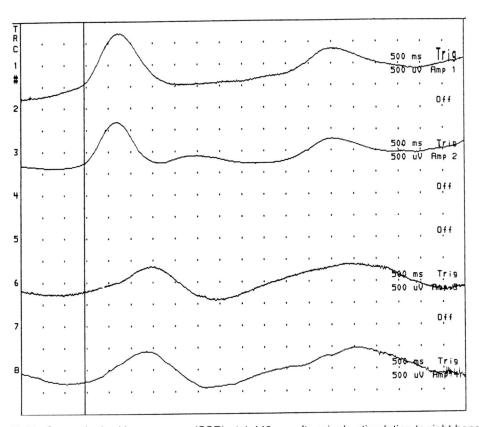

FIG. 13.12. Sympathetic skin responses (SSR) at 1,440 ms after single stimulation to right hand at 23 mA. *Trace 1,* SSR from right perineum. *Trace 2,* SSR from left perineum. *Trace 6,* SSR from right foot. *Trace 8,* SSR from left foot. Machine parameters: 500 ms, 500 µV, 0.1-ms pulse duration, 100-Hz and 0.2-Hz high and low cut filters, respectively.

Sympathetic Skin Response

A suprabulbar somatosympathetic reflex may be recorded in response to stimuli (e.g., electrical), a loud noise, or skin stroking. The source of the response is electrical activity in sweat glands. Typically recorded over palms or soles, it can also be recorded over the perineum (Fig. 13.12). The test correlates with QSART, although it is not as sensitive. The variability of the test precludes its general use clinically.

Systemic Vasoconstrictor Function

During upright tilt, normal individuals undergo transient reduction in BP, recovering within 1 minute. Patients with adrenergic failure have more reduction and less recovery.

Heart Rate Response to Deep Breathing

Afferent and efferent pathways are vagal. A Valsalva ratio, the maximal HR divided by the minimal HR response within 30 seconds of the peak HR, may be obtained while the patient is undergoing controlled Valsalva expiration. The ratio primarily reflects cardiovagal function but is also dependent on cardiac sympathetic function.

Response to Standing

Upon standing, resultant tachycardia occurs that is maximal at the fifteenth heartbeat after standing and relative bradycardia at about the thirtieth beat. The RR interval at beat 30 divided by the RR interval at beat 15 can be used as an index of cardiovagal function.

Autonomic testing is indicated when distal small fiber neuropathy is suspected or when generalized autonomic disorders, including postural hypotension, sympathetically maintained pain, or bladder and bowel dysfunction, are present.

Bethanechol Test for Vesical Denervation

A cystometrogram (CMG) (gas-filling acceptable) is recorded as a baseline control, recording pressure, and volume at 100 mL.

Bethanechol chloride, 0.05 mg/kg, is injected subcutaneously, and postinjection CMGs are collected at 10, 20, and 30 minutes, performed in the same manner as the control CMG. A positive test is an intravesical pressure increase of more than 15 cm H_2O over the control CMG at 100-mL bladder volume.

CONCLUSIONS

Bladder and bowel dysfunction can accompany neuromuscular disease, metabolic problems, and orthopedic difficulties. With increasing willingness to discuss and seek help for such problems, associated with a vast improvement in therapeutic choices, there is more need for thorough evaluation. Information derived from clinical neurophysiologic testing is unique in that it relates to function. It therefore acts complementary to imaging studies, so that clinical decisions regarding treatment of anatomic disorders may be more properly made.

Patients particularly helped by electrophysiologic testing include the following: those being evaluated for anal sphincter repair; those with voiding disorders, detrusor sphincter dyssynergia, overflow incontinence, stress incontinence (especially where intrinsic sphincter deficiency is suspected), spinal myelopathies, or peripheral or autonomic neuropathies; diabetic patients with bladder or bowel symptoms, pelvic floor trauma from childbirth or other sacral injuries; and patients with unexplained perineal numbness or pain or with failure of diagnosis on standard evaluations for bladder or rectal dysfunction.

The suggestions of the Clinical Neurophysiology Committee at the 2nd International Consultation on Incontinence (19), on Organization of Clinical Neurophysiology Service for Neurourology/Uroneurology include the following:

The information gained by clinical examination (and urodynamic testing) may be enhanced by uroneurophysiological tests in selected patient groups. It seems that tests have often been performed by non-neurophysiologists in research but for routine diagnostics, an established service would seem necessary, and the physicians performing the tests should be appropriately trained, as required by national policies. As a rule, the service should be in liaison with general clinical neurophysiology. It seems optimal to create interdisciplinary programs between urology, urogynecology and neurology departments. Eventually, 'neurourology' or 'uroneurology' sections should provide the appropriate setting for testing of the individual patient to be performed within a wider scope of clinical evaluation, and treatment. Such specialized teams, sections, or even departments within larger institutions are as yet few, but the organization of such teams in (university) medical centres should be encouraged.

ALGORITHM FOR PELVIC CLINICAL NEUROPHYSIOLOGIC STUDY IN CONJUNCTION WITH OTHER PELVIC FLOOR STUDIES

Baseline

Lower Limb Motor

Peroneal nerve: response at extensor digitorum brevis (EDB) or tibialis anterior if EDB is absent. Stimulate ankle, knee, and F waves

Tibial nerve: response at abductor halluces brevis with stimulation at ankle, knee, and F waves

Lower Limb Sensory

Sural nerve sensory action potential: superficial peroneal sensory or other sensory nerves if sural absent

Needle Electromyography

Pelvic girdle, paraspinal, and limb muscles if indicated by physical findings and/or nerve conduction studies

Somatic Motor Abnormalities

Anal–Rectal

Manometry with rectal–anal inhibitory reflex
Balloon expulsion test for constipation disorders

Imaging

Ultrasound for sphincteroplasty
Dynamic cystoproctography for pubococcygeus function
External anal sphincter surface EMG—resting and maximum voluntary activity
Pudendal (inferior hemorrhoidal) motor conduction study—latency, amplitude
Clitoral–anal reflex: latency, suppressibility, threshold
Needle EMG anal sphincter, puborectalis, and pubococcygeus if clinically indicated

Urethral

Manometry: cystometrics with urethral lead for pressure and surface EMG
Urethral pressure profile and/or leak point pressure
Urethral surface EMG—resting and maximum voluntary activity
Perineal motor conduction study—latency, amplitude
Sacral reflexes
Urethral–anal reflex: threshold, latency, suppressibility
Clitoral–anal reflex: threshold, latency, suppressibility
Needle EMG: periurethral skeletal muscle

Somatic Sensory Abnormalities

Anal–Rectal

Rectal and anal canal balloon distention test
Manometry with rectal–anal inhibitory reflex testing
If mixed nerve (motor and sensory) abnormality suspected, repeat motor algorithm for motor.
Clitoral–anal reflex: threshold, latency, suppressibility
Current perception threshold: paraanal
Pudendal and/or posterior tibial somatosensory evoked potentials

Urethral

Cystometrics: includes urethral pressure profile and surface EMG

If mixed nerve (motor and sensory) abnormality is suspected, repeat motor algorithm for motor sacral reflexes.

Clitoral–anal reflex: threshold, latency, suppressibility

Urethral–anal reflex: threshold, latency, suppressibility

Current perception threshold: paraclitoral

Proximal urethral evoked potentials: if abnormal or if unobtainable, pudendal somatosensory evoked potentials

Visceral Motor

Anal–Rectal

If clinical indications are present:

Balloon expulsion test

Dynamic proctography

Anal manometry with rectal–anal inhibitory reflex

Colon transit studies

Sacral reflexes

Urethral–anal reflex: threshold, latency, suppressibility

Clitoral–anal reflex: threshold, latency, suppressibility

Autonomic studies added adjunctively if clinically indicated

Lower Urinary Tract

Cystometry study, voiding study

Bethanechol stimulation test if no detrusor contraction on urodynamics

Sacral reflexes

Urethral–anal reflex: threshold, latency, suppressibility

Clitoral–anal reflex: threshold, latency, suppressibility

Autonomic tests added adjunctively if clinically indicated

Visceral Sensory

Anal–Rectal

Visceral motor studies plus balloon distention studies

Evoked potential studies

Pudendal and/or posterior tibial

Paraanal current perception threshold studies plus urethral evoked potentials

Sacral reflexes

Lower Urinary Tract

Visceral motor studies plus urethral evoked potentials

Paraclitoral current perception threshold

Sacral reflexes

REFERENCES

1. Thind P. The significance of smooth and striated muscles in the sphincter function of the urethra in healthy women. *Neurourol Urodyn* 1995;14:585–618.
2. Daunser H, Thor K. Spinal 5-HT2 receptor-mediated facilitation of pudendal nerve reflexes in the anaesthetized cat. *Br J Pharmacol* 1996;118:150–154.
3. Rempen A, Kraus M. Measurement of head compression during labor. J Perinat Med 1991;19:115–120.
4. Lundberg G. *Nerve injury and repair.* New York: Churchill Livingstone, 1988:54.
5. Hetzel DJ, Stanhope CR, O'Neill BP, et al. Gynecologic cancer in patients with subacute cerebellar degeneration predicated by anti-Purkinje cell antibodies. *Mayo Clin Proc* 1990;65:1558–1563.
6. Ropper AH, Wijdicks EFM, Truaz BT. Guillain-Barré syndrome. *Contemporary neurology sciences.* Philadelphia: FA Davis, 1991.
7. Torens MJ, Hald T. Bladder denervation procedure. *Urol Clin North Am* 1979;6:283–284.
8. Cheng CL, Liu JC, Chang SY, et al. Effect of capsaicin on the micturition reflex in normal and chronic spinal cord-injured cats. *Am J Physiol* 1999;277(3 Pt 2): R786–794.
9. Yoshimura N. Bladder afferent pathway and spinal cord injury: possible mechanisms inducing hyperreflexia of the urinary bladder. *Prog Neurobiol* 1999;57(6):583–606.
10. Vizzard MA. Increased expression of spinal cord Fos protein induced by bladder stimulation after spinal cord injury. *Am J Physiol Regul Integr Comp Physiol* 2000; 279(1):R295–305.
11. Callsen-Cencic P, Mense S. Increased spinal expression of c-Fos following stimulation of the lower urinary tract in chronic spinal cord-injured rats. *Histochem Cell Biol* 1999;112(1):63–72.
12. Vizzard MA. Alterations in spinal cord Fos protein ex-

pression induced by bladder stimulation following cystitis. *Am J Physiol Regul Integr Comp Physiol* 2000;278 (4):R1027–1039.

13. Steers WD, Creedon DJ, Tuttle JB. Immunity to nerve growth factor prevents afferent plasticity following urinary bladder hypertrophy. *J Urol* 1996;155(1):379–385.

14. Doggweiler R, Jasmin L, Schmidt RA. Neurogenically mediated cystitis in rats: an animal mode. *J Urol* 1998; 160(4):1551–1556.

15. Steers WD, Kolbeck S, Creedon D, et al. Nerve growth factor in the urinary bladder of the adult regulates neuronal form and function. *J Clin Invest* 1991;88 (5):1709–1715.

16. Chancellor MB, Chartier-Kastler EJ. Principles of sacral nerve stimulation (SNS) for the treatment of bladder and urethral sphincter dysfunctions. *Neuromodulation* 2000;3(1):15–26.

17. Shaker H, Wang Y, Loung D, et al. Role of C-afferent fibers in the mechanism of action of sacral nerve root neuromodulation in chronic spinal cord injury. *Br J Urol* 2000;85(7):905–910.

18. Stewart JD, Low PA, Fealey RD. Distal small fiber peripheral neuropathy: results of tests of sweating and autonomic cardiovascular reflexes. *Muscle Nerve* 1992; 15:661–665.

19. Fowler C, Benson T, Vodusek DB, et al. Electrodiagnostic testing: clinical neurophysiology. In: Abrams S, Cardoy L, Khoury S, Wein A, eds. *Incontinence*. Paris: 2nd International Consultation on Incontinence; Plymouth, UK: Plymbridge Distributors Ltd., 2001.

20. Kenton K, FitzGerald MP, Brubaker L. *Role of urethral EMG in predicting outcome of Burch retropubic urethropexy.* Paper 30, American Urogynecologic Society 21st annual meeting, October 2000.

21. Dorfman LJ, Howard JE, McGill KC. Influence of ADEMG analysis. *J Neurol Sci* 1988;86:125–136.

22. Mastropietro M, Fuller E, Benson JT. *Electrodiagnostic features of responders and non-responders to sacral neuromodulation test stimulation.* Paper 47, American Urogynecologic Society annual meeting, October 2000.

23. Rushworth G. Diagnostic value of the electromyographic study of reflex activity in man. *Electroencephalogr Clin Neurophysiol* 1967;25[Suppl]:65–73.

24. Dyro FM, Yalla SV. Refractoriness of urethral striated sphincter during voiding: studies with afferent pudendal reflex arc stimulation. *J Urol* 1986;135:732–736.

25. Bradley WE. Urethral electromyelography. *J Urol* 1972; 108:563–564.

26. Fowler CJ. *Methods in clinical neurophysiology.* Denmark: Dantec Elektronik, 1991:1–17.

27. Low PA. Autonomic nervous system function. *J Clin Neurophysiol* 1993;10:14–27.

*Ostergard's Urogynecology and Pelvic Floor
Dysfunction, Fifth Edition.* edited by A.E. Bent, et al.
Lippincott Williams & Wilkins, Philadelphia © 2003.

14

Imaging of the Pelvic Floor

Harpreet Pannu,* Mikio Albert Nihira,** and Rene Genadry†

*Russell H. Morgan Department of Radiology and Radiology Sciences, Johns Hopkins Medical
Institutions, Baltimore, Maryland
**Department of Obstetrics and Gynecology, Division of Urogynecology and Reproductive Pelvic
Surgery, University of Texas Southwestern Medical Center, Dallas, Texas
† Department of Gynecology and Obstetrics, Johns Hopkins Medical Institutions,
Baltimore, Maryland

Dysfunction of the pelvic floor disrupts the normal function of the pelvic organs. The result of these displacements and dysfunctions may present as pelvic pain, symptoms of herniation, voiding dysfunction, urinary incontinence, sexual dysfunction, defecatory dysfunction, and fecal incontinence. The goal of this chapter is to review the current role of imaging in the evaluation of pelvic organ prolapse and associated dysfunction.

IMAGING MODALITIES

The pelvic floor has been divided conceptually into the anterior, apical, and posterior segments. The anterior compartment has received the most attention of, and benefits from, imaging. Conventional imaging of the anterior compartment has included abdominal x-rays, intravenous and retrograde pyelograms, lateral cystograms with and without bead chains, and voiding cystourethrograms. For the posterior compartment, barium enema has classically been used, and defecating proctograms are a relatively recent addition. The pelvic floor itself has been difficult to evaluate. Pelvimetry assesses the bony pelvis and its diameters, although its contribution has generally been ignored in favor of examinations of the soft tissue and musculature of the pelvic floor.

Conventional Studies

Conventional imaging techniques are of low cost, simple to perform, and readily available. The limitations to fluoroscopic techniques relate mainly to (a) examination of specific organs, (b) limited ability to visualize soft tissue detail, and (c) radiation exposure.

Abdominal Plain Film

An abdominal plain x-ray, in addition to identification of skeletal abnormalities, provides an excellent means of visualizing radiopaque foreign bodies, soft tissue calcification, and calculi potentially responsible for abnormal function. A recent example was a misplaced bone anchor responsible for significant pain, vulvodynia, and dyspareunia with persistent voiding dysfunction. Constipation or fecal incontinence secondary to fecal impaction may be easily diagnosed. The study of constipation can be augmented by evaluation of colorectal motility using radiopaque markers.

Intravenous Urogram

An intravenous urogram remains the best screening study of the entire urinary tract. It provides anatomic as well as functional information. In patients with symptoms of bladder irritability, suspected fistulas or ectopic ureters, hematuria, suburethral diverticulum, malignancy, or obstruction, it remains the mainstay of evaluation of the urinary tract. In the evaluation of the pelvic floor, it is mostly helpful in cases of suspected genitourinary fistula or ectopic ureter, obstructive uropathy, and previous reconstructive surgery.

Urethrogram

A special double-balloon catheter was developed to improve visualization of a small communicating suburethral diverticulum during a positive-pressure urethrogram (PPUG) (1). This catheter has a Foley balloon that is held tight at its proximal end against the internal urethral meatus while an adjustable sliding outer balloon can be positioned to obstruct the external urethral meatus. An opening between the two balloons allows for the injection of dye under pressure to outline a suburethral diverticulum or a communicating ectopic ureter. It can localize suburethral diverticula and identify the relationship to the bladder neck (see Figs. 17.4 through 17.6 in Chapter 17). Newer technologies, including ultrasonography and magnetic resonance imaging (MRI), may obviate the need for this test.

Cystogram

Cystography is visualization of the bladder contour and anatomy by retrograde filling. It helps to identify diverticular or fistulous pathology. Historically, it has been used to assess urethral mobility and bladder neck position in relation to the symphysis pubis at rest and with straining. Straining cystograms may identify ureteral reflux and funneling of the upper urethra. Voiding cystograms can elucidate the degree of emptying and the presence of communicating suburethral diverticulum.

Bead chain cystography was introduced by Hodgkinson (2). The placement of a radiopaque bead chain in the urethra and bladder base drew particular attention to the anatomy and function of the bladder neck, including urethral position, closure, and mobility. The lateral straining cystogram has re-placed this technique. A lateral static and dynamic chain cystogram permits the evaluation of the bladder and bladder neck, including its shape, mobility, and position in relation to the symphysis pubis. The addition of fluoroscopic images with simultaneous manometric recordings, including intraabdominal and intravesical pressures (videourodynamic studies), to such a technique permits simultaneous evaluation of the anatomy as well as the function of the bladder.

Complex Imaging Modalities

Complex investigative procedures bridge the gap between the anterior and posterior compartments in the evaluation of the pelvic floor. Newer imaging modalities rely on newer applications of ultrasound, fluoroscopy, and magnetic imaging technology. Their respective roles in clinical management remain to be defined, and the lack of standardization of nomenclature and technique limits their current utility. These techniques continue to stimulate new theories as they challenge current concepts and paradigms in the evaluation and management of pelvic organ prolapse and dysfunction. The ideal imaging modality should include the following characteristics: (a) real-time imaging, (b) adequate visualization of soft tissue detail within the pelvic floor, (c) multiplanar and global relationships and detail, (d) ability to obtain functional studies, (e) nonionizing radiation, (f) short duration and minimal discomfort, and (g) low cost, simplicity, and accessibility.

Real-time Ultrasound

Ultrasound uses sound energy to penetrate tissue and produce an image. There is a direct relationship between frequency and image resolution and an inverse relationship between frequency and penetration such that the higher the frequency, the lower the penetration and the higher the resolution. Newly designed transducers and real-time capability provide the ability to visualize anatomic detail in actual function from a variety of angles and distances. Lack of ionizing radiation, as well

TABLE 14.1. *Ultrasound transducer parameters*

	Transducer	Probe	Position	Technique
Evaluation of postvoid residual (PVR)	Sector, B mode, 3.5 MHz	Suprapubic	Supine	Transverse and longitudinal measurements of bladder. Volume formula for an ellipsoid ($V = 4/3\pi \times r1 \times r2 \times r3$)
Urethral mobility	Linear array, 2.4–3.5 mHZ	Transabdominal (suprapubic)	Supine, lithotomy or standing	Transducer placed on labia, aimed cranially.
	5 mHz	Transperineal	Lithotomy	The 5-mHz transducer is superior to the 7.5-mHz transducer to observe dynamic changes of the bladder with straining. Translabial scanning is superior to transrectal ultrasound for measurements of anterior vaginal wall prolapse due to placement of transducer in rectum may limit movement of anterior vaginal wall.
	7.5 mHz	Endovaginal	Lithotomy or sitting	Transducer placed in introitus, directed anteriorly. The 7.5-mHz transducer is superior for imaging intraperitoneal structures. Visualization of the urethra is limited with significant anterior vaginal wall prolapse due to the presence of transducer in the vagina, which may distort the endogenous anatomic relationships or may interfere with the movement of urethra by its direct contact.
Anal sphincters and anal canal	7-mHz rotating ultrasound transducer with sonolucent plastic cone (1.7-cm external diameter) filled with degassed water for acoustic coupling	Endoanal	Left lateral decubitus position	Exam of upper, middle, and lower zones of anal canal. Exams performed at rest and with squeeze.

as the ability to combine its measurements with intraabdominal pressure measurements, permits repetitive assessment without undue risk to the patient or the investigator.

The type of transducer used, ultrasound frequency, angle of projection, and type of technique employed depend on the area of investigation (Table 14.1). In addition to imaging the various urogenital organs, ultrasound is useful in the evaluation of postvoid residual, urethral anatomy and mobility, anal sphincter anatomy and pathology, and imaging of the urogenital organs.

Fluoroscopy

Pelvic fluoroscopy goes by several different names, including colpocystoproctography, defecography, and defecating proctography, depending on the precise technique used. Pelvic fluoroscopy is an established test to evaluate pelvic organ prolapse and measure defects in the pelvic floor (3). The technique takes advantage of increased abdominal and pelvic pressure during rectal evacuation to demonstrate organ descent. Rectal emptying in patients with constipation is simultaneously evaluated. The degree of prolapse can be quantified relative to bony landmarks, such as the pubic symphysis, or relative to soft tissue structures, such as the anal canal. It also provides a simultaneous assessment of all the compartments of the pelvis, so that all pelvic defects can be recognized (3,4). Patients who present with symptoms related to one compartment frequently have abnormalities in other compartments when examined with fluoroscopy. Because of this high degree of overlap and presence of global pathology, evaluation of the entire pelvis is recommended when fluoroscopy is performed (5). This technique remains highly dependent on both patient and operator and requires patience and careful attention to technical detail. It is limited in its ability to visualize soft tissue detail despite significant radiation exposure.

Fluoroscopy has been described as a useful adjunct to the physical examination in patients who have severe pelvic organ prolapse with vaginal eversion (6). Imaging helps to distinguish the various components of prolapse, such as cystocele, rectocele, and enterocele, in this group of patients. Fluoroscopy has also been shown to be superior to clinical examination in the diagnosis of enterocele (4). Two possible reasons for the higher sensitivity of fluoroscopy are (a) the higher pelvic pressures generated with rectal evacuation during fluoroscopy compared with straining during physical examination and (b) easier filling of the cul-de-sac with bowel once the rectum has emptied and is no longer a space-occupying structure in the pelvis. Most importantly, fluoroscopy facilitates identification of the soft tissues that herniate through defects in the vaginal wall connective tissue. This permits the contents of the cul-de-sac to be separated into enterocele and sigmoidocele, which is relevant in patients with constipation in whom sigmoid resection may be considered. Because fluoroscopy depends on soft tissue opacification for visualization, it is a poor modality for imaging the pelvic floor musculature.

Magnetic Resonance Imaging

Interest in using MRI to evaluate pelvic organ prolapse stems primarily from the superior soft tissue contrast resolution that permits visualization of the lumens of the pelvic organs, as with fluoroscopy, but also provides information on the internal architecture of the viscera and the surrounding soft tissues (7). Because this is a relatively new and emerging application of MRI, much work remains to be done in defining normal and abnormal criteria, in determining sensitivity, and in optimizing protocols for performing studies.

There are a variety of MRI scanners available. The most common type consists of a closed cylindric bore in which patients are imaged in the supine position. Another common type is the open-bore magnet, in which patients lie supine but are not enclosed by the imaging apparatus. There is also a vertical configuration scanner that is primarily designed for interventional MRI research and is available in only a handful of centers worldwide. A vertical gap is present in the center of the magnet in which a commode can be placed to image the patient in the seated position. This scanner combines the advantages of MRI, including superior contrast resolution, with the advantages of fluoroscopy, including physiologic evaluation of patients, but is not presently a viable clinical modality because of the limited availability of this type of scanner.

CLINICAL APPLICATIONS

Imaging technologies are highly variable in their usefulness and accuracy in the assessment of urinary incontinence, pelvic organ prolapse, fecal incontinence, and defecatory dysfunction.

Urinary Incontinence

The progressive integration of functional cystometric studies to fluoroscopic imaging led to the videourodynamic study. The real-time advantage of this study of the functional anatomy of the bladder and urethra has helped it maintain its status as the gold standard for the evaluation of urinary incontinence and dysfunction.

Real-time ultrasonography, with its significantly improved soft tissue resolution of anatomic detail, provides another modality to capture the events related to the bladder and bladder neck during episodes of function and dysfunction. It provides a good alternative for the real-time evaluation of urethral anatomy and function. Dynamic ultrasound has been recommended for first-line imaging of bladder support because bladder neck hypermobility diagnosed with ultrasound correlated better with stress incontinence than bladder morphology diagnosed during static cystography (8). Good correlation has been reported between voiding cystourethrogram (VCUG) and ultrasound for the anatomic assessment of

the bladder neck in urinary incontinence (9). Ultrasound presents the advantages of lower cost of procedure and equipment with no radiation exposure or reaction to contrast medium. In addition to assessing postvoid bladder volume and degree of mobility of the urethra during straining, the anatomic detail of the urethra provided by ultrasound makes it useful for the diagnosis of periurethral cysts, neoplasms, and diverticular disease (10).

Preliminary reports on the use of suprapubic ultrasound to evaluate the mobility of the urethra were published in the 1980s. Such studies were limited by their inability to evaluate other components of the pelvic floor and even the urethra in overweight patients because of their limited field of view. Quinn and colleagues used transvaginal endosonography in 1988 (11) for the evaluation of the lower urinary tract anatomy in stress incontinence. They noted that in 18 of 23 patients with primary stress incontinence and in 12 of 14 patients with recurrent stress incontinence, the urethra was situated below the midsymphysis at rest, with opening and descent of the bladder neck during cough (Fig. 14.1).

Conversely, Peschers and co-workers using perineal ultrasound noted that the location of the bladder neck at rest was significantly below the symphysis pubis in primigravidas compared with age-matched nulligravidas (12). Furthermore, bladder neck mobility was increased in primiparous and multiparous patients delivered vaginally.

Johnson and associates placed a transurethral calcium alginate swab to better identify the urethrovesical junction (13), and Schaer and colleagues found that the introduction of ultrasound contrast material into the bladder improved the ability to identify bladder neck funneling (14). Whether this has any advantage over clinical assessment of urethral mobility remains to be shown.

Nishizwa and coauthors advocated transrectal ultrasound examination of the urethra because with this approach, the probe did not seem to change the urethrovesical junction mobility (15,16). Saunders and co-workers described their experience with transrectal ex-

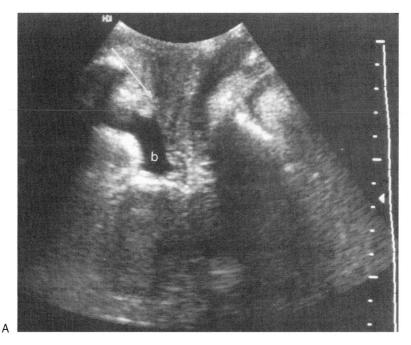

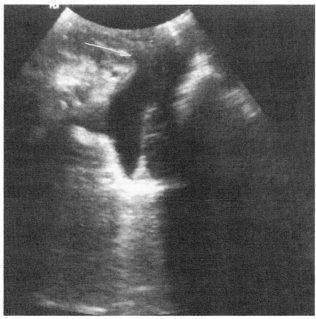

FIG. 14.1. Funneling of the urethra. Translabial ultrasound of the pelvis with longitudinal views. The head of the patient is to the left of the image. **A:** Image obtained with the patient at rest. The bladder (b) has a small amount of urine. The proximal urethral lumen is closed (*arrow*). **B:** Image obtained with the patient straining down. The proximal urethral lumen is open (*arrow*) compatible with funneling.

amination of the pelvic floor in which they used a specially designed chair and side fire transrectal transducer, so that measurements could be made with the patient in an upright, seated position with views obtained at rest and with straining as if to defecate (17). They suggested that of the various ultrasonic features of stress, "funneling has been found to correlate much better with incontinence than urethral angle changes or urethral movement." They further concluded "the combination of translabial and transrectal approaches has proved most helpful with the transvaginal approach as a useful backup if the transrectal approach is impractical" (17).

Intraurethral ultrasonography appears to afford a direct visualization of the sphincter mechanism. With a 12.5-mHz endoluminal ultrasound, loss of sphincter function was detected in patients with stress incontinence that correlated with urodynamic studies (18). Heit correlated decreasing rhabdosphincter thickness with intrinsic sphincter deficiency and reduced maximal urethral closure pressure (19). Such reduction in rhabdosphincter thickness was also reported in patients with stress incontinence using a 7.5-mHz transrectal probe transvaginally (20). On three-dimensional ultrasound, the rhabdosphincter was also of smaller volume in women with genuine stress incontinence (21). Intraurethral ultrasound is presently an experimental modality but has significant promise as a clinical tool.

Fluoroscopic studies of the bladder neck and urethra provide little information on the anatomic details of the urethra, bladder neck, pelvic floor, and surrounding tissue. For this, static MRI provides unsurpassed detail. In its dynamic form, it currently lacks sufficient resolution to allow the visualization of the alteration in urethral anatomy during movement and function. Because the urethra and urethrovesical junction are extremely well visualized with MRI, including surface, endovaginal, and intraurethral coil, it is particularly useful in assessing urethral wall abnormalities such as are seen with congenital and traumatic anomalies, neoplasms, periurethral cysts, and diverticula. In the evaluation of

suburethral diverticulum, MRI was more sensitive than VCUG and PPUG (22,23). Because of cost considerations, Kim and associates recommend it only when urethroscopic and urethrographic findings are inconclusive but urethral diverticula remains clinically suspected (24). In some reports, PPUG appears more sensitive than VCUG in detecting suburethral diverticula (25). Transperineal and transvaginal ultrasonography at 5 MHz represent a noninvasive mean of diagnosis, whereas endoluminal ultrasound at 12.5 or 20 MHz has been used intraoperatively to facilitate surgical repair (26). Its effectiveness deserves further investigation.

Pelvic Organ Prolapse

Pelvic organ prolapse (POP) results from global weakness of the pelvic floor, focal musculo-fascial defects, or both. Yang and coworkers introduced the critical concepts of compartmentality, focality, threshold, and sequence in their evaluation of pelvic floor defects (27–29). Fluoroscopy helps visualize the pelvic viscera and their relationship to each other, where dynamic MRI with cine loop reconstruction affords a more complete demonstration of the pelvic floor and its content.

The imaging of the pelvic floor is clinically useful in the evaluation of pelvic organ prolapse when there is discordance between the history and the physical findings and in circumstances of prior failed repair.

Fluoroscopy can be used as an adjunct to physical examination when there is severe prolapse and the distinction needs to be made between enterocele and sigmoidocele. MRI can be used for assessment of the pelvic floor, whereas ultrasound has a limited role in prolapse in the middle and posterior compartments.

Ultrasound

Nguyen and colleagues evaluated the sensitivity to detect paravaginal defects with suprapubic ultrasonography (30). They performed examinations on 15 women with stage 4 POP with coexisting paravaginal defects on physical examination and 15 nulliparous control women. They observed that in both the study and control groups, the size of the apparent paravaginal defects observed was related to the size of the balloon placed in the vagina as contrast. Furthermore, there were no differences in the size of the paravaginal defects measured at different known bladder volumes. They concluded that transabdominal ultrasound is not useful in the detection of paravaginal defects.

Beverly and colleagues examined retrospectively the records of 323 patients evaluated for POP for evidence of hydronephrosis and concluded that a rate of less than 1% did not justify routine intravenous pyelography (IVP) for the assessment of POP (31). However, renal imaging would be prudent in the evaluation of a patient with a previously unsuccessful repair.

Pelvic Fluoroscopy

Contrast studies offer some advantages over physical examination alone in the detection of enteroceles and particularly sigmoidoceles. Although the clinical significance of this finding is not always clear in the absence of symptoms, Kelvin and associates concluded that dynamic pelvic fluoroscopy imaging improved the detection of POP by 2% to 3% in a retrospective review of 170 patients (32).

Contrast is administered into the small bowel, bladder, vagina, and rectum in order to evaluate all the compartments in the pelvis (3) (Fig. 14.2). The concept of competition for space in the limited area of the pelvic hiatus has been stressed when performing imaging studies for pelvic organ prolapse (33). Overdistention or dominant prolapse in one compartment of the pelvis may limit prolapse in another compartment, resulting in a false-negative diagnosis. Failure to recognize all abnormalities may predispose the patient to recurrent prolapse after surgery. Once the contrast has been administered, the patient is imaged while voiding on a commode. Fluoroscopy is performed after complete voiding to identify small enteroceles because bladder distention may hinder the small bowel from prolapsing (33). The bladder should also be assessed before placing rectal contrast, which may mask a cystocele (34). After voiding and the initial fluoroscopic evaluation, the patient

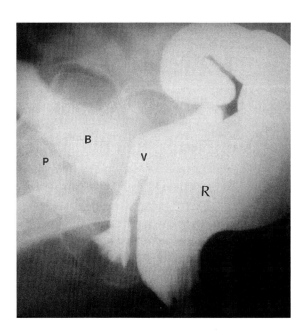

FIG. 14.2. Normal pelvis on fluoroscopy. Lateral fluoroscopic image of the pelvis obtained with the patient at rest and seated on a commode. There is contrast in the rectum (R), vagina (V), and bladder (B), which appear normal with the patient at rest. P, pubis.

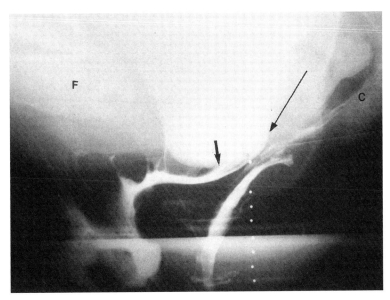

FIG. 14.3. Cystocele and vaginal vault prolapse. Lateral fluoroscopic image of the pelvis obtained during defecation with the patient seated on a commode. The bladder is low in the pelvis and creates an impression on the anterior wall of the vagina (*short arrow*) compatible with a cystocele. The apex of the vagina (*long arrow*) is also low in the pelvis compatible with vault prolapse. C, coccyx; F, femur.

is imaged while defecating on a commode. Continuous imaging is necessary to understand the dynamics of prolapse and rectal function and is usually performed by videotaping the study (34).

Descent of the bladder base below the pubic symphysis is the radiologic definition of cystocele (3) (Fig. 14.3). If the patient is able to void, urethral axis change with urethral hypermobility can also be demonstrated. Vaginal topography on frontal views can be used to assess indirectly the integrity of the pelvic floor (35). Downward sagging of the proximal vagina is suggestive of weakness of the cardinal ligaments and loss of lateral indentations in the distal vagina has been suggested to reflect weakness of the levator muscles. Herniation of the cul-de-sac between the rectum and vagina constitutes an enterocele. Descent of the small bowel may be seen with descent of the vaginal vault or widening of the rectovaginal space (Fig. 14.4). Widening of this space without bowel is due to presence of fat or unopacified bowel loops. Peritoneal contrast

has been used to identify an abnormal cu-de-sac, which may not contain bowel loops, and this increases the sensitivity of fluoroscopy by identifying 60% more enteroceles (3) but requires the intraperitoneal injection of contrast. In this technique, 60 mL of water-soluble contrast is injected into the peritoneal cavity inferior to the umbilicus for peritoneography. Sigmoid descent into the cul-de-sac has been divided into three degrees: (a) sigmoid colon is above the pubococcygeal line (3), (b) it descends below the pubococcygeal line, and (c) it descends below the ischiococcygeal line. Pelvic fluoroscopy is the preferred technique for objectively measuring perineal descent. This is measured as the movement of the anorectal junction during straining with respect to the ischial tuberosity.

Magnetic Resonance Imaging

With the addition of rectal contrast, abnormalities of rectal evacuation, such as rectal intussusception, which previously were only

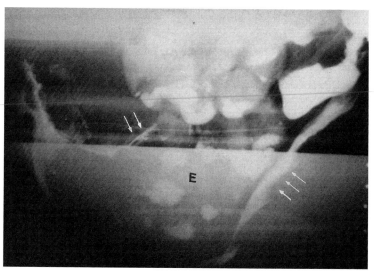

FIG. 14.4. Enterocele. Lateral fluoroscopic image of the pelvis obtained during defecation with the patient seated on a commode. There are multiple contrast filled loops of small bowel between the vagina (*double arrows*) and rectum (*triple arrows*) in this patient with an enterocele (E).

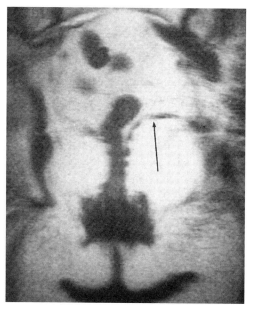
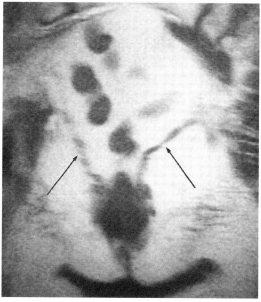

A   B

FIG. 14.5. Caudal angulation and bulging of the levator ani muscles on magnetic resonance imaging (MRI). Coronal T_2-weighted MRI of the pelvis. **A:** Image at rest shows relatively normal configuration of the left levator muscle (*arrow*). **B:** With patient straining, there is bulging outward and caudal angulation of both levator muscles (*arrows*).

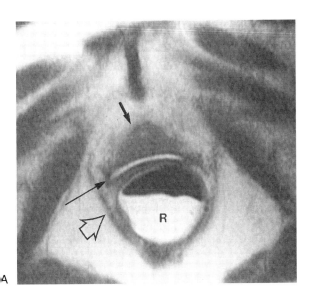

A

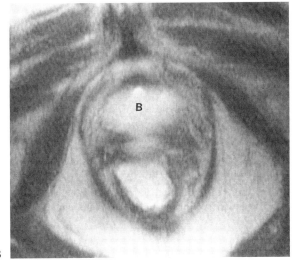

B

FIG. 14.6. Increase in pelvic hiatus area and organ descent on axial images. Axial T_2-weighted magnetic resonance imaging of the pelvis. **A:** Image at rest shows vagina (*long arrow*), urethra (*short arrow*), rectum (R), and surrounding levator ani muscle (*open arrow*). **B:** With patient straining, there is descent of the bladder (B) and increase in the area of the pelvic hiatus.

evaluated with fluoroscopy, can be visualized with MRI (27,36). The distinction between enteroceles and rectoceles can also be made reliably on MRI in patients with posthysterectomy vaginal prolapse (37). A major advantage of MRI is the ability to visualize the pelvic floor musculature and soft tissue. For example, MRI has shown that bladder and uterine descent and ballooning of the levator muscle are more common in patients with constipation, whereas anorectal descent is greater in patients with fecal incontinence (38) (Figs. 14.5 and 14.6).

The appearance of the pelvis can also be studied with MRI after vaginal delivery and surgery. The signal intensity of the levator ani muscle is increased after delivery, and this suggests muscle edema (39). The muscle recovers with time, and the size of the pelvic hiatus decreases. On static imaging, the distances between pelvic structures does not change appreciably (40). Decrease in organ prolapse after surgical correction and the sacral colpopexy site can also be determined with MRI (41,42).

With the instillation of contrast into the vagina and rectum, visualization of the viscera is enhanced (Fig. 14.7). The axis of the vagina is straightened in patients with prolapse, and the normal backward angulation

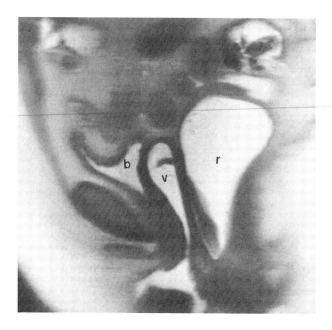

FIG. 14.7. Normal appearance of the pelvic organs on magnetic resonance imaging (MRI) with luminal contrast. Sagittal T$_2$-weighted MRI of the pelvis with the patient at rest. Urine in the bladder (b) provides natural contrast. Lubricating jelly in the vagina (v) and rectum (r) fills the lumens of these structures.

over the levator muscle is lost (43). With straining, the vaginal vault descends, and the vagina may evert (Fig. 14.8). Uterine descent can also be diagnosed because the cervix is easily visualized. With an enterocele, fat, small bowel or sigmoid colon (sigmoidocele) is seen in the rectovaginal space. An anterior rectocele appears as an abnormal bulge in the anterior rectal wall and posterior rectoceles appear as protrusions in areas of focally defi-

cient levator support. Stretching and descent of the perineal body is seen with large rectoceles and enteroceles.

Direct evidence of paravaginal defects appears to be possible with endovaginal MRI (44,45). The appearance of the posterior pubourethral and paravaginal attachments has been described using this technique. Attenuation or detachment of these structures was seen in a small group of incontinent women.

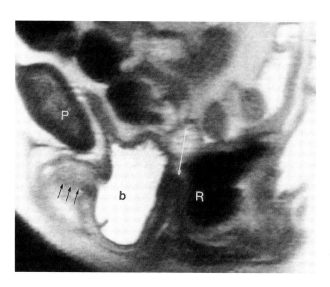

FIG. 14.8. Cystocele, urethral hypermobility, and vault prolapse on magnetic resonance imaging (MRI). Sagittal T$_2$-weighted MRI of the pelvis during patient straining. The bladder (b) and urethra (*short arrows*) are below the pubis (P). The axis of the urethra is horizontal. The vaginal vault is low in the pelvis (*long arrow*), and there is a small anterior bulge of the rectum (R).

The space of Retzius was also larger and asymmetric in this group compared with that in continent volunteers (44).

Magnetic Resonance Imaging Versus Fluoroscopy

When MRI has been compared with fluoroscopy, investigators have reported conflicting results, and this is likely due to differences in how the MRI studies were performed (Table 14.2). When studies have been performed with rectal evacuation of contrast, the number of pelvic floor defects detected by fluoroscopy or MRI has been similar or greater with MRI, and patient preference for both studies was also equal (36,46). Uterine prolapse and enterocele were detected more often on MRI than on fluoroscopy because of better soft tissue contrast. The detection of cystocele and

vaginal vault prolapse was similar with both imaging modalities.

When MRI has been done without luminal contrast or rectal evacuation, it has not compared favorably with fluoroscopy (47,48). When compared with surgery, the sensitivity of MRI has been reported as 100% for cystocele, 87% for enterocele, and 76% for rectocele (49). The supine position of the patient for the MRI scan is the main drawback regarding the use of this modality. Imaging while the patient is seated on a commode will likely continue to be necessary in patients with predominantly posterior complaints.

Criteria for Diagnosing Pelvic Organ Prolapse on Imaging

Although there are no standardized criteria for diagnosing prolapse on MRI or fluoroscopy, it is usually measured relative to the

---

TABLE 14.2. *Comparison of fluoroscopy and magnetic resonance imaging (MRI)*

Patient position
    Fluoroscopy: sitting; patient defecates on commode
    MRI: supine; patient strains or defecates in supine position
Rectal contrast
    Fluoroscopy: administered; provides dynamic assessment of rectal evacuation
    MRI: variable; rectal contrast may more reliably increase abdominal pressure during study to demonstrate prolapse; allows assessment for rectal intussusception
Imaging plane
    Fluoroscopy: sagittal; frontal views may be performed in patients with small body habitus
    MRI: multiplanar; coronal, sagittal, axial, oblique images can be obtained; lateral prolapse easier to identify
Ionizing radiation
    Fluoroscopy: dose depends on study time
    MRI: none
Study time
    Both studies average 30–60 min
    Fluoroscopy: operator dependent
    MRI: operator dependent
Soft tissue contrast
    Fluoroscopy: low
    MRI: excellent
    (a) Visualization of pelvic organs
        Fluoroscopy: rectal/bladder/vaginal contrast necessary to visualize; only lumens of structures seen
        MRI: contrast often given but not necessary to visualize pelvic organs; see lumen of viscera and surrounding soft tissues; can distinguish fat/fluid/muscle
    (b) Visualization of cervix
        Fluoroscopy: indirect assessment of cervix by edge of contrast column in vagina
        MRI: cervix and uterus can be directly visualized
    (c) Diagnosis of abnormal rectovaginal space
        Fluoroscopy: herniating contrast-filled small bowel or peritoneal contrast necessary to see abnormal space
        MRI: peritoneal fat in rectovaginal space can be recognized; small bowel herniation not necessary
    (d) Visualization of pelvic floor structures
        Fluoroscopy: cannot see pelvic floor muscles/anal sphincter
        MRI: pelvic floor muscles, ligaments, urethral wall, anal sphincter can be visualized

---

bony landmarks of the pelvis. The pubococcygeal line from the inferior pubic symphysis to the last coccygeal joint is the usual reference line on MRI because it is reproducible (27) (Fig. 14.9). In general, if the bladder base and cervix or vaginal vault lie below the pubococcygeal line, it is considered to be abnormal. On fluoroscopy, descent of the bladder below the pubic symphysis is abnormal. If small bowel in the rectovaginal septum is below the junction of the proximal one third and distal two thirds of the vagina, an enterocele is diagnosed (50). A rectocele is diagnosed if the anterior bulge of the rectal wall is larger than 2 cm relative to a line drawn along the anterior margin of the anal canal. Because there is a wide range of normal descent of the pelvic organs and rectal bulging with straining, pelvic organ prolapse is considered to be clinically significant only if the patient is symptomatic (50). Other measurements on MRI are the angle of the levator plate relative to the pubococcygeal line and the width and area of the pelvic hiatus at rest and with straining.

Imaging is useful in the evaluation of POP in patients with symptoms unexplained by the clinical evaluation, those with defecatory and voiding disorders, and those with recurrence or a failed previous repair.

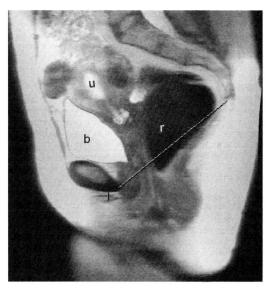

FIG. 14.9. Pubococcygeal line on magnetic resonance imaging (MRI). Sagittal T$_2$-weighted MRI of the pelvis with the patient at rest. The pubococcygeal line extends from the inferior pubis to the last coccygeal joint. Bladder (b), uterus (u), and rectum (r) are normal in position.

Fecal Incontinence

Fecal incontinence often results from a dysfunctional anal sphincteric mechanism or rectal reservoir or from a bypass of the normal continence system (fistula). Double incontinence (incontinence of feces and urine) or fecal incontinence due to two mechanisms is even more challenging in defining a causative factor for each dysfunction, whereas recurring incontinence requires the utmost care in diagnosis and management (51). Fluoroscopy, ultrasound, and MRI are useful in addition to functional studies to evaluate patients with fecal incontinence. Radiographic imaging with or without contrast aims at identifying or excluding impaction and congenital, inflammatory, and neoplastic processes. More recently, fluoroscopy has been employed to study the real-time and dynamic interaction between the anorectum and the adjacent pelvic organs during defecation. However, fluoroscopy offers little information on soft tissue or muscle anatomy and function. MRI provides an unsurpassed advantage, particularly as regards the anatomy of the anal sphincters. Ultrasound also provides excellent imaging detail of anatomy and focal pathology.

During the 1980s, the gold standard for the identification of anal sphincter defects was electromyographic mapping of the anal sphincters. In 1990, Law and coworkers evaluated 15 patients with fecal incontinence subsequent to perineal trauma by anal endosonography and concentric needle electromyography (52). In the 12 patients with electromyographic muscle defects, endoanal ultrasound identified sphincter defects in the same quadrants. Meyenberger and colleagues validated the accuracy of endoanal ultrasound to identify internal and external anal sphincter defects and found it to be more accurate for internal than external anal sphincter tears (53). Endoanal ultrasound provides more accurate information regarding the internal anal sphincter because it tends to overestimate external anal sphincter volume (54,55). It has been recommended in all patients with fecal incontinence to detect occult sphincter defects or muscular hypotrophy of structurally intact sphincters (56,57). Although not an optimal tool for the diagnosis of rectovaginal fistula, it has been recommended to identify and map out occult sphincter defects (58).

Endoanal ultrasound is the principal method to examine the morphology of the internal anal sphincter (IAS), external anal sphincter (EAS), the puborectalis, and the rectovaginal septum. It may be used to look for cryptoglandular abscesses and has been used to evaluate the relative bulk of the sphincters in the upper, middle, and lower portions of the anal canal (59).

Some clinicians have sought to avoid the cost of the endoanal ultrasound probe through the use of transvaginal ultrasound imaging of the anal sphincters, although its utility is controversial (60). Assessment of the perineal body and perineal inflammation may be more accurate with the transvaginal approach.

The internal and external anal sphincters are also visible on MRI (61). MRI is more accurate than ultrasound in the evaluation of the anal sphincters and in particular the external anal sphincter while also providing an excellent visualization of pelvic floor structures (62). Hussain and co-workers conclude that endoanal MRI is superior to endoanal ultrasound in the detection and the classification of fistula in ano (63).

Defecatory Dysfunction

Defecatory dysfunction results from bowel dysmotility or outlet dysfunction. The latter is seen in pelvic floor dyssynergia in which the patient looses the ability to relax during rectal evacuation and with poor anatomic support as seen in significant rectocele, sigmoidocele, and enterocele with or without rectal intussusception.

The evaluation of colonic dysmotility is hindered by its relative inaccessibility. The colon transit time represents about 75% of mouth-to-anus transit. The oral ingestion of radiopaque markers retrieved by radiographs of the stools provides a good approximation. Further simplifications have been introduced with the use of serial abdominal films to localize the markers in the colon and then three doses of markers and a single x-ray (64). Y-scintigraphy provides a means of assessing regional transit along the course of the colon by using a pH-sensitive radiolabel capsule.

Rectal evacuation depends on a colonic contraction as well as sphincter and pelvic floor relaxation for a full evacuation of a well-supported anorectum. Contraction of the levator ani or abnormal angulation of the enteric viscera as a result of herniation or deficient support will interfere with a normal and complete evacuation. This can also be seen in extrinsic compression of the pelvic floor and organs by prolapsing loops of bowel.

Pelvic fluoroscopy is the accepted imaging test to evaluate rectal evacuation. Pelvic fluoroscopy can demonstrate obstructive defecation disorders (65). The results of the test must be used in conjunction with symptoms and clinical examination, because patients without symptoms have been demonstrated to have rectoceles and minor degrees of intussusception (33).

Mahieu and associates recorded findings in normal subjects and defined five criteria for normal: (a) decrease in the anorectal angle, (b) obliteration of the puborectalis impression, (c) widening of the anal canal, (d) complete rectal evacuation, and (e) normal resistance of the pelvic floor. Rectoceles have been graded as less than 2 cm, 2 to 4 cm, and

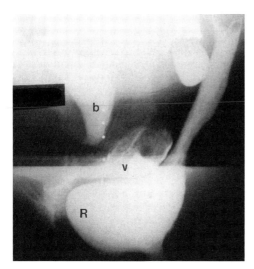

FIG. 14.10. Anterior rectocele. Lateral fluoroscopic image of the pelvis obtained during defecation with the patient seated on a commode. There is an abnormal anterior bulge of the rectum compatible with a rectocele (R). There is also prolapse of the vagina (v) and bladder (b).

greater than 4 cm. Anterior rectal bulges relative to the anal canal 2 cm or smaller are considered normal and only clinically relevant in patients with symptoms (66). The size of the rectocele and barium retention can be estimated on pelvic fluoroscopy (Fig. 14.10).

Pelvic fluoroscopy is the definitive test for diagnosing intrarectal intussusception (33) (Fig. 14.11). This can be anterior or annular and starts at the anterior wall of the rectum 6 to 8 cm from the anorectal junction (33). Pelvic fluoroscopy can also demonstrate incomplete relaxation of the puborectalis (also known as paradox or anismus) and delayed initiation of rectal emptying, which is incomplete in patients with a spastic pelvic floor (33).

On MRI, rectal evacuation can be determined if rectal contrast is administered. Imaging can be performed along the plane of the rectum and sigmoid colon. Rectoceles usually appear as an anterior bulge in the contour of the rectum. Typically, a line is extrapolated upward from the anterior wall of the anal canal, and a rectal bulge of greater than 2 cm anterior to this line is described as a rectocele (36) (Fig. 14.12). If the rectocele is large, it is seen as a circular structure inferior to the bladder on coronal images of the anterior pelvis. The rectum can also appear to fold on itself with anterior displacement. Lateral and posterior bulging of the rectum can also be seen with anterior displacement. Lateral and posterior bulging of the rectum can also occur in areas where there is weakness in the levator ani muscle.

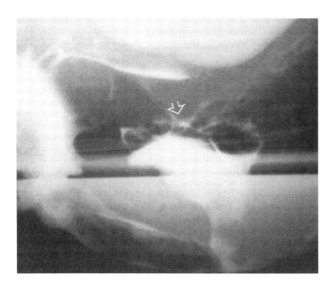

FIG. 14.11. Intrarectal intussusception. Lateral fluoroscopic image of the pelvis obtained during defecation with the patient seated on a commode. There is circumferential infolding of the rectal mucosa (*open arrow*) compatible with intussusception in the rectum.

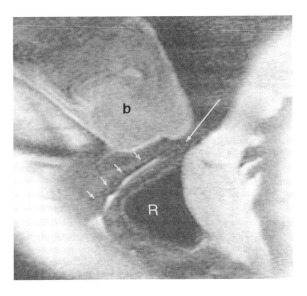

FIG. 14.12. Rectocele on magnetic resonance imaging (MRI). Sagittal T$_2$-weighted MRI of the pelvis during patient defecation. Contrast in the anal canal and rectum is bright in signal intensity. There is an anterior bulge of the rectum relative to the anus compatible with anterior rectocele (R). The apex of the vagina is also low in the pelvis (*long arrow*). The vagina is outlined by luminal contrast (*short arrows*). There is also minimal prolapse of the bladder (b).

Upright Magnetic Resonance Imaging Studies

Lamb and associates studied 40 patients with defecatory dysfunction in a vertical configuration magnet using mashed potatoes mixed with gadolinium as rectal contrast (67). Patients evacuated contrast on a commode, and rectoceles, animus, and rectal intussusception were demonstrated in addition to anterior pelvic prolapse. MRI defecography in a vertical configuration magnet has been found to be comparable to fluoroscopy for detecting anorectal pathology and also provides additional information on the pelvic soft tissues (68).

CONCLUSIONS AND FUTURE RESEARCH

In summary, current imaging modalities offer an improved opportunity to evaluate the pelvic floor and organs in displacement and dysfunction. Real-time ultrasound is appropriate for evaluation of bladder volume, particularly postvoid residual, imaging of urethral mobility, and anal sphincter assessment. Dynamic fluoroscopy is useful for the evaluation of the pelvic viscera and their dysfunction, voiding and defecatory. MRI is optimal for POP as well as urethral and anal sphincter definition.

Improved clinical applications of imaging requires an urgent and cooperative effort at standardizing nomenclature, reporting, and techniques as well as multimodality investigation of the various components of the pelvic floor and organs. The exact contribution of the architecture of the bony pelvis needs elucidation. The future will rely on combined anatomic and functional studies using ultrasound and MRI modalities to answer some basic and critical questions. The role and function of recognized anatomic structures, and the mechanisms of functional or surgical correction need to be defined.

Advances in technology have allowed a better appreciation of the functional anatomy of the pelvic floor. Initially, various modalities have documented that what can be seen during a thorough examination can also be visualized. With more refined understanding of the unitary and global interaction of the pelvic floor and its contents, it has become possible to image what could only be determined on physical examination in the upright position. Now, upright MRI, sitting ultrasound, and dynamic fluoroscopy are helping to visualize what lies behind what is seen on examination. This allows the role of imaging to extend beyond documentation of what is visible to the exploratory uncovering of the invisible. Recognizing that imaging is important not only to visualize what is not obvious but also to visualize what is evident but not recognized, one may wonder about whether the current value of imaging does not reside more in the questions it raises than in the answers it actually provides. Its role in clinical management remains to be defined.

Technology is driving progress. Ultimately, not only should imaging document what is seen, it also should allow us to see the critical part that cannot be otherwise appreciated. For this, technologic progress should be matched by clinical progress and understanding of all the extraordinary data afforded us by the new universe of the pelvic floor that remains to be explored and understood.

Until then, technology offers various modalities, each revealing certain aspects of the pelvic floor better than others. Attention to their judicious use and the individual patient's condition, not simply the latest technology, should guarantee our best results. Clinical management should continue to rely on historical and clinical evaluation of the patient with symptoms using currently established imaging to address the individual circumstance with the aim of minimizing risk for failure, recurrence, and dysfunction while maximizing resolution and ultimately cure.

REFERENCES

1. Davis HJ, Cian LG. Positive pressure urethrography: a new diagnostic method. *J Urol* 1956;75:753–757.
2. Hodgkinson CP. Relationship of female urethra and bladder in urinary stress incontinence. *Am J Obstet Gynecol* 1953;65:560.
3. Maglinte DDT, Kelvin FM, Hale DS, et al. Dynamic cystoproctography: a unifying diagnostic approach to pelvic floor and anorectal dysfunction. *AJR Am J Roentgenol* 1997;169:759–767.
4. Hock D, Lombard R, Jehaes C, et al. Colpocystodefecography. *Dis Colon Rectum* 1993;36:1015–1021.
5. Halligan S, Spence-Jones C, Kamm MA, et al. Dynamic cystoproctography and physiological testing in women with urinary stress incontinence and urogenital prolapse. *Clin Radiol* 1996;51:785–790.
6. Brubaker L, Retzky S, Smith C, et al. Pelvic floor evacuation with dynamic fluoroscopy. *Obstet Gynecol* 1993;82:863–868.
7. Siegelman ES, Outwater EK, Banner MP, et al. High-

8. Mouritsen L. Techniques for imaging bladder support. *Acta Obstet Gynecol Scand Suppl* 1997;166:48–49.
9. Dietz HP, Wilson PD. Anatomical assessment of the bladder outlet and proximal urethra using ultrasound and videocystourethrography. *Int Urogynecol J Pelvic Floor Dysfunct* 1998;9:365–369.
10. Roehrborn CG, Peters PC. Can transabdominal ultrasound estimation of postvoiding residual replace catheterization? *Urology* 1988;16:445–449.
11. Quinn MJ, Benyon J, Mortensen NJ, et al. Transvaginal endosonography to study the anatomy of the lower urinary tract in urinary stress incontinence. *Br J Urol* 1988;62:414–418.
12. Peschers U, Schaer G, Anthuber C, et al. Changes in vesical neck mobility following vaginal delivery. *Obstet Gynecol* 1996;88:1001–1006.
13. Johnson JD, Lamensdorf H, Hollander IN, et al. Use of transvaginal endosonography in the evaluation of women with stress urinary incontinence. *J Urol* 1992;147:421.
14. Schaer GN, Koechli OR, Schuessler B, et al. Improvement of perineal sonographic bladder neck imaging with ultrasound contrast medium. *Obstet Gynecol* 1995;86:950–954.
15. Nishizwa O, Moriya I, Satoh S, et al. A new video urodynamics: combined ultrasonotomography and urodynamic monitoring. *Neurourol Urodyn* 1982;1:295–301.
16. Bergman A, Ballard CA, Platt LD. Ultrasonic evaluation of urethrovesical junction in women with stress urinary incontinence. *J Clin Ultrasound* 1988;16:295.
17. Sanders R, Genadry R, Yang A, et al. Imaging of the female urethra. *Ultrasound Q* 1994;12:167–183.
18. Frauscher F, Helweg G, Strasser H, et al. Intraurethral ultrasound: diagnostic evaluation of the striated urethral sphincter in incontinent females. *Eur Radiol* 1998;8(1):50–53.
19. Heit M. Intraurethral ultrasonography: correlation of urethral anatomy with functional urodynamic parameters in stress incontinent women. *Int Urogynecol J Pelvic Floor Dysfunct* 2000;11(4):204–211.
20. Kondo Y, Homma Y, Takahashi S, et al. Transvaginal ultrasound of urethral sphincter at the mid urethra in continent and incontinent women. *J Urol* 2001;165(1):149–152.
21. Athanasiou S, Khullar V, Boos K, et al. Imaging the urethral sphincter with three-dimensional ultrasound. *Obstet Gynecol* 1999;94(2):295–301.
22. Neitlich JD, Foster HE Jr, Glickman MG, et al. Detection of urethral diverticula in women: comparison of a high resolution fast spin echo technique with double balloon urethrography. *J Urol* 1998;159(2):408–410.
23. Wang AC, Wang CR. Radiologic diagnosis and surgical treatment of urethral diverticulum in women: a reappraisal of voiding cystourethrography and positive pressure urethrography. *J Reprod Med* 2000;45(5):377–382.
24. Kim B, Hricak H, Tanagho EA. Diagnosis of urethral diverticula in women: value of MR imaging. *AJR Am J Roentgenol* 1993;161(4):809–815.
25. Jacoby K, Rowbotham RK. Double balloon positive pressure urethrography is a more sensitive test than voiding cystourethrography for diagnosing urethral diverticulum in women. *J Urol* 1999;162(6):2066–2069.
26. Chancellor MB, Liu JB, Rivas DA, et al. Intraoperative

resolution MR imaging of the vagina. *Radiographics* 1997;17:1183–1203.

endo-luminal ultrasound evaluation of urethral diverticula. *J Urol* 1995;153(1):72–75.

27. Yang A, Mostwin JL, Rosenshein NB, et al. Pelvic floor descent in women: dynamic evaluation with fast MR imaging and cinematic display. *Radiology* 1991;179:25–33.

28. Yang A, Mostwin JL, Genadry R, et al. Patterns of prolapse demonstrated with dynamic fast scan MRI, reassessment of conventional concepts of pelvic floor weaknesses. *Neurourol Urodyn* 1993;12:310–311.

29. Genadry, R Yang A, Mostwin JL, et al. Dynamics of pelvic relaxation: early observations. *Int Urogynecol J Pelvic Floor Dysfunct* 1993;4:395.

30. Nguyen JK, Hall CD, Bhatia NN. Sonographic diagnosis of paravaginal defects: A standardization of technique. *Int Urogynecol J Pelvic Floor Dysfunct* 2000;11:341–345.

31. Beverly CM, Walters MD, Weber AM, et al. Prevalence of hydronephrosis in patients undergoing surgery for pelvic organ prolapse. *Obstet Gynecol* 1997;90:37–41.

32. Kelvin FM, Hale DS, Maglinte DD, et al. Female pelvic organ prolapse: diagnostic contribution of dynamic cystoproctography and comparison with physical examination. *AJR Am J Roentgenol* 1999;173:31–37.

33. Kelvin FM, Maglinte DD, Hornback JA, et al. Pelvic prolapse: assessment with evacuation proctography (defecography). *Radiology* 1992;184:547–551.

34. Stoker J, Halligan S, Bartram CI. Pelvic floor imaging. *Radiology* 2001;218:621–641.

35. DeLancey JOL. The anatomy of the pelvic floor. *Curr Opin Obstet Gynecol* 1994;6:313–316.

36. Lienemann A, Anthuber C, Baron A, et al. Dynamic MR colpocystorectography assessing pelvic-floor descent. *Eur Radiol* 1997;7:1309–1317.

37. Tunn R, Paris S, Taupitz M, et al. MR imaging in posthysterectomy vaginal prolapse. *Int Urogynecol J Pelvic Floor Dysfunct* 2000;11:87–92.

38. Healy JC, Halligan S, Reznek RH, et al. Patterns of prolapse in women with symptoms of pelvic floor weakness: assessment with MR imaging. *Radiology* 1997;203:77–81.

39. Tunn R, DeLancey JOL, Howard D, et al. MR imaging of levator ani muscle recovery following vaginal delivery. *Int Urogynecol J Pelvic Floor Dysfunct* 1999;10:300–307.

40. Hayat SK, Thorp JM, Kuller JA, et al. Magnetic resonance imaging of the pelvic floor in the postpartum patient. *Int Urogynecol J Pelvic Floor Dysfunct* 1996;7:321–324.

41. Goodrich MA, Webb MJ, King BF, et al. Magnetic resonance imaging of pelvic floor relaxation: dynamic analysis and evaluation of patients before and after surgical repair. *Obstet Gynecol* 1993;82:883–891.

42. Lienemann A, Sprenger D, Anthuber C, et al. Functional cine magnetic resonance imaging in women after abdominal sacrocolpopexy. *Obstet Gynecol* 2001;97:81–85.

43. Osaza H, Mori T, Togashi K. Study of uterine prolapse by magnetic resonance imaging: topographical changes involving the levator ani muscle and the vagina. *Gynecol Obstet Invest* 1992;34:43–48.

44. Aronson MP, Bates SM, Jacoby AF, et al. Periurethral and paravaginal anatomy: an endovaginal magnetic resonance imaging study. *Am J Obstet Gynecol* 1995;173:1702–1710.

45. Tan IL, Stoker J, Lameris JS. Magnetic resonance imaging of the female pelvic floor and urethra: body coil vs endovaginal coil. *Magma* 1997;5:59–63.

46. Kelvin FM, Maglinte DDT, Hale DS, et al. Female pelvic organ prolapse: a comparison of triphasic dynamic MR imaging and triphasic fluoroscopic cystoproctography. *AJR Am J Roentgenol* 2000;174:81–88.

47. Vanbeckevoort D, Van Hoe L, Oyen R, et al. Pelvic floor descent in females: Comparative study of colpocystodefecography and dynamic fast MR imaging. *J Magn Reson Imaging* 1999;9:373–377.

48. Delemarre JBVM, Kruyt RH, Doornbos J, et al. Anterior rectocele: assessment with radiographic defecography, dynamic magnetic resonance imaging, and physical examination. *Dis Colon Rectum* 1994;37:249–259.

49. Gousse AE, Barbaric ZL, Safir MH, et al. Dynamic half Fourier acquisition, single shot turbo spin-echo magnetic resonance imaging for evaluating the female pelvis. *J Urol* 2000;164:1606–1613.

50. Goh V, Halligan S, Kaplan G, et al. Dynamic MR imaging of the pelvic floor in asymptomatic subjects. *AJR Am J Roentgenol* 2000;174:661–666.

51. Genadry R, Nichols D. Recurrent anal incontinence. In: Nichols D, ed. *Reoperative gynecologic and obstetric surgery.* St. Louis: Mosby, 1997:240–260.

52. Law PJ, Kamm MA, Bartram CI. A comparison between electromyography and anal endosonography in mapping external anal sphincter defects. *Dis Colon Rectum* 1990;33:370–373.

53. Meyenberger C, Bertschinger P, Zala GF, et al. Anal sphincter defects in fecal incontinence: correlation between endosonography and surgery. *Endoscopy* 1996;28:217–224.

54. Konerding MA, Dzemali O, Gaumann A, et al. Correlation of endoanal sonography with cross-sectional anatomy of the anal sphincter. *Gastrointest Endosc* 1999;50:804–810.

55. Bartram C. Radiologic evaluation of anorectal disorders. *Gastroenterol Clin North Am* 2001;30:55–75.

56. Rieger NA, Sweeney JL, Hoffmann DC, et al. Investigation of fecal incontinence with endoanal ultrasound. *Dis Colon Rectum* 1996;39:860–864.

57. Sailer M, Leppert R, Fuchs KH, et al. [Endo-anal sonography in diagnosis of fecal incontinence] [article in German]. *Zentralbl Chir* 1996;121:639–644.

58. Yee LF, Birnbaum EH, Read TE, et al. Use of endoanal ultrasound in patients with rectovaginal fistulas. *Dis Colon Rectum* 1999;42:1057–1064.

59. Keighley MRB, Williams NS. Faecal incontinence. In: Keighley MRB, Williams NS, eds. *Surgery of the anus rectum and colon.* London: WB Saunders, 1993:516–608.

60. Frudlinger A, Bartram CI, Kamm MA. Transvaginal versus anal ultrasound for detecting damage to the anal sphincter. *AJR Am J Roentgenol* 1997;168:1435–1438.

61. Peschers UM, Delancey JO, Fritsch H, et al. Cross sectional imaging anatomy of the anal sphincter. *Obstet Gynecol* 1997;90:839.

62. Stoker J, Rociu E. Endoluminal MR imaging of diseases of the anus and rectum. *Semin Ultrasound CT MRI* 1999;20:47–55.

63. Hussain SM, Stoker J, Schouten WR, et al. Fistula in ano: endoanal sonography versus endoanal MR imaging in classification. *Radiology* 1996;200:475–481.

64. Phillips SF. Techniques of assessment of colonic motility in humans. In: Schuster MM, ed. *Atlas of gastrointestinal motility in health and disease.* Baltimore: Williams & Wilkins, 1993:215–218.

65. Kelvin FM, Maglinte DDT, Benson JT. Evacuation proctography (defecography): an aid to the investigation of pelvic floor disorders. *Obstet Gynecol* 1994;83: 307–314.

66. Yoshioka K, Matsui Y, Yamada O, et al. Physiologic and anatomic assessment of patients with rectocele. *Dis Colon Rectum* 1991;34:704–708.

67. Lamb GM, De Jode MG, Gould SW, et al. Upright dynamic MR defaecating proctography in an open configuration MR system. *Br J Radiol* 2000;73:152–155.

68. Schoenenberger AW, Debatin JF, Guldenschuh I, et al. Dynamic MR defecography with a superconducting, open-configuration MR system. *Radiology* 1998;206: 641–646.

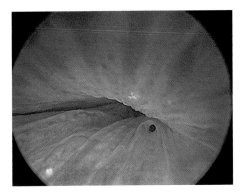

Color Plate 1. Normal urethra. There is pink, lush epithelium in folds. (See Figure 12.4.)

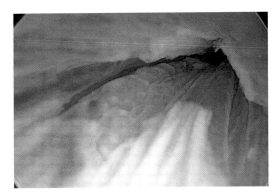

Color Plate 2. Urethral crest and squamous epithelium of normal urethra. The urethral crest runs posteriorly as a longitudinal ridge, and over it is white epithelium. (See Figure 12.5.)

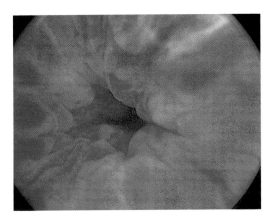

Color Plate 3. Acute urethritis. The urethra is reddened along its length. (See Figure 12.6.)

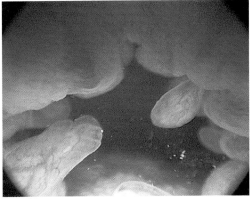

Color Plate 4. Polyps and fronds at the urethrovesical junction. (See Figure 12.7.)

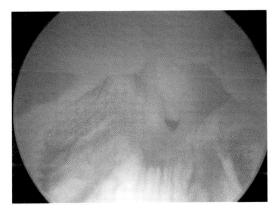

Color Plate 5. Urethrovaginal fistula. The urethral canal is in the upper right of the photograph, and the opening from the urethra to the vagina is clearly seen as a small opening in the center of the picture. (See Figure 12.8.)

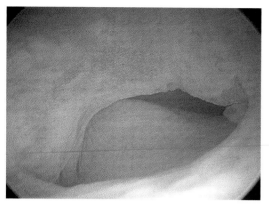

Color Plate 6. Functionless urethra. The urethra is very short and remains passively open, with the urethroscope barely inside the meatus. The epithelium is smooth, and there is no movement with hold or strain maneuvers. (See Figure 12.9.)

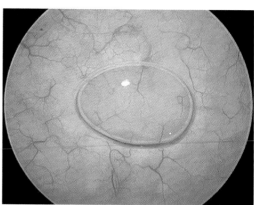

Color Plate 7. Normal bladder. The air bubble is at the dome of the bladder and serves as a reference marker. The epithelium of the bladder wall is smooth and pale pink and has fine vasculature. (See Figure 12.10.)

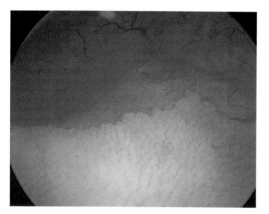

Color Plate 8. Metaplasia of trigone. The white membrane covers much of the trigone leading up to the ureters. Biopsy reveals squamous metaplasia. (See Figure 12.11.)

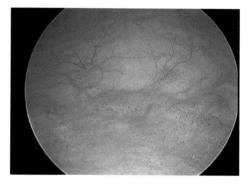

Color Plate 9. Trigone. The trigone is formed by the urethrovesical junction inferiorly and the ureteral orifices superiorly. The trigone is frequently reddened and granular. (See Figure 12.12.)

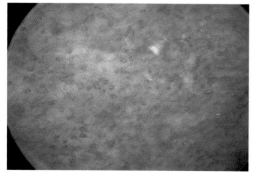

Color Plate 10. Acute cystitis. The bladder mucosa is reddened and edematous, making it difficult to see clearly. There is often active bleeding further compromising the view. (See Figure 12.13.)

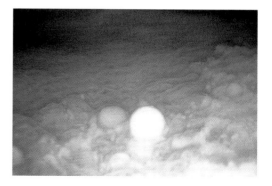

Color Plate 11. Cystitis cystica. The 1- to 2-mm cysts at the bladder base are smooth-walled and are clear or sometimes pigmented. (See Figure 12.14.)

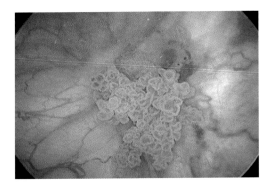

Color Plate 12. Bladder cancer. The pedunculated papillary lesion is a transitional cell carcinoma. (See Figure 12.15.)

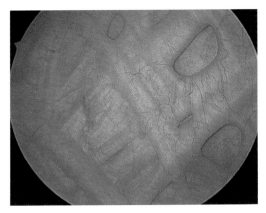

Color Plate 13. Trabeculation. The muscle bundles appear as prominent ridges with intervening pockets or cellules. (See Figure 12.16.)

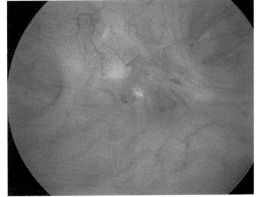

Color Plate 14. Vesicovaginal fistula. The openings in the bladder with a posthysterectomy fistula occur superior to the trigone in the posterior aspect of the bladder, and there are two distinct holes to the vagina in this picture. (See Figure 12.17.)

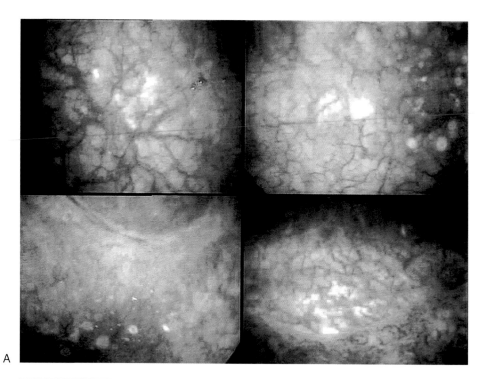

A

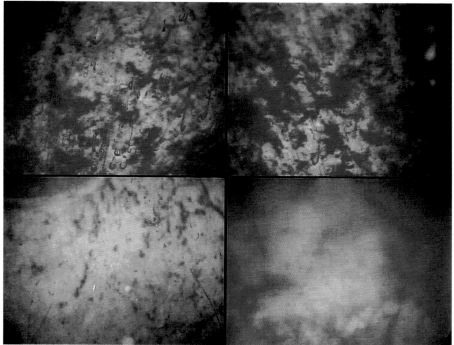

B

Color Plate 15. A: Interstitial cystitis (IC) before hydrodistention. The initial filling of the bladder appears normal. **B:** IC after hydrodistention in same patient. Numerous petechiae and glomerulations appear after the bladder has been distended and emptied, then refilled, indicating a diagnosis of interstitial cystitis. Eventually, enough blood accumulate to cloud the picture in bottom right of figure. (See Figure 21.3.)

Ostergard's Urogynecology and Pelvic Floor
Dysfunction, Fifth Edition. edited by A.E. Bent, et al.
Lippincott Williams & Wilkins, Philadelphia © 2003.

15

Evaluation of Colorectal Dysfunction

Marc R. Toglia

Department of Obstetrics and Gynecology, Thomas Jefferson Medical College, Philadelphia,
Pennsylvania; and Subdivision of Gynecology, Department of Obstetrics and Gynecology, Riddle
Memorial Hospital, Media, Pennsylvania

Colorectal disorders occur commonly among adult women and are associated with diverse symptoms, including abdominal pain and bloating, constipation, incomplete defecation, and fecal incontinence. Clinicians caring for women with pelvic floor dysfunction need to have an adequate understanding of the physiology and pathophysiology of the colon and anorectum.

OVERVIEW OF NORMAL COLORECTAL FUNCTION

Stool Formation and Colonic Transit

Voluntary storage and defecation of the rectal contents is a complex neuromuscular mechanism that involves many physiologic processes. Intestinal transit and absorption, colonic transit, rectal compliance, anorectal sensation, and sphincteric mechanism are among the variables involved. An understanding of how each of these variables affects continence is essential in the proper diagnosis and treatment of women with colorectal disorders.

A major function of the colon is the final regulation of water and electrolyte balance in the intestine. The colon is capable of absorbing up to 5 L of water and associated electrolytes in 24 hours. Stool content is propelled along the large intestine through contractile waves know as peristalsis. Colonic motility is complex, with great regional heterogeneity. Functionally, the colon can be divided into three segments: the proximal colon; the segment from the middle transverse colon to the proximal rectosigmoid; and the rectosigmoid. The rectosigmoid is uniquely adapted for sodium and water absorption. The transit of the stool content is significantly delayed in this region to permit complete reabsorption of fecal water and electrolytes before final elimination.

Anorectal Continence

The voluntary storage and evacuation of solid waste is a complex physiologic process involving learned social behavior, voluntary cortical control, and a series of involuntary reflexes. When stool content first enters into the rectal vault, several physiologic events take place. The arrival of stool in the rectum is associated with a transient decrease in internal anal sphincter tone and an increase in external sphincter activity; this is known as the rectoanal inhibitory reflex. This allows the sensory-rich anal canal to come in contact with the rectal contents to determine whether it contains solid, liquid, or gas. This physiologic event is known as sampling. This is followed by a relaxation of the rectum to contain the increased rectal volume in a process known as accommodation. The rectum, like the bladder, is a highly compliant reservoir that facilitates storage of waste. As rectal volume increases, an urge to defecate is experienced. If this urge is voluntarily suppressed, the rectum relaxes to continue the accommodation of stool.

Rectal compliance may be decreased in certain disease states such as ulcerative proctitis or radiation proctitis. A loss in compliance may decrease the ability of the rectal wall to stretch (i.e., accommodate); as a result, rectal pressure remains high. This may compromise this first part of the continence mechanism and place an increased demand on the continence mechanism of the anorectum.

The continence mechanism of the anorectum is primarily responsible for preventing leakage of the rectal contents during the stage of storage. The anal canal maintains a high-pressure zone as the result of the interactions between three distinct muscles: the puborectalis portion of the levator ani, the external anal sphincter, and the internal anal sphincter. The puborectalis and external anal sphincter

are composed of a unique type of striated muscles that is capable of maintaining a constant resting tone, which is proportional to the volume of the rectal content and relaxes at the time of defecation. Both of these muscles contain a majority of type I (slow-twitch) muscle fibers, which are ideally suited to maintaining a constant tone over time. Each muscle group also contains a smaller proportion of type II (fast-twitch) fibers, which allows them to respond quickly during sudden increases in intraabdominal pressures (1).

Continence of solid stool is maintained primarily by the actions of the puborectalis. This muscle originates from the pubic rami on either side of the midline at the level of the arcus tendineus levator ani. The muscle fibers pass laterally to the vagina and form a U-shaped sling that cradles the rectum. The constant resting tone of the puborectalis pulls the anorectal junction toward the pubic symph-

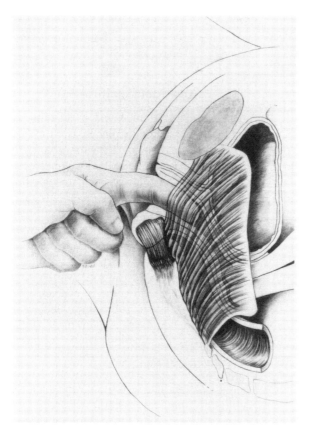

FIG. 15.1. Lateral view of the external anal sphincter and levator ani muscles showing palpation of the medial border of the levator ani muscle (puborectalis-pubococcygeus portion). Note the approximately 90-degree angle between the anal canal and the axis of the rectum. (From Toglia MR, DeLancey JOL. Anal Incontinence and the Obstetrician Gynecologist. *Obstet Gynecol* 1994;84; 4(2):731–740, with permission.)

ysis creating a near 90-degree angle between the anal and rectal canals referred to as the anorectal angle (Fig. 15.1). This angulation is easily palpated on digital rectal examination. It was once proposed that this acute angulation creates a flap-valve effect in which an increase in intraabdominal pressure compresses the anterior rectal wall against the pelvic floor and that this action was critical to maintaining continence. However, more recent physiologic studies have failed to demonstrate that such a mechanism exists (2,3), and successful surgical restoration of anal continence does not appear to depend on the restoration of this angle (4,5).

Defecation of solid stool is initiated by the voluntary relaxation of this muscle, which together with intestinal peristalsis, voluntary increase in intraabdominal pressure, and relaxation of the external and internal anal sphincters, allows for the passage of stool downward through the anal canal. The effectiveness of the puborectalis muscle in maintaining continence without the external or internal anal sphincter is illustrated by the relative continence that women with a chronic fourth-degree laceration have over solid stool.

The internal and external anal sphincters maintain continence below the level of the puborectalis (Fig. 15.2). These two structures are critical in the control of flatus and liquid feces because the puborectalis mechanism is ineffective in this regard. The shape of the combined internal and external sphincter complex is nearly cylindrical as it encircles the anal canal and, measured in the midline, is about 18-mm thick and 28-mm long (6). It is critical that clinicians recognize that 50% of the anterior thickness of the sphincter complex is attributable to the internal anal sphincter. The anatomic and functional importance of the internal anal sphincter is often underappreciated in most textbooks on obstetrics and gynecologic surgery but is critical in the proper repair of obstetric sphincter lacerations as well as the surgical correction of anal incontinence.

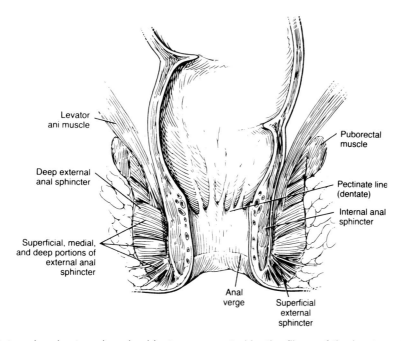

FIG. 15.2. Internal and external anal sphincters, separated by the fibers of the levator ani muscles, seen in coronal section. (From Lee RA. *Atlas of Gynecologic Surgery*. Philadelphia, PA: WB Saunders, 1992:313, by permission of the Mayo Foundation.)

The internal anal sphincter is a thickened, downward continuation of the circular smooth muscle layer of the colon and is innervated by sympathetic nerves from the presacral complex. Unlike the external anal sphincter and puborectalis muscle, the internal anal sphincter is not under voluntary control, and its function is mediated largely by reflex arcs at the spinal cord level. At rest, the anal canal is kept closed by the constant tonic activity of both the internal and external anal sphincters. Physiologic studies suggest that the internal anal sphincter is responsible for 75% to 85% of the resting tone of the anal canal (7,8). As the intestinal content passes into the rectum, the internal anal sphincter relaxes reflexively to allow the upper anal canal to "sample" the contents and to discriminate between solid, liquid, and gas. Once the intestinal contents have been determined, the internal anal sphincter contracts again to augment closure of the anal canal. Thus, it is currently believed that continence at rest (particularly for liquid stool and flatus) is largely the responsibility of the internal anal sphincter, whereas continence during sudden distention of the anal canal is principally maintained by the external anal sphincter (9).

Anal sensation is also thought to play a critical role in the normal continence mechanism. Sensory receptors located within the anal canal and within the levator ani muscles detect the presence of stool in the rectum as well as the degree of rectal distention. The upper anal canal is capable of distinguishing between solid, liquid, and gaseous forms of stool, and feedback from these sensory organs is important in coordinating the actions of the sphincteric musculature.

The anal canal cushions (hemorrhoids) are thought to assist in the continence mechanism by facilitating mucosal coaptation. These vascular channels fill with blood and may occlude the lower anal canal. Supporters of this theory suggest that the loss of these structures after hemorrhoidectomy may account for the reported incidence of incontinence following this procedure.

Defecation

Defecation is a complex act that involves neuromuscular regulation by the central nervous system. Rectal distention by the stool content initiates the rectoanal inhibitory reflex discussed previously and allows the sensory-rich upper anal canal to sample stool content. The act of defecation is initiated by a Valsalva maneuver to raise intraabdominal and intrarectal pressure. Voluntary inhibition of the external anal sphincter and puborectalis enables the rectum to empty. This is assisted by coordinated peristaltic activity of the rectosigmoid. When evacuation is completed, the external anal sphincter and puborectalis contract (termed the closing reflex), and the continence mechanism is initiated again.

SYMPTOM-BASED APPROACH TO COLORECTAL DISORDERS

Clinicians who care for women with pelvic floor disorders are commonly asked to evaluate patients with two separate syndromes involving colorectal disorders. The first syndrome involves symptoms suggestive of disordered defecation, and the second syndrome involves symptoms of fecal incontinence.

Disordered Defecation

Women with disordered defecation typically refer to their symptoms as "constipation." Constipation frequently has different meanings to different people. Commonly accepted definitions include: infrequent stools (less than three per week); passing stool that is too hard or too small; difficulty or prolongation of the act of defecation (straining); and a feeling of rectal fullness or incomplete evacuation. Abdominal pain and bloating are frequently the predominant complaint in constipated patients. Therefore, the first step in managing constipation is to understand what the patient means by using that term. It may be helpful to classify patients with constipation into one of three categories: (a) those with colonic motility disorders, (b) those with pelvic outlet obstructive symptoms, and (c) those with a combination of both (10) (Table 15.1). History, examination, and ancillary testing can distinguish them.

Clinicians should question the patient carefully to determine the following historical data: number of bowel movements a week; length of time spent on the commode; pain associated with defecation; sensation of incomplete evacuation or a false sense of the need to evacuate; need to assist defecation digitally by either splinting the perineum or vagina, or extracting feces from the anus directly; presence of a bulge either vaginal or rectal. Physical examination may reveal the presence of the following: uterovaginal prolapse, including a rectocele, rectal prolapse, fecal impaction, poor sphincter tone, or spasm of the puborectalis muscle. Proctoscopy is helpful in the detection of anal fissures, edema, internal hemorrhoids, or a solitary rectal ulcer. Ancillary testing is discussed in detail later.

Systemic Factors

After inadequate dietary fiber, drug therapy is probably the most common cause of constipation. Common prescription and over-the-counter medications that may cause constipa-

TABLE 15.2. *Drugs commonly associated with constipation*

Over-the-counter medication
Antidiarrheals such as loperamide and kaopectate®
Antacids (calcium and aluminum products)
Iron therapy
Prescription medication
Antidepressants
Anticholinergics
Anticonvulsants
Calcium-channel blockers
β-Blockers
Diuretics
Opiates
Nonsteroidal antiinflammatory agents
Phenothiazines
Psychotherapeutic agents

tion are listed in Table 15.2. Many systemic factors may also affect normal colonic factors and cause constipation. The prevalence of constipation during pregnancy is well recognized. Hypothyroidism, diabetes, hyperparathyroidism, and severe electrolyte abnormality can also cause constipation. Uncommon diseases such as scleroderma and amyloidosis can cause structural changes in the intestine that can lead to constipation. Central neurologic diseases, such as multiple sclerosis and Parkinson's disease, are frequently associated with constipation.

Colonic Motility Disorders

A deficiency in dietary fiber has long been thought to be an important cause of constipation. Fiber may shorten whole-gut transit and increase stool weight. Primary therapy for constipation consists of a diet trial with about 30 g of dietary fiber per day for 4 to 6 weeks coupled with an adequate intake of fluid.

Colonic inertia, or slow-transit constipation, is a condition of chronic idiopathic constipation in which patients are found to have no organic cause for their symptoms and to have diffuse, pancolonic marker delay on transit study. Megacolon or megarectum may or may not be present in association with colonic inertia. Colonic inertia is found almost exclusively in women, and some studies suggest an unusually high prevalence of psy-

TABLE 15.1. *Causes of constipation*

Systemic factors
Drug therapy
Metabolic and endocrine disorders
Neurologic disease
Pregnancy
Motility disorders
Inadequate fiber intake
Colonic inertia
Global motility disorder
Anorectal outlet obstruction
Intrarectal prolapse
Rectocele
Enterocele
Paradoxical puborectalis syndrome
Descending perineum
Irritable bowel syndrome

chiatric disturbances among these patients (11). Some patients with megacolon have a loss of the normal myenteric plexus ganglion cells, which is considered diagnostic of Hirschsprung's disease and usually presents in childhood or early adulthood.

Anorectal Outlet Obstruction Syndromes

Functional outlet obstruction is a common cause of constipation in women. These patients typically have no obvious organic cause of their symptoms. Colonic transit studies reveal normal pancolonic transit time but delayed transit through the rectum. Anorectal outlet obstruction may be the manifestation of a variety of pelvic floor disorders listed in Table 15.1.

Intrarectal prolapse, also referred to as rectal intussusception, is characterized by a circumferential intussusception of the upper rectal wall into the rectal ampulla. It occurs most commonly among women with an age of onset between 40 and 50 years. Symptoms include a sensation of obstruction, incontinence, pain on defecation, bleeding, and a mucus discharge (12). Patients with obstructive defecation typically complain of the sensation of incomplete evacuation and often have normal stool frequency and consistency. Bleeding is usually related to localized proctitis or a solitary rectal ulcer that occurs as the result of the intussusception. Diagnosis is most reliably confirmed by cinedefecography and proctosigmoidoscopy.

A rectocele represents a detachment of the rectovaginal fascia and subsequent herniation of the rectum and anal canal anteriorly against the posterior vaginal wall. Breaks in the rectovaginal fascia can occur transversely at its attachment to the perineal body or at the vaginal apex. Longitudinal breaks may exist laterally at the point that the lateral vagina attaches to the capsule of the levator ani or in the midline. Many rectoceles are clinically asymptomatic; however, in some patients they are the cause of obstructed defecation (13). Patients typically complain of incomplete evacuation and "pocketing" of stool into the vagina during attempts at defecation. Patients often re-

port using their fingers to splint the vagina during defecation or applying pressure to the posterior vaginal wall to complete evacuation. It is important to rule out other causes of constipation before contemplating surgical repair because as many as 54% of women continue to have significant constipation postoperatively in several published series (14,15). Most rectoceles can be characterized by vaginal and rectal examination, but cinedefecography is the preferred method of imaging the rectocele radiographically as well as of confirming that the rectocele is responsible for trapping the stool. It should be kept in mind that a rectocele by itself is not a common cause of constipation but rather presents as obstructed defecation. Therefore, a proper evaluation for other causes of anorectal outlet obstruction should be considered before proceeding with surgical correction.

Enterocele may be best described as a herniation of a peritoneal sac through the fibromuscular layer at the apex of the vagina. It is typically located posterior to the uterus and anterior to the rectum. On examination, the sac is typically filled with small intestine, omentum, or sigmoid colon. Enteroceles are thought to be a significant cause of symptoms after hysterectomy and anterior urethropexies. The best way to diagnose an enterocele is with the patient standing and straining. The examiner should place one finger in the vagina and another in the rectum. Although radiologic studies are often unnecessary, they may help to distinguish a true enterocele from a high rectocele or large cystocele. Symptoms include pelvic pressure, low back pain, and a feeling of perineal protrusion. In general, enteroceles are an uncommon cause of constipation.

Descending perineal syndrome is often associated with pronounced difficulty with defecation leading to prolonged straining efforts. First described by Sir Alan Parks, the syndrome is now clinically defined as when the plane of the perineum (at the level of the anal verge) descends beyond the ischial tuberosities during Valsalva maneuvers (16). Excessive descent of the perineum is typically readily apparent on physical examination and can be objectively quantified by defecography. Patients with this syndrome may also complain of deep-seated pain that is precipitated by prolonged standing and relieved by lying down. Neurologic damage to the pudendal nerve is thought to occur as the result of stretching, which may eventually result in denervation of the anal sphincter and may, in time, lead to anal incontinence.

Constipated patients who have no structural abnormalities of the anorectum or dysfunction of colonic motility may experience dysfunction of the pelvic floor musculature. Electromyography (EMG) and anal manometry studies have identified a subgroup of patients who complain of constipation that experience a paradoxical contraction of the anal sphincter and pelvic floor at the time of attempted defecation (17,18). This syndrome has been termed anismus, pelvic floor dyssynergia, and paradoxical puborectalis syndrome. The failure of the pelvic floor to relax at the time of straining to defecation results in a physiologic anorectal outlet obstruction. The typical patient is a young woman who suffers from constipation who fails to respond to fiber therapy and laxatives. Symptoms include pain with defecation, excessive straining, and the sensation of incomplete evacuation. Patients with anismus frequently use digital evacuation of the rectum to assist defecation. Definitive diagnosis can be made by anorectal manometry, EMG, or cinedefecography. Patients with anismus who undergo cinedefecography are unable to evacuate barium and retain a prominent impression of the puborectalis muscle on lateral films during attempts to evacuate the rectum. This suggests that the pelvic floor remains contracted during straining and prevents rectal emptying. Anal manometry uses a balloon expulsion test in which the patient attempts to evacuate a 30-cc intrarectal balloon. EMG studies actually measure neuromuscular action potentials, looking for normal silencing before defecation. Anal manometry and EMG studies are superior to cinedefecography because they show evidence of nonrelaxation of the anal

sphincters and pelvic diaphragm with straining or attempted defecation. EMG studies are generally considered the most sensitive technique for diagnosing anismus.

Functional Bowel Disorders

Constipation is a frequent symptom in patients with irritable bowel syndrome (IBS). IBS is thought by many to be the most common disorder of the digestive tract. About two thirds of those affected are women, and it occurs most commonly in younger patients. One study suggests that 5% to 11% of patients with IBS present with constipation (19). Stress has long been thought to contribute to the symptoms of IBS, and patients with IBS frequently have a history of depression.

The Rome Criteria for functional bowel disorders have established criteria for the diagnosis of IBS listed in Table 15.3 (20). Irritable bowel syndrome is a symptom-based diagnosis, and the physical examination in these patients is primarily directed at ruling out other etiologies of disordered defecation. Key symptoms include abdominal pain usually relieved by bowel movement as well as a subjective change in bowel frequency or consistency. Supporting symptoms include bloating and passage of mucus. Complaints of blood in the stool or nocturnal stool are highly unlikely

TABLE 15.3. *Rome criteria for irritable bowel syndrome [20]*

At least 12 weeks or more, which need not be consecutive, in the preceding 12 months, of abdominal discomfort or pain that has two out of three features:
  Relieved with defecation; and/or
  Onset associated with a change in frequency of
    stool; and/or
  Onset associated with a change in form of stool
  Supportive Symptoms
  • Abnormal stool frequency (greater than 3
    bowel movements a day or less than 3
    bowel movements a week);
  • Abnormal stool form (lumpy/hard or
    loose/watery stool);
  • Abnormal stool passage (straining, urgency, or
    feeling of incomplete evacuation);
  • Passage of mucus;
  • Bloating or feeling of abdominal distention.

with IBS. Episodes of IBS are often associated with stress, including anxiety or depression. Patients should be referred for a thorough gastrointestinal workup including rigid or flexible sigmoidoscopy.

A growing body of evidence links constipation with psychological factors in some patients. Personality factors, self-esteem, psychological distress, and anxiety have all been linked to stool frequency and constipation. Studies have suggested that constipation is responsive to psychological intervention, further supporting the theory that not all constipation has an organic cause.

Fecal Incontinence

Fecal incontinence, the involuntary loss of flatus or feces, is rapidly gaining recognition as a more prevalent condition that occurs more frequently than previously thought. In most studies, it is reported to occur most frequently in multiparous women and has its highest incidence in adults older than 65 years of age, although some recent studies have shown a surprisingly high prevalence in men (21). Unfortunately, the symptoms of anal incontinence are frequently underreported by patients and commonly unrecognized by the clinician. The emotional, psychological, and social problems created by this condition can be both devastating and debilitating.

The most common cause of fecal incontinence in healthy women is related to obstetric trauma. It is widely recognized that vaginal delivery can damage the anal continence mechanism by direct injury to the anal sphincter muscles or damage to the motor innervation of the sphincters and pelvic floor. Recent studies have reported that injury to the anal continence mechanism is much more common following a vaginal delivery than previously recognized. In a prospective study of 200 pregnant women evaluated both before and after delivery, Sultan and colleagues (22) reported that 13% of women develop incontinence or urgency following their first vaginal delivery and that 30% have unrecognized structural injury to the internal and external anal sphincter detected by anal endosonography. Women who suffered a traumatic rupture of the anal sphincter at the time of vaginal delivery appear to have a greater risk for anal incontinence than previously recognized. Several investigators have reported that 36% to 63% of women develop symptoms of incontinence following primary sphincter repair (23–26).

There is strong evidence to suggest that vaginal delivery results in significant injury to the innervation of the pelvic floor muscles. Snooks and colleagues (27) noted a significant increase in the mean pudendal nerve motor terminal latencies (PNMTLs) 48 hours after delivery in primiparous women who had a forceps delivery compared with controls and with multiparous patients. In a study of 128 women in whom PNMTLs were measured both during pregnancy and after delivery, PNMTLs were significantly prolonged 6 weeks postpartum in 32% of women who delivered vaginally (28). Two thirds of those women with an abnormally prolonged PNMTL had PNMTL within the normal range when restudied after 6 months, suggesting that nerve damage is permanent in 19% of women.

Although obstetric trauma is a leading cause of fecal incontinence in women, it can also result from a variety of other conditions (Table 15.4). Several operations performed frequently by colorectal surgeons can result in fecal incontinence, including internal sphincterotomy, fistulectomy, and fistulotomy. Several disease states have been associated with fecal incontinence. These include diabetes, multiple sclerosis, Parkinson's disease, spinal cord injury, and myotonic dystrophy. Fecal impaction is a leading cause of fecal incontinence among elderly and institutionalized individuals.

Illnesses causing diarrhea are another important cause of fecal incontinence. Irritable bowel syndrome is frequently associated with incontinence, as is inflammatory bowel disease. Infectious diarrheal states are also commonly associated with incontinence. Radiation proctitis can lead to fecal incontinence through a variety of mechanisms, including decreases in rectal compliance and neurogenic injury to the sphincter complex.

TABLE 15.4. *Causes of fecal incontinence*

Obstetric
   Rupture of anal sphincter
   Chronic third- and fourth-degree laceration
   Rectovaginal fistula
Surgical
   Internal sphincterotomy
   Fistulectomy
   Low anterior resection
Traumatic sphincter rupture
Diarrheal states
   Inflammatory bowel disease
   Radiation enteritis
   Infectious enteritis
   Laxative abuse
Neurologic conditions
   Congenital anomalies
   Multiple sclerosis
   Parkinson's disease
   Systemic sclerosis
   Spinal cord injury
   Stroke
   Dementia
   Diabetic neuropathy
Congenital anorectal malformation
Pelvic floor denervation
   Rectal prolapse
   Chronic straining
   Descending perineum syndrome

From Toglia MR. Pathophysiology of anorectal dysfunction. *Obstet Gynecol Clin North Am* 1998;25: 771–781, with permission.

ELEMENTS OF THE PHYSICAL EXAMINATION

The basis for evaluating colorectal dysfunction begins with a good history taking and careful physical examination. The clinician must specifically address colorectal symptoms because patients seldom offer this information voluntarily. It is important to ask specific questions regarding the onset, duration, and frequency of symptoms and to identify associated exacerbating factors such as diet and activity.

The evaluation of colorectal dysfunction requires a focused examination of the abdomen and pelvis. Routine examination of the abdomen involves inspection, palpation, and auscultation to rule out the presence of masses, organomegaly, and areas of peritoneal irritation. This should be followed by a detailed evaluation of the vagina and anorectum. Visual and digital inspection of the vagina and anus identifies structural abnormalities such as prolapse, fistulas, fissures, hemorrhoids, or prior trauma. A simple neurologic examination should test for the intactness of the motor component of S-2 to S-4. The anal wink, bulbocavernosus, and cough reflexes all test the integrity of the motor innervation of the external anal sphincter. Sensation over the inner thigh, vulva, and perirectal areas should be tested for symmetry by light touch and pinprick. Pelvic muscle strength can be subjectively graded by digital palpation of the puborectalis sling with voluntary contraction.

The integrity of the external anal sphincter and puborectalis muscle can be evaluated by observation and palpation of these structures during voluntary contraction. When a patient is asked to contract her pelvic floor, two motions should be present. First the external anal sphincter should contract concentrically, and the anal verge should be pulled inward. These actions should also be readily apparent on digital rectal examination. The firm and resilient muscular sling of the puborectalis should be readily palpable posteriorly because it creates a 90-degree angle between the anal and rectal canals. Voluntary contraction of this muscle "lifts" the examining finger anteriorly toward the insertion of this muscle on the pubic rami. An external anal sphincter muscle that is intact but lax at rest, as well as a weak voluntary contraction of this muscle, often indicates pudendal neuropathy. Neuropathy affecting the puborectalis can likewise be recognized if the anorectal angle is obtuse and if there is a palpable weakness with voluntary contraction. The presence of fecal material in the anal canal may suggest fecal impaction or neuromuscular weakness of the anal continence mechanism. Finally, defects in the anterior aspects of the external anal sphincter may be detected by digital examination. The patient should then be asked to strain or bear down with a finger still within the anus. Both the puborectalis and external anal sphincter should relax during such activity. Patients suffering from anismus may have a paradoxical contraction of these muscles during straining.

ANCILLARY TESTING

Disordered Defecation

Patients presenting with symptoms suggestive of disordered defecation should undergo a standard gastrointestinal evaluation, including a barium enema or colonoscopy to eliminate colorectal malignancy from the differential diagnosis. Anoscopy should be included as part of the routine examination because it may reveal anorectal pathology, such as prolapsing hemorrhoids. Rigid proctosigmoidoscopy should also be performed to exclude intrarectal prolapse, ulcerative or radiation proctitis, or a solitary rectal ulcer.

In most cases, referral to an anorectal physiology laboratory is necessary to differentiate between patients with colonic motility disorders and those with predominant pelvic outlet symptoms. Standard evaluation in these laboratories includes colonic transit studies, cinedefecography, anorectal manometry, and EMG.

Cinedefecography is a radiologic examination of the anatomy and function of the pelvic floor and anorectum. It is useful in the diagnosis of the following conditions: intrarectal prolapse, rectocele, enterocele, paradoxical puborectalis syndrome (anismus), and perineal descent. A series of lateral still films and, in some laboratories, cinevideography, are made with fluoroscopy while the patient sits on a radiolucent commode. The patient is filmed at rest, during defecation, and while squeezing the anal sphincters. Measurements are taken, including the size of the rectal ampulla, length of the anal canal, size of the anorectal angle, motion of the puborectalis, and degree of pelvic floor descent. The procedure is more fully described in Chapter 14.

Anal manometry is performed as described earlier to determine maximum resting pressure, maximum squeeze pressure, and rectal sensation. The role of manometry is to evaluate sphincteric function, although it is also helpful in diagnosing Hirschsprung's disease. Surface EMG of the anal sphincter is helpful in excluding anismus as a cause of obstructed defecation. Normally, the anal sphincter relaxes at the time of defecation. Patients with anismus typically show an increase in electrical activity in both the external sphincter and the puborectalis with attempted defecation (29).

Colonic transit studies involve the use of ingested radiopaque markers followed by abdominal radiographs or scintigraphic studies performed serially over a period of several days. Patients are asked to observe a high-fiber diet over the test period. Twenty to 24 markers are ingested initially, and abdominal radiographs are taken either daily or on the fourth day, the seventh day, and every 3 days until all the markers are gone. Segmental transit times are then calculated using a mathematical formula. On the basis of colonic transit studies, patients suffering from constipation can be divided into those with delayed colonic transit, those with anorectal outlet obstruction, and those who are normal.

Fecal Incontinence

Sophisticated diagnostic testing is currently being used in clinical research and in anorectal physiology laboratories to quantify the function of the colon and anorectum.

Transanal ultrasonography is a recently introduced technique that allows for the accurate imaging of both the internal and external anal sphincters. Transanal ultrasound is currently the single best method of identifying defects in the anal sphincters. In this technique, continuity of the muscle is assessed, as is the thickness of the muscle. Transanal ultrasound is performed using a Bruel-Kjaer (Copenhagen, Denmark) ultrasound scanner with a 360-degree rectal endoprobe (type 1850) with a 7.0 MHz transducer (focal length, 2 to 5 cm) housed within a plastic cone (Fig. 15.3). The normal internal anal sphincter is observed as a continuous hypoechoic band. A thick layer of mixed echogenicity outside of the internal anal sphincter is the

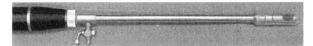

FIG. 15.3. Bruel-Kjaer (Copenhagen, Denmark) ultrasound probe (type 1850) with a 7.0 MHz transducer (focal length, 2 to 5 cm) housed within a plastic cone.

striated layer of the normal external anal sphincter (Fig. 15.4). Discontinuity of the muscle bands is considered evidence of a sphincteric defect. Defects can be measured in degrees of circumference as well as distance from the anal verge (Fig. 15.5A,B).

EMG has been used to evaluate the integrity of external anal sphincter innervation following a traumatic injury such as childbirth as well as to document the presence of pelvic floor neuropathy (30). EMG is a study of electrical activity arising in muscle fibers during contraction and at rest. Many different electrodes may be used to measure electrical activity in the muscles. Surface electrodes applied near or within the anal canal record electrical activity within the area adjacent to

the electrode and can give a general record of anal sphincter activity. Surface electrodes are typically used in conjunction with biofeedback therapy. Concentric needle electrodes are most commonly used in anorectal physiology labs. The recording electrode consists of a thin steel wire contained within a thin, needle-like cannula. The area surveyed by the electrode is small and therefore records selectively from individual muscles. Single-fiber EMG electrodes contain extremely small electrodes and record the activity of single muscle fibers. Quantification of single-fiber EMG results allows for calculation of fiber density.

Denervation injury to a muscle is accompanied by subsequent reinnervation of the ef-

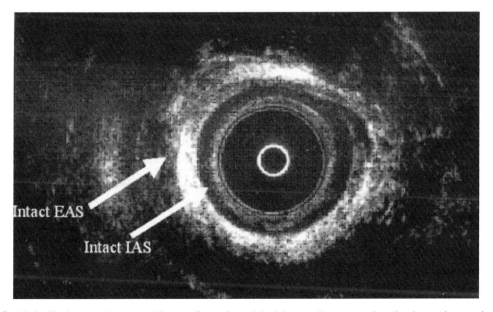

FIG. 15.4. Endoanal ultrasound image from the midsphincter demonstrating the intact hypoechoic internal anal sphincter and hyperechoic external anal sphincter.

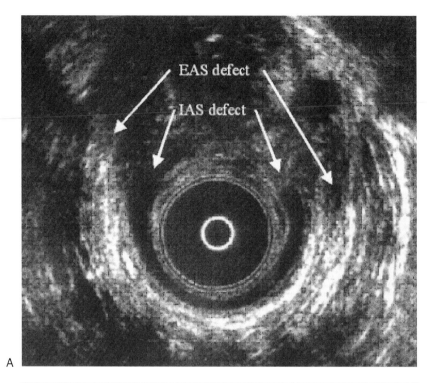

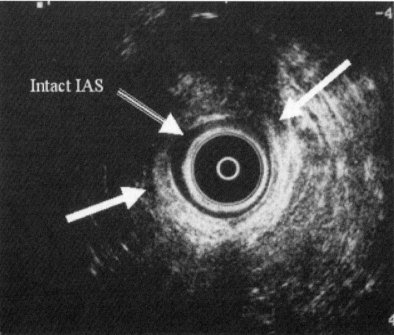

FIG. 15.5. A: Endoanal ultrasound image from the midsphincter demonstrating defects in both the internal and external anal sphincters from 10 to 2 o'clock. **B:** Endoanal ultrasound image from cranial sphincter demonstrating an intact internal anal sphincter (*broken arrow*) and defect in external anal sphincter from 8 to 2 o'clock (*solid arrows*).

fected motor unit, which is reflected by an increase in fiber density. Thus, single-fiber EMG studies provide indirect evidence of neurologic injury by measuring the amount of reinnervation. Single EMG can be used to map the external anal sphincter and to identify areas of injury. Unfortunately, this requires multiple needle punctures around the anus and can be uncomfortable for the patient. This technique has largely been replaced by transanal ultrasound in clinical practice for the detection of disruption to the external anal sphincter based both on increased patient comfort and more reliable results.

Motor nerve conduction studies offer a way of measuring neuropathic injury to the muscles of the pelvic floor. These studies are performed by stimulating the axon of a nerve and measuring the speed that it takes the action potential to reach the muscle supplied by the nerve. The delay between stimulation and the response is called the nerve latency. PNMTL can be determined by transrectal stimulation of the pudendal nerve (31). These studies are performed using a nerve stimulator mounted on an examination glove at the fingertip (Fig. 15.6). The nerve stimulator is positioned transrectally over the pudendal nerve at each ischial spine. A transrectal stimulus of 0.1-ms duration and up to 50 mV is given, and the latency of the external anal sphincter muscle contraction is measured. A value of 2.2 ms or less is considered normal. Prolongation of the pudendal nerve terminal motor latency is indicative of damage to that nerve or a demyelinating condition. A normal or near-normal PNMTL study is a significant predictor for successful surgical repair of traumatic sphincter injuries (32).

Anal manometry can be used to quantify function of the anal sphincter mechanism. Pressures in the anal canal can be measured by a variety of techniques and catheters. Water-perfused manometry catheters and water-filled balloons are the most commonly used method (Fig. 15.7). Resting anal canal pressure is mostly a reflection of the activity of the internal anal sphincter, and mechanical defects in this structure can be inferred indirectly from the measurement of a low resting anal pressure. Anorectal pressures measured in the lower anal canal during maximal voluntary contraction reflect external anal sphincter function. Vector analysis of the manometric pressures consists of computerized analysis of data and can be used to determine symmetry or asymmetry within the anal sphincter. The pressure measurements obtained by anal

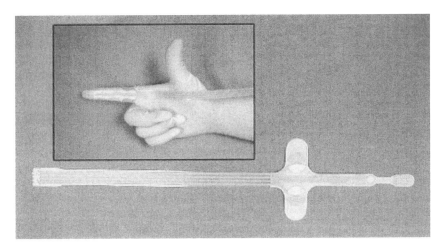

FIG. 15.6. St. Mark's electrode used for measuring pudendal nerve motor terminal latency. The stimulating electrode is on the fingertip and the receiving electrode is on the proximal finger near the knuckle (*inset*).

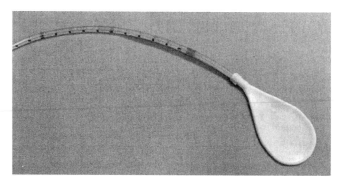

FIG. 15.7. Manometry catheter with balloon.

manometry provide indirect evidence of sphincter injury—a low resting tone is often an indication of subclinical injury to the internal anal sphincter, whereas a decrease in the maximum squeezing pressure tends to reflect activity of the external anal sphincter. A variety of factors influence anal pressure measurements, including tissue compliance and muscular tone. These measurements do not distinguish between the activities of the individual sphincter muscles and often lack specific anatomic correlation. Interpretation of anal canal pressures is difficult, and the range of normal pressures varies widely with age and parity. There is a wide overlap between manometric values obtained from incontinent patients and normal controls. Anal manometry may therefore be of limited value in helping the clinician determine proper therapy.

REFERENCES

1. Gosling JA, Dixson JS, Critchey HOD, et al. A comparative study of the human external sphincter and periurethral levator ani muscles. *Br J Urol* 1983;53:35–41.
2. Bartolo DCC, Roe AM, Locke-Edmunds JC, et al. Flap-valve theory of anorectal continence. *Br J Surg* 1986; 73:1012–1014.
3. Bannister JJ, Gibbons C, Read NW. Preservation of faecal continence during rises in intraabdominal pressure: is there a role for the flap valve? *Gut* 1987;28: 1241–1245.
4. Miller R, Bartolo DCC, Locke-Edmunds JC, et al. Prospective study of conservative and operative treatment of faecal incontinence. *Br J Surg* 1988;75: 101–105.
5. Miller R, Orrom WJ, Cornes H, et al. Anterior sphincter plication and levatorplasty in the treatment of faecal incontinence. *Br J Surg* 1989;76:1058–1060.
6. Aronson MP, Lee RA, Berquist TH. Anatomy of anal sphincters and related structures in continent women studied with magnetic resonance imaging. *Obstet Gynecol* 1990;76:846–851.
7. Sweiger M. Method for determining individual contributions of voluntary and involuntary anal sphincters to resting tone. *Dis Colon Rectum* 1979;22:415-6.
8. Frenckner B, Euler CV. Influence of pudendal block on the function of the anal sphincters. *Gut* 1975;16: 482–489.
9. Read NW, Bartolo DCC, Read MG. Differences in anal function in patients with incontinence to solids and in patients with incontinence to liquids. *Br J Surg* 1984; 71:39–42.
10. Modesto VL, Gold RP, Gottesman L. Pelvic floor abnormalities. In: Mazler WP, Levien DH, Luchtefeld MA, et al., eds. *Surgery of the colon, rectum, and anus.* Philadelphia: WB Saunders, 1995:1075–1090.
11. Varma JS, Smith AM. Neurophysiological dysfunction in young women with intractable constipation. *Gut* 1988;29:963–968.
12. Ihre T, Seligson U. Intussusception of the rectum: internal procedentia. *Dis Colon Rectum* 1975;18:391–396.
13. Weber AM, Walters MD, Ballard LA, et al. Posterior vaginal prolapse and bowel function. *Am J Obstet Gynecol* 1998;179(6 Pt 1):1446–1449; discussion, 1449–1450.
14. Arnold MW, Stewart WR, Aquilar PS. Rectocele repairs: four year's experience. *Dis Colon Rectum* 1990;3: 684–687.
15. Kodner IJ, Fry RD, Fleshman JW. Rectal prolapse and other pelvic floor abnormalities. *Surg Annu* 1992;2: 157–190.
16. Henry MM. Descending perineum syndrome. In: Henry MM, Swash M, eds. *Coloproctology and the pelvic floor,* 2nd ed. Oxford, UK: Butterworth-Heinemann, 1992:299–305.
17. Turnbull GK, Lennard-Jones JE, Bartrum CI. Failure of rectal expulsion as a cause of constipation: why fiber and laxatives sometimes fail. *Lancet* 1986;1:767–769.
18. Read NW, Timms JM, Barfield LJ, et al. Impairment of defecation in young women with severe constipation. *Gastroenterology* 1986;90:53–60.
19. Everhart JE, Renault PF. Irritable bowel syndrome in office-based practice in the United States. *Gastroenterology* 1991;100:998–1005.

20. Thompson WG, Longstreth G, Drossman DA, et al. Functional bowel disorders and functional abdominal pain. In: Drossman DA, ed. *ROME II: the functional gastrointestinal disorders,* 2nd ed. McLean, VA: Degnon Associates, 2000:360.

21. Campbell AJ, Reinken J, McCosh L. Incontinence in the elderly: Prevalence and prognosis. *Age Ageing* 1985;14: 65–70.

22. Sultan AH, Kamm MA, Hudson CN, et al. Anal sphincter disruption during vaginal delivery. *N Engl J Med* 1993;329:1905–1911.

23. Sorenson M, Tetzschner T, Rasmussen OO, et al. Sphincter rupture in childbirth. *Br J Surg* 1993;80:393–394.

24. Bek KM, Laurberg S. Risks of anal incontinence from subsequent vaginal delivery after a complete obstetric anal sphincter tear. *Br J Obstet Gynaecol* 1992;99:724–726.

25. Haadem K, Dahlstrom JA, Ling L, et al. Anal sphincter function after delivery rupture. *Obstet Gynecol* 1987; 70:53–56.

26. Haadem K, Ohrlander S, Lingman G. Long-term ailments due to anal sphincter rupture caused by delivery—a hidden problem. *Eur J Obstet Gynecol Reprod Biol* 1988;27:27–32.

27. Snooks SJ, Swash M, Henry MM, et al. Risk factors in childbirth causing damage to the pelvic floor innervation. *Int J Colorect Dis* 1986;1:20–24.

28. Sultan AH, Kamm MA, Hudson CN. Pudendal nerve damage during labour: prospective study before and after childbirth. *Br J Obstet Gynaecol* 1994;101:22–28.

29. Preston DM, Lennard-Jones JE. Is there a pelvic floor disorder in slow transit constipation? *Gut* 1981;22:A890.

30. Swash M. Electromyography in pelvic floor disorders. In: Henry MM, Swash M, eds. *Coloproctology and the pelvic floor,* 2nd ed. Oxford, UK: Butterworth-Heinemann, 1992:184–195.

31. Swash M, Snooks SJ. Motor nerve conduction studies of the pelvic floor innervation. In: Henry MM, Swash M, eds. *Coloproctology and the pelvic floor,* 2nd ed. London: Butterworth, 1992:196–206.

32. Laurberg S, Swash M, Henry MM. Delayed external sphincter repair for obstetric tear. *Br J Surg* 1988;75: 786–788.

SECTION III

Pathology and Treatment

PART A
Urinary Tract Dysfunction

*Ostergard's Urogynecology and Pelvic Floor
Dysfunction, Fifth Edition.* edited by A.E. Bent, et al.
Lippincott Williams & Wilkins, Philadelphia © 2003.

16

The Urinary Tract in Pregnancy

Roger P. Goldberg,* Robert W. Lobel,** and Peter K. Sand†

*Evanston Continence Center, Northwestern University Medical School, Evanston, Illinois
**Division of Urogynecology, Albany Medical College, Albany, New York
† Evanston Continence Center, Department of Obstetrics & Gynecology,
and Division of Urogynecology, Northwestern University Medical School, Evanston, Illinois

During pregnancy, morphologic and physiologic changes occur throughout the urinary tract. These alterations can cause an array of symptoms and pathologic conditions. Although some of these conditions are benign and compensatory in nature, others can adversely affect mother, fetus, or both. Some may persist long after the pregnancy is over, with important repercussions on a woman's postreproductive health and quality of life. In this chapter, we review these alterations of the urinary tract in pregnancy and examine their pathophysiologic consequences.

MORPHOLOGIC AND PHYSIOLOGIC CHANGES

Urethra

The urethral mucosa appears hyperemic and congested as pregnancy progresses. Within an increasingly estrogen-rich hormonal milieu, the transitional epithelium becomes more squamous in character. The urethra passively lengthens as the bladder is drawn farther cephalad and anterior by the enlarging uterus. Several investigators have documented an increase in total urethral length ranging from 4 to 7 mm and an average increase in functional length of 5 mm. Both total and functional urethral lengths decrease slightly below their first-trimester values after vaginal delivery, but not after cesarean section. Iosif and colleagues (1) showed the urethral closure pressure to increase an average of 12 cm H_2O, from 61 to 73 cm H_2O during pregnancy—a change that promotes continence in pregnancy. The wide prevalence of stress incontinence in pregnancy must result from alternative mechanisms. At the urethral level, some investigators have suggested that progesterone-mediated effects may inhibit estrogen-induced changes and in some way negatively influence pressure transmission and coaptation within the urethral walls during moments of increased intraabdominal pressure. Altered smooth muscle tone may represent one important mechanism behind this alteration in urethral tone, as suggested by decreased responsiveness to α-agonists in pregnant rabbit bladder bases (2). The resulting diminished intrinsic urethral function, at the level of the urethrovesical junction and proximal urethra, may provide at least a partial explanation for the high incidence of stress incontinence associated with pregnancy.

Bladder

As noted previously, the urinary bladder is displaced anteriorly and superiorly as pregnancy progresses, becoming more an abdominal organ than a pelvic one by the third trimester. The base of the bladder enlarges, and the trigone appears convex rather than concave, beside the expanding lower uterine segment. Although detrusor hypertrophy occurs in response to the increased estrogen stimulation of pregnancy, elevated progesterone levels cause hypotonia of the detrusor smooth muscle, leading to an increased bladder capacity exceeding 1 L in some studies (3). With engagement of the fetal head, bladder capacity typically decreases as a result of anatomic crowding, only to rise again in the early postpartum period (4). In one postpartum study, 86% of the patients had reduced bladder sensation and tone associated with volumes greater than 865 mL (5). Despite this progesterone-induced detrusor smooth muscle relaxation, anatomic factors cause the average supine bladder pressure to increase from 9 cm H_2O in early pregnancy to 20 cm H_2O at term; normal levels then resume during the postpartum period.

Descent of the bladder neck and increased vesical neck mobility at Valsalva maneuver commonly occur during pregnancy (6) and tend to persist after delivery. Even before delivery, bladder neck position at rest differs from its average position in nulligravidas (7). In one series of 117 women in their first pregnancy, it was found that lowering of the urethrovesical junction may occur as early as 12 to 16 weeks of gestation (8). However, among the 35% of women in this series who reported

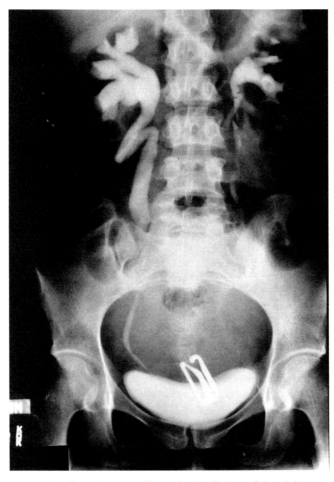

FIG. 16.1. Hydroureter in the first trimester. Physiologic dilation of the right ureter and renal pelvis above the pelvic brim at 12 weeks' gestation before physical compression by the gravid uterus.

urinary incontinence, no relationship was found between subjective and objective incontinence data and the position and mobility of the urethrovesical junction.

Ureter

Hydroureter is the most dramatic anatomic response of the urinary tract to pregnancy. Dilation usually has an abrupt onset after 21 weeks of gestation (9) but can be seen as early as the first trimester (Fig. 16.1)—a pattern that reflects, respectively, its dual physical and hormonal etiologies. The major hormonal effect is a progesterone-mediated inhibition of ureteral motility, owing to the hypotonic effects of this pregnancy hormone on smooth muscle. Later in pregnancy, mechanical compression by the enlarging uterus probably accounts for most ureteral dilation (10), with al-

most 90% of patients demonstrating some degree of hydroureter at term. Anatomically, the ureters are displaced laterally and assume a more tortuous appearance. The right ureter is affected more than the left in 86% of cases (11)—an asymmetry that most likely results from the left-sided cushioning effect of the sigmoid colon, dextrorotation of the uterus, and the greater potential for right-sided ureteral obstruction by the crossing right ovarian vein and iliac vessels. Physiologic dilation is typically restricted to the renal pelvis and the upper two thirds of the ureters.

Ureteral dilation is associated with a large increase in ureteral volume (50 to 200 mL). This reservoir effect, together with decreased ureteral motility, leads to nearly a fivefold delay in excretion from the right ureter. Ureteral changes resolve by 4 weeks postpartum in most patients (Fig. 16.2).

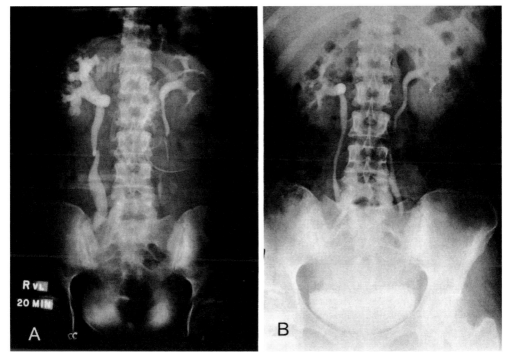

FIG. 16.2. Postpartum resolution of hydroureter. **A:** Right hydroureter above the pelvic brim at 29 weeks of gestation. **B:** Intravenous pyelogram performed 3 weeks after cesarean section shows resolution of these physiologic changes.

Kidney

Dilation of the renal pelvis, calyces, and parenchyma lengthen the kidney by 1.5 cm during pregnancy. Contributing factors include those outlined above for hydroureter as well as a 40% to 50% increase in the glomerular filtration rate (GFR) and a 60% to 80% increase in the effective renal plasma flow (ERPF) (12).

The GFR increases steadily during pregnancy and normalizes in the puerperium (13). The ERPF increases to a greater degree and then falls abruptly in the last month of pregnancy. It may remain depressed for up to 6 months after delivery. Thus, the filtration fraction (GFR/ERPF) remains slightly elevated after the first trimester, and the amount of solute filtered by the kidney increases dramatically while reabsorptive capacity remains constant. The net effect is an increased loss of many solutes. Both the blood urea nitrogen and serum creatinine values fall 30% below normal; the mean serum urea nitrogen in the pregnant woman is 8.7 mg/dL, and the mean plasma creatinine is 0.46 mg/dL (14). Increased excretion of glucose and amino acids can lead to physiologic glycosuria and aminoaciduria. There is some resolution of these changes later in pregnancy. Significant proteinuria (300 mg per 24 hours) is not seen in normal pregnancy.

Despite the increase in GFR, tubular reabsorption of salt and water increase, resulting in gradual retention of sodium ions (20 to 30 mEq/wk) and consequently, increased thirst. Increased thirst during gestation leads to further intake of free water and the eventual retention of 950 mEq of sodium and 7 L of water (15). This excess fluid is thought to be distributed between the fetal and reproductive tissues (80%) and the maternal extracellular space (20%) (16). Interestingly, studies of limb volume in pregnancy show that edema of the lower extremities accounts for no more than 500 mL (17). Therefore, most excess water, on the maternal side, must be stored elsewhere.

URINARY PROBLEMS IN PREGNANCY

Frequency

Frequency of urination is a common complaint and occurs in 46% to 95% of gravidas, beginning in the first trimester (18) (Table 16.1). Normal nonpregnant females urinate between four and six times during the day and rarely at night; thus, frequency is defined as voiding more than seven times during the day and more than once at night. Frequency usually begins early in pregnancy, increases progressively in each trimester, and rapidly resolves postpartum. Some authors describe higher incidences in primigravidas, whereas others show no influence of parity on frequency (19). The postpartum incidence (10% to 20%) is equal to that found before pregnancy.

Bladder capacity increases in pregnancy and cannot be inferred as a cause of frequency until late in gestation, when uterine enlargement and engagement of the fetal head create a space-occupying effect and mechanically compress the bladder. Serial uroflowmetry measurements, at various points throughout pregnancy, have documented significantly smaller voided volumes in the third trimester compared with the first two trimesters (20). During early gestation, the more plausible explanation for urinary frequency is the polydipsia and polyuria of pregnancy. As noted previously, both fluid intake and urine output rise rapidly in the first trimester and remain constant until the third trimester, when decreased sodium excretion eventually leads to a decline in urine output. Transient diabetes insipidus is a less commonplace etiology behind excessive urine

TABLE 16.1. *Prevalence of lower urinary tract symptoms in pregnancy*

Symptom	Prevalence (%)
Urgency	60–70
Frequency	45–95
Nocturia	55–65
Stress incontinence	30–70
Urge incontinence	20–40
Incomplete emptying	30–35

output in late pregnancy but can occur either alone or in association with preeclampsia or acute fatty liver of pregnancy. Excessive vasopressinase activity is one suggested etiology for this disorder. Treatment with desmopressin (DDAVP) has been used successfully for achieving a reduction in urine output in the third trimester and can typically be discontinued within the first postpartum month (21). However, a strategy of aggressive fluid restriction should be avoided in gravid women because of their elevated risk for dehydration.

Nocturia

The polyuria of pregnancy is in large part a nocturnal diuresis; the increase in nocturnal urine flow is double that which occurs in the daytime. Clinically evident as edema in the lower extremities, daytime fluid retention is mobilized at night when the woman reclines. Most of this nocturnal diuresis is nonosmotically obligated water, most likely due to the reduction in renal concentrating ability in pregnancy. The mean nocturnal urine flow and solute excretion are 60% to 70% greater

in the first and second trimesters than before pregnancy (22). Although both urine flow and solute excretion decline somewhat in the third trimester, the incidence of nocturia continues to rise. As previously discussed, this paradox results from the apparent decrease in functional bladder capacity that follows fetal descent and engagement in the third trimester.

Urinary Retention

Although the symptoms of incomplete emptying and postvoid fullness are common, antepartum urinary retention is rare and usually associated with uterine retroversion early in the second trimester (23). Asymptomatic retroversion occurs in up to 20% of first-trimester pregnancies, with spontaneous resolution by 16 weeks of gestation in most cases. For symptomatic cases, successful manual reduction of the incarcerated uterus usually requires drainage of the bladder, adequate anesthesia, and knee–chest positioning. Presentation at term with incarceration (Fig. 16.3) has been reported and generally requires a vertical cesarean section (24,25). Pelvic neoplasms, including fibroids

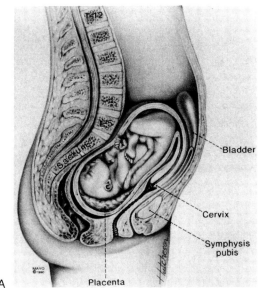
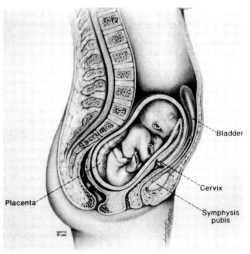

FIG. 16.3. A: Incarcerated uterus with fetal vertex. **B:** Incarcerated uterus with fetal breech. (From Van Winter JT, Ogburn PL, Ney JA, et al. Uterine incarceration during the third trimester: a rare complication of pregnancy. *Mayo Clin Proc* 1991;66:608–613, with permission.)

(26), may also cause retention by interfering with bladder neck relaxation; after the retroversion is reduced or the tumor removed, resolution of this interference can be demonstrated by cystourethrography (4). A similar etiology could account for urinary retention associated with marked uterine prolapse early in pregnancy. With both retroversion and prolapse, a Smith or Hodge pessary can serve to maintain uterine position after reduction.

Postpartum retention is far more common. After spontaneous vaginal delivery, bladder dysfunction is noted in 9% to 14% of patients; after forceps deliveries, this number rises to 38% (27). This retention is usually due to a detrusor–sphincter dyssynergia voiding pattern, with incomplete urethral relaxation secondary to pain and edema. Conversely, patients unable to void after cesarean section usually have an acontractile or underactive detrusor muscle. Kerr-Wilson and McNally (28) showed that epidural analgesia caused acute retention of more than 850 mL of urine after cesarean section in up to 44% of patients whose catheters were removed at the end of the operation. Tapp and colleagues (29) found epidurals to be associated with a significant increase in postpartum residual urine but noted spontaneous resolution in all cases by 6 weeks postpartum.

Cystometry after vaginal delivery demonstrates that 86% of patients have decreased bladder sensation and tone, leading to an increased bladder capacity (30). These changes are associated with edema and congestion of the bladder base. Most of these findings are asymptomatic and resolve spontaneously in the early postpartum period.

Significant postpartum urinary retention requires prompt establishment of adequate drainage to avoid chronic detrusor damage. This is most easily achieved by placement of a Foley catheter for 24 to 72 hours. Retention due to a failure of urethral and periurethral skeletal muscle relaxation after vaginal delivery is best treated by "tincture of time," but ice to the perineum and analgesics are also helpful to relieve increased afferent sensation. Persistent retention due to an underactive de-

trusor beyond the early puerperium is best treated by clean intermittent self-catheterization. Use of bethanechol or α-blockers is usually unrewarding in these patients.

Incontinence

The symptom of stress incontinence has been reported to occur in 32% to 85% of pregnant women (31,32). It is usually mild and affects multiparas more often than nulliparas. Francis showed an intrapartum prevalence of 85% in multiparas, compared with 53% in nulliparas (32). Nearly half of these patients noted some degree of incontinence before the observed pregnancy. The new onset of incontinence during pregnancy was divided equally among the trimesters. Although Francis noted no new incidence of stress incontinence in the puerperium, other investigators have estimated that antepartum stress incontinence may fail to resolve in a substantial number of cases. Stanton and colleagues (33) prospectively studied 181 women in the third trimester and through the puerperium. Of the 83 nulliparas, 38% had stress incontinence in the third trimester and 6% had persistent postpartum stress incontinence. Of the 98 multiparas, 10% had a history of stress incontinence before pregnancy, 42% had stress incontinence in the third trimester, and 11% had persistent postpartum stress incontinence. Meyer and associates (34) examined 149 women during pregnancy and at about 9 weeks postpartum. The rates of stress urinary incontinence were 31% and 7%, respectively, meaning that 22% of patients with stress incontinence during pregnancy had persistence after delivery.

Incontinence usually increases in severity as pregnancy progresses, and mode of delivery appears to have a profound impact on its persistence for the long term. Viktrup and coauthors (35) performed a prospective study questioning 305 primiparous women about their urinary incontinence symptoms before, during, and after pregnancy. In their multivariate analysis, they found that length of the second stage, head circumference, episiotomy, and birth weight were associated with postpartum stress incontinence, whereas cesarean section was protective against stress incontinence. Of those women without stress incontinence during pregnancy, 21 of 167 (13%) had persistent incontinence postpartum compared with none of the 35 delivered by cesarean section ($p < 0.05$). Three months postpartum, only 4% of these women had persistent stress incontinence complaints, and at 1 year, only 3% still had stress incontinence. However, in subsequent pregnancies, these patients are at greater risk for more severe incontinence with earlier onset and persistence beyond the puerperium. In a 5-year follow-up study, Vikrup and Lose (36) questioned 278 of the 305 women (91%) in their original study and found a 30% prevalence of stress incontinence. Nineteen percent of these women who were not incontinent in the original trial developed stress incontinence in the ensuing 5 years. They thought this might have been the consequence of worsening pudendal neuropathy following the initial vaginal delivery. Again, cesarean section was found to decrease the risk for stress incontinence significantly.

Vaginal delivery can produce neurologic changes in the pelvic floor, resulting in adverse effects on pudendal nerve conduction velocities, vaginal contraction strength, and urethral closure pressures. These changes are not seen after cesarean section. Presumably, these changes allow for the persistence or onset of genuine stress incontinence in women after vaginal delivery. Looking at the physiologic changes of pregnancy and delivery, Van Geelen and co-workers (37) urodynamically studied pregnant women before and after delivery. They found a significant decrease in urethral closure pressure and functional length. No change was found in the women who had cesarean sections. Meyer and associates (34) found similar changes in functional urethral length as well as decreases in intravaginal and intraanal pressure 9 weeks after vaginal delivery compared with antepartum values in their prospective study of 149 women. None of these changes was found in the 33 women who had cesarean sections. Consistent with these differences in physiologic measures, these investigators found that only 1 of the 33 women delivered by cesarean section had persistence of stress incontinence postpartum compared with 36% of the 25 women delivered by forceps and 21% of the 91 women who delivered spontaneously.

Peschers and colleagues (38) studied the anatomic effects of vaginal delivery and found that bladder neck support was significantly worse after vaginal delivery than after cesarean section ($p < 0.001$) or compared with a group of 25 nulliparous controls ($p < 0.001$). They also found that bladder neck descent during Valsalva maneuver was significantly increased after vaginal delivery than after cesarean section in both primiparous and multiparous women ($p < 0.001$).

Whether or not the pelvic floor damage leading to persistent urinary stress incontinence is cumulative in multiparas is controversial. Mallett and colleagues (39) demonstrated that absolute parity and further childbearing did not further affect pelvic floor neurophysiology and concluded that most pudendal nerve damage occurs during the first vaginal delivery. However, several population-based trials since 1998 have been consistent with the prospective trials in showing strong associations between vaginal delivery, and increasing parity, with stress incontinence. Hojberg and colleagues (40) studied 1,781 primiparas at 16 weeks of gestation and showed an odds ratio of 5.7 for stress incontinence after vaginal delivery compared to 1.3 with cesarean delivery. Persson and associates (41) studied 10,074 women in Sweden having surgery for stress incontinence and found that the odds ratio of prior cesarean section versus vaginal delivery was 0.21. They also found a strong association with stress incontinence and parity. Moller and coauthors (42) studied 502 women with lower urinary tract symptoms and 742 controls. They found an association of parity and stress incontinence with an odds ratio of 2.2 after one vaginal delivery, 3.9 after a second vaginal delivery, and 4.5 after a third delivery. Marshall and associates

(43) studied 7,771 women early in the puerperium and found a strong association between stress incontinence and constipation with parity. Continued straining at bowel movements would theoretically further increase urethral hypermobility with concomitant stress incontinence and prolapse in these constipated women.

Iosif and colleagues (1) showed that cesarean section might also be related to the development of stress incontinence, but much less commonly than after vaginal birth. In 1982, they performed a retrospective trial of 204 of 264 women who had an elective cesarean section 1 to 6 years earlier. They found that 4.7% of these women had persistent stress incontinence after primary cesarean section and 4.1% after a second cesarean section. At present, there are no data allowing us to conclude the proper role of elective cesarean, for the purpose of avoiding stress incontinence or pelvic prolapse.

Finally, urge incontinence is also more prevalent during and after pregnancy. The prepregnancy incidence of urge incontinence is about 5% and can increase to 43% by the third trimester (44). After pregnancy, the incidence remains nearly twice that noted before pregnancy. Urodynamic evaluation of the incontinent gravida has shown that detrusor instability is reliably identified in patients complaining of urge incontinence, but less reliably among women with urgency and frequency in the absence of leakage. Not surprisingly, the symptom of stress incontinence (32%) is far more prevalent than urodynamically diagnosed genuine stress incontinence (7%) (45).

Urinary Tract Infections

Asymptomatic Bacteriuria

Asymptomatic bacteriuria, a pathologic entity that occurs in up to 10% of the general female population, is defined as the presence of 10^5 bacteria/mL of urine in a clean-catch specimen from patients without symptoms of a bladder infection. The prevalence is higher in patients with lower socioeconomic status, sickle cell trait, and Lewis blood group. Race, age, and parity have no relationship to increased infection rates.

In 1960, Kass first recognized that up to 40% of pregnant patients with bacteriuria develop pyelonephritis, compared with 1% of patients without bacteriuria at the time of the initial culture (46). This has been consistently borne out in numerous studies, showing that symptomatic infection develops in 12% to 43% of patients with bacteriuria during pregnancy compared with 0% to 14% of patients who did not have bacteriuria at their initial prenatal visit (Table 16.2). Antibiotic treatment of asymptomatic bacteriuria in

TABLE 16.2. *Development of symptomatic infection after asymptomatic bacteriuria*

Investigators	Positive initial culture		Negative initial culture	
	No. of patients	Symptomatic infection	No. of patients	Symptomatic infection
Kass, 1962 (82)	95	18 (0.12%)	1,000	0 (0%)
Sleigh et al., 1965 (83)	100	43 (43%)	100	14 (14%)
Kincaid-Smith & Bullen, 1964 (84)	55	20 (37%)	4,000	48 (1.2%)
Norden, Kass, 1968 (85)	110	25 (23%)	105	1 (1.0%)
Whalley, 1967 (86)	179	46 (26%)	179	0 (0%)
Little, 1966 (87)	141	35 (25%)	4,735	19 (0.4%)
Brumfitt, 1975 (88)	179	55 (31%)		
Chung & Hall, 1982 (89)	212	25 (12%)	1,575	51 (3.2%)
Campbell-Brown, et al., 1987 (90)	226	18 (16%)	4,244	1/226 (0.4%)
Golan et al., 1989 (91)	67	16 (24%)	1,063	17 (1.6%)
Gratacos et al., 1994 (92)	77	2/7 (28%)	1,575	5 (0.31%)
Total	1,441	333 (23%)	18,576	174 (0.94%)

pregnancy reduces this risk for pyelonephritis to 5% of patients; for this reason, urine culture is recommended at the first prenatal visit. Although controversial, there also appears to be a potentially strong link between untreated asymptomatic bacteriuria and both preterm labor and low birth weight. A meta-analysis review of 19 published studies found that treatment significantly reduced the risks for low birth weight and prematurity (47). A recent Cochrane review of 14 studies on asymptomatic bacteriuria in pregnancy agreed that antibiotic treatment is effective in reducing the incidence of pyelonephritis (odds ratio, 0.24; 95% confidence interval, 0.19 to 0.32) and also appears to be associated with reduced rates of preterm delivery and low birth weights (odds ratio, 0.60; 95% confidence interval, 0.45 to 0.80) (48). Experimental gestational pyelonephritis has been shown to be capable of inducing preterm birth and low birth weight in a mice model (49).

By definition, the diagnosis of asymptomatic bacteriuria is made on the basis of urine culture rather than urinalysis or dipstick tests. Attention must be given to collection and storage methods to minimize false-positive results. The most common bacterial isolates in asymptomatic pregnant women include *Escherichia coli, Klebsiella pneumoniae, Proteus mirabilis, Pseudomonas aeruginosa,* and *Enterobacter, Enterococcus, Streptococcus,* and *Staphylococcus* species. *E. coli* is responsible for more than 70% of these infections, with *Klebsiella pneumoniae, Enterobacter* species, and enterococci accounting for most of the remaining isolates.

Treatment should be based on the results of sensitivity testing, and a 3-day course is usually sufficient. Single-dose therapy has attracted some interest, but cure rates are overall not as high (65% to 88%) as with more extended therapy (50). Additionally, failure to respond to single-dose therapy has been identified as a high-risk factor that indicates a 50% risk for subsequent reinfection, compared with only 5% of those pregnant women who respond to single-dose therapy (51). Single-dose therapy therefore acts not only as an effective treatment with minimal side effects but also as a test to identify those patients at high risk for subsequent reinfection. It is postulated that these women who fail to respond to single-dose therapy have renal bacteriuria as demonstrated by antibody-coated bacteria. This subgroup of patients might be better treated after initial therapy by low-dose antibiotic suppression rather than by surveillance.

Enthusiasm for ampicillin has waned in recent years because of widespread resistance, reportedly up to 30% with *E. coli* and almost universal with *K. pneumoniae* (52). However, when indicated by sensitivity testing, ampicillin is an excellent choice because it is inexpensive, and safe for use during all pregnancy trimesters in nonallergic patients. Amoxicillin has a simpler dosing schedule and potentially fewer side effects; the addition of clavulanic acid to amoxicillin greatly increases gram-negative coverage, making it useful for recurring or resistant infections. Cephalexin is safe throughout pregnancy and equally effective to higher-generation cephalosporins for treating urinary tract infection. Although cross-reactivity to cephalosporins had historically raised concern for patients with a history of penicillin allergy, the actual incidence of adverse reactions is minimally, if at all, increased in those patients (53).

Nitrofurantoin is an excellent choice for initial therapy because of its safety, broad coverage of uropathogens, and high concentration in the urine. However, nausea and vomiting have been reported in up to 8% of patients. Nitrofurantoin has also rarely been associated with pulmonary hypersensitivity reactions and can cause hemolytic anemia in patients with a deficiency in glucose-6-phosphate-dehydrogenase (G6PD). Notably, people of African descent have a 10% risk for G6PD deficiency. Theoretically, nitrofurantoin should not be used in pregnant patients at term or in labor because of the risk to the neonate of hemolytic anemia, but such an effect has never been reported.

Sulfonamides, including sulfisoxazole and sulfamethoxazole, should not be used in patients near term because of their tendency to displace bilirubin from fetal albumin-binding sites. Toxicities reported in neonates after *in utero* exposure to sulfonamides include severe jaundice and hemolytic anemia but, surprisingly, not kernicterus (54). Trimethoprim may interfere with folic acid metabolism and is relatively contraindicated in the first trimester of pregnancy, although an increase in fetal abnormalities has not been demonstrated.

Nalidixic acid is safe in pregnancy but frequently causes side effects of nausea, vomiting, rash, headache, and drowsiness, limiting its usefulness. It should also not be given to patients with G6PD deficiency. Because of its limited spectrum and excellent urinary concentration, however, it can work well for patients with multiple allergies or recurrent infections.

Tetracyclines and fluoroquinolones should not be used in pregnancy. Tetracycline causes staining of fetal decidual teeth after 20 weeks of gestation and has been associated with maternal hepatic toxicity. Fluoroquinolones, although very effective in nonpregnant women, can erode fetal cartilage within weight-bearing joints, causing permanent arthropathy.

After initial treatment, close follow-up with biweekly cultures is as effective as suppressive medication in preventing pyelonephritis, even though the patients without suppressive therapy have a higher incidence of recurrent bacteriuria. Suppressive therapy may thus be reserved for resistant infections, patients with pyelonephritis in pregnancy, patients who failed single-dose therapy, and those for who close outpatient follow-up may be difficult. Suppressive therapy is usually accomplished with nitrofurantoin, ampicillin, or cephalexin in a once-daily dose at bedtime.

Recurrent bacteriuria in pregnancy is associated with underlying structural disease in 40% of patients. Up to 50% of all patients with asymptomatic bacteriuria have positive fluorescent antibody tests for antibody-coated bacteria, implying renal infection (55). The fluorescent antibody test is nearly as effective as direct methods (ureteral catheterization and bladder washout techniques) in the determination of renal bacteriuria. These patients often have decreased kidney function, with mildly elevated blood urea nitrogen and serum creatinine levels; creatinine clearance values of less than 100 mL/min are discovered in 45%. These abnormalities revert to normal within 6 weeks after treatment in most patients.

Long-term follow-up shows that 38% of patients with asymptomatic bacteriuria in pregnancy have bacteriuria 10 to 14 years later (56). Those with recurrent bacteriuria in pregnancy have a 10% incidence of chronic pyelonephritis. In subsequent pregnancies, 38% of asymptomatic bacteriuric patients have symptomatic infections (57).

Cystitis

Cystitis, or uncomplicated urinary tract infection, is a syndrome of urinary urgency, frequency, and dysuria in the absence of systemic symptoms. The incidence in pregnancy ranges from 1% to 3%. Diagnosis can be made with as few as 10^2 colonies from a catheterized specimen. Pathogens are similar to those in asymptomatic bacteriuria; *E. coli* is the most common isolate by far. Only 6% of these patients have antibody-coated bacteria.

Initial antepartum screening is of limited effectiveness for predicting which pregnant women will develop cystitis. Two thirds of patients who ultimately develop cystitis, in fact, demonstrate negative initial urine cultures. This differs markedly from the reliability of urine culture in predicting an elevated risk for pyelonephritis during pregnancy; only one fifth of patients who develop upper tract infection have negative cultures initially. Moreover, recurrent infection after treatment is far less common in patients with cystitis (17%)

than in patients with pyelonephritis (75%) or asymptomatic bacteriuria (33%).

Treatment for cystitis is identical to that used for asymptomatic bacteriuria and broadly successful with little risk for subsequent pyelonephritis. Only 9% of these patients will have recurrent bacteriuria. The low recurrence risk is probably a result of the low incidence of renal involvement (6%) in these patients.

Pyelonephritis

Pyelonephritis complicates 1% of all pregnancies. Although pregnancy does not increase the incidence of asymptomatic bacteriuria, it does increase the risk for pyelonephritis. The normal dilation of the ureters and subsequent urinary stasis, as well as enhanced growth of coliform bacteria in pregnant urine, are largely responsible for this increased risk. Three quarters of kidney infections in pregnant women are predated by asymptomatic bacteriuria. Conversely, less than 5% of women whose bacteriuria is successfully treated develop pyelonephritis.

The onset of symptoms of pyelonephritis usually occurs during the second or third trimester (67%) or intrapartum or postpartum (27%) and rarely presents in the first trimester. The most frequent signs and symptoms among patients with pyelonephritis are costovertebral tenderness (97%), temperature higher than 38.3°C (84%), flank pain and chills (82%), dysuria, frequency, urgency (40%), and nausea and vomiting (24%). Urinalysis reveals pyuria, bacteriuria, and white cell casts. Identification of white blood cells and bacteria on a drop of unspun urine correlates well with a positive culture (58). Temporary renal dysfunction leads to an elevation in blood urea nitrogen and creatinine in 20% of patients with active infection and to a decrease in creatinine clearance below 100 mL/min in 46% (56). If not treated, up to 10% of women may develop septic shock and multi-organ failure. Respiratory distress with pulmonary edema occurs in 2% of cases, rarely before the third trimester (59). Unrecognized pyelonephritis has also been associated with spontaneous rupture of the urinary tract during pregnancy (60).

Pyelonephritis during pregnancy may also result in anemia for between 25% and 60% of women, resulting from endotoxin-mediated hemolysis. Prospective controlled studies have not confirmed suspected associations between upper urinary tract infection and pregnancy-induced hypertension or low birth weight. Premature labor requiring tocolysis occurs in about 4% of patients with pyelonephritis, with only those patients presenting in labor being at increased risk for premature delivery. Appropriately treated patients are at low risk for preterm labor requiring tocolysis.

Treatment generally consists of hospital admission, intravenous fluid hydration, antibiotics, and close observation. Because of widespread hospital resistance to ampicillin, a first-generation cephalosporin such as cefazolin is the preferred empiric treatment and is successful in 75% of patients. Because 95% of these patients are afebrile in 72 hours, patients not responding by this time should have gentamicin or aztreonam, added with drug levels monitored to ensure adequate therapy and prevent toxicity. A renal ultrasound or "one-shot" intravenous pyelogram should also be obtained to evaluate the possibility of urolithiasis or obstruction.

Once the patient has been afebrile for 24 to 48 hours, she may be changed to oral therapy for 7 to 14 days, followed by suppressive therapy as outlined previously for the duration of the pregnancy. This reduces the risk for recurrent pyelonephritis to about 5%. Surveillance with biweekly cultures, rather than antibiotic suppression, is an alternative for reliable patients; however, one third of women followed in this manner develop positive cultures.

At least two prospective randomized studies suggest that selected patients with pyelonephritis may be safely treated as outpatients. Angel and associates (61) found that oral antibiotic therapy (cephalexin) and intravenous therapy (cephalothin) were equally effective. Millar and colleagues (62) later showed that for women at less than 24 weeks of gestation, outpatient therapy with ceftriaxone and cephalexin is safe and equally effective to inpatient therapy. Patients treated as outpatients should be reliable and able to return to the hospital quickly if their condition worsens.

Follow-up studies reveal that up to 30% to 45% of women with pyelonephritis in pregnancy demonstrate radiologic evidence of renal disease or anomalies (Fig. 16.4). These patients are at higher risk (40%) for developing recurrent pyelonephritis in subsequent pregnancies.

Postpartum Urinary Infection

Recurrent pyelonephritis occurs postpartum in as many as 10% of patients who have antepartum infection. Many of these infections may be iatrogenic after routine intrapartum catheterization; indeed, bacteriuria develops twice as often among women who are catheterized before or during delivery (9.1% versus 4.7%). Indwelling catheters increase the risk for bacteriuria to nearly 25%. Catheterization is often necessitated during labor and delivery but should not be performed as a routine procedure.

Bladder Injuries and Fistulas

Moderate amounts of urine in the bladder do not have a deleterious effect on the course

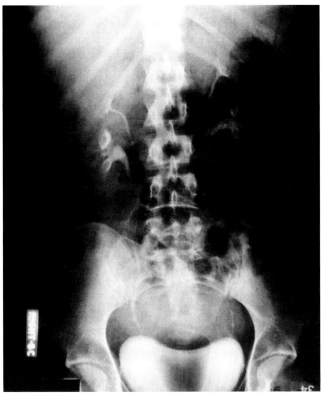

FIG. 16.4. Urinary anomalies in pyelonephritis patients. Intravenous pyelogram performed 6 weeks after a pregnancy complicated by recurrent pyelonephritis shows bifid collecting systems to the pelvic brim.

of labor (63). Epidural anesthesia, however, can eliminate the urge to void and result in overdistention of the bladder (64). For this reason, patients selecting an epidural are often subjected to either intermittent catheterization or continuous bladder drainage, throughout labor. A rapid ultrasound assessment can estimate bladder volume and reduce or eliminate the need for catheterization in many cases.

Minor trauma to the bladder during spontaneous vaginal delivery is common, with urinary retention occurring in 10% to 15% of all postpartum patients. Obstructed labor leading to necrosis of the anterior vaginal wall and bladder (and thus vesicovaginal fistula) has been essentially eradicated in Western countries but remains a significant problem in underdeveloped nations.

The abdominal position of the bladder during pregnancy subjects it to a higher risk for injury at laparotomy. The incidence of urinary tract injury at cesarean section is overall less than 1% (65) but increases with Pfannenstiel incision, lower segment uterine incision, prior cesarean section, prolonged second stage of labor, uterine rupture, and cesarean hysterectomy. Barclay (66) reported bladder and ureteral injury in the latter case to be 4.8% and 0.5%, respectively. Outlet forceps should confer little increased risk, but several studies document increased risk for urinary tract injury with midpelvic maneuvers such as Kielland forceps and Scanzoni rotation. Kibel and associates (67) reported a bladder perforation in a primigravid patient with no history of pelvic surgery. Although the laceration occurred during the vacuum-assisted delivery of a 4,200-g infant, it was not detected until 3 days postpartum when the patient presented with renal failure and ascites.

Most bladder injuries involve laceration of the bladder dome, which can be easily repaired in two layers using 0-0 or 0-00 chromic or polyglactin suture. Injuries extending onto the trigone or close to the ureteral orifices demand more careful attention because ureteral reimplantation is some-times necessary. Infant feeding tubes or umbilical artery catheters available in the delivery room can be passed retrograde to ensure patency of the ureters.

Urinary fistulas are rare and usually result from unrecognized injury at the time of operative delivery. Vesicovaginal fistula is the most common, with an incidence of 0.7% in Barclay's study. Fistula formation is classically heralded by continuous incontinence 7 to 14 days after injury. Patients with vesicouterine or vesicocorporeal fistulas (Fig. 16.5A) have cyclic hematuria as the menstrual flow empties into the bladder (menouria). Finally, the patient presenting with normal menses but loss of urine from the external cervical os may have a vesicocervical fistula (Fig. 16.5B).

If a fistula is identified, it should be evaluated by cystoscopy and intravenous pyelography to rule out other fistulous tracts and ureteral compromise. Drainage and decompression above the site of the fistula may result in the resolution of some small fistulas. The remainder will ultimately require surgical repair, although the most optimal timing and operative route remain subjects of debate.

Vesicoureteral Reflux

Vesicoureteral reflux can cause radiating flank pain with urination and occurs in up to 3.5% of pregnancies but is rarely found before the third trimester except in patients with bacteriuria, who have a 50% incidence of reflux. Many of these latter patients probably have reflux before pregnancy. In normal pregnancy, ureteral catheter studies demonstrate an increase in resting basal pressure but somewhat decreased ureteral contractility. This increase in ureteral pressure offsets a similar increase in bladder pressure until the third trimester, when detrusor pressure is often higher than 25 cm H_2O. This increase in pressure may lead to a further reduction of ureteral ejaculation of urine, with total stasis occurring at pressures above 41 cm H_2O. Pressures this high are usually only reached in

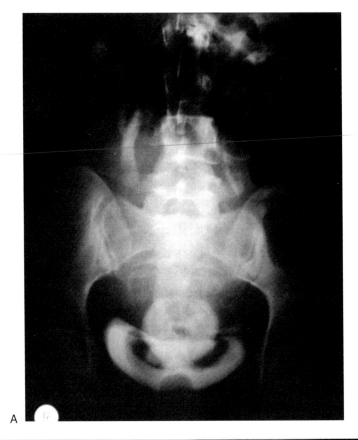

A

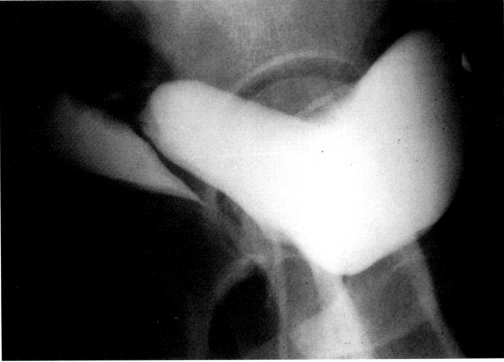

B

FIG. 16.5. A: Vesicouterine fistula discovered during investigation of cyclic hematuria after cesarean section. **B:** Lateral view of a vesicovaginal fistula masquerading as a vesicocervical fistula in a patient presenting with continuous leakage of urine 3 days after emergent cesarean section for a ruptured uterus while attempting a vaginal birth after cesarean section. (**A** courtesy of Dr. Allan Shanberg.)

the third trimester with a full bladder and predispose to reflux.

Urolithiasis

Urolithiasis in pregnancy is rare, with an incidence of 0.03% to 0.44%, a rate similar to that in the general population (Table 16.3). The higher incidences are found in the Southeast and mid-Atlantic "stone belt" in the United States. Urolithiasis is twice as common in multiparous women, but this may be largely due to the increase in urinary calculi with advancing age.

Pregnancy does not influence calculus disease unless nausea and vomiting prevent treatment of preexisting stones. For unknown reasons, calculus disease is four times as common in women who spontaneously abort as in pregnant and nonpregnant controls.

The onset of symptomatic urolithiasis occurs predominantly (88%) after 20 weeks of gestation when ureteral dilation is prominent. The composition of these stones is the same as found in nonpregnant patients, with the exception of an increased incidence of struvite stones ("infection stones") in pregnant patients.

The signs and symptoms of urolithiasis in pregnancy are identical to those in the nonpregnant patient. In the presence of physiologic hydroureter, however, colic and hematuria are frequently absent. Stones should be suspected in any patient presenting with lateralizing flank pain and tenderness without fever. They should also be suspected in those patients with pyelonephritis who do not respond to parenteral antibiotics within 48 to 72 hours.

Patients with suspected urolithiasis should be initially evaluated by ultrasonography; renal stones as small as 0.5 mm can sometimes be visualized with this technology (68). However, a recent review of a 13-year study period at Parkland Hospital (69) found that among 57 pregnant women with symptomatic nephrolithiasis, calculi were visualized in only 60% of renal ultrasonographic examinations. In contrast, single-shot intravenous pyelography identified the stone in 93% of cases. Therefore, a negative ultrasonogram, in the context of strong clinical suspicion, should be followed up with a one-shot intravenous pyelogram 20 minutes after dye injection may be done, followed by a 1-hour film if necessary. This results in less than 1 cGy to the fetus. A dose of 5 to 15 cGy in the first trimester is associated with an increased risk for congenital anomalies of 1% to 3%. The risk for carcinogenesis is less than 1% at doses less than 10 cGy, and the risk for leukemia in these infants is 1.5 cases per million people exposed to 1 cGy. These risks are far lower than those associated with failure to diagnose and treat urolithiasis. Finally, magnetic resonance urography, with strongly T_2-weighted images, may identify the site and type of obstruction without contrast administration or x-ray exposure (70). However, the cost-effectiveness of ultrasound justifies its use before either intravenous pyelography or magnetic resonance imaging.

Initial treatment of urolithiasis should always be conservative because 60% to 80% of all stones pass spontaneously. Stones 4 mm or less in diameter pass 80% of the time, but stones greater than 7 mm have a spontaneous

TABLE 16.3. *Urolithiasis in pregnancy*

Investigators	Incidence	Spontaneous passage
Harris & Dunnihoo, 1967 (93)	19/11,977 (0.16%)	10/19 (53%)
Strong et al., 1978 (94)	14/22,495 (0.06%)	11/14 (79%)
Coe et al., 1978 (95)	20[a]	20/20 (100%)
Cumming & Taylor, 1979 (96)	13/21,277 (0.06%)	5/13 (38%)
Lattanzi & Cook, 1980 (97)	11/11,292 (0.09%)	7/11 (64%)
Butler, 2000 (98)	1/3300 (0.03%)	43/57 (75%)

passage rate of only 20% (71). For patients in whom the composition of the stone is unknown, initial therapy consists of aggressive hydration, analgesia, and bed rest. Experimental work suggests that a bolus of 250 mg of hydroxyprogesterone results in the prompt passage of stones in nonpregnant patients (72). This may be due to an acute progestational effect that simulates the hormonal milieu of pregnancy.

Where conservative management fails—or in cases of bilateral ureteric obstruction, obstruction of a solitary kidney, or sepsis—surgical intervention may be necessary. Procedures such as cystoscopy with basket extraction, or draining the obstructed collecting system with passage of a ureteral stent or nephrostomy tube may be all that is necessary until after delivery. Although reports of extracorporeal shock-wave lithotripsy used inadvertently in pregnancy appear to indicate a low risk for adverse effects (73), the technique should still be considered experimental in the absence of outcome data (74). Ureteroscopic lithotripsy and stone extraction may represent a safer alternative. When major procedures such as ureterolithotomy, pyelolithotomy, or the very rare nephrectomy are necessary, they have been accomplished with minimal complications to either the mother or the fetus.

Determination of the exact etiology can usually be deferred until the postpartum period. When a previous etiology is known, specific therapy and aggressive hydration should be used. D-Penicillamine and allopurinol have both been used successfully and safely in pregnancy for cysteine and uric acid stones, respectively. Likewise, thiazide diuretics have been useful in curtailing calcium stone formation in hypercalciuric patients. Whenever possible, these medications should be avoided in the first trimester.

Hematuria

Hematuria in pregnancy is usually caused by catheterization or trauma at the time of labor and delivery. Outside of these, it is decidedly abnormal and must be investigated. Causes include urinary tract infection, calculi, trauma, urologic cancer, and placenta percreta. Infection and calculus disease are discussed above. Trauma complicates 7% of all pregnancies, with half occurring during the third trimester; most of these are blunt abdominal injuries incurred in motor vehicle accidents. Although rare, the gravida with a full bladder may experience extraperitoneal rupture of the bladder with sudden blood loss and shock. The lower urinary tract is injured in 15% of pelvic fractures. Hematuria, gross or microscopic, warrants prompt investigation in the trauma setting.

Renal adenocarcinoma is the most common urologic cancer of pregnancy, causing hematuria in almost half of patients (75). A palpable abdominal mass, however, is present in most patients. Transitional cell carcinoma of the bladder has been reported in a small series of pregnant patients (76), most presenting with painless hematuria. Ultrasound evaluation of the urinary tract, combined with cystoscopy and biopsy, is usually sufficient for diagnosis. When the patient presents late in pregnancy, definitive treatment in most cases can be delayed until after delivery. Placenta percreta is a rare condition in which the placenta penetrates the myometrium and uterine serosa and can invade adjacent structures such as the bladder. It is most commonly associated with placenta previa and a history of prior cesarean section. In the past, diagnosis was made at the time of delivery, but antepartum diagnosis can now be made in most cases with ultrasound or magnetic resonance imaging; cystoscopy can be a valuable adjunct. For cases involving profuse bleeding during delivery, cesarean hysterectomy and partial cystectomy are mandated. If the patient is not actively bleeding, the placenta may be left *in situ* with high ligation of the umbilical cord, followed by observation along with antibiotic therapy to minimize risk for infection. Methotrexate may be useful for accelerating the reabsorption of the trophoblastic tissue but is not universally effective (77).

Pregnancy Complicated by Prior Bladder Surgery

Pregnancy is not contraindicated in patients having had surgery on the bladder or bladder neck. Successful outcomes have been reported in patients who have undergone continent urinary diversion (78), augmentation cystoplasty, and artificial urinary sphincter placement. These patients are at high risk for urinary tract infection, and antibiotic suppression may be indicated. Most patients can deliver vaginally. For patients with previous antiincontinence surgery on the bladder neck, some practitioners have recommended a classic cesarean section to minimize damage to the surgical site; this decision, however, should be individualized. The potential benefits of this procedure should be carefully weighed against the increased morbidity and necessity for future cesarean sections. Data are lacking regarding the effects of vaginal delivery for women with prior anti-incontinence procedures, but scattered case reports (79) and small series indicate that it may be safe, with the efficacy of the original surgery maintained in some cases. A recent survey of more than 300 members of the American Urogynecology Society accumulated data on 40 vaginal deliveries and 47 cesarean sections following stress incontinence surgery. Although the study design poses serious limitations regarding the conclusions that can be drawn, 95% of women who delivered by cesarean were reported as continent postnatally versus only 73% of those who underwent a vaginal birth. One retrospective review found that 11 of 13 (85%) pregnant patients with an artificial urinary sphincter were able to have vaginal deliveries, with no intrapartum or postpartum complications (80). Another report suggests that vaginal delivery is possible after pelvic floor reconstruction (81). Determining the effects of vaginal birth on long-term surgical outcomes will require further longitudinal study. In the absence of established guidelines, we evaluate patients during pregnancy to reassess their anatomic support and urodynamic parameters before deciding on mode of delivery. The patient should be an active participant in this decision.

REFERENCES

1. Iosif S, Ingemarsson I, Ulmsten U. Urodynamic studies in normal pregnancy and in puerperium. *Obstet Gynecol* 1980;137:696–700.
2. Tong Y, Wein AJ, Levin RM. Effects of pregnancy on adrenergic function in the rabbit urinary bladder. *Neurourol Urodyn* 1992;11:525–533.
3. Brown ADG. The effects of pregnancy on the lower urinary tract. *Clin Obstet Gynaecol* 1978;5:151–168.
4. Francis WJA. Disturbances of bladder function in relation to pregnancy. *J Obstet Gynaecol Br Emp* 1960;67: 353–366.
5. Bennetts FA, Judd GE. Studies of the postpartum bladder. *Am J Obstet Gynecol* 1941;42:419–427.
6. Meyer S, Bachlard O, DeGrandi P. Do bladder neck mobility and urethral sphincter function differ during pregnancy compared with during the non-pregnant state? *Int Urogynecol J Pelvic Floor Dysfunct* 1998;9(6): 397–404.
7. Peschers U, Schaer G, Anthuber C, et al. Changes in vesical neck mobility following vaginal delivery. *Obstet Gynecol* 1996;88:1001–1006.
8. Wijma J, Weis Potters AE, deWolf BT, et al. Anatomical and functional changes in the lower urinary tract during pregnancy. *Br J Obstet Gynaecol* 2001;108(7):726–732.
9. Schulman A, Herlinger H. Urinary tract dilatation in pregnancy. *Br J Radiol* 1975;48:638–645.
10. Pitkin RM. Morphologic changes in pregnancy. In: Buchsbaum HJ, Schmidt JD, eds. *Gynecologic and obstetric urology,* 3rd ed. Philadelphia: WB Saunders, 1993:586.
11. Schulman A, Herlinger H. Urinary tract dilatation in pregnancy. *Br J Radiol* 1975;48:638–645.
12. Dafnis E, Sabatini S. The effect of pregnancy on renal function: physiology and pathophysiology. *Am J Med Sci* 1992;303:184–205.
13. Davison JA, Dunlop W. Renal hemodynamics and tubular function in normal human pregnancy. *Kidney Int* 1980;18:152–161.
14. Sims EAH, Krantz KE. Serial studies of renal function during pregnancy and the puerperium in normal women. *J Clin Invest* 1958;37:1764–1774.
15. Dafnis E, Sabatini S. The effect of pregnancy on renal function: physiology and pathophysiology. *Am J Med Sci* 1992;303:184–205.
16. Little B. Water and electrolyte balance during pregnancy. *Anesthesiology* 1965;26:400–408.
17. Hytten FE, Taggart N. Limb volumes in pregnancy. *J Obstet Gynaecol Br Commonw* 1967;74:663–668.
18. Cutner A, Cardozo LD, Benness CJ. Assessment of urinary symptoms in early pregnancy. *Br J Obstet Gynaecol* 1991;98:1283–1286.
19. Stanton SL, Kerr-Wilson R, Harris VG. The incidence of urological symptoms in normal pregnancy. *Br J Obstet Gynaecol* 1980;87:897–900.
20. Hong PL, Leong M, Seltzer V. Uroflowmetric observations in pregnancy. *Neurourol Urodyn* 1988;7:61–70.
21. Kennedy S, Hall PM, Seymour AE, et al. Transient diabetes insipidus and acute fatty liver of pregnancy. *Br J Obstet Gynaecol* 1994;101(5):387–391.

22. Parboosingh J, Doig A. Studies of nocturia in normal pregnancy. *J Obstet Gynaecol Br Commonw* 1973;80: 888–895.

23. Myers DL, Scotti RJ. Acute urinary retention and incarcerated, retroverted, gravid uterus. *J Reprod Med* 1995; 40:487–490.

24. Jackson D, Elliot JP, Pearson M. Asymptomatic uterine retroversion at 36 weeks gestation. *Obstet Gynecol* 1988;71:466–468.

25. Van Winter JT, Ogburn PL, Ney JA, et al. Uterine incarceration in the third trimester: a rare complication of pregnancy. *Mayo Clin Proc* 1991;66:608–613.

26. Monga AK, Woodhouse CR, Stanton SL. Pregnancy and fibroids causing simultaneous urinary retention and ureteric obstruction. *Br J Urol* 1996;77(4):606–607.

27. Ramsay IN, Torbet TE. Incidence of abnormal voiding parameters in the immediate postpartum period. *Neurourol Urodyn* 1993;12:179–183.

28. Kerr-Wilson RHJ, McNally S. Bladder drainage for caesarean section under epidural analgesia. *Br J Obstet Gynaecol* 1986;93:28–30.

29. Tapp AJS, Meire H, Cardozo LD. The effect of epidural analgesia on post-partum voiding. *Neurourol Urodyn* 1987;6:235–237.

30. Bennetts FA, Judd GE. Studies of the postpartum bladder. *Am J Obstet Gynecol* 1941;42:419–427.

31. Viktrup L, Lose G, Rolff M, et al. The symptom of stress incontinence caused by pregnancy or delivery in primiparas. *Obstet Gynecol* 1992;79:945–949.

32. Francis WJA. The onset of stress incontinence. *J Obstet Gynaecol Br Emp* 1960;67:899–903.

33. Stanton SL, Kerr-Wilson R, Harris VG. The incidence of urological symptoms in normal pregnancy. *Br J Obstet Gynaecol* 1980;87:897–900.

34. Meyer S, Schreyer A, DeGrandi P, et al. The effects of birth on urinary continence mechanisms and other pelvic floor characteristics. *Obstet Gynecol* 1998;92: 613–618.

35. Viktrup l, Lose G, Rolff M, et al. The symptom of stress incontinence caused by pregnancy or delivery in primiparas. *Obstet Gynecol* 1992;79:945–949.

36. Viktrup L, Lose G. The risk of stress incontinence 5 years after first delivery. *Am J Obstet Gynecol* 2001; 185:82–87.

37. Van Geelen JM, Lemmens WAJG, Eskes TK, et al. The urethral pressure profile in pregnancy and after delivery in healthy nulliparous women. *Am J Obstet Gynecol* 1982;144:636–649.

38. Peschers U, Schaer G, Anthuber C, et al. Changes in vesical neck mobility following vaginal delivery. *Obstet Gynecol* 1996;88:1001–1006.

39. Mallett V, Hosker G, Smith ARB, et al. Pelvic floor damage and childbirth: a neurophysiologic follow up study. *Neurourol Urodyn* 1994;13:357–358.

40. Hojberg KE, Salvig JD, Winslow NA, et al. Urinary incontinence: prevalence and risk factors at 16 weeks of gestation. *Br J Obstet Gynaecol* 1999;106(8):842–850.

41. Persson J, Wolner-Hanssen PAL, Rydhstroem H. Obstetric risk factors for stress urinary incontinence: a population-based study. *Obstet Gynecol* 2000;96:440–445.

42. Moller LA, Lose G, Jorgensen T. Risk factors for lower urinary tract symptoms in women 40 to 60 years of age. *Obstet Gynecol* 2000;96:446–451.

43. Marshall K, Thompson KA, Walsh DM, et al. Incidence of urinary incontinence and constipation during pregnancy and postpartum: survey of current findings at the rotunda lying-in hospital. *Br J Obstet Gynaecol* 1998;105:400–402.

44. Cutner A, Cardozo LD, Benness CJ. Assessment of urinary symptoms in the second half of pregnancy. *Int Urogynecol J* 1992;3:30–32.

45. Cutner A, Cardozo LD, Benness CJ. Assessment of urinary symptoms in the second half of pregnancy. *Int Urogynecol J* 1992;3:30–32.

46. Kass EH. Bacteriuria and pyelonephritis of pregnancy. *Arch Intern Med* 1960;105:194–198.

47. Romero R, Oyarzun E, Mazor M, et al. Meta-analysis of the relationship between asymptomatic bacteriuria and preterm delivery/low birth weight. *Obstet Gynecol* 1989;73:576–582.

48. Smaill F. Antibiotics for asymptomatic bacteriuria in pregnancy. *Cochrane Database Syst Rev* 2001;2: CD000490.

49. Schaeffer AJ. Experimental gestational pyelonephritis induces preterm births and low birth weights in C3H/HeJ mice. *J Urol* 2000;164:260–261.

50. Vercaigne LM, Zhanel GG. Recommended treatment for urinary tract infection in pregnancy. *Ann Pharmacother* 1994;28:248–251.

51. Jakobi P, Neiger R, Merzbach D, et al. Single-dose antimicrobial therapy in the treatment of asymptomatic bacteriuria of pregnancy. *Am J Obstet Gynecol* 1987; 156:1148–1152.

52. Dunlow S, Duff P. Prevalence of antibiotic-resistant uropathogens in obstetric patients with acute pyelonephritis. *Obstet Gynecol* 1990;76:241–244.

53. Anne S, Reisman RE. Risk of administering cephalosporin antibiotics to patients with histories of penicillin allergy. *Ann Allergy Asthma Immunol* 1995; 74(2):167–170.

54. Briggs GG, Freeman RK, Yaffe SJ. *Drugs in lactation and pregnancy,* 4th ed. Baltimore: Williams & Wilkins, 1994:796–847.

55. Harris RE, Thomas VL, Shelokov A. Asymptomatic bacteriuria in pregnancy: antibody-coated bacteria, renal function, and intrauterine growth retardation. *Am J Obstet Gynecol* 1976;126:20–25.

56. Zinner SH, Kass EH. Long-term (10 to 14 years) follow-up of bacteriuria of pregnancy. *N Engl J Med* 1971; 285:820–824.

57. Gilstrap LC III, Cunningham FG, Whalley PJ. Acute pyelonephritis in pregnancy: an anterospective study of 656 women. *Obstet Gynecol* 1981;57:409–413.

58. Kunin CM. The quantitative significance of bacteria visualized in the unstained urinary sediment. *N Engl J Med* 1961;265:589–590.

59. Cunningham FG, Lucas MJ, Hankins GDV. Pulmonary injury complicating antepartum pyelonephritis. *Am J Obstet Gynecol* 1987;156:797–807.

60. Meyers SJ, Lee RV, Munschauer RW. Dilatation and nontraumatic rupture of the urinary tract during pregnancy: a review. *Obstet Gynecol* 1985;66:809–815.

61. Angel JL, O'Brien WF, Finan MA, et al. Acute pyelonephritis of pregnancy: a prospective study of oral versus intravenous antibiotic therapy. *Obstet Gynecol* 1990;76:28–32.

62. Millar LK, Wing DA, Paul RH, et al. Outpatient treatment of pyelonephritis in pregnancy. *Obstet Gynecol* 1995;86:560–564.

63. Read JA, Miller FC, Yeh SY, et al. Urinary bladder dis-

tention: effect on labor and uterine activity. *Obstet Gynecol* 1980;56:565–570.

64. Weil A, Reyes H, Rottenberg RD, et al. Effect of lumbar epidural analgesia on lower urinary tract function in the immediate postpartum period. *Br J Obstet Gynaecol* 1983;90:428–432.

65. Evrard JR, Gold EM, Cahill TF. Cesarean section: a contemporary assessment. *J Reprod Med* 1980;24:147–152.

66. Barclay DL. Cesarean hysterectomy: thirty years' experience. *Obstet Gynecol* 1970;35:120–131.

67. Kibel AS, Staskin DR, Grigoriev VE. Intraperitoneal bladder rupture after normal vaginal delivery. *J Urol* 1995;153:725–727.

68. Swanson SK, Heilman RL, Eversman WG. Urinary tract stones in pregnancy. *Surg Clin North Am* 1995;75: 123–142.

69. Butler EL, Cox SM, Eberts EG, et al. Symptomatic nephrolithiasis complicating pregnancy. *Obstet Gynecol* 2000;96:753–756.

70. Grenier N, Pariente JL, Trillaud H, et al. Dilatation of the collecting system during pregnancy: physiologic vs obstructive dilatation. *Eur Radiol* 2000;10(2):271–279.

71. Swanson SK, Heilman RL, Eversman WG. Urinary tract stones in pregnancy. *Surg Clin North Am* 1995;75: 123–142.

72. Perlow DL. The use of progesterone for ureteral stones: a preliminary report. *J Urol* 1980;124:715–716.

73. Asgari MA, Safarinejad MR, Hosseini SY, et al. Extracorporeal shock wave lithotripsy of renal calculi during early pregnancy. *Br J Urol Int* 1999;84(6):615–617.

74. Evans HJ, Wollin TA. The management of urinary calculi in pregnancy. *Curr Opin Urol* 2001;11(4):379–384.

75. Walker JL, Knight EL. Renal cell carcinoma in pregnancy. *Cancer* 1986;58:2343–2347.

76. Loughlin KR, Ng B. Bladder cancer during pregnancy. *Br J Urol* 1995;75:421–422.

77. Jaffe R, DuBeshter B, Sherer DM, et al. Failure of methotrexate treatment for term placenta percreta. *Am J Obstet Gynecol* 1994;171:558–559.

78. Fenn N, Barrington JW, Stephenson TP. Clam enteroplasty and pregnancy. *Br J Urol* 1995;75:85–86.

79. Iskander MN, Kapoor D. Pregnancy following tension-free vaginal taping. *Int Urogynecol J* 2000;11:199–200.

80. Creagh TA, McInerney PD, Thomas PJ, et al. Pregnancy after lower urinary tract reconstruction in women. *J Urol* 1995;154:1323–1324.

81. Kovac SR, Cruikshank SH. Successful pregnancies and vaginal deliveries after sacrospinous uterosacral fixation in five of nineteen patients. *Am J Obstet Gynecol* 1993;168:1778–1786.

82. Kass EH. Pyelonephritis and bacteriuria. *Ann Intern Med* 1962;56:46–53.

83. Sleigh JD. Detection of bacteriuria by a modification of the nitrite test. *BMJ* 1965;1:765–767.

84. Kincaid-Smith P, Bullen M, Mills J, et al. The reliability of screening tests for bacteriuria in pregnancy. *Lancet* 1964;2:61–62.

85. Norden CW, Kass EH: Bacteriuria of pregnancy—a critical appraisal. *Ann Rev Med* 1968;19:431–470.

86. Whalley P. Bacteriuria of pregnancy. *Am J Obstet Gynecol* 1967;97(5):723–738.

87. Little PJ. The incidence of urinary infection in 5000 pregnant women. *Lancet* 1966;29:925–928.

88. Brumfitt W. The effects of bacteriuria in pregnancy on maternal and fetal health. *Kidney Int Suppl* 1975;Suppl 4:S113–S119.

89. Chung PK, Hall MH. Antenatal prediction of urinary tract infection in pregnancy. *Br J Obstet Gynaecol* 1982;89:(1):8–11.

90. Campbell-Brown M, McFadyen IR, Seal DV, et al. Is screening for bacteriuria in pregnancy worth while? *Br Med J* (Clin Res Ed) 1987;20;294(6587):1579–1582.

91. Golan A, Wexler S, Amit A, et al. Asymptomatic bacteriuria in normal and high-risk pregnancy. *Eur J Obstet Gynecol Reprod Biol* 1989;33(2):101–108.

92. Gratacos E, Torres PJ, Vila J, et al. Screening and treatment of asymptomatic bacteriuria in pregnancy prevent pyelonephritis. *J Infect Dis* 1994;169(6):1390–1392.

93. Harris RE, Dunnihoo DR. The incidence and significance of urinary calculi in pregnancy *Am J Obstet Gynecol* 1967;99(2):237–241.

94. Strong DW, Murchison RJ, Lynch DF. The management of ureteral calculi during pregnancy. *Surg Gynecol Obstet* 1978;146(4):604–608.

95. Coe FL, Parks JH, Lindheimer MD. Nephrolithiasis during pregnancy. *N Engl J Med* 1978;298(6):324–326.

96. Cumming DC, Taylor PJ. Urologic and obstetric significance of urinary calculi in pregnancy. *Obstet Gynecol* 1979;53(4):505–508.

97. Lattanzi DR, Cook WA. Urinary calculi in pregnancy. *Obstet Gynecol* 1980;56(4):462–466.

98. Butler EL, Cox SM, Eberts EG, et al. Symptomatic nephrolithiasis complicating pregnancy. *Obstet Gynecol* 2000;96(5 Pt 1):753–756.

Ostergard's Urogynecology and Pelvic Floor Dysfunction, Fifth Edition. edited by A.E. Bent, et al. Lippincott Williams & Wilkins, Philadelphia © 2003.

17

Disorders Affecting the Urethra

Alfred E. Bent

Department of Gynecology and Obstetrics, Johns Hopkins School of Medicine;
and Department of Gynecology, Greater Baltimore Medical Center, Baltimore, Maryland

The role of the urethra in pelvic floor dysfunction in women, along with the varied insults it has suffered since the mid-20th century, is a mystery in continuous evolution. Most recently, there are those who ascribe all urethral complaints to the painful bladder disorders, mainly interstitial cystitis. There are many patients who can benefit from reasonable treatment of a variety of urethral conditions that does not expose the urethra to traumatic manipulation or the patient to prolonged, frustrating medical therapy. The sections discussed in this chapter include the following:

- Urethral pain syndrome
- Atrophic urethritis
- Acute urethritis
- Meatal abnormalities
- Urethral diverticulum

URETHRAL PAIN SYNDROME

Sensory disorders of the urethra are both distressing and disabling conditions. They can be defined as a symptom complex including urinary frequency, urgency, dysuria, suprapubic pain, postvoid fullness, urinary hesitancy, dyspareunia, and urge incontinence, in the absence of significant bacteriuria or structural urinary tract abnormality. Most patients think they have a urinary tract infection, and many have been treated on several occasions for this problem, either without resolution or with rapid recurrence. Often, the patient responds after 1 or 2 days of antibiotic therapy and then relapses very soon after the course is complete. Other patients present with a history of recurrent yeast infections, for which they now self-medicate almost weekly with very poor relief. Many patients have a combination of recurrent antibiotic therapy, followed by a history of recurrent yeast infections. Many physicians still use the term urethral syndrome, as devised by Gallagher and colleagues (1), to describe the condition. The most recent terminology, adopted by the International Continence Society, is urethral pain syndrome (2), which is defined as the occurrence of persistent or recurrent episodic urethral pain usually on voiding, with daytime frequency and nocturia, in the absence of proven infection or other obvious pathology. The diagnosis implies longevity of symptoms, and 6 months is a minimal duration of the problem.

Incidence

The incidence and prevalence of the condition is not known, but of patients presenting with lower urinary tract symptoms in the absence of infection, 15% to 30% were diagnosed with urethral syndrome (3–4). A more likely number is in the range of less than 5%. In a questionnaire to 792 members of the American Urogynecologic Society, with a 31% response rate, most practitioners saw zero to five patients per month with this condition (5). The age groups more commonly affected are 20 to 30 years and 50 to 60 years.

Etiology

The etiology has previously been explored, and in the numerous explanations of causality, the pathophysiology has been developed for each proposed cause. The etiology at best is unclear. The more common factors implicated are as follows: (a) infectious—low growth of common organisms often detectable only in the urethra (6); (b) fastidious organisms—*Chlamydia trachomatis, Mycoplasma hominis, Ureaplasma urealyticum* (7,8); (c) early manifestation of interstitial cystitis (9,10); (d) response to stress (11,12); (e) hypersensitivity dysfunction (10,13,14); and (f) levator myofascial syndrome (15–17). Other causes include allergy, trauma, anatomic features, coexisting medical conditions (18,19), urethral instability, external urethral spasm (20), and urethral obstruction (21).

Evaluation

The evaluation requires the basic evaluation for an incontinent patient, which includes history, physical examination, urinalysis and culture, residual urine determination, and 24-hour voiding diary (22). The rest of the workup is a means to exclude other causes of the irritation. The differential diagnosis includes urethral pain syndrome, urinary tract infection, and vaginitis. Other conditions to be ruled out include atrophic urethral changes, acute or subacute urethritis, unstable or overactive bladder, local urethral anatomic pathology, suburethral diverticulum, bladder stone, bladder cancer, and painful bladder syndrome (interstitial cystitis). Additional studies may include wet preparations for vaginal infections, urethral culture, cervical culture for sexually transmitted disease, cystourethroscopy, and cystometrogram.

Treatment

The treatment for urethral pain syndrome is not specific and requires a persistent approach with frequent patient follow-up and reassessment of progress. Most patients are improved over time, with a treatment course lasting up to 2 years for resolution. Much effort is expended in explanation of the condition, its interaction with many body functions, and its gradual road to recovery given the duration of its course to this point. Although many patients have had several years of discomfort before commencing therapy, the treatment course is productive, and there is little connection of this specific focus of urethral pain with the more profound diagnosis of interstitial cystitis.

Because much of this process is trial and error, and there is considerable difference of opinion regarding efficacy, the treatment approaches are described in the order in which I would proceed in dealing with a refractory patient. Less well-defined modalities are included as areas of last resort (Table 17.1).

The first step is to explain that the nerve endings supplying sensation of pain and discomfort to the urethra and pelvic area have probably been hypersensitized by some process, and these patients have a low sensation threshold (23). The source of this inciting agent may never be determined, but the important treatment theory is to interrupt the cycle of pain or discomfort and allow the patient to return gradually to normal function. There is no question regarding the validity, severity, and physical nature of the symptoms. The treatment may take as long to reverse the process as the process itself has been present. A lot of effort is expended in how the patient can assist her own recovery by doing certain things, or avoiding certain things, during an exacerbation. The most comprehensive approach is a multidisciplinary one that includes pain medication, local treatment regimens, physical therapy, and psychological support (13). However, the patient does best in a single office setting with an understanding therapist (physician) who is able to direct management in all these areas, while being the major support figure for the patient.

TABLE 17.1. *Treatment of urethral pain syndrome*

Extensive explanation of the condition and potential etiology
Dietary changes
Fluid intake
Manage acute or subacute urethral infection
Treat documented urinary tract infection
Prophylaxis against recurrent urinary tract infections
Antispasmodic/analgesic
Antiinflammatory medication trial
Antidepressant medication
Urethral muscle relaxants
Pelvic floor muscle rehabilitation
Urethral dilation and massage
Steroid periurethral injection
Acupuncture
Overactive bladder medication
Sacral nerve neuromodulation
Urethroplasty

The importance of diet and fluid intake is difficult to determine, and most of the time is by patient experimentation. Generally, caffeine products and alcoholic beverages should be avoided. The effect of high acid or spicy foods is uncertain. A modest fluid intake is desirable, and water is best because it is devoid of additives.

Many of the inciting factors for initiating the disease process are infection related, with a subsequent poor resolution of accompanying symptoms. Patients often report quick response with antibiotic therapy the first several times they had what they thought was an infection, but gradually the treatment courses are less effective, and the episodes are more frequent. It is still important to be certain that there is no residual of acute or subacute infective source, and at least one full course of doxycycline or azithromycin should be given (Table 17.2). If this has been done previously, there is no need to repeat an adequate course of therapy unless the patient found the previous treatment effective in correcting symptoms for an extended time period. The next object of therapy is to prevent recurring urinary tract infections, particularly if these have been documented and considered causal in the disease process (18,24). If the patient was treated for infections that were not proven by microscopy or culture, the first two episodes should be managed by seeing the patient and obtaining urine for microscopy and culture. Treatment of documented infection with a standard 5-day course of trimethoprim-sulfamethoxazole, nitrofurantoin (Macrobid), or cephalosporin is adequate.

The patient will need something for days when symptoms are ganging up on her or for when she has symptoms she calls a urinary tract infection that you have excluded by microscopy or culture. The antispasmodic-analgesic preparations may be administered for a 1- to 3-day course to get over this episode and then reserved for future need. Some patients can get through the day with only one dose of the medication, but they require it each day. This is appropriate therapy for a few months while awaiting the impact of other definitive therapy. Concurrently, a course of an antiinflammatory such as celecoxib (Celebrex) or ibuprofen (Motrin) may be initiated.

The selection of the next agent carries a wide array of opinions. Amitriptyline is a tricyclic antidepressant from a generation ago that has been found to have pain-modulating effects and is extensively used in chronic pain syndromes, interstitial cystitis, and urethral pain syndrome (25). The medication must be given at the time of the evening meal

TABLE 17.2. *Pharmacologic management of urethral pain syndrome*

Antibiotics
  Subacute
    Azithromycin (Zithromax), 500 mg/d for 6 d
    Doxycycline, 100 b.i.d. for 14 d
  Chronic (suppression)
    Nitrofurantoin, 50 mg/d
    Trimethoprim/sulfamethoxazole (TMP/SMZ) (40/200), 1 tablet daily
    Cephalosporin, 250 mg/d
    Norfloxacin (Noroxin), 400 mg/d
Antispasmodic/analgesic
  Pyridium plus 1 tablet t.i.d.
  Methenamine hippurate (Urised), 1–2 tablets q.i.d.
Antiinflammatory
    Celecoxib (Celebrex), 200 mg b.i.d.
    Ibuprofen (Motrin), 800 mg t.i.d.
Antidepressants—chronic pain modulators
    Amitriptyline HCl (Elavil), 12.5–100 mg/d at 6 p.m.
    Doxepin HCl, 12.5–100 mg/d
  Nortriptyline HCl, 12.5 to 100 mg/d
  Selective serotonin reuptake inhibitors (SSRIs), usual antidepressant dose
Urethral smooth muscle relaxants
  Doxazosin mesylate (Cardura), 1–8 mg/d
  Prazosin HCl (Minipress), 1–2 mg b.i.d.
  Terazosin HCl (Hytrin), 1–5 mg once daily
  Phenoxybenzamine HCl (Dibenzyline), 10–20 mg once or twice daily
Urethral skeletal muscle relaxant
  Diazepam (Valium), 2–5 mg t.i.d.
Anticonvulsant
  Gabapentin (Neurontin), 300 to 1,200 mg t.i.d.
Frequency-urgency symptoms (overactive bladder)
  Oxybutynin chloride (Ditropan XL), 5–30 mg/d
  Tolterodine tartrate (Detrol LA), 4 mg/d

or earlier to avoid the severe drowsiness that ordinarily hits the next morning. It should be commenced in a very low dose of 10 to 12.5 mg, and increased in 2- to 6-week intervals to ensure lack of serious side effects. Efficacy cannot usually be determined for at least 6 to 8 weeks. Patients still get dry mouth and may have some alteration or slowing of bowel function. After 3 months of therapy, the side effects become much less pronounced, although a prolonged low-dosage level may be required before increasing the dose to determine efficacy. The course duration is 1 to 3 years. Some patients sensitive to amitriptyline are able to tolerate doxepin, and some therapists prefer the latter agent. The selective serotonin reuptake inhibitors have been suggested and used, but the effect may be more for the antidepressant properties and perhaps even the mood-ele-vating properties associated with some of these preparations (Table 17.2).

The combination of urethral skeletal and smooth muscle relaxants has been used for a long time, and many physicians find this effective as an initial approach (26). The dose of diazepam should be kept low and the course of therapy not prolonged beyond 1 year because of risk for dependency. The choice of smooth muscle relaxant has some options, and although phenoxybenzamine was originally used, the safer products now are doxazosin mesylate (Cardura) (27), prazosin, and terazosin HCl (Hytrin) (Table 17.2).

As part of a multidisciplinary approach, pelvic floor muscle exercises and bladder-retraining drills with or without biofeedback may provide a form of bladder physiotherapy to which some patients respond. The bladder retraining is especially helpful in patients with urinary frequency. The pelvic floor exercises are useful for coordinating pelvic floor muscles, but the relaxation component of the exercise program may help with relieving overactive pelvic muscles. The extension of this program is in the area of myofascial trigger points, which can be manually released for symptom relief (16).

The use of urethral dilation and massage is declining as older physicians stop practice. The once common initial treatment is mostly used now in patients who have had and request continuing dilation therapy and in occasional refractory patients (5,28). Often used in association with dilation was the periurethral injection of long-acting local anesthetic agents and a steroid. This procedure is also no longer commonly used (29). Another procedure performed infrequently is urethroplasty (30). Acupuncture use may be considered before invasive therapy (31,32).

Sacral neuromodulation in the treatment of overactive bladder symptoms and some pelvic pain conditions has been established. The frequency-urgency symptoms of interstitial cystitis have also responded to this intervention. It makes sense that the urethral pain syndrome and its myriad of symptoms may also be treated by this modality (33–35). There is a paucity of information on neuromodulation for urethral pain syndrome, but the expanded use of this modality and its modifications should provide continuing additions to the literature over the next few years.

ATROPHIC URETHRITIS

The urethra is an estrogen-sensitive organ (36,37). Atrophic changes result from lack of estrogen, which normally occurs in varying degrees of severity after spontaneous or surgical menopause in the absence of hormone replacement therapy. Sometimes, oral replacement is not sufficient to prevent local vaginal or urethral changes.

Evaluation

Presenting symptoms include dyspareunia, vaginal discharge, urgency, frequency, dysuria, recurrent urinary tract infections, and urinary stress incontinence. Diagnosis is by clinical examination of the vagina and pelvic organs. Saline wet preparations may be prepared from a gentle scrape of the lateral vaginal wall and the slide observed for mature versus immature epithelial cells. Vaginal pH may be increased from a normal of 4 to between 6 and 7. Blood values of follicle-stimulating hormone and estradiol may not reflect local estrogen effects. Urethroscopy may reveal a pale urethra or one that is easily irritated by movement of the scope through it.

Treatment

Urogenital tissues are more sensitive to estrogen than other tissues, and absorption of low-dose topical applications is highest when the vaginal epithelium is atrophic and decreases as the epithelium matures (38), but not to zero. Oral preparations are used according to appropriate indications and contraindications. Atrophic changes respond to topical therapy (39–41), such as one fourth to one third of an applicator of vaginal cream two to three times per week (Table 17.3). The medication should be continued indefinitely

TABLE 17.3. *Vaginal estrogen preparations*

Estradiol (Estrace), 0.1 mg/g 42.5-g tube	1–2 g one to three times per week
Premarin, 0.625 mg/g 42-g tube	1–2 g one to three times per week
Estropipate (Ogen), 1.5 mg/g 42-g tube	1–2 g one to three times per week
Estradiol vaginal tablets (Vagifem), 25 μg	1–2 tablets weekly
Estradiol vaginal ring (Estring), 2 mg	1 ring every 3 months

at a maintenance dose. The usual precautions are to be followed for initiating therapy, with risk and benefit determined in those patients with relative contraindications (42). Abnormal vaginal bleeding should be evaluated appropriately. An alternative to vaginal cream preparations is an estradiol-releasing vaginal ring (43).

ACUTE URETHRITIS

This condition is more common in young patients and generally implies one of the sexually transmitted disease entities. The onset of symptoms is recent, and the duration of the problem is generally less than 1 month before consultation. The incubation period for gonorrhea is as short as 1 day and usually within 2 weeks, whereas the incubation period for chlamydia is 1 to 2 weeks, and may be up to 5 weeks. Occasionally a low-grade infection may persist, and symptoms may suggest the urethral pain syndrome. The infection may also persist in an asymptomatic state.

Evaluation

Symptoms are usually dysuria, urgency, and frequency. Urethral discharge is uncommon in female patients. The differential diagnosis must include urinary tract infection, vulvovaginal inflammation, primary and recurrent herpes simplex virus inflammation, and local trauma. Vaginal examination is performed. Wet preparations are made for trichomonal infections, yeast, and clue cells. Primary herpetiform lesions are cultured. Specimens are taken for chlamydia and gonorrhea isolation. Urine microscopy or culture is performed to rule out urinary tract infection. Patients diagnosed with a sexually transmitted disease should have serologic testing for syphilis. Cystourethroscopy is indicated for treatment failures and persisting symptoms (see Fig. 12.6 in Chapter 12).

Treatment

Gonorrhea is managed according to Centers for Disease Control and Prevention recommendations, which can be a single dose of cephalosporin or fluoroquinolone followed by 7 days of doxycycline to cover chlamydia, or a single dose of azithromycin, 1 g given orally. The usual recommendation for nongonococcal urethritis is treatment for 7 days with tetracycline, 500 mg given four times a day, or doxycycline, 100 mg twice daily. Alternative therapies include azithromycin, 1 g as a single dose; erythromycin, 500 mg four times daily for 7 days or 250 mg four times daily for 14 days; and ofloxacin, 300 mg twice daily for 7 days (44). More recent information suggests that a 6-day course of azithromycin, 500 mg once daily, or a 14-day course of doxycycline, 100 mg twice daily, is more effective (45).

MEATAL ABNORMALITIES

The urethral lesions that are often disturbing to the patient include caruncle, prolapse, and polyps.

A caruncle is an inflammatory lesion on the posterior aspect of the urethral meatus. It is red in color and measures 5 to 10 mm in size. Symptoms may not be present or may include pain and bleeding. Treatment includes topical estrogen therapy and occasionally local removal using cryosurgery, laser, or excision. A pillar block is useful analgesia for doing the procedure in the office or clinic setting (46) (Fig. 17.1).

Urethral prolapse is a circumferential red mucosal eversion extending outside the urethral meatus. It is seldom painful but may bleed, especially in children. Treatment is by topical estrogen application for a 2- to 3-month course. It is seldom necessary to perform surgical removal, but the techniques described previously can be used.

Urethral polyps are virtually always benign, but occasionally they protrude from inside the urethra canal and present as a lump or with bleeding. Urethroscopy is used to deter-

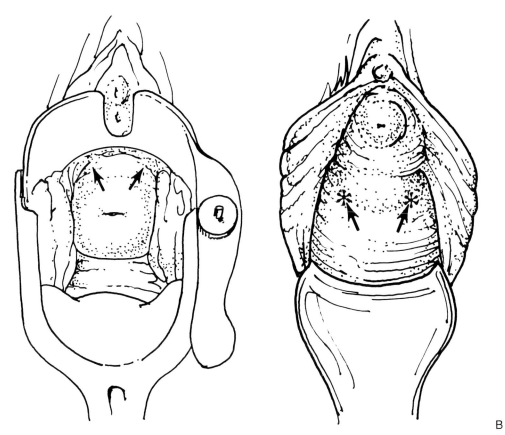

FIG. 17.1. Bladder pillar block. **A:** With speculum in place, bladder pillars are at the 2- and 10-o'clock positions (*arrows*), at the attachment to the cervix. **B:** If there is no cervix, the urethrovesical junction is visualized and the injections are placed at 5- and 7-o'clock (*arrows*). (From Ostergard DR. Bladder pillar block anesthesia for urethral dilatation in women. *Am J Obstet Gynecol* 1980;136:187–188, with permission.)

mine the extent of the abnormality. Treatment is seldom required, but usually an endoscopic maneuver is required to sever the polyp at the base.

URETHRAL DIVERTICULUM

A diverticulum is a branch or sac pouching out from a hollow organ. A urethral diverticulum is generally located posteriorly anywhere along the urethra, and there may be more than one. The etiology is thought to be obstruction of the duct from a paraurethral gland, although congenital defects have been postulated.

Evaluation

Some diverticula are asymptomatic, but common symptoms (47) include recurrent urinary tract infections, suburethral cyst, painful intercourse, and urinary incontinence (Table 17.4). The size of the diverticular ostia may determine symptoms in that large-necked diverticula are more apt to be associated with incontinence, and small-necked diverticula are more frequently associated with pain or recurrent infections. During vaginal examination, a cyst may be seen under the urethra, and pus may be able to be expressed by compression and movement of the examining finger distally along the

TABLE 17.4. *Clinical symptoms of urethral diverticula*

Asymptomatic recurrent urinary tract infection
Vaginal mass
Dyspareunia
Incontinence
Postmicturition dribbling
Dysuria
Hematuria
Frequency, urgency
Pain
Urinary retention

urethra. A sound or a catheter placed in the urethra may facilitate this examination. Urine is obtained for examination and culture. Frequently, the clinical examination is benign.

Urethroscopy may show one or more posterior openings along the urethra that on compression are associated with extrusion of pus material (Fig. 17.2). The openings can be difficult to differentiate from urethral fistulas (see Fig. 12.8 in Chapter 12), except that urine escapes through these latter openings.

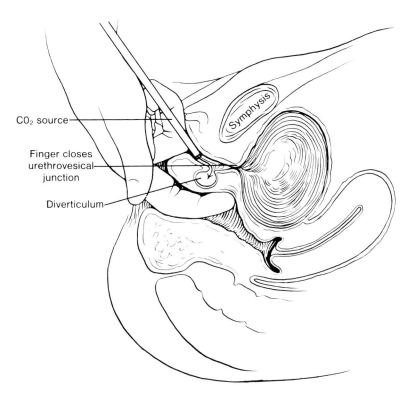

FIG. 17.2. Urethroscopy with occlusion of bladder neck. The bladder is distended with fluid, and the urethrovesical junction is occluded with the examining finger. The fluid is allowed to run briskly, and as the urethroscope is slowly withdrawn, the diverticular opening distends and is visible.

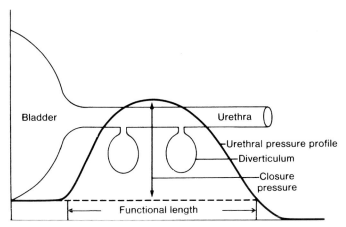

FIG. 17.3. Urethral closure pressure profile with superimposed diverticular orifices proximal and distal to peak urethral closure pressure.

Urodynamics should be performed to determine concurrent presence of genuine stress incontinence and the quality of the urethral sphincter mechanism. The urethral closure pressure can have a biphasic profile, and the position of the pressure drop reflects the location of the diverticulum related to high urethral pressure zone (Fig. 17.3). This has been important in determining the type of surgical repair because a distal diverticulum could be treated by a marsupialization procedure; however, the pressure depression in the profile may not accurately indicate the position of the diverticulum opening into the urethra (48).

Transvaginal or endoluminal ultrasonography may accurately predict multiple diverticula (49,50). Positive-pressure urethrography with a Davis or Tratner catheter has been a longstanding technique for identifying urethral diverticula (Figs. 17.4 through 17.6). A voiding cystourethrogram may also be performed for diagnosis. Recently, magnetic resonance imaging has been used (51). The accuracy of the various

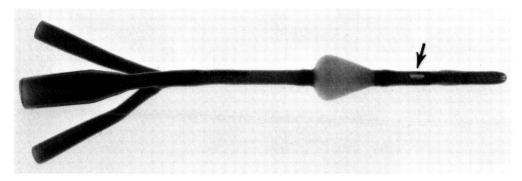

FIG. 17.4. The Tratner catheter. The triple-lumen catheter has a distal balloon that is filled with air to keep it in the bladder by resting against the bladder neck. The proximal balloon is inflated with air and then slides along the catheter to fit snugly against the urethra to prevent escape of dye from the urethral meatus. The third lumen is injected with contrast material, which egresses through an opening between the two air-filled balloons and distends the urethra and urethral diverticulum.

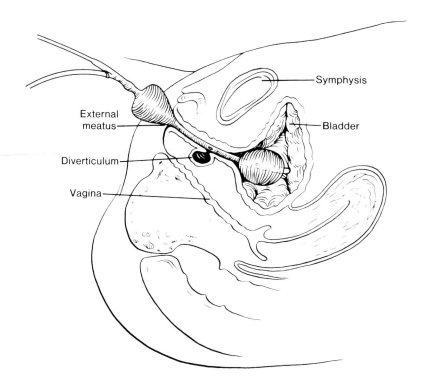

FIG. 17.5. The Tratner catheter in place in the urethra.

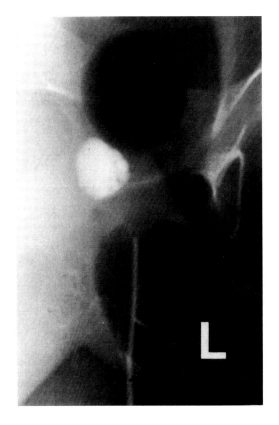

FIG. 17.6. Radiologic view of urethral diverticulum. The diverticulum is filled with contrast material, which shows nicely between the two air-filled balloons.

TABLE 17.5. *Efficacy of diagnostic modalities in diagnosing urethral diverticula*

Technique	Accuracy (%)
Radiologic	
Voiding cystourethrography	65–77
Positive-pressure urethrography	90
Ultasound	
Transvaginal	90
Intraluminal	100
Urodynamics	
Urethral pressure profile	72
Endoscopy	
Urethroscopy	90

From Cundiff DW. Urethral diverticula. In: Cundiff GW, Bent AE, eds. *Endoscopic diagnosis of the female lower urinary tract.* London: WB Saunders, 1999: 43–51, with permission.

methods of diagnosis is summarized in Table 17.5 (47,52).

Treatment

The Spence procedure is used for diverticula when the sac is located distally below the midurethral pressure peak. The diverticulum is marsupialized and the defect closed with 4-0 polyglycolic acid suture (Fig. 17.7).

A midurethral diverticulum or one located more proximally requires excision (51–53). The principles are to dissect carefully, creating several layers to be closed later over the repair. A Martius graft may be beneficial to prevent wound breakdown and fistula. Intraoperative urethroscopy is helpful in localizing the diverticulum, and sometimes, a Fogarty catheter can be placed transurethrally into the diverticular opening and inflated, if there is not a palpable cyst structure. An inverted U incision is used over the diverticulum and the vaginal epithelium is reflected inferiorly. A vertical incision is next made in the pubocervical fascia, which is gradually dissected to reveal the cyst. It is often possible to create one vertical and one horizontal fascial plane before entering the cyst structure. The cyst structure is opened and a Foley catheter placed into the bladder to help determine the

nature and size of the connection of the diverticulum to the urethra. Sometimes, a pediatric Foley catheter can also be placed externally into the diverticular sac to make complete dissection easier. The diverticulum is excised sharply while leaving the floor of the urethra as undamaged as possible. The urethral defect is closed transversely over the urethral Foley catheter with 4-0 polyglycolic acid suture (Fig. 17.8). The fascial tissue flaps are closed in one or two layers over the repaired defect in the urethra. The vaginal epithelium is then closed. Alternatively, to obtain an extra layer for closure, the excess portion of vaginal epithelium can be used to obtain another fascial layer by stripping off the epithelial covering, either in a transverse or longitudinal incision. If an inverted U incision was made, the fascia can be folded under the remaining epithelium. If a vertical incision was made in the vaginal epithelium, the fascia from one flap can be sutured over the urethra and the full-thickness flap pulled over the top of it (Fig. 17.9). The catheter is left in place for 1 week and removed in an office setting to be sure the patient is able to void.

The partial ablation technique (54) is commenced in similar fashion to the previous description. The diverticular sac is opened longitudinally, and excess sac tissue is excised. The sac is then sutured side-to-side to cover the urethral defect using fine suture. A second imbricating layer is placed. The remaining diverticular wall is closed in double-breasted fashion. The vaginal mucosa is closed, and usually a gentle pack is placed overnight to prevent hematoma under the incisions (Fig. 17.10).

If stress incontinence has been identified preoperatively or if the diverticulum is very large or is located near the bladder neck, a concomitant suburethral fascial sling should be performed to prevent stress incontinence (55).

Complications include urethral stricture and urethrovaginal fistula. Antibiotic therapy is recommended intraoperatively and during initial healing while the catheter is in place.

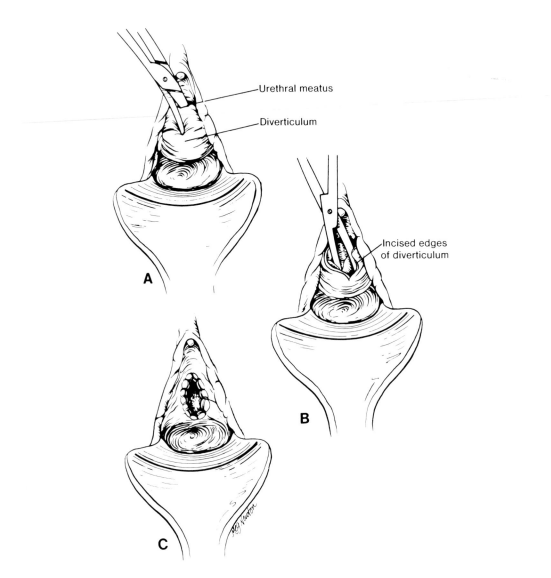

FIG. 17.7. Spence procedure. The scissors are placed into the diverticulum (**A**) and incise full-thickness through to vagina (**B**). **C:** A running locked suture secures the edges to prevent bleeding.

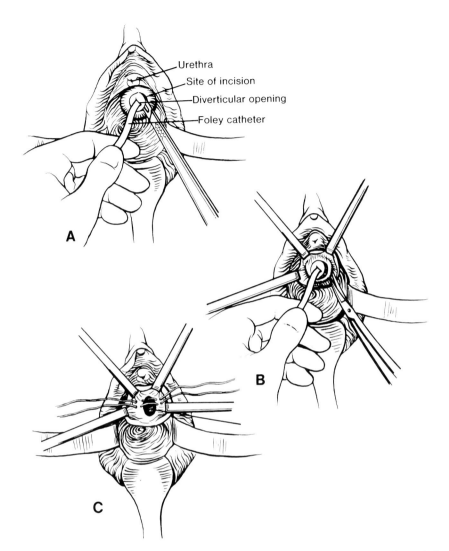

FIG. 17.8. Excision of urethral diverticulum. **A:** The vaginal incision has been made and dissection of fascia completed to expose the diverticulum sac, which has been opened and a pediatric Foley catheter placed for traction. **B:** The diverticular sac is sharply dissected free from surrounding attachments and the urethra mucosa. **C:** Closure of the urethral defect is started, generally a transverse closure, to prevent urethral stricture. (From Glenn JF. *Urologic surgery.* Hagerstown, MD: Harper & Row, 1975, with permission.)

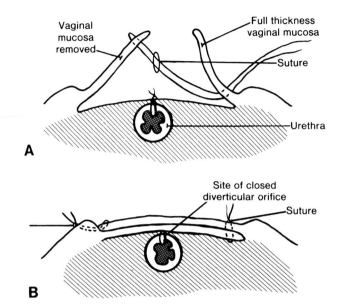

FIG. 17.9. Vaginal flap technique for closure over urethral defect. **A:** One vaginal flap is denuded of epithelium and sutured underneath the full thickness flap. **B:** The full-thickness flap then is sutured over top of the first flap. (From Judd GE, Marshall JR. *Repair of urethral diverticulum or vesicovaginal fistula by vaginal flap technique.* Obstet Gynecol 1976;47:627–629, with permission.)

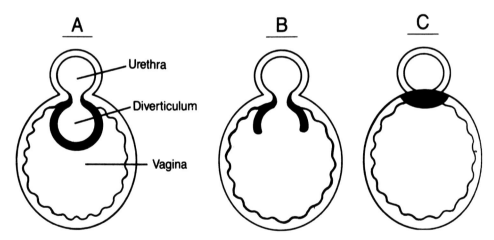

FIG. 17.10. Partial ablation of diverticulum. **A:** The technique is especially useful when there is considerable inflammation in the tissues. The diverticulum is exposed and isolated from surrounding structures. **B:** The sac is opened and excess amount of tissue removed. **C:** The urethral defect is closed by suturing the opening in the sac side to side. The diverticular wall is closed, and vaginal mucosa closed. (From Sanz L. *Gynecologic surgery.* Oradell, NJ: Medical Economics Company, Inc. Copyright 1988. All rights reserved.)

Patient stay is generally limited to 1 day unless sling surgery or other procedures are performed. Catheter drainage is for 1 week. Successful outcome is the rule.

REFERENCES

1. Gallagher DJ, Montgomery JZ, North JD. Acute infections of the urinary tract and the urethral syndrome in general practice. *BMJ* 1965;543:622–626.
2. Abrams P, Cardozo L, Fall M, et al. The standardisation of terminology of lower urinary tract function: report from the standardisation sub-committee of the International Continence Society. *Neurourol Urodyn* 2002;21:167–178.
3. Tait J, Peddie BA, Bailey RR, et al. Urethral syndrome (abacterial cystitis): search for a pathogen. *Br J Urol* 1985;57:522–526.
4. Gurel H, Gurel SA, Atilla MK. Urethral syndrome and associated risk factors related to obstetrics and gynecology. *Eur J Obstet Gynecol Reprod Biol* 1999;83:5–7.
5. Blomquist JL. Personal communication, 2001.
6. Cox CE. The urethra and its relationship to urinary tract infection: the flora of the normal female urethra. *South Med J* 1966;59:621–626.
7. Mutlu B, Mutlu N, Yucesoy G. The incidence of Chlamydia trachomatis in women with urethral syndrome. *Int J Clin Pract* 2001;55:525–526.
8. Vitoratos N, Gregoriou O, Papadias C, et al. Sexually transmitted diseases in women with urethral syndrome. *Int J Gynaecol Obstet* 1988;27:177–180.
9. Parsons CL, Zupkas P, Parsons JK. Intravesical potassium sensitivity in patients with interstitial cystitis and urethral syndrome. *Urology* 2001;57:432–433.
10. Bologna RA, Tu LM, Whitmore KE. Hypersensitivity disorders of the lower urinary tract. In: Walters MD, Karram MM, eds. *Urogynecology and reconstructive surgery*. St. Louis: Mosby, 1999:320–321.
11. Baldoni F, Ercolani M, Baldaro B, et al. Stressful events and psychological symptoms in patients with functional urinary disorders. *Percept Mot Skills* 1995;80:605–606.
12. McCauley AJ, Stern RS, Nomes DM, et al. Micturition and the mind: psychological factors in the etiology and treatment of urinary symptoms in women. *BMJ* 1987;294:540–543.
13. Wesselmann U, Burnett A, Heinberg LJ. The urogenital and rectal pain syndromes. *Pain* 1997;73:269–294.
14. Price WE. The urethral syndrome: myth or reality? A commentary. *Minn Med* 1990;73:33–34.
15. Summit RL. Urogynecologic causes of chronic pelvic pain. *Obstet Gynecol Clin North Am* 1993;20:685–698.
16. Weiss JM. Pelvic floor myofascial trigger points: manual therapy for interstitial cystitis and the frequency-urgency syndrome. *J Urol* 2001;166:2226–2231.
17. Bernstein AM, Phillips HC, Linden W, et al. A psychophysiological evaluation of female urethral syndrome: evidence for a muscular abnormality. *J Behav Med* 1992;15:299–312.
18. Hamilton-Miller JM. The urethral syndrome and its management. *J Antimicrob Chemother* 1994;33[Suppl A]:63–73.
19. Paira SO. Fibromyalgia associated with female urethral syndrome. *Clin Rheumatol* 1994;13:88–89.
20. Barbalia G, Meares E. Female urethral syndrome: clinical and urodynamic perspectives. *Urology* 1984;23:208–212.
21. Lyon RT, Smith DR. Distal urethral stenosis. *J Urol* 1963;8:414–421.
22. Urinary Incontinence Guideline Panel. *Urinary incontinence in adults: clinical practice guideline update*. AHCPR Pub. No. 96-0686. Rockville, MD. Agency for Health Care Policy and Research, Public Health Service, U.S. Department of Health and Human Services, March 1996.
23. Kellner R. Psychosomatic syndromes, somatization and somatoform disorders. *Psychother Psychosom* 1994;61:4–24.
24. Parziani S, Costantini E, Petroni PA, et al. Urethral syndrome: clinical results with antibiotics alone or combined with estrogen. *Eur Urol* 1994;26:115–119.
25. Pranikoff K, Constantino G. The use of amitriptyline in patients with urinary frequency and pain. *Urology* 1998;51[Suppl 5A]:179–181.
26. Raz S, Smith RB. External sphincter spasticity syndrome in female patients. *J Urol* 1976;115:443–446.
27. Serels S, Stein M. Prospective study comparing hyoscyamine, doxazosin, and combination therapy for the treatment of urgency and frequency in women. *Neurourol Urodyn* 1998;17:31–36.
28. Lemack GE, Foster B, Zimmern PE. Urethral dilation in women: a questionnaire-based analysis of practice patterns. *Urology* 1999;54:37–43.
29. Altman BL. Treatment of urethral syndrome with triamcinolone acetonide. *J Urol* 1976;116:583–584.
30. Richardson FH. External urethroplasty in women: technique and clinical evaluation. *J Urol* 1969;101:719–721.
31. Zheng H, Wang S, Shang J, et al. Study on acupuncture and moxibustion therapy for female urethral syndrome. *J Tradit Chin Med* 1998;18:122–127.
32. Chang PL, Wu CJ, Huang MH. Long-term outcome of acupuncture in women with frequency, urgency, and dysuria. *Am J Chin Med* 1993;21:231–236.
33. Hassouna MM. Sacral neuromodulation in the treatment of urgency-frequency symptoms: a multicenter study on efficacy and safety. *J Urol* 2000;163:1849–1854.
34. VanBalken MR, Vanoninck V, Gisolf K, et al. Posterior tibial nerve stimulation as neuromodulative treatment of lower urinary tract dysfunction. *J Urol* 2001;166:914–918.
35. Hasan ST, Neal DE. Neuromodulation in bladder dysfunction. *Curr Opin Obstet Gynecol* 1998;10:395–399.
36. Youngblood VH, Tomlin EM, Williams JO, et al. Exfoliative cytology of the senile female urethra. *J Urol* 1958;79:110–113.
37. Ingleman-Sundberg A, Rosen J, Gustafsson SA, et al. Cytosol estrogen receptors in the urogenital tissues in stress-incontinent women. *Acta Obstet Gynaecol Scand* 1981;60:585–586.
38. Samsioe G. Urogenital aging: a hidden problem. *Am J Obstet Gynecol* 1998;178:S245–249.
39. Manonai J, Theppisai U, Suthutvoravut S, et al. The effect of estradiol vaginal tablet and conjugated estrogen cream on urogenital symptoms in postmenopausal women: a comparative study. *J Obstet Gynaecol Res* 2001;27:255–260.

40. Bernier F, Jenkins P. The role of vaginal estrogen in the treatment of urogenital dysfunction in postmenopausal women. *Urol Nurs* 1997;17:92–95.

41. Stenberg A, Heimer G, Ulmsten U. The prevalence of urogenital symptoms in postmenopausal women. *Maturitas* 1995;22[Suppl]:S17–S20.

42. Pritchard KI. The role of hormone replacement therapy in women with a previous diagnosis of breast cancer and a review of possible alternatives. *Ann Oncol* 2001; 12:301–310.

43. Henriksson L, Stjernquist M, Boquist L, et al. A one-year multicenter study of efficacy and safety of a continuous, low-dose, estradiol-releasing vaginal ring (Estring) in postmenopausal women with symptoms and signs of urogenital aging. *Am J Obstet Gynecol* 1996; 174:85–92.

44. McCormack WM, Rein MF. Urethritis. In: Mandell GL, Bennett JE, Dolin R, eds. *Mandell, Douglas, and Bennett's principles and practice of infectious diseases,* 5th ed. Philadelphia: Churchill Livingstone, 2000:1208–1218.

45. Skerk V, Schonwald S, Strapac Z, et al. Duration of clinical symptoms in female patients with acute urethral syndrome caused by Chlamydia trachomatis treated with azithromycin or doxycycline. *Chemotherapy* 2001; 13:176–181.

46. Ostergard DR. Bladder pillar block anesthesia for urethral dilatation in women. *Am J Obstet Gynecol* 1980; 136:187–188.

47. Cundiff GW. Urethral diverticula. In: Cundiff GW, Bent AE, eds. *Endoscopic diagnosis of the female lower urinary tract.* London: WB Saunders, 1999:43–51.

48. Summitt RL, Stovall TG. Urethral diverticula: evaluation by urethral pressure profilometry, cystourethroscopy, and voiding cystourethrogram. *Obstet Gynecol* 1992;80: 695–699.

49. Lee TG, Keller FS. Urethral diverticulum: diagnosis by ultrasound. *AJR Am J Roentgenol* 1977;128:690–694.

50. Chancellor MB, Liu JB, Rivas DA, et al. Intraoperative endoluminal ultrasound evaluation of urethral diverticula. *J Urol* 1995;153:72–75.

51. Nezu FM, Vasavada SP. Evaluation and management of female urethral diverticulum. *Tech Urol* 2001;7:169–175.

52. Jacoby K, Rowbotham RK. Double balloon positive pressure urethrography is a more sensitive test than voiding cystourethrography for diagnosing urethral diverticulum in women. *J Urol* 1999;162:2066–2069.

53. Fortunato P, Schettini M, Gallucci M. Diagnosis and therapy of the female urethral diverticula. *Int Urogynecol J Pelvic Floor Dysfunct* 2001;12:51–57.

54. Tancer ML, Mooppan MM, Pierre-Louis C, et al. Suburethral diverticulum: treatment by partial ablation. *Obstet Gynecol* 1983;62:511–513.

55. Romanzi LJ, Groutz A, Blaivas JG. Urethral diverticulum in women: diverse presentations resulting in diagnostic delay and mismanagement. *J Urol* 2000;164:428–433.

56. Faerber G. Urethral diverticulectomy and pubovaginal sling for simultaneous treatment of urethral diverticulum and intrinsic sphincter deficiency. *Tech Urol* 1998; 4:192–197.

*Ostergard's Urogynecology and Pelvic Floor
Dysfunction, Fifth Edition.* edited by A.E. Bent, et al.
Lippincott Williams & Wilkins, Philadelphia © 2003.

18

Lower Urinary Tract Infection

Mickey M. Karram* and Steven D. Kleeman**

** Department of Obstetrics and Gynecology, University of Cincinnati; and Department of Obstetrics
and Gynecology, Good Samaritan Hospital, Cincinnati, Ohio
** Department of Obstetrics and Gynecology, Wright State University, Miami Valley Hospital, Dayton,
Ohio; and Department of Obstetrics and Gynecology, Good Samaritan Hospital, Cincinnati, Ohio*

Urinary tract infections in women produce significant health problems. They are among the most common infections dealt with by primary care physicians. Although rarely followed by severe sequelae, they sometimes lead to acute pyelonephritis and bacteremia and become a major cause of morbidity and time lost from work. The health care expenditures necessitated by the diagnosis, antimicrobial treatment, and subsequent management of women with urinary tract infections has been estimated to exceed $1 billion annually (1).

The proper management of these patients, although often simple, has recently been challenged by several occurrences: (a) the introduction of new antimicrobial agents, (b) the advent of single-dose therapy, (c) the recognition of additional lower urinary tract pathogens such as *Staphylococcus saprophyticus* and *Chlamydia trachomatis*, (d) the realization that many women with symptomatic cystitis may have less than 10^5 organisms/mL in urine cultures; and (e) the understanding that certain patients with infection-like symptoms will be termed urethral syndrome, painful bladder, or even interstitial cystitis because they have no apparent cause for their symptoms.

PREVALENCE

About 5 million cases of acute cystitis occur annually in the United States, resulting in an estimated 6 million office visits (2). Urinary tract infections are much more prevalent among women than men (ratio of 8:1). This is probably secondary to an anatomically short urethra in proximity to a large bacterial reservoir within the introital tract and along the vaginal vestibule (3).

The incidence of urinary tract infections rises with age. At 1 year of age, there is an approximate 1% to 2% incidence of bacteriuria in females; pathology directly correlates with these infections. As many as 50% of patients show abnormalities on intravenous pyelogram (IVP) that is scarring and either ipsilateral reflux or some obstructive disease (4,5). After 1 year of age, the infection rate decreases to about 1% and continues to decrease until puberty. The incidence of urologic pathology associated with these infections also continues to decrease progressively. With the introduction of sexual activity and pregnancy, the incidence starts to rise and continues to increase progressively with age. Between the ages of 15 and 24 years, the prevalence of bacteriuria is about 2% to 3% and increases to about 10% at the age of 60 years, 20% after the age of 65 years, and 25% to 50% after the age of 80 years (6) (Fig. 18.1).

About 2% of all patients admitted to a hospital acquire a urinary tract infection during their stay, which accounts for 500,000 hospital-acquired urinary tract infections per year. One percent (5,000) of these infections become life-threatening. Instrumentation or catheterization

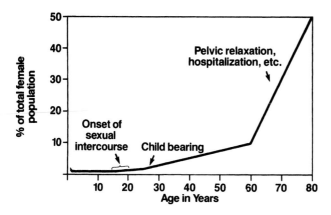

FIG. 18.1. Prevalence of bacteriuria in females as a function of age.

of the urinary tract is a precipitating factor in at least 80% of these nosocomial infections (7,8).

DEFINITIONS

Before discussing urinary tract infection, an understanding of generally accepted definitions is essential because the commonly used terminology can, at times, be confusing.

Cystitis indicates inflammation of the bladder whether used as a histologic, bacteriologic, cystoscopic, or clinical description. Most commonly, it produces symptoms of urinary frequency and dysuria. Bacterial cystitis needs to be differentiated from nonbacterial cystitis (i.e., radiation, interstitial, and so on).

Urethritis refers to inflammation of the urethra and usually requires an adjective for modification (i.e., chlamydial, nonspecific, and so on). In female patients, symptoms of urethritis are impossible to distinguish from those of cystitis.

Trigonitis is inflammation or localized hyperemia of the trigone. This term is commonly used to describe the normal cobblestone or granular appearance of the trigone and floor of the vesical neck. The failure to recognize that this epithelium is part of the normal embryologic development, and the lack of experience in cystoscopic examinations of normal women without bladder symptoms, are probably responsible for the terms trigonitis and granular urethral trigonitis.

Bacteriuria implies the presence of bacteria in the bladder urine and not contaminants that have been added to sterile bladder urine. The term includes both renal and bladder bacteria. Symptomatic bacteriuria can have as few as 10^2 colony-forming units per milliliter (cfu/mL), whereas asymptomatic bacteriuria requires the growth of 10^5 cfu/mL or more.

Urethral syndrome is a poorly defined syndrome of frequency, urgency, dysuria, suprapubic discomfort, and voiding difficulties in the absence of any organic pathology. This term needs clarification, and it should not be used to describe urine with bacteria counts of less than 10^5 organisms/mL or chlamydial infection of the urethra or a hypoestrogenic urethra. When we use the term urethral syndrome, we have ruled out detrusor and urethral dysfunction as well as any lower urinary tract infection. Thus, it is basically a "wastebasket" diagnosis of lower urinary tract symptoms without any discernable pathology (9,10).

PATHOGENESIS

The pathogenesis of urinary tract infection in female patients has been postulated to involve three primary mechanisms: hematogenous, lymphatic spread, or ascending extension of organisms directly from the rectum (Fig. 18.2). Retrograde (ascending) infection is the most widely accepted mechanism and appears to be important in the management of infections. Hematogenous dissemination is the principal route by which staphylococcal organisms seed the kidney. This leads to pyelonephritis and may be an important route

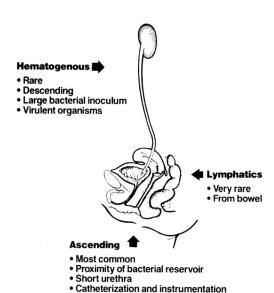

Hematogenous ▶
- Rare
- Descending
- Large bacterial inoculum
- Virulent organisms

◀ **Lymphatics**
- Very rare
- From bowel

Ascending ▲
- Most common
- Proximity of bacterial reservoir
- Short urethra
- Catheterization and instrumentation

FIG. 18.2. Pathways of bacterial entry into the urinary tract.

for *Escherichia coli* in patients who do not have vesicoureteral reflux.

The normal female urinary tract is remarkably resistant to infection. Although certain risk factors for developing urinary tract infections have been identified (Table 18.1), it remains unclear why certain women are more

TABLE 18.1. *Known risk factors for urinary tract infection*

Advanced age
Inefficient bladder emptying
Pelvic relaxation
Large cystocele with high residuals
Uterovaginal prolapse resulting in obstructive voiding
Neurogenic bladder, i.e., diabetes, multiple sclerosis, spinal cord injury, etc.
Drugs with anticholinergic effects
Decreased functional ability
Dementia
Cardiovascular accidents
Fecal incontinence
Neurologic deficits
Nosocomial infections
Indwelling catheters
Hospitalized patients
Physiologic changes
Decreased vaginal glycogen and increased vaginal pH in women

prone to infection. Susceptibility probably also depends on the inoculum size, the virulence properties of the invading microorganism, and, most importantly, the status of the defense mechanisms of the host. These host mechanisms are found in the urine, the vagina, and throughout the female urinary tract.

The Enterobacteriaceae are responsible for about 80% of bacteriuria in urinary tract infections. *E. coli* accounts for about 80% of the community-acquired infections; other organisms are responsible for a disproportionate number of infections, considering their frequency in stool flora. *Klebsiella* species cause about 5% of infections, whereas *Enterobacter* and *Proteus* species each cause about 2% of infections outside the hospital (11). *Serratia marcescens* and *Pseudomonas aeruginosa* are almost always hospital acquired and are due to omission of infection control practices, usually after urethral catheterization or manipulation. Although anaerobes are present in abundance in the feces of normal individuals, they are rarely the cause of urinary tract infection. The oxygen tension in the urine probably prevents their growth and persistence within the urinary tract. *S. saprophyticus* is the second most common pathogen isolated from young women with acute cystitis and accounts for about 10% of these cases (9,10, 12–16). *Staphylococcus epidermidis* is a frequent cause of nosocomial urinary tract infection in catheterized patients and is frequently resistant to antibacterial agents (17). Other gram-positive organisms, including the group B and group D streptococci, cause 1% to 2% of urinary tract infections.

HOST DEFENSE MECHANISMS

Urine

Urine has certain defense mechanisms against infection. The most important inhibitory factors include a very high or low osmolality, a high urea concentration, a high organic acid concentration, and a low pH. A very dilute urine, as well as urine with a high osmolality, especially when associated with a low pH, inhibits bacterial growth by inhibiting phagocytosis and decreasing the reactivity of complement. In general, anaerobic bacteria and other fastidious organisms that make up most of the urethral flora do not multiply in urine. However, urine usually supports growth of nonfastidious bacteria (18,19).

Vaginal, Periurethral, and Perineal Colonization

There is accumulating evidence that the antibacterial defense mechanisms of the vaginal walls and periurethral area are important in preventing the progression of microorganisms from the rectum to the bladder. Normally, this area is colonized by gram-positive bacteria, lactobacillus, and diphtheroids (organisms that grow very poorly in urine and do not cause urinary tract infections). A number of studies have shown that females with recurrent cystitis first colonize their vaginal introitus and periurethral area with enterobacteria before the onset of the symptoms of cystitis and then are at risk for infection until this colonization reverses to a normal situation (3, 18,20). Acidity of vaginal secretions may contribute to vaginal resistance to coliform bacteria. In premenopausal females, the vaginal pH is usually near 4.0. This low acidic pH prohibits the growth of organisms such as *E. coli* but promotes the growth of the normally present organisms (e.g., lactobacillus) that will interfere with the growth of uropathogens (21,22). High vaginal pH appears to be associated with the growth of enterobacteria (23).

Normal Periodic Voiding

Periodic voiding is one of the most important known bladder defense mechanisms. One study noted the introduction of 10 million bacteria into normal male bladders failed to establish infection because the organisms were rapidly cleared by voiding, diluting with fresh urine, and voiding again (24). Another study noted that postmenopausal patients with recurrent urinary tract infections had significantly fewer urinary tract infections while

maintaining low urine osmolality (25). Voiding displaces infected urine with sterile urine and flushes out bacteria attached to desquamated uroepithelial cells.

Prevention of Bacterial Adherence

The ability of an organism to bind to the epithelial cell has been shown to correlate with its ability to infect the urinary tract. The ascending loop of Henle secretes Tamm-Horsfall protein, which is a uromucoid, rich in mannose. This protein may inhibit bacterial adherence and trap bacteria in the urine, allowing them to be flushed from the urinary tract (26). Also, the presence of urinary immunoglobulin and the lining of the bladder with a glycosaminoglycan may be important factors in the blocking of bacterial adherence. The reduction of glycosaminoglycan probably plays a role in recurrent cystitis (27,28).

HOST SUSCEPTIBILITY FACTORS

Bacterial Adherence

Adherence of microorganisms to mucosal cells is considered to be a prerequisite to colonization and infection (29). As previously mentioned, when these organisms enter the urethra and bladder in most women, they do not adhere and are easily washed away. In patients who are susceptible to urinary tract infections, the organisms will quickly lock into the defective epithelial cells. The fecal flora is almost invariably the source of the infecting organisms. *E. coli* is the major pathogen, although *S. epidermidis* and *Enterococcus, Klebsiella,* and *Proteus* species can sometimes be identified (Fig. 18.3). The interaction of the mucosal and bacterial cells is probably dependent on both receptors on the mucosa and some type of attachment mechanism used by the bacteria. *E. coli* has been shown to possess surface organelles that mediate attachment to specific host receptors. These structures are called pili and can be present in large numbers on the microbial cell. Two types that appear to be important in

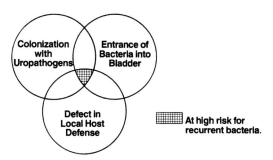

FIG. 18.3. Factors determining host risk and susceptibility to bacterial cystitis in normal females with anatomically normal urinary tracts.

urinary infections have been identified. Type I pili seek mannose as a receptor and are isolated from individuals with cystitis. They tend to bind with a low affinity, and their presence is not correlated highly with pathogenicity. Type II pili are mannose-negative or "p pili" and adhere to the P blood group. *E. coli* strains possessing p fimbriae are more virulent and more likely to cause pyelonephritis than strains without them (30–32).

Schaeffer and colleagues (33) studied the adherence of *E. coli* to vaginal epithelial cells in control subjects and in women who had experienced at least three urinary tract infections in the past year. They found adherence to be greater in the study patients than in the controls. The vaginal cells of those receiving a sustained course of antimicrobial showed less adherence than the vaginal cells of patients who were not taking antibiotics. If the antibiotics were discontinued, adherence returned, and reinfection usually occurred (33). In another study, Schaeffer and colleagues (34) noted that adherence tended to be higher during the early estrogen-dependent phase of the menstrual cycle.

Furthermore, women at high risk for recurrent urinary tract infections may be more genetically prone to recurrent infection because they have a higher prevalence of the human leukocyte antigen A3 subtype than do women who have never had urinary tract infections (35). Other work also suggests that women of blood group B or AB who are nonsecretors of blood group substances are at significantly higher risk for developing infections than are women of other blood groups (36). In addition, patients with Lewis blood group types who are considered secretors have a lower incidence of urinary tract infections. The Lewis blood groups exists at two genetic loci: Le_a and Le_b. Secretors are $Le_{(a+,b+)}$ and $Le_{(a-,b+)}$, whereas nonsecretors are $Le_{(a-,b-)}$. Evidence suggests that bacteria are unable to adhere to the urothelial cell because of alterations to the uromucoid, which inhibits binding (37–41).

Thus, these genetic differences at the cellular level appear to influence bacterial adherence and make certain women more prone to urinary tract infections. These differences also influence the anatomic level of the infections.

Sexual Intercourse

In women, sexual intercourse appears to be a major determinant for bacterial entry into the bladder. Prospective studies have shown that many urinary tract infections develop the day after sexual intercourse (42). Both the frequency and recency of sexual intercourse increase the risk for urinary tract infection. It has been shown that women who have engaged in sexual intercourse within the prior 48 hours have a risk for infection 60 times greater than women who have not (42). This appears to occur through inoculation of periurethral bacteria into the bladder during active intercourse. Women who have not colonized their vaginal and periurethral areas with coliform bacteria will have introduction of normal vaginal flora (e.g., lactobacillus, diphtheroid, or *S. epidermidis*), which will not produce infection and are rapidly cleared with voiding. However, in the colonized women, the pathogenic organisms, such as *E. coli,* will infect the bladder.

Another commonly overlooked factor is the use of diaphragms. A number of studies have confirmed that diaphragm users are at increased risk for urinary tract infection even after statistically controlling for sexual activity and history of previous urinary tract infection (43,44). The mechanism is unknown; it is believed that it may be related to urethral obstruction caused by the diaphragm (45,46). Also, diaphragm users have reduced vaginal colonization with lactobacillus, but coliforms are isolated three times more often than in women using other contraceptive methods (44).

Systemic Factors

Diabetic patients are prone to develop neurogenic bladder dysfunction and severe vascular disease, both of which can predispose to urinary tract infections. Other genetic problems that are commonly associated with urinary tract infections are gouty nephropathy, sickle cell trait, and cystic renal disease.

It must be understood that the explanations mentioned for the pathogenesis of urinary tract infections only apply to those females who have normal urinary tracts. Bacteria in the presence of obstructions, stones, or a neurogenic bladder does not need to have special invasive properties other than the ability to grow in urine.

CLINICAL PRESENTATION

The signs and symptoms of urinary tract infection in females can be diverse. It is helpful to distinguish lower urinary tract infection (cystitis) from upper tract infection (pyelonephritis) to aid in the selection of proper antimicrobial therapy and to plan appropriate follow-up.

Cystitis and associated urethral irritation are usually manifested by lower urinary tract irritative symptoms in the form of dysuria, frequency of small amounts of urine, urgency, nocturia, suprapubic discomfort, and low backache and flank pain. Occasionally, there may be mild incontinence and hematuria at the end of voiding. Rarely, the urine is grossly bloody. Systemic symptoms in the form of fever, chills, and so on are usually absent in lower urinary tract infections.

Upper urinary tract infections involving the renal pelvis, calyces, and parenchyma commonly present with fever, chills, malaise, and, occasionally (especially in elderly patients), nausea and vomiting. Costovertebral angle tenderness and flank pain are usually present.

There is colicky pain if acute pyelonephritis is complicated by either a renal calculus or a sloughed renal papilla secondary to diabetic or analgesic nephropathy.

DIAGNOSIS OF BACTERIURIA

Before performing tests to document the presence or absence of pathogenic bacteria in the urine, the method of urinary collection must be considered. Considerable care must be taken in the collection of urine from ambulatory females. Kass (47,48) published results demonstrating that one whole voided urine specimen with a colony count of greater than 10^5 cfu/mL has only an 80% chance of representing true infection. Three specimens increased the odds to 95% (47,48). Even when intelligent, educated patients are given clear, detailed instructions for collection of urine, errors can occur. Certain patients, because of physical disability or obesity, are simply unable to obtain a clean voided specimen without assistance. When necessary to avoid these limitations, specimens can be obtained by urethral catheterization, the patient can lie in the lithotomy position on an examining table and void after the perineum is cleaned with soap and water while the nurse collects a midstream specimen, or bladder urine can be aspirated suprapubically (49). Although urethral catheterization is the most time-honored method, it should be kept in mind that catheterization is not without risks. Reports have noted that catheter-induced infection rates range from 1% in young, healthy females to as high as 20% in hospitalized females (50,51).

Urine Microscopy

Microscopic analysis of urine is an easy and valuable method of evaluating women with symptoms of urinary tract infection. A thorough microscopic examination of an uncentrifuged sample of urine can detect the presence of significant bacteria, leukocytes, and red blood cells. If infection with greater than 10^4 cfu/mL is present, the finding of one or more bacteria on a Gram stain specimen of urine correlates highly with the presence of urinary tract infection, having a sensitivity of 80% and a specificity of 90% with a positive predictive value of about 85% (52). Thus, a Gram stain of the urine is useful in detecting abundant bacteriuria but is of little help in infection with colony counts of less than 10^4 cfu/mL.

Fresh, unspun urine should also be quantitatively assessed with a hemocytometer for the number of white blood cells. The hemocytometer is positioned on the microscope stage. The number of leukocytes is counted in each of nine large squares, divided by 9 and multiplied by 10 to yield the number of white blood cells per milliliter. Pyuria is defined as greater than 10 leukocytes/mL. Pyuria is present in nearly all women with acute urinary tract infection. Studies note the presence of pyuria to be 80% to 95% sensitive (even when bacteria counts are less than 10^4) and 50% to 75% specific for the presence of urinary tract infection. However, a study of pregnant patients presenting acutely to a labor ward showed that only 17% of patients with significant pyuria had a significant urine culture (53). It is also of value to ascertain whether red blood cells are present or to perform a urine dipstick for blood. Microscopic hematuria can be found in about 50% of women with acute urinary tract infection and is rarely present in patients who have dysuria from other causes (54,55).

Office Urine Kits

If expertise for office microscopy is not available or feasible, it is reasonable to substitute a rapid diagnostic test for bacteriuria, pyuria, and hematuria, although, in general, these lead to less accurate results than microscopy. The most common rapid detection test is the nitrite test. This test depends on the conversion of urinary nitrate to nitrite by bacterial action. Numerous test kits are available (Multistix®10 SG, Bayer, West Haven, CT) (56). The test is often integrated with a test for esterase that suggests the presence of pyuria by a substrate color change caused by the esterase found in leukocytes. The sensitivity of these tests is directly related to the bacterial counts.

Wu and colleagues (57) showed a sensitivity of only 22% in infections with 10^4 to 10^5 cfu/mL versus 60% for those with greater than 10^5 cfu/mL. The test should be performed on concentrated first-morning voided specimens. It has been suggested that false-negative results are more likely if the test is used as a sampling technique at other times during the day (58). False-negative results can also occur in infections due to enterococci because they do not convert nitrate to nitrite and also in the presence of certain dyes such as bilirubin, methylene blue, or phenazopyridine that may interfere with the interpretation of the test (59,60). Some believe that these are good screening tests for asymptomatic bacteriuria (58–60), whereas others believe that the high false-negative rate limits their value (57).

Other rapid detection tests, such as filter methods (e.g., Back-T-Screen, Marion Laboratories, Inc., Kansas City, MO), concentrate a specific quantity of urinary sediment on a filter of controlled pore size. One milliliter of urine is mixed with 3 mL of a diluent containing glacial acetic acid and other ingredients that dissolve crystals and increase adherence of bacteria and leukocytes. The diluted mixture is then passed through the filter and rinsed with a diluent. A safranin dye is then used to stain the bacteria and leukocytes, and a decolorizer is added to remove excess dye. Resulting colors are compared with a reference to quantitate the presence of bacteria and leukocytes. The sensitivity of these tests for urine infected with 10^4 to 10^5 cfu/mL is from 34% to 65%. As the number of organisms increases to greater than 10^5, the sensitivity also increases to 79% to 85%. The specificity of this test at lower bacterial counts is about 75% (57,61). The main advantage of these tests is a more reliable detection of smaller numbers of bacteria at the expense of lower specificity (62). The test is believed by some to be a good screening method because it detects both bacteria and pyuria.

Urine Culture

In the patient who has clinical signs of acute lower urinary tract infection and is noted to have pyuria, bacteriuria, or hematuria on one of the previously mentioned office tests, it is reasonable to initiate antibiotic therapy without obtaining a urine culture. However, if one of the screening techniques is deemed inappropriate or inconclusive, if the patient has recurrent infection that has not been subjectively relieved with previous antibiotics, or if signs and symptoms are consistent with upper urinary tract infection, a bacterial culture and sensitivity should be performed. The traditional approach to the interpretation of a urinary culture has been that there must be growth of at least 10^5 cfu/mL to consider it positive. This criterion is based on studies demonstrating that the finding of at least 10^5 cfu/mL on two consecutive urine cultures distinguishes women with asymptomatic bacteriuria or pyelonephritis from those with contaminated specimens (47, 48,52). The use of this cutoff, however, has two limitations for the clinician who treats these patients. First, 20% to 24% of women with symptomatic urinary infections present with less than 10^5 bacteria/mL of urine (49,63–65). This is probably secondary to a slow doubling time of bacteria in urine combined with frequent bladder emptying from persistent irritation. Stamm and associates (66) proposed that the best diagnostic criterion for culture detection in young symptomatic women is 10^2 cfu/mL, not 10^5 cfu/mL. The second limitation of the 10^5 cutoff is one of overdiagnosis. In the original studies by Kass (47,48,67), a single culture of at least 10^5 cfu/mL had a 20% chance of representing contamination. Because patients who are susceptible to infection often carry large numbers of pathogenic bacteria on the perineum, contamination of an otherwise sterile urine can occur. For this reason, care in the collection of the urine specimen must again be emphasized. Most health care workers spend much time and effort to explain adequately how a patient should collect a midstream urine clean-catch specimen. A recent study showed contamination rates to be similar among patients whose urine samples were collected with traditional instructions (midstream urine sample, perineal cleansing and spreading of the labia) compared with urine samples of patients told to urinate into a clean container without cleansing (68).

Although methods of obtaining cultures in the office are available, most clinicians use commercial laboratories. One should be familiar with the individual laboratory policy of reporting culture results. Some laboratories report any culture of less than 10^5 cfu/mL as negative and often report only the predominant organism in mixed cultures.

Sensitivity testing is also usually obtained using a commercial laboratory even though office tests have been described. The disadvantages of sensitivity testing include the time involved, which is typically 24 to 48 hours; the absence of control of processing by the referring physician; and the relatively high cost.

CYSTOURETHROSCOPY

Indications for endoscopic evaluation in females with urinary tract infection have been a controversial issue. Fowler and Pulaski (69) reported on 74 cystoscopies performed in women with two or more previous infections and noted the only abnormality that altered treatment was the presence of a urethral diverticulum in three cases. Engel and associates (70) reviewed 153 women who had undergone cystoscopy for urinary tract infection. Although abnormalities were noted in 62% of the cases, 84% of these abnormalities were inflammatory in nature and presumably secondary to prior infection. Only one abnormality, a colovesical fistula, had an effect on treatment (70). Cystoscopy under local anesthesia has basically no risk and occasionally reveals findings useful in subsequent patient management. Therefore, it should be considered in patients with recurrent or persistent urinary tract infection or asymptomatic hematuria.

RADIOLOGIC STUDIES

Although it has long been believed that urinary tract infection constitutes one of the important indications for urography, the use of routine IVPs in women with otherwise uncomplicated infection has been challenged. The minimal (1% to 2%) yield of the IVP makes it an inefficient and expensive method of identifying underlying disease (69–74). The cost of detecting a single significant and treatable urologic disorder has been estimated at $9 thousand (74). However, the IVP is a valuable diagnostic test when properly indicated. The indications for obtaining an IVP for urinary tract infection are (a) a history of previous upper urinary tract infection; (b) a history of childhood urinary tract infections; (c) a history of recurrent infections caused by the same organism, particularly if the organism is urea splitting, such as *Proteus mirabilis*, because this is frequently associated with infected stones (Fig. 18.4); (d) all cases of infection associated with painless hematuria; (e) women with a history of stones or obstruction; and (f) patients with bacterial evidence of rapid recurrence, suggesting bacterial persistence or the presence of an enterovesical fistula.

A voiding cystourethrogram or a double-balloon catheter study should be performed if a urethral diverticulum is thought to be contributing to recurrent infections. Signs and symptoms of urethral diverticulum include leakage of urine and the finding of pus or pain on palpation and massage of the urethra.

URODYNAMIC STUDIES

Urodynamic studies involving a range of procedures from a simple cystometrogram and flow studies to complicated video-urodynamic studies are sometimes useful to demonstrate abnormal contraction and emptying of the bladder. A vicious cycle of repeated lower urinary tract infections can lead to an obstructed voiding pattern, with high residuals resulting from spasm of the external striated urethral sphincter secondary to infection or to the pain of the acute cystitis (75). These tests can prove

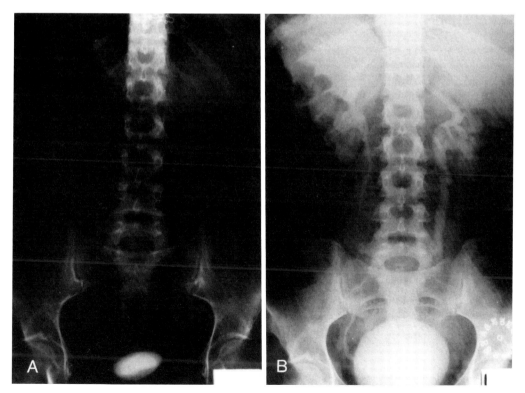

FIG. 18.4. Flat plate and intravenous pyelogram of a young female who presented with persistent urinary tract infection secondary to *Klebsiella pneumoniae*. **A:** Large intravesical bladder calculi. **B:** Bilateral hydronephrosis and hydroureter.

helpful in patients with recurrent urinary tract infection who have neurologic disease or a history of pelvic or spinal surgery.

DIFFERENTIAL DIAGNOSIS

In women whose history or laboratory findings are not consistent with urinary tract infection, other causes of their lower urinary tract symptoms must be considered.

Vaginitis is a major cause of lower urinary tract symptoms, with *Trichomonas* and *Candida* species being the most commonly implicated organisms. Nonspecific urethritis is a term that has been used by some to describe patients with dysuria secondary to what is believed to be an inflamed urethra. Several organisms have been proposed as potential pathogens in such cases. These have included *C. trachomatis*, lactobacilli, *S. saprophyticus*,

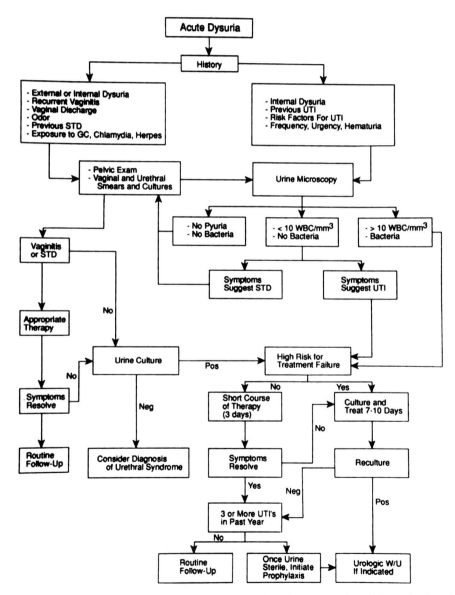

FIG. 18.5. Algorithm for diagnosis and management of females presenting with acute dysuria.

and corynebacteria as well as other fastidious organisms, such as *Ureaplasma urealyticum,* and *Mycoplasma hominis.* However, data to substantiate correlation between clinical symptoms and the presence of these organisms are lacking (76,77). Trauma related to intercourse or other activities may also produce symptoms of urinary tract infection. Unfortunately, many of these patients are unnecessarily treated with repetitive courses of antibiotics. Dysuria is also a common presenting symptom in sexually transmitted diseases, particularly *C. trachomatis* and, less commonly, herpes simplex virus or *Neisseria gonorrhoeae.*

Some patients can distinguish internal from external dysuria. Discomfort that is centered inside the body is more commonly associated with urinary tract infection or urethritis due to *C. trachomatis*; pain that starts when the urine flows across the perineum is more commonly associated with vaginitis or herpetic infection. Frequency, urgency, and voiding small amounts of urine are common in urinary tract infection and in sexually transmitted diseases and rare in vaginitis. Virtually all women with acute symptomatic urinary tract infection have pyuria, and about half have microscopic hematuria. Pyuria can also exist in patients with urethritis secondary to sexually transmitted diseases. It is not present in vaginitis. Hematuria is not a feature of either sexually transmitted diseases or vaginitis; therefore, its presence is a strong clue toward the diagnosis of cystitis. Postmenopausal women may have dysuria secondary to desiccation of the urethra and the vaginal mucosa caused by estrogen deficiency (78). A group of women exists who are not estrogen deficient and who complain of persistent lower urinary tract symptoms despite negative urine, vaginal, and urethral cultures. The term urethral syndrome (76–79) has been introduced to describe these patients, and a full discussion of this condition is presented elsewhere. A suggested approach to the evaluation and management of women with dysuria is shown in Fig. 18.5.

MANAGEMENT OF LOWER URINARY TRACT INFECTION

General measures, such as rest and hydration, should always be emphasized in women with urinary tract infection. Hydration dilutes bacterial counts and may destroy cell wall–deficient bacterial strains. Acidification of the urine is only helpful in recurrent infections and in patients taking methenamine compounds, which demonstrate maximal antibacterial activity at a pH of 5.5 or less. Urinary analgesic agents such as phenazopyridine hydrochloride (Pyridium) help relieve pain and burning on urination. If prescribed, they should be used for only 2 or 3 days along with a specific antibacterial agent. It has also been noted that the ingestion of cranberry juice may be protective against the development of cystitis by inhibiting bacterial adherence (80).

With regard to the therapeutic management of this condition, certain factors should be kept in mind. Because the fecal flora is the reservoir for most of the organisms causing the infection, a drug that has little or no effect on these microbes should ideally be prescribed. The reason to avoid altering these bacteria is that 20% of female patients with simple cystitis have a recurrence shortly after stopping medication. A drug can alter bacteria in the bowel either by passing through the gastrointestinal tract without being absorbed or by having a high serum level. It is also important that a drug maintain a low serum level to avoid disrupting the flora in other parts of the body, such as the vagina. If a drug appropriately matched to bacterial sensitivity causes a yeast vaginitis, the subsequent therapy for the vaginitis will increase patient morbidity and raise the cost of therapy. In addition, the vaginitis set up by the antibiotic could lead to a vaginitis–cystitis circle that may be difficult to treat. These therapeutic goals should be kept in mind when treating these infections because there are many misconceptions about commonly prescribed antibiotics. For example, ampicillin and tetracycline are both frequently prescribed for simple cystitis, despite the fact that they have an incidence of yeast vaginitis that may approach 25% and 70% to 80%, respectively, because both drugs are excreted in the fecal stream unchanged and have a stool level three times the urine level (81–83). Nitrofurantoin, on the other hand, has excellent activity against *E. coli* and has no significant serum level. It has a 19-minute serum half-life and is metabolized in every tissue in the body, resulting in no significant changes in fecal or vaginal flora, which is why no increase in bacterial resistance to nitrofurantoin is seen after 30 years of use in the United States (83–88). The most common sulfonamide preparation used in the management of urinary tract infection is the combination of trimethoprim and sulfamethoxazole (TMP-SMX, Bactrim, Septra). These drugs have become very popular in the management of urinary tract infections because of their broad range of activity against uropathogens, low incidence of adverse effects, twice-daily dosage, and infrequent occurrence of bacterial resistance. However, these agents have been shown to have a moderate effect on bowel and vaginal wall flora (89,90).

A group of synthetic quinoline derivatives, which are related chemically to nalidixic acid, has recently been introduced as antibacterial agents for urinary tract infections. Derivatives include norfloxacin (Noroxin), ciprofloxacin, enoxacin, ofloxacin, levofloxacin, and amifloxacin. These agents are more active than nalidixic acid against gram-negative urinary tract pathogens (e.g., *E. coli*). In addition, they have an expanded antibacterial spectrum that includes *Pseudomonas aeruginosa* and gram-positive bacteria (e.g., staphylococci, enterococci). All of these agents are administered orally, and parenteral formulations are available for some (e.g., ciprofloxacin and levofloxacin). Adverse effects have been infrequent; however, their cost limits their routine use. Because they have no advantage over more standard agents (e.g., nitrofurantoin, TMP-SMX) for uncomplicated infections, they should be reserved for use in patients with resistant infections or as an alternative to parenteral antibiotics in certain complicated infections and cases of pyelonephritis (91–97). Unfortunately, their attractiveness has lead to widespread use, making ciprofloxacin the fourth most commonly prescribed antibiotic in the United States. This overuse has been accompanied by an increase in bacterial resistance; already, strains of *E. coli* are resistant to ciprofloxacin.

Listed in Tables 18.2 and 18.3 are the dosage, toxicity, and spectrum of antimicrobial activity of some of the commonly prescribed oral antibiotics.

TABLE 18.2. *Dosage and toxicity of antibiotics commonly used in the treatment of urinary tract infections*

Drug	Oral dose and frequency	Minor toxicity	Major toxicity
TMP-SMX	1 tablet b.i.d.	Allergic	Serious skin reactions, blood dyscrasia
Nitrofurantoin	50–100 mg q 6–8 h	Gastrointestinal upset	Peripheral neuropathy, pneumonitis
Ampicillin	250–500 mg q 6 h	Allergic candidal overgrowth	Allergic reactions, pseudomembranous colitis
Tetracycline	250–500 mg q 6 h	Gastrointestinal upset, skin rash, candidal overgrowth	Hepatic dysfunction, nephrotoxicity
Cephalexin	250–500 mg q 6 h	Allergic	Hepatic dysfunction
Norfloxacin	400 mg q 12 h	Nausea, vomiting, diarrhea, abdominal pain, skin rash	Convulsions, psychoses, joint damage
Levofloxacin	250–500 mg q 24 h	Disturbance of blood glucose, allergic, photosensitivity, nausea, headache	Allergic reactions, tendon rupture, pseudomembranous colitis
Ciprofloxacin	100–500 mg q 12 h	Anosmia, taste loss, myalgia, dyspepsia, central nervous system effects	Theophylline interactions, pseudomembranous colitis, anaphylactic reaction

TABLE 18.3. *Spectrum of antimicrobial activity against common lower urinary tract pathogens*

Organism	TMP-SMX	Nitro-furantoin	Ampi-cillin	Tetra-cycline	Cepha-lexin	Carben-icillin	Genta-micin	Nor-floxacin	Levo-floxacin	Cipro-floxacin
Escherichia coli	++	++	++	±	++	++	++	++	++	++
Pseudomonas sp.	—	—	—	—	—	++	++	++	++	++
Klebsiella sp.	++	±	—	±	++	—	++	++	++	++
Proteus sp.	++	—	++	—	++	++	++	++	++	++
Enterobacter sp.	++	—	—	—	—	++	++	++	++	++
Enterococcus sp.	—	±	++	++	±	—	—	++	±	±
Staphylococcus sp.	—	±	++	+	++	++	+	++	++	++
Serratia marcescens	+	—	—	—	—	—	++	++	++	++

++, excellent; +, good; ±, occasionally effective; —, resistant.

Asymptomatic Bacteriuria in Patients without Catheters

By definition, asymptomatic bacteriuria is the recovery of at least 10^5 cfu/mL of a single bacterial species in at least two consecutive clean-voided urine specimens in the absence of clinical symptoms (47). Little is known about the natural history of untreated bacteriuria in women because most are treated once the diagnosis is made. Two studies have, however, compared antibiotic treatment with placebo in women with asymptomatic bacteriuria. They noted that 60% to 80% of these patients spontaneously clear their infection whether they are treated or receive placebo (98,99). Although the long-term effects of asymptomatic bacteriuria are not completely known, there appears to be no association with renal scarring, hypertension, or progressive renal azotemia.

Screening for asymptomatic bacteriuria has little apparent value in adults, with two exceptions: before urologic surgery and during pregnancy. Postoperative complications, including bacteremia, are reduced by recognizing and treating asymptomatic bacteriuria before urologic surgery (100). All pregnant women should be screened for bacteriuria in the first trimester and should be treated if bacteriuria is present to reduce their markedly increased risk for acute pyelonephritis and the accompanying risks for prematurity and low birth weight in their infants (101,102).

To date, there is no definite advantage to treating asymptomatic bacteriuria in nonpregnant female patients. There are, however, recent studies that have shown a significant association between asymptomatic urinary tract infection and overall mortality (103,104). Whether this mortality is a false-positive result or whether the bacteriuria is serving as a marker for a chronic disease that was the actual cause of death needs to be confirmed by further studies.

First Infections or Infrequent Reinfections

Many treatment regimens have been reported for initial therapy of simple cystitis, ranging from one dose to 2 or more weeks of medication. The longer treatment regimens were instituted in an attempt to prevent the relapse rate that occurs in about 20% of patients treated for cystitis. Almost all of these relapses are attributable to the colonization of the vaginal walls and urethra with gram-negative bacteria that have continued to grow on the perineum or reappeared when the drug was stopped. It does not indicate that the prescribed drug has failed to eradicate the bacteriuria.

There are numerous studies in the literature evaluating single-dose therapy in the management of acute uncomplicated cystitis (105–114). When single-dose therapy was compared with 10 days of TMP-SMX, there was a significantly higher treatment failure rate with single-dose therapy (114). Further concern has been raised that single-dose regimes are less likely to be effective in treatment of infections when an unrecognized complicating factor is present, such as pregnancy, diabetes, or an anatomic or functional abnormality of the urinary tract. Single-dose therapy has also been noted to be suboptimal in the treatment of occult upper urinary tract infection (115).

A plethora of studies has been conducted in recent years to define the optimal antimicrobial agent and length of treatment for uncomplicated cystitis in women. With most antimicrobial agents, 3-day regimes appear optimal, with efficacy comparable with 7-day regimes but with fewer side effects and lower cost. Nitrofurantoin, cefadroxil, amoxicillin, and TMP-SMX have been shown to be effective in 3-day regimes, either in open trials or in comparative trials with longer regimes. A recent prospective randomized trial compared these four antimicrobial agents in a 3-day regime in young women with acute cystitis (116). The findings demonstrated that a 3-day regime of twice-daily TMP-SMX was more effective than 3 days of nitrofurantoin, cefadroxil, or amoxicillin. Moreover, TMP-SMX was the least expensive of the four regimes, mainly because, compared with the other regimes, patients were less likely to have to return for evaluation of persistent or recurrent urinary tract infection or for yeast vaginitis (116). We, therefore, favor the use of TMP-SMX as our first-line agent for empiric treatment of acute uncomplicated cystitis in women.

Alternate regimes that can be used in women who have a history of intolerance to TMP-SMX are nitrofurantoin, 100 mg four times daily, or TMP, 100 mg twice daily. We try to avoid the use of amoxicillin or first-generation cephalosporins because we have experienced a relatively high failure rate with these agents in our clinic. Single-dose therapy or a short course of therapy should only be considered in patients who are at very low risk for treatment failures. Thus, patients who have (a) systemic diseases, such as diabetes mellitus; (b) a history of acute pyelonephritis; (c) a history of a treatment failure in the last 6 months; (d) a history of childhood urinary tract infections; or (e) known structural abnormalities of the urinary tract should be given a longer 7- to 10-day course of therapy.

For patients with acute simple cystitis who have complete resolution of their symptoms, it is not necessary to perform any routine post-treatment urinary assessment. However, in those patients whose urinary symptoms persist beyond the 3 days of therapy, a urine culture and sensitivity should be obtained. Persistence of symptoms should suggest the possibility that either the initial diagnosis of urinary tract infection was in error or that the patient's infection is secondary to a resistant organism that was present from the onset of therapy or has developed during initial therapy. In cases of resistance, a 7- to 10-day course of a sensitive antibiotic should then be prescribed.

A recent study evaluated the use of phone triage of patients with symptoms of acute uncomplicated urinary tract infection. Eligible patients were offered antibiotics without an office visit, urinalysis, or urine culture. There were no significant increases in potential adverse outcomes, namely, subsequent visits for cystitis, sexually transmitted diseases, or pyelonephritis, during the 60 days after diagnosis (117).

Recurrent Infections

About 75% of all women who experience a urinary tract infection subsequently experience less than one infection per year (118). However, the other 25% of women develop reinfections at a rate of almost three infections per year. These women compose 50% of all women presenting with acute urinary tract infections (118–121).

Once the urine has been sterilized by appropriate antimicrobial therapy, the pattern of culture-documented reinfection or recurrence is very helpful in the subsequent management of these patients (Fig. 18.6). It can also be used to classify patients with different infectious etiologies to identify those who may be at increased risk or require further urologic evaluation. The most common type of recurrence is reinfection by bacteria different from the initially infecting strain. Even though the infections may be caused by the same species (e.g., *E. coli*), the organisms can usually be differentiated on the basis of colonial morphology and antimicrobial sensitivities. These infections are almost invariably due to a re-

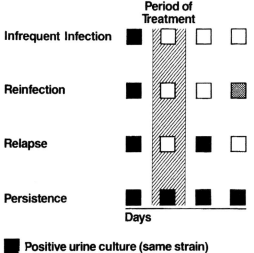

FIG. 18.6. Natural history of urinary tract infection.

TABLE 18.4. *Correctable urinary tract abnormalities causing persistent bacteriuria*

Urethral diverticulum
Infected stone
Significant anterior vaginal wall relaxation
Papillary necrosis
Foreign body
Duplicated or ectopic ureter
Atrophic pyelonephritis (unilateral)
Medullary sponge kidney

current ascending infection from the vaginal introital area. It has been shown that the same strain can exist in the introital area for many months and cause multiple reinfections. Sexual intercourse and occult urinary tract abnormalities may also facilitate reinfection and must always be considered in these patients.

Relapsing infection from an upper urinary tract source of an infected stone should be suspected if the same organism is repeatedly isolated 7 to 10 days after treatment with an antimicrobial agent to which the organism is sensitive. In many of these patients, one cannot obtain sterile urine, and thus these cases are termed bacterial persistence (causes are listed in Table 18.4). Endoscopic and radiographic evaluations must be selectively performed in cases of relapse or persistence of infection.

The goal of the management of reinfected urine is to achieve sterile urine; this is the basis for subsequent successful use of antimicrobial agents. To eradicate urinary tract infections successfully, antimicrobial agents should be administered in sufficient doses to exceed by a wide margin the minimal concen-

tration required to inhibit growth. Lower dosages lead to the selection of resistant organisms from the original population in about 10% of the cases, complicating the treatment of these already difficult patients.

Recurrent cystitis should be documented by culture at least once and then managed by one of three strategies: continuous prophylaxis, postcoital prophylaxis, or therapy initiated by the patient (self-start therapy). Continuous prophylaxis has been shown to be highly cost-effective and is recommended as the initial form of therapy in women who have frequent reinfections (122,123). Its success depends on using the minimal dosage of an antimicrobial agent that has minimal or no adverse effect on the fecal flora. Once the urine has been completely sterilized by a full-dose course of therapy, nightly therapy is begun with one of many different drugs (Table 18.5). Nitrofurantoin (122), 100 mg, or cephalexin (123), 250 mg, is effective therapy. These drugs do not cause resistance in the fecal flora; however, vaginal colonization with sensitive bacteria does continue. Their efficacy depends on nightly bactericidal activity in the bladder urine against sensitive reinfecting organisms. The efficacy of cephalexin

TABLE 18.5. *Oral antimicrobial agents useful for prophylactic prevention of recurrent urinary tract infections*

Agent	Dosage
Nitrofurantoin	100 mg
Cephalexin	250 mg
TMP-SMX[a]	1 tablet
Cinoxacin	250–500 mg

[a]Each regular tablet contains 80 mg trimethoprim and 400 mg sulfamethoxazole.

is dependent on use of a minimal dosage. If it is given 4 times a day in full dosages, it gives rise to resistant strains. When it is given in a dose of 250 mg nightly, it does not. TMP-SMX (124) is active not only because of bactericidal activity against urinary bacteria but also because TMP diffuses into the vaginal fluid at a concentration bactericidal to most urinary pathogens (125). Low-dose TMP-SMX or TMP alone causes resistance in about 10% of rectal cultures (124). Most of these patients continue to maintain sterile urine while receiving prophylactic therapy, although breakthrough infections may infrequently occur and should be treated with full-dose sensitive antimicrobial therapy. We empirically continue the prophylactic therapy for about 6 months and, at that time, follow the patient off therapy with frequent cultures. About 30% of women have a spontaneous remission for at least the following 6 months (121). Unfortunately, a remission does not necessarily reflect a complete cure. If reinfection occurs, it must be managed by reinstitution of low-dose nightly prophylaxis.

Self-start intermittent therapy can be an alternative to continuous prophylactic therapy in patients with recurrent urinary tract infections. When this regimen is used, the patient is given a dip-slide device and instructed to perform a urine culture when she has symptoms consistent with a recurrent urinary tract infection. She then empirically starts a 3-day course of full-dose antimicrobial therapy, usually with one of the previously mentioned antibiotics. Full-dose nitrofurantoin, cinoxacin, or norfloxacin is usually successful. Norfloxacin appears to be an ideal drug for self-start therapy. It has a broader spectrum of activity than any other oral agent and is comparable with or better than most available parenteral antimicrobial agents. In addition, it has activity against multiple-resistance bacteria, and bacteria exposed to this agent have a low rate of spontaneous mutation to resistant organisms. In a multicenter comparative study of more than 350 patients with urinary tract infection, the percentage of strains susceptible to norfloxacin was 99%. This was significantly greater than the percentage of strains susceptible to TMP-SMX, which was

about 90%. Also, the percentage of bacteriologic cures was significantly higher with the norfloxacin (than TMP-SMX), and side effects were minimal (126). Self-start therapy has proved to be safe, effective, reliable, and economical in women with recurrent urinary tract infections (127,128).

If a patient's history suggests that reinfections are preceded by intercourse, she may take a single antimicrobial tablet before or after intercourse (129). Vosti (130) first demonstrated that nitrofurantoin given after coitus prevented recurrent urinary tract infection. More recently, Pfau and colleagues (131) showed that TMP-SMX, nalidixic acid, nitrofurantoin, and sulfonamide were all effective in preventing recurrent urinary tract infections when given to young sexually active women whose infections occurred postcoitally. In a recent study, 135 sexually active premenopausal women with recurrent urinary tract infections were randomly assigned to receive daily prophylaxis of ciprofloxacin, 125 mg, or a single dose of 125 mg after intercourse. Results for the two groups were similar, with the postintercourse group consuming only one third the amount of drug (132). If feasible, a woman who has recurrent urinary tract infections and uses a diaphragm as her mode of contraception should consider another method. If she is unable or unwilling to change to another method, she should be closely questioned about symptoms of urinary obstruction occurring with the diaphragm in place. If such symptoms occur, it should be ascertained if the fit of the diaphragm is too large. Women in this category of intercourse-related infection should also be advised to void as promptly as possible after intercourse. Postmenopausal women may also have frequent reinfections. These infections are sometimes attributable to residual urine after voiding, which is often associated with pelvic organ prolapse. In addition, the lack of estrogen causes marked changes in the vaginal microflora, including loss of bacilli and increased colonization by *E. coli* (133). Antimicrobial prophylaxis or topically applied estrogen cream can be used as an alternative preventive measure in such women.

It has been shown that in addition to antibiotic prophylaxis, postmenopausal women with recurrent urinary tract infections using an estradiol-releasing silicone vaginal ring had significantly fewer recurrent urinary tract infections than women without estrogen treatment (134).

Complicated Infections

Complicated urinary tract infections occur in patients with a functionally, metabolically, or anatomically abnormal urinary tract or are caused by pathogens that are resistant to antibiotics. The clinical spectrum can range from mild cystitis to life-threatening urosepsis. In addition, there may be long periods of asymptomatic bacteriuria. Urine cultures, therefore, must be obtained in patients suspected of having complicated infection to identify the infecting pathogen and perform susceptibility testing. The wide variety of underlying conditions and diverse spectrum of possible etiologic agents make generalizing about antimicrobial therapy difficult. For empiric therapy in patients with mild to moderate illness who can be treated as outpatients, the fluoroquinolones provide a broad spectrum of antimicrobial activity covering most expected pathogens and achieve high levels in the urine. At least 10 to 14 days of therapy is usually necessary. Pseudomonas and enterococcal infections are especially difficult to treat and may warrant more prolonged therapy. Without correction of the underlying anatomic, functional, or metabolic defect, infection often recurs. For this reason, a urine culture should be repeated 1 to 2 weeks after the completion of therapy.

Catheter-associated Infection

Catheter-associated urinary tract infection is the most common hospital-associated infection and is the most frequent source of bacteremia in hospitalized patients (135). One study showed a threefold increase in mortality in these patients (136). In another study of 1,497 newly catheterized patients at a university hospital, 235 new cases of catheter-associated urinary tract infection were discovered. However, greater than 90% of the infected patients were symptom free, and only one patient developed a secondary bloodstream infection (137). The mechanism through which bacteriuria is related to mortality is uncertain. Risk factors of catheter-associated infection are advanced age, female sex, and an increasing degree of underlying illness (138). The pathogenesis of catheter-associated urinary infection has not been studied as well as urinary tract infection of noncatheterized patients. Points of bacterial entry, however, have been well defined and include introduction of bacteria residing in the urethra into the bladder at the time of catheterization, subsequent entry of bacteria colonizing the urethra meatus along the mucus sheath external to the catheter, and ascent of bacteria within the catheter lumen itself. The relative proportion of infections occurring through these different routes of entry have not been clearly defined. Prospective studies demonstrated that organisms causing infection in catheterized patients can be identified in the urethral or rectal flora 2 to 4 days before the onset of bacteriuria in 70% of women (139). Another prospective study of 1,497 newly catheterized patients found 235 new urinary tract infections and determined that 66% were extraluminal and 34% were derived from intraluminal contaminants (140). Until more is known about the pathogenesis of nosocomial bacteriuria, the bulk of preventive efforts should continue to focus on aseptic care of the urinary catheter (141) (Table 18.6). There has been no demonstrable efficacy of local antimicrobial ointments applied to the meatal junction despite the apparent association of meatal colonization with subsequent infection (142, 143). The use of antimicrobial irrigants has also been ineffective in reducing the preva-

TABLE 18.6. *Prevention of bladder infection in elderly long-term catheterized patients*

Monitor urine level in bag every 4 h; exchange catheter if cessation of flow for 4 h
Fluid intake of 1.5 L/d
Avoid catheter manipulations
Exchange catheter if infection is suspected
Exchange catheter every 8–12 wk

lence of bacteriuria (144). Although systemic antimicrobial agents reduce the occurrence of bacteriuria for the first few days of catheterization, their use cannot be widely recommended at this time because the benefit accrued, that is, reduction of asymptomatic bacteriuria, may not be worth the cost and attendant risk for development of resistant microorganisms (145).

The diagnosis and management of these urinary tract infections in elderly nursing home patients with long-term catheterization (greater than 3 months) can present a challenge. All patients with indwelling catheters for any length of time will develop bacteria in their urine (Fig. 18.7). However, as long as the catheter system is a closed functioning system

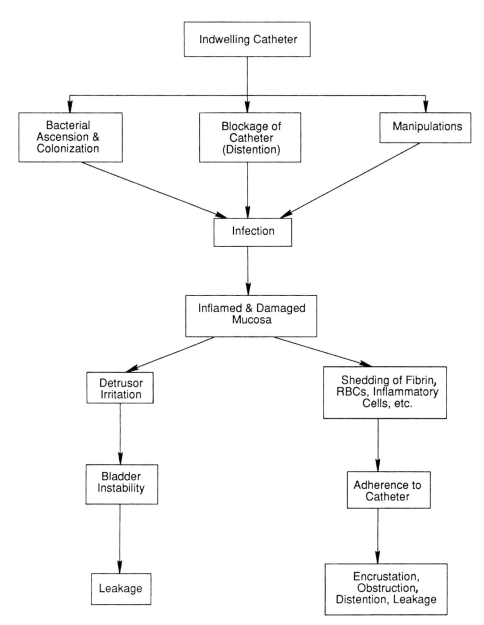

FIG. 18.7. Pathogenesis of infection and clinical picture of females with long-term indwelling catheters.

and the patient has no local or systemic symptoms or signs, there is no advantage to empiric systemic antibiotics. On the other hand, 10% of elderly patients with indwelling catheters develop bacteremia and gram-negative septicemia, a serious disease with a 20% to 50% mortality rate. These patients must be promptly identified because they require hospitalization and vigorous systemic antibiotic therapy. A traumatic event consisting of obstruction, manipulation, or removal of an inflated indwelling bladder catheter often precedes the onset of urosepsis. In addition to antibiotic therapy, it is essential to establish free flow of urine for the catheterized patient with acute urosepsis. The complications of concomitant bacteremia (shock, adult respiratory distress syndrome, disseminated intravascular coagulation, and gastric hemorrhage) must be readily recognized and managed appropriately. Certain measures can be taken to prevent these life-threatening complications in patients with chronic indwelling catheters (Table 18.6). Catheters should be checked every 4 hours by experienced personnel to ensure proper drainage and to prevent formation of any encrustation within the tubing of the catheter; indwelling catheters should be changed every 8 to 12 weeks, depending on whether they are silicon- or Teflon-coated catheters.

LOWER URINARY TRACT INSTRUMENTATION

Whether patients undergoing lower urinary tract instrumentation for diagnostic or therapeutic purposes need prophylactic antibiotics is, currently, an unresolved issue. A recent prospective double-blind placebo-controlled study by Cundiff and colleagues (146) compared nitrofurantoin with placebo in patients undergoing urodynamics and cystourethroscopy. Although the power of the study was limited, they found no significant difference in bacteriuria between the two groups. Also, the prevalence of significant bacteriuria before instrumentation was low at 5%, and the overall incidence of significant bacteriuria after instrumentation was 6% for both groups (146). For this reason, we do not routinely give antibiotics to low-risk patients after lower urinary tract instrumentation. In patients undergoing intermittent catheterization, bacteriuria may be reduced by bladder irrigation with a solution of neomycin or polymyxin or by oral methenamine, nitrofurantoin, or TMP-SMX prophylaxis (147).

ACUTE PYELONEPHRITIS

Pyelonephritis is defined as inflammation of the kidney and renal pelvis, even though the diagnosis is based on clinical findings. Patients with acute pyelonephritis have chills, fever, and unilateral or bilateral costovertebral angle tenderness. These upper tract signs are often accompanied by dysuria, increased urinary frequency, and urgency. The urine is usually cloudy and malodorous, and in very rare cases, acute renal failure may be present.

Urinalysis notes the urinary sediment to show increased white blood cells, white blood cell casts, and red blood cells. Bacteria rods or chains of cocci are also often seen. Urine cultures grow various amounts of bacteria. Systemic blood tests may show polymorphonuclear leukocytosis, increased erythrocyte sedimentation rate, elevated C-reactive protein, and elevated creatinine if renal failure is present. The most common bacteria to cause acute pyelonephritis are those of the Enterobacteriaceae family. These include *E. coli* and species of *Klebsiella*, *Proteus*, *Enterobacter*, *Pseudomonas*, *Serratia*, and *Citrobacter*.

Only recently, the radiologic findings characteristic of acute pyelonephritis have been emphasized. It was previously thought that the intravenous urograms in these patients were normal; however, in 24% to 28% of patients with acute pyelonephritis, abnormal urograms have been attributed to the acute disease (148,149). Findings on intravenous urogram in patients with acute pyelonephritis have included renal enlargement, impaired contrast excretion, nonobstructive dilation of the urinary collecting system, cortical striations in the nephrogram, and ureteral striations. Although renal ultrasound is useful to show renal size in most infected kidneys, no findings are seen on ultrasound that are not seen on the urogram. Contrast-enhanced computed tomography (CT) is very sensitive for detection of renal enlargement, attenuated parenchyma, and compressed collecting systems characteristic of acute pyelonephritis. CT scans, however, are not indicated unless the diagnosis cannot be established on urogram or renal ultrasound or if the patient does not respond to therapy.

The treatment of acute pyelonephritis should be subdivided into three categories: patients who have mild symptoms and do not warrant hospitalization; patients who are ill enough to warrant hospitalization for parenteral antibiotics; and infection associated with hospitalization, catheterization, urologic surgery, or urinary tract abnormalities. For patients needing parenteral therapy, ampicillin and aminoglycoside have proven efficacy and offer effectiveness against most of the Enterobacteriaceae family, *Pseudomonas* species, and other gramnegative bacilli. In non–hospital-acquired infections, a third-generation cephalosporin is an effective alternative. Both oral fluoroquinolones and TMP-SMX have been proved efficacious in patients receiving outpatient therapy. It is important that the patient understand that fever and flank pain may persist for several days after the initiation of successful antimicrobial therapy. However, if symptoms persist beyond this time, the possibility of underlying renal or urinary tract abnormalities should be considered, and radiologic investigation with ultrasound, urography, or CT should be performed. The duration of therapy for acute pyelonephritis should be 14 days (150). Repeat urine culture should be performed 5 to 7 days after initiation of therapy and 4 to 6 weeks after discontinuation of antimicrobial therapy to ensure that the urinary tract remains free of infection. Between 10% and 30% of patients with acute pyelonephritis relapse after a 14-day course of therapy. Patients who relapse usually are cured by a second 14-day course of therapy, but occasionally, a 6-week course of therapy is necessary.

REFERENCES

1. Fihn SD. Urinary tract infections in primary care obstetrics and gynecology. *Clin Obstet Gynecol* 1988; 31:1003–1016.
2. National Center for Health Statistics. Ambulatory medical care rendered in physicians offices. United States 1975. *Adv Data* 1977;12:1–8.
3. Cox LE, Lacy SS, Hinman F. The urethra and its relationship to urinary tract infection. II. The urethral flora of the female with recurrent urinary tract infection. *J Urol* 1968;99:632–638.
4. Winberg J, Anderson HJ, Bergstrom T, et al. Epidemiology of symptomatic urinary tract infection in childhood. *Acta Paediatra Scand* 1974;252[Suppl]: 3–21.
5. Rolleston GL, Shannon FT, Utley WLF. Relationship of infantile vesico-ureteric reflux to renal damage. *Br Med J* 1970;1:460–464.
6. Mulholland SG. Controversies in management of urinary tract infection. *Urology* 1986;27[Suppl]:3–8.
7. Mayer TR. UTI in the elderly: how to select treatment. *Geriatrics* 1980;35:67–73.
8. Turck M, Stamm W. Nosocomial infection of the urinary tract. *Am J Med* 1981;70:651–659.
9. Maskell R. Importance of coagulase-negative Staphylococci as pathogens in the urinary tract. *Lancet* 1974; 1:1155–1159.
10. Sellin M, Cooke DI, Gillespie WA, et al. Micrococcal urinary tract infections in young women. *Lancet* 1975; 2:570–572.
11. Cunha B. Urinary tract infections. I. Pathophysiology and diagnostic approach. *Postgrad Med* 1981;70: 141–158.
12. Hovelius B. Urinary tract infections caused by *Staphylococcus saprophyticus* recurrences and complications. *J Urol* 1979;122:645–650.
13. Marrie T, Kwan C, Noble M, et al. *Staphylococcus saprophyticus* as a cause of urinary tract infections. *J Clin Microbiol* 1982;6:427–432.
14. Bailey RR. Significance of coagulase-negative Staphylococcus in urine. *J Infect Dis* 1973;127:179–183.
15. Wallmark G, Arremark I, Telander B. *Staphylococcus saprophyticus*: a frequent cause of acute urinary tract infection among female outpatients. *J Infect Dis* 1978; 138:791–794.
16. Lewis JF, Brake SR, Anderson DJ, et al. Urinary tract infection due to coagulase-negative Staphylococcus. *Am J Clin Pathol* 1982;77:736–742.
17. Nicolle LE, Hoban SA, Harding GKM. Characterization of coagulase-negative Staphylococci from urinary isolates. *J Clin Microbiol* 1983;17:267–271.
18. Bryant RE, Sutcliffe MC, McGee FE. Human polymorphonuclear leukocyte function in urine. *Yale J Biol Med* 1973;46:113.
19. Kaye D. Antibacterial activity of human urine. *J Clin Invest* 1968;47:2374–2390.
20. Stamey TA. Urinary tract infections in women. In: Stamey TA, ed. *Pathogenesis and treatment of urinary tract infections.* Baltimore: Williams and Wilkins, 1980; 122–209.
21. Eden CS, Eriksson B, Hanson LA. Adhesion of *Escherichia coli* to human uroepithelial cells in vitro. *Infect Immunol* 1977;18:767–773.
22. Stamey TA, Timothy MM. Studies of introital colo-

nizations in women with recurrent urinary infections. I. The role of vaginal pH. *J Urol* 1975;114:261–265.

23. Parsons DL, Schmidt JD. Control of recurrent lower urinary tract infections in the postmenopausal women. *J Urol* 1982;128:1224.

24. Cox CE, Hinman F. Experiments with induced bacteriuria, vesical emptying and bacterial growth on the mechanism of bladder defense to infection. *J Urol* 1961;86:739.

25. Eckford SD, Keane DP, Lamond E, et al. Hydration monitoring in the prevention of recurrent idiopathic urinary tract infections in pre-menopausal women. *Br J Med* 1995;76:90–93.

26. Orskov I, Ferencz A, Orskov F. Tamm-Horsfall protein or uromucoid is the normal urinary slime that traps type I fimbriated *Escherichia coli*. Lancet 1980;1:887–893.

27. Parsons CL. Prevention of urinary tract infection by the exogenous glycosaminoglycan sodium pentosan-polysulfate. *J Urol* 1982;127:167–169.

28. Parsons CL, Greenspan C, Moore SW, et al. Role of surface mucin in primary antibacterial defense of bladder. *Urology* 1977;9:48–52.

29. Reid G, Sobol JD. Bacterial adherence in the pathogenesis of urinary tract infection: a review. *Rev Infect Dis* 1987;9:470–487.

30. Kallonius G, Mollby R, Svenson SB, et al. The P^k antigen as receptor for the haemagglutinin of pyelonephritic *Escherichia coli*. *FEMS Microbiol Lett* 1980; 7:297.

31. Vaisanen V, Elo J, Tallgreen LG, et al. Mannose-resistant haemagglutination and P antigen recognition are characteristic of *Escherichia coli* causing primary pyelonephritis. *Lancet* 1981;2:1366–1371.

32. Iwahi T, Abe Y, Nakao M, et al. Role of type I fimbriae in the pathogenesis of ascending urinary tract infection induced by *Escherichia coli* in mice. *Infect Immunol* 1983;39:1307–1315.

33. Schaeffer AJ, Jones JM, Dunn JK. Association of in vitro *Escherichia coli* adherence to vaginal and buccal epithelial cells with susceptibility of women to recurrent urinary tract infections. *N Engl J Med* 1981;304: 1062–1066.

34. Schaeffer AJ, Amundsen SK, Schmidt LN. Adherence of *Escherichia coli* to human urinary tract epithelial cells. *Infect Immunol* 1979;24:753–757.

35. Schaeffer AJ, Radvany RM, Chmiel JS. Human leukocyte antigens in women with recurrent urinary tract infections. *J Infect Dis* 1983;148:604–610.

36. Kinane DF, Blackwell CC, Brettle RP, et al. ABO blood group, secretor state and susceptibility to recurrent urinary tract infection in women. *Br Med J* 1982; 285:7–11.

37. Gaffney RA, Schaeffer AJ, Anderson BE, et al. Effect of Lewis blood group antigen on antigen expression on bacterial adherence to COS-1 cells. *Infect Immunol* 1994;62:3022–3026.

38. Hopkins WJ, Heisey DM, Lorentzen DF, et al. A comparative study of major histocompatibility complex and red blood cell antigens phenotypes as risk factors for recurrent urinary tract infections in women. *J Infect Dis* 1998;177:1296–1301.

39. Jantausch BA, Criss VR, O'Donnell R, et al. Association of Lewis blood groups phenotypes with urinary tract infection in children. *J Pediatr* 1994;124: 863–868.

40. May SJ, Blackwell CC, Brettle RP, et al. Non-secretion of ABO blood group antigens: a host factor predisposing to recurrent urinary tract infections and renal scarring. *FEMS Microbiol Immunol* 1989;1(6–7):383–387.

41. Sheinfeld J, Schaeffer AJ, Cordon-Cardo C, et al. Association of the Lewis blood group phenotype with recurrent urinary tract infections in women. *N Engl J Med* 1989;320:773–777.

42. Nicolle LE, Harding GKM, Preiksaitis J, et al. The association of urinary tract infection with sexual intercourse. *J Infect Dis* 1982;146:579–584.

43. Strom BL, Collins M, West SL, et al. Sexual activity, contraceptive use, and other risk factors for symptomatic and asymptomatic bacteriuria. *Ann Intern Med* 1987;107:816–823.

44. Fihn SD, Latham RH, Roberts P, et al. Association between diaphragm use and urinary tract infection. *JAMA* 1985;253:240–244.

45. Foxman B, Frerichs RR. Epidemiology of urinary tract infection. I. Diaphragm use and sexual intercourse. *Am J Public Health* 1985;75:1308–1315.

46. Fihn SD, Johnson L, Pinkstaff C, et al. Diaphragm use and urinary tract infection: analysis of urodynamic and microbiologic factors. *J Urol* 1986;136:853–856.

47. Kass EH. Asymptomatic infections of the urinary tract. *Trans Assoc Am Physicians* 1956;69:56.

48. Kass EH. Bacteriuria and diagnosis of infections of the urinary tract. *Arch Intern Med* 1967;100:709–714.

49. Stamey TA, Govan DE, Palmer JM. The localization and treatment of urinary tract infections: the role of bactericidal urine levels as opposed to serum levels. *Medicine* 1965;44:1–8.

50. Turck M, Goffe B, Petersdorf RG. The urethral catheter and urinary tract infection. *J Urol* 1962;88: 834–837.

51. Thiel G, Spuhler O. Urinary tract infection by catheter and the so-called infectious (episomal) resistance. *Schweiz Med Wochenschr* 1965;95:1155.

52. Fihn SD, Stamm WE. Management of women with acute dysuria. In: Rund D, Wolcott BW, eds. *Emergency medicine annual.* Norwalk, CT: Appleton-Century-Crofts, 1983;2:225.

53. MacDermott RJ. The interpretation of midstream urine microscopy and culture results in women who present acutely to the labour ward. *Br J Obstet Gynecol* 1994; 101:712–713.

54. Stamm WE. Measurement of pyuria and its relation to bacteriuria. *Am J Med* 1983;75:53.

55. Johnson JR, Stamm WE. Diagnosis and treatment of acute urinary tract infection. *Infect Dis Clin North Am* 1987;1:773–779.

56. Free AH, Free HM. Urinalysis: its proper role in the physician's office. *Clin Lab Med* 1986;6:253–259.

57. Wu TC, Williams EC, Koo SY, et al. Evaluation of three bacteriuria screening methods in a clinical research hospital. *J Clin Microbiol* 1985;21:796–814.

58. Kunin CM. *Detection, prevention and management of urinary tract infection,* 4th ed. Philadelphia: Lea & Febiger, 1987:195–234.

59. Schaeffer AJ. The office laboratory. *Urol Clin North Am* 1980;7:29–58.

60. Reid G. The office microbiology laboratory. *Urol Clin North Am* 1986;13:569–576.

61. Bixler-Forell E, Bertram MA, Bruckner DA. Clinical evaluation of three rapid methods for the detection of

significant bacteriuria. *J Clin Microbiol* 1985;22: 62–68.

62. Needham CA. Rapid detection methods in microbiology: are they right for your office? *Med Clin North Am* 1987;71:591–605.

63. Kraft JK, Stamey TA. The natural history of symptomatic recurrent bacteriuria in women. *Medicine* 1977;56:55–61.

64. Mabeck CE. Studies in urinary tract infections. I. The diagnosis of bacteriuria in women. *Acta Med Scand* 1969;186:35–41.

65. Kunz HH, Sieberth HG, Freiberg J, et al. Zur Bedeutung der Blasenpunktion fur den sicheren Nachweis einer Bacteriurie. *Dtsch Med Wochenschr* 1975;100: 2252.

66. Stamm WE, Counts GW, Running KR, et al. Diagnosis of coliform infection in acutely dysuric women. *N Engl J Med* 1982;307:463–467.

67. Kass EH. The role of asymptomatic bacteriuria in the pathogenesis of pyelonephritis. In: Quinn EL, Kass EH, eds. *Biology of pyelonephritis.* Boston: Little, Brown, 1960:399.

68. Lifshitz E, Kramer L. Outpatient urine culture: does collection technique matter? *Arch Intern Med* 2000; 160:2537–2540.

69. Fowler JE Jr, Pulaski T. Excretory urography, cystography, and cystoscopy in the evaluation of women with urinary tract infection. *N Engl J Med* 1981;304: 462–468.

70. Engel G, Schaeffer AJ, Grayhack JT, et al. The role of excretory urography and cystoscopy in the evaluation and management of women with recurrent urinary tract infection. *J Urol* 1980;123:190–198.

71. DeLange HE, Jones B. Unnecessary intravenous urography in young women with recurrent urinary tract infections. *Clin Radiol* 1983;34:551–556.

72. Fair WR, McClennan BL, Jost RG. Are excretory urograms necessary in evaluating women with urinary tract infections? *J Urol* 1979;121:313.

73. Mogensen P, Hansen LK. Do intravenous urography and cystoscopy provide important information in otherwise healthy women with recurrent urinary tract infection? *Br J Urol* 1983;55:261.

74. Newhouse JH, Rhea JT, Murphy RX, et al. Yield of screening urography in young women with urinary tract infection. *Urol Radiol* 1982;4:187.

75. Tanagho EA, Miller ER, Lyon HP, et al. Spastic striated external sphincter and urinary tract infection in girls. *Br J Urol* 1971;43:69.

76. Gallagher DJ, Montgomerie JZ, North JD. Acute infections of the urinary tract and the urethral syndrome in general practice. *Br Med J* 1965;1:622.

77. Gillespie WA, Henderson EP, Linton KB, et al. Microbiology of the urethral (frequency and dysuria) syndrome: a controlled study with 5 year review. *Br J Urol* 1989;64:270–274.

78. Bergman A, Karram MM, Bhatia NN. Urethral syndrome: a comparison of different treatment modalities. *J Reprod Med* 1989;34:157–160.

79. Stamm WE, Running K, McKevitt M, et al. Treatment of acute urethral syndrome. *N Engl J Med* 1981;304: 956–960.

80. Sobota AE. Inhibition of bacterial adherence by cranberry juice: potential use for the treatment of urinary tract infections. *J Urol* 1984;131:1013–1017.

81. Kunin CM, Finland M. Clinical pharmacology of the tetracycline antibiotics. *Clin Pharmacol Ther* 1961; 2:51.

82. Francke EL, Neu HC. Chloramphenicol and tetracyclines. *Med Clin North Am* 1987;71:1155–1168.

83. Parsons CL. Urinary tract infections in the female patient. *Urol Clin North Am* 1985;12:355–361.

84. Reed MD, Blumer JL. Urologic pharmacology in the office setting. *Urol Clin North Am* 1988;15:737–751.

85. Conklin JD. The pharmacokinetics of nitrofurantoin and its related bioavailability. *Antimicrob Agents Chemother* 1978;25:233–237.

86. Mayrer AR, Andriole VT. Urinary tract antiseptics. *Med Clin North Am* 1982;66:199–216.

87. Hoener B, Patterson SE. Nitrofurantoin disposition. *Clin Pharmacol Ther* 1981;29:808–815.

88. Kalowski S, Rudford N, Kincaid-Smith P. Crystalline and macrocrystalline nitrofurantoin in the treatment of urinary tract infection. *N Engl J Med* 1974;290:385–389.

89. Reed MD, Besunder JB, Blumer JL. Sulfonamides. In: Koren G, Prober CG, Gold R, eds. *Antimicrobial therapy in infants and children.* New York: Marcel Dekker, 1988:153–172.

90. Weinstein L, Madoff MA, Samet CM. The sulfonamides. *N Engl J Med* 1960;263:793–801.

91. Hooper DC, Wolfson JS. The fluoroquinolones: pharmacology, clinical uses and toxicities in humans. *Antimicrob Agents Chemother* 1985;28:716–722.

92. Neu HC. Quinolones: a new class of antimicrobial agents with wide potential uses. *Med Clin North Am* 1988;72:623–636.

93. Wise R, Griggs D, Andrews JM. Pharmokinetics of the quinolones in volunteers: a proposed dosing schedule. *Rev Infect Dis* 1988;10[Suppl 1]:S83–S89.

94. Wolfson JS, Hooper DC. The fluoroquinolones: structures, mechanisms of action and resistance, and spectra of activity in vitro. *Antimicrob Agents Chemother* 1985;28:581–590.

95. Childs SJ, Goldstein EJ. Ciprofloxacin as treatment for genitourinary tract infection. *J Urol* 1989;141:1–5.

96. Goldstein EJ, Alpert ML, Najem A. Norfloxacin in the treatment of complicated and uncomplicated urinary tract infections: a comparative multicenter trial. *Am J Med* 1987;82:65–69.

97. Lee C, Ronald AN. Norfloxacin: its potential in clinical practice. *Am J Med* 1987;82:27–34.

98. Guttmann D. Follow-up of urinary tract infection in domiciliary patients. In: Brumfitt W, Asscher AW, eds. *Urinary tract infection.* London: Oxford University Press, 1973:62.

99. Mabeck CE. Treatment of uncomplicated urinary tract infection in non-pregnant women. *Postgrad Med* 1972;48:69–81.

100. Zhanel GG, Handing GRM, Guay DRP. Asymptomatic bacteriuria: which patients should be treated? *Arch Intern Med* 1990;150:1389–1396.

101. Andreole VT, Patterson TF. Epidemiology, natural history, and management of urinary tract infections in pregnancy. *Med Clin North Am* 1991;75:359–373.

102. Kass EH, Platt R. Urinary tract and genital mycoplasmal infection. In: Wald NJ, ed. *Antenatal and neonatal screening,* 1st ed. New York: Oxford University Press, 1984:345–357.

103. Platt R. Adverse consequences of acute urinary tract infections in adults. *Am J Med* 1987;82[Suppl 6B]:47–52.

104. Evans DA, Kass EH, Hennekens CH, et al. Bacteriuria and subsequent mortality in women. *Lancet* 1982;1: 156–161.

105. Fihn SD. Single-dose antimicrobial therapy for urinary tract infections: "less is more?" or "reductio ad absurdum?" *J Gen Intern Med* 1986;1:62–65.

106. Brumfitt W, Faiers MC, Franklin INS. The treatment of urinary infection by means of a single dose of cephaloxidine. *Postgrad Med* 1970;46:65–72.

107. Buckwold FJ, Ludwid P, Godfrey KM, et al. Therapy for acute cystitis in adult women: randomized comparison of single-dose sulfasoxazole vs trimethoprim-sulfamethoxazole. *JAMA* 1982;247:1839–1843.

108. Rubin RH, Fang LST, Jones SR, et al. Single-dose amoxicillin therapy for urinary tract infection. *JAMA* 1980;244:561–564.

109. Greenberg RN, Sanders CV, Lewis AC, et al. Single-dose cefaclor therapy of urinary tract infection: evaluation of antibody-coated bacteria test and C-reactive protein assay as predictors of cure. *Am J Med* 1981;71: 841–847.

110. Bailey RR, Abbott GD. Treatment of urinary tract infection with a single dose of amoxicillin. *Nephron* 1977;18:316–321.

111. Ireland D, Tacchi D, Bint AJ. Effect of single-dose prophylactic cotrimoxazole on the incidence of gynaecological postoperative urinary tract infection. *Br J Obstet Gynaecol* 1982;89:578–585.

112. Tolkoff-Rubin NE, Weber D, Fang LST, et al. Single dose therapy with trimethoprim-sulfamethoxazole for urinary tract infection in women. *Rev Infect Dis* 1982; 4:443–447.

113. Fang LST, Tolkoff-Rubin NE, Rubin RH. Efficacy of single-dose and conventional amoxicillin therapy in urinary tract infection localized by the antibody-coated bacteria technic. *N Engl J Med* 1978;298:413–418.

114. Fihn SD, Johnson C, Roberts PL, et al. Trimethoprim-sulfamethoxazole for acute dysuria in women: a double-blind, randomized trial of single-dose versus 10-day treatment. *Ann Intern Med* 1988;108:350–357.

115. Ronald AR, Boutros P, Mourtada H. Bacteriuria localization and response to single-dose therapy in women. *JAMA* 1976;235:1854–1858.

116. Hooten TM, Winter C, Tiu F, et al. Randomized comparative trial and cost analysis of 3-day antimicrobial regiments for treatment of acute cystitis in women. *JAMA* 1995;273:41–45.

117. Saint S, Scholes D, Fihn SD, et al. The effectiveness of a clinical practice guideline for the management of presumed uncomplicated urinary tract infection in women. *Am J Med* 1999;106:636–641.

118. Wathne B, Hovelius B, Mardh PA. Causes of frequency and dysuria in women. *Scand J Infect Dis* 1987;19:223.

119. Kraft JK, Stamey TA. The natural history of symptomatic recurrent bacteriuria in women. *Medicine* 1977; 56:55–64.

120. Stamm WE, McKevitt M, Counts GW, et al. Is antimicrobial prophylaxis of urinary tract infections cost effective? *Ann Intern Med* 1981;94:251–256.

121. Nicolle LE, Ronald AR. Recurrent urinary tract infections in adult women. *Infect Dis Clin North Am* 1987;1:793–814.

122. Stamey TA, Condy M, Mihara G. Prophylactic efficacy of nitrofurantoin macrocrystals and trimetho-prim-sulfamethoxazole in urinary infections: biologic effects on the vaginal and rectal flora. *N Engl J Med* 1977;296:780–788.

123. Martinez FC, Kindrachuk RW, Thomas E, et al. Effect of prophylactic low dose cephalexin on fecal and vaginal bacteria. *J Urol* 1985;133:994–998.

124. Stamm WE, Counts GW, McKevitt M, et al. Urinary prophylaxis with trimethoprim and trimethoprim-sulfamethoxazole: efficacy, influence on the natural history of recurrent bacteriuria, and cost control. *Rev Infect Dis* 1982;4:450–461.

125. Stamey TA, Condy M. The diffusion and concentration of trimethoprim in human vaginal fluid. *J Infect Dis* 1975;131:261–268.

126. Sabbaj J, Hoagland VL, Shih WJ. Multiclinic comparative study of norfloxacin and trimethoprim-sulfamethoxazole for treatment of urinary tract infections. *Antimicrob Agents Chemother* 1985;27:297–302.

127. Schaeffer AJ, Stuppy BA. Efficacy and safety of self-start therapy in women with recurrent urinary tract infections. *J Urol* 1999;161:207–211.

128. Gupta K, Hooton TM, Roberts PL, et al. Patient-initiated treatment of uncomplicated recurrent urinary tract infections in young women. *Ann Intern Med* 2001;135:9–16.

129. Wong ES, McKevitt M, Running K, et al. Management of recurrent urinary tract infections with patient-administered single-dose therapy. *Ann Intern Med* 1985; 102:302–309.

130. Vosti KL. Recurrent urinary tract infections: prevention by prophylactic antibiotics after sexual intercourse. *JAMA* 1975;231:934–938.

131. Pfau A, Sacks T, Englestein D. Recurrent urinary tract infections in premenopausal women: prophylaxis based on an understanding of the pathogenesis. *J Urol* 1983; 129:1152–1160.

132. Melekos MD, Asbach HW, Gerharz E, et al. Post-intercourse versus daily ciprofloxacin prophylaxis for recurrent urinary tract infections in premenopausal women. *J Urol* 1997;157:935–939.

133. Raz R, Stamm WE. A controlled trial of intravaginal estriol in postmenopausal women with recurrent urinary tract infections. *N Engl J Med* 1993;320:753–756.

134. Eriksen BC. A randomized, open, parallel-group study on the preventive effect of an estradiol-releasing vaginal ring (Estring) on recurrent urinary tract infections in postmenopausal women. *Am J Obstet Gynecol* 1999;180:1072–1079.

135. Kreger DE, Creven DE, Carling PC, et al. Gram negative bacteremia. III. Reassessment of etiology, epidemiology and ecology in 612 patients. *Am J Med* 1980;68:332–338.

136. Platt R, Polk BF, Murdock B, et al. Mortality associated with nosocomial urinary tract infection. *N Engl J Med* 1982;307:736–745.

137. Tambyah PA, Maki DG. A prospective study of 1497 catheterized patients. *Arch Intern Med* 2000;160: 678–682.

138. Garibaldi RA, Burke JP, Dickman ML, et al. Factors predisposing to bacteriuria during indwelling urethral catheterization. *N Engl J Med* 1974;291:215–221.

139. Garibaldi RA, Burke JP, Britt MR, et al. Meatal colonization and catheter-associated bacteriuria. *N Engl J Med* 1980;303:316–321.

140. Tambyah PA, Halvorson KT, Maki DG. A prospective

study of pathogenesis of catheter-associated urinary tract infections. *Mayo Clin Proc* 1999;74:131–136.

141. Wong ES, Hooton TM. Guidelines to prevention of catheter-associated urinary tract infection. *Infect Control* 1980;2:125–136.

142. Burke JP, Jacobson JA, Garibaldi RA, et al. Evaluation of daily meatal care with poly-antibiotic ointment in prevention of urinary catheter-associated bacteriuria. *J Urol* 1983;129:331–334.

143. Burke JP, Garibaldi RA, Britt MR, et al. Prevention of catheter-associated urinary tract infections. *Am J Med* 1981;70:655–661.

144. Warren JW, Platt R, Thomas RJ, et al. Antibiotic irrigation and catheter-associated urinary tract infections. *N Engl J Med* 1978;299:570–576.

145. Britt MR, Garibaldi RA, Miller WA, et al. Antimicro-bial prophylaxis for catheter-associated bacteriuria. *Antimicrob Agent Chemother* 1977;11:240–246.

146. Cundiff GW, McLennan MT, Bent AE. Randomized trial of antibiotic prophylaxis for combined urodynamics and cystourethroscopy. *Obstet Gynecol* 1999;93:749–752.

147. Kuhlemeier K, Stover SL, Lloyd LK. Prophylactic antibacterial therapy for preventing urinary tract infections in spinal cord injury patients. *J Urol* 1985;134:514–518.

148. Little PJ, McPherson DR, Wardener HE. The appearance of the intravenous pyelogram during and after pyelonephritis. *Lancet* 1965;1:1186–1190.

149. Silver TM, Kass EM, Thornburg JR, et al. The radiological spectrum of acute pyelonephritis in adults and adolescents. *Radiology* 1976;118:65–69.

150. Ronald AR. Optimal duration of treatment for kidney infection. *Ann Intern Med* 1987;106:467–468.

Ostergard's Urogynecology and Pelvic Floor Dysfunction, Fifth Edition. edited by A.E. Bent, et al. Lippincott Williams & Wilkins, Philadelphia © 2003.

19

Urinary Retention and Overflow Incontinence

Michelle M. Germain

Greater Baltimore Medical Center, Towson, Maryland

The lower urinary tract has two main functions: storage and elimination of urine. Overflow incontinence, as defined by the International Continence Society (ICS), is the involuntary loss of urine associated with overdistention of the bladder (1). The term overdistention, however, has not been clearly defined. Overflow incontinence results from voiding dysfunction and urinary retention caused by abnormalities of bladder elimination. Overflow incontinence is one end point on a continuum from voiding dysfunction to urinary retention.

As with most types of lower urinary tract dysfunction, it is difficult to determine the true incidence of urinary retention and overflow incontinence because of variation in study populations and definitions. Gender differences are also difficult to determine accurately, but there is a higher incidence of urinary retention and overflow incontinence due to urethral obstruction in men, secondary to prostatic hypertrophy. The literature on female overflow incontinence remains sparse. Most likely, this is because the true clinical problem is urinary retention and its associated morbid sequelae and not the incontinence (2). In this chapter, the clinical presentation, evaluation, etiology, and management options of urinary retention and overflow incontinence are presented.

SYMPTOMS

Patients with overflow incontinence have a variety of urinary symptoms. They may report urine loss without awareness, intermittent dribbling of urine, or constant wetness. In some cases, these women may report symptoms consistent with stress incontinence and urine loss with position change. These patients often report frequent urinary tract infections, presumably secondary to large residual urine volumes. In addition, the urinary retention can precipitate symptoms of voiding dysfunction, including difficulty initiating urination; a weak, slow, or intermittent stream; a sensation of incomplete emptying; and the need to strain or use suprapubic pressure to void.

It is important to remember, however, that history alone may not be an accurate tool in determining the etiology of incontinence. Symptoms of voiding difficulty are not always a reliable guide to the final urodynamic diagnosis or to the severity of the voiding dysfunction. One study reported that the most valuable symptoms for the prediction of voiding dysfunction are poor urinary stream, incomplete bladder emptying, straining to void, and nocturia (3).

EVALUATION

For any patient with lower urinary tract complaints, a thorough history and physical examination, with a pelvic examination, neurologic examination, 24-hour voiding diary, urinalysis and urine culture, and measurement of the postvoid residual urine volume, are essential. A firm definition of abnormal volumes for postvoid residual urine has not been universally accepted. A postvoid residual urine volume less than or equal to 50 mL is considered normal, whereas a residual urine volume above 200 mL is unquestionably abnormal and consistent with urinary retention. However, it is the significance of volumes between 50 and 199 mL that is debated (4). Perhaps more important than the absolute volume of the residual is the percentage of the total bladder volume the residual represents. A postvoid residual of 100 mL is of much more concern if the voided volume is only 50 mL, compared with a 100-mL residual if the voided volume is 300 mL. A postvoid residual of 25% of the total bladder volume is an acceptable residual.

Complaints of constantly feeling wet and of urine loss without awareness suggest the presence of a fistula or an ectopic ureter, which is located beyond the urethral continence mechanism; in these cases, cystourethroscopy is necessary. In addition, evaluation of bladder capacity and bladder wall compliance, with multichannel urodynamic equipment, is essential. Voiding function should also be investigated, whether by uroflowmetry, pressure voiding studies, or voiding cystourethrography. Finally, because urinary retention, decreased bladder compliance, and increased intravesical pressure can result in ureteral reflux, it is crucial to image the kidneys and ureters to rule out hydronephrosis, either by ultrasound or intravenous pyelography. In most cases, urinary retention and overflow incontinence indicate underlying major pathology; thus, after the diagnosis is made, careful investigation for the etiology is imperative.

ETIOLOGY

The normal act of micturition involves urethral relaxation followed by detrusor contraction. Voiding is centrally controlled in the pontine and sacral micturition centers. Impaired bladder emptying may occur as a result of defective functioning in the central or pe-

TABLE 19.1. *Causes of overflow incontinence*

Urinary retention
Iatrogenic
Surgery
Obstetric trauma
Infectious
Neurologic
Cerebral cortical lesions
Spinal cord trauma
Nerve root damage
Demyelinating diseases
Peripheral neuropathy
Anatomic urethral obstruction
Extrinsic compression
Pharmacologic
Psychiatric disorders
Decreased bladder compliance
Urethral sphincter dysfunction

ripheral nervous systems or in the genital and lower urinary tracts.

In women, urinary retention is the major cause of overflow incontinence; there are both acute and chronic causes of urinary retention. If the acute causes are not promptly resolved, more permanent damage can result, presumably because the detrusor muscle, or the parasympathetic ganglia in the bladder wall, becomes compromised. In cases of chronic urinary retention, there is special concern for the increased intravesical pressure causing ureteral reflux, upper urinary tract disease, and a reduction in renal function. The following is a discussion of the various conditions that can lead to urinary retention, as outlined in Table 19.1.

Iatrogenic

Postoperative and postpartum patients account for the major proportion of women with acute urinary retention. This phenomenon may result from bladder trauma and edema secondary to surgery or obstetric delivery, epidural anesthesia, narcotic pain medications, pelvic nerve stretching or trauma, pelvic hematoma, or episiotomy and abdominal incision pain, especially for patients who void mainly by Valsalva maneuver.

Any type of pelvic reconstructive surgery or antiincontinence surgery can cause urinary retention postoperatively, whether from tissue edema, pain resulting in the inability to relax the pelvic floor, or bladder outlet obstruction. Women identified preoperatively with a history of urinary retention or abnormal voiding mechanisms, such as Valsalva voiding or detrusor hyporeflexia, are at higher risk for postoperative voiding difficulty (5). Many postoperative problems and patients' anxieties can be relieved by adequate preoperative education of all patients. It is often easiest to teach patients intermittent catheterization preoperatively, when discomfort and anxiety are at a minimum. Postoperative urinary retention usually improves with time and adequate bladder drainage.

Infectious

Severe dysuria, either because of urethritis or cystitis, can be associated with acute urinary retention. Infection and inflammation of the bladder and urethra may interfere with the normal micturition reflex. Acute urinary retention may also occur in women with primary anogenital herpes simplex virus infections. This may be secondary to pain or pelvic neuritis involving the bladder (6). Herpes zoster has also been implicated in urinary retention, presumably as a result of invasion of the sacral spinal ganglia by the virus (7).

Neurologic Disease

Neurologic disease is one of the most common causes of urinary retention in women. In fact, voiding dysfunction may be the first indication of neurologic disease. However, the severity of urinary symptoms does not necessarily correlate with the degree of urinary tract dysfunction (8). When evaluating women for neurologic causes of urinary retention, it is important to remember that the location of the lesions in the nervous system (brain, spinal cord, or peripheral and autonomic nerves) determines the degree and characteristics of the voiding dysfunction.

The pontine micturition center, located in the brain stem, controls the motor neuronal input to the bladder and external urethral sphincter and coordinates voluntary voiding. Input from suprapontine centers is mainly inhibitory. Lesions above the brain stem cause loss of inhibition to the pontine micturition center, and detrusor hyperreflexia can result. The duration of a detrusor contraction is controlled by efferent fibers from the brain stem to the sacral micturition center. Disruption of the spinal pathway from the brain stem to the sacral micturition center causes detrusor hyperreflexia and detrusor sphincter dyssynergia, simultaneous contraction of the bladder and external urethral sphincter.

The sacral micturition center is located at S-2 through S-4 and allows the bladder to contract without cortical or pontine input. Patients with interruption of this pathway lose motor and sensory control of the bladder. They classically have detrusor areflexia with impaired sensation and thus develop high-volume, high-compliance bladders with overflow incontinence. Lumbosacral disc disease, lesions of the sacral spinal cord or nerve roots, and "spinal shock" secondary to trauma can cause these voiding abnormalities. Nontraumatic conditions include spinal cord tumors, vascular disease, and demyelinating diseases, like multiple sclerosis.

Peripheral innervation of the lower urinary tract is through the pudendal, pelvic, and hypogastric nerves. The autonomic nerves, with afferent fibers through S-2 to S-4, carry information from tension receptors and nociceptors within the bladder wall to initiate micturition. The pudendal nerves carry somatic input from S-2 through S-4 to the external sphincter and pelvic floor muscles and provide the circuitry for coordination of detrusor and urethral muscular activity during voiding. The pelvic nerves, from S-2 through S-4, carry parasympathetic efferent fibers to the bladder for the principle excitatory input necessary for micturition. The hypogastric nerves carry efferent sympathetic fibers from T-11 through L-2 to the bladder and urethra. The hypogastric nerves provide inhibitory input to the bladder and excitatory input to the urethra, thus promoting urine storage. In addition to spinal cord lesions discussed in the previous paragraph, diseases that result in peripheral neuropathy, such as diabetes, hypothyroidism, alcoholism, and tabes dorsalis secondary to syphilis, can destroy the coordinating functions of the peripheral nerves. Patients with these diseases can have loss of sensation and bladder contractility. Depending on the extent of the peripheral nerve damage, the pelvic floor and external sphincter may also be affected, resulting in detrusor sphincter dyssynergia and obstructive voiding symptoms or uninhibited urethral relaxation.

Anatomic Urethral Obstruction

Bladder neck obstruction is an uncommon cause of urinary retention and overflow incontinence in women. However, there have been reports of pelvic tumors, both benign leiomyomas and malignant neoplasms, that compressed and obstructed the urethra. Vaginal mesonephric or paramesonephric remnant cysts have been reported to cause obstruction (9). There has also been a report of bladder neck obstruction due to circular smooth muscle hypertrophy, although the underlying etiology of this was not addressed (10). Chronic inflammation can result in urethral stricture, as can prior surgery for urethral diverticula or fistula repair.

Additionally, malposition of the uterus and vagina can cause significant problems. An entrapped, retroverted, gravid, or nongravid uterus can result in urethral obstruction (11). Women with uterovaginal prolapse can also have voiding dysfunction, diminished peak flow rates, and elevated postvoid residuals, which are most likely due to urethral kinking. This obstruction is usually intermittent and is relieved when the patient reduces the prolapse or lies down. The sever-

ity of voiding dysfunction does not always correlate with the severity of the prolapse. Rosenzweig and colleagues found that women with large cystoceles did not have significantly different voiding patterns from those with small cystoceles (12). However, Gardy and associates demonstrated that the dysfunctional voiding seen in women with significant genital prolapse often resolves when the prolapse is surgically repaired (13). Even though genital prolapse can cause some voiding dysfunction, acute urinary retention is rare (14).

Pharmacologic Agents

A number of medications for cardiovascular, neurologic, psychological, and allergic disorders can affect voiding function. These drugs can affect bladder contractility and urethral resistance. In patients with preexisting voiding disorders, the addition of one of these drugs can lead to significant urinary retention (15).

Agents with anticholinergic properties, including neuroleptics, anticonvulsants, phenothiazines, antidepressants, and medications for Parkinson's disease, can cause urinary retention. In addition, these agents have been associated with frequency, hesitancy, and irritative bladder symptoms. Morphine by epidural or parenteral administration is a well-known cause of urinary retention, most likely owing to its detrusor relaxant effects. An α-adrenergic agonist, such as ephedrine, can impair bladder emptying by increasing urethral resistance. Diospyramide, an antiarrythmic, and pindolol, a β-blocking agent, can also cause retention. Finally, there are a number of chemotherapeutic agents that can cause peripheral neuropathy, resulting in impaired bladder function. These include vincristine and cisplatin.

Psychiatric Disorders

Urinary retention resulting from psychiatric disorders is difficult to diagnose and should be considered a diagnosis of exclusion. Urodynamics with electromyography can aid in the diagnosis. This type of urinary retention can be seen with conversion disorders, hysteria, and depression, to name a few. Voiding dysfunction is thought to result from subconscious inhibition, by the central nervous system, of normal detrusor and urethral function. However, psychotropic drugs, such as tricyclic antidepressants, must be excluded as a contributing factor (3).

Bladder and Urethral Dysfunction

Injury to the bladder wall as a result of radiation therapy, surgery, or inflammation can result in a small-volume, low-compliance bladder. Decreased bladder compliance places the upper urinary tract at high risk secondary to vesicoureteral reflux and chronic pyelonephritis; this may subsequently lead to renal failure (16). The loss of bladder wall compliance results in an increase in intravesical pressure with increased volume, although the bladder volume may not be excessive. Eventually, the intravesical pressure exceeds the intraurethral pressure, and urinary incontinence results (2). Finally, in women with intrinsic sphincter deficiency, overflow incontinence can occur at lower bladder volumes, before the bladder is technically overdistended. In these women, intravesical pressure exceeds resting urethral pressure at smaller bladder volumes than in women with normal urethral function or urethral obstruction.

TREATMENT

Acute Urinary Retention

In patients presenting with acute urinary retention, the immediate treatment should be bladder drainage. Because of the risk for bladder hemorrhage, hypotension, and postobstructive diuresis, rapid bladder decompression is usually discouraged. However, in review of the literature from 1920 to 1997, no studies were found to support this practice; in fact, most studies supported quick and complete drainage of the bladder. In cases in which one of the complications described ear-

lier did occur, the complication was not clinically significant (17). There are no randomized trials comparing rapid and gradual bladder drainage. In most cases, continuous drainage, by Foley catheter or intermittent self-catheterization (ISC), may be necessary until bladder function normalizes, usually within 48 to 72 hours. The numerous advantages to ISC are discussed later. One main advantage of ISC in women with an episode of acute urinary retention is that the voiding trials can be done before self-catheterization. For short-term bladder drainage, antibiotic therapy is not necessary unless there is a documented urinary tract infection.

Chronic Urinary Retention

In cases of chronic urinary retention, intervention is essential if the patient has recurrent urinary tract infections or evidence of upper tract disease. Additionally, patients with irritative bladder symptoms or urinary incontinence may seek medical evaluation and request medical intervention to relieve these symptoms.

Long-term management of patients with urinary retention should be directed at preventing renal damage and correcting the underlying cause of urinary retention, by normalizing voiding and urethral pressures. All urinary tract infections should be treated before initiating a diagnostic evaluation and proceeding with other therapy for urinary retention. More specific therapeutic interventions are outlined in Table 19.2 and discussed in the following sections.

TABLE 19.2. *Treatment of overflow incontinence and urinary retention*

Acute urinary retention
  Bladder drainage
  Antibiotic therapy
Chronic urinary retention
  Pharmacologic agents
  Intermittent self-catheterization
  Sacral root neuromodulation
  Behavioral modification
  Surgical intervention

Pharmacologic Therapy

Pharmacologic treatment should be initiated only after urodynamic evaluation. Urinary retention due to detrusor hypoactivity or areflexia is difficult to treat. Most studies with pharmacologic agents are uncontrolled, and there are contradictory results reported about their efficacy. Drugs to increase intravesical pressure, cholinergic agonists, and β-adrenergic antagonists have not proved effective. Acetylcholine agonists are promoted as detrusor contractility enhancers. These drugs have been used with limited success, most likely because they do not increase the strength of detrusor contractions but merely increase the resting tone of the detrusor muscle (18). Bethanechol chloride has both muscarinic and nicotinic effects. It has been a longstanding drug in the treatment of retention; however, controlled studies have not proved it beneficial in the treatment of urinary retention (19).

For women with detrusor hyperreflexia, the goal is to obtain a sustained and coordinated detrusor contraction at the time of desired micturition and to decrease outlet resistance in the presence of detrusor sphincter dyssynergia. Parasympathomimetic drugs have been used, including anticholinergic agents, smooth muscle relaxants, calcium-channel blockers, and β-adrenergic agonists. Tricyclic antidepressants may also be used, although these do have α-agonist properties and thus may increase urethral tone. However, in patients with decreased bladder compliance or urethral sphincter dysfunction, tricyclic antidepressants are the drug of first choice. In cases of detrusor–sphincter dyssynergia, skeletal sphincter spasm is most commonly seen with detrusor hyperreflexia. Diazepam can be used in these patients to decrease outlet resistance. α-Adrenergic blocking agents, like prazosin hydrochloride and phenoxybenzamine, have been used to decrease the contractility of the smooth muscle component of the urethral sphincter (20). Once again, however, the reports on clinical efficacy of α-blockers are contradictory.

Intermittent Self-catheterization

Continuous bladder catheter drainage is best avoided in cases of urinary retention because of the high complication rate from infections, ulcerations, calculi, malignancies, and bladder spasms. Over the long term, permanent drainage can result in a small-volume low-compliance bladder, with subsequent upper urinary tract damage (21). Intermittent catheterization is a much less morbid treatment intervention and is an acceptable option for women with sufficient mobility and manual dexterity. The incidence of cystitis is low and, if necessary, can be controlled by antibiotic prophylaxis. Bacteriuria is common in patients using catheterization for extended periods of time; however, only symptomatic infections should be treated.

Sacral Root Neuromodulation

Sacral neuromodulation is a U.S. Food and Drug Administration–approved treatment option for refractory bladder storage and voiding dysfunction (see Chapter 22). It is indicated for the treatment of nonobstructive chronic urinary retention. One study of 20 patients reported an improvement in the voided volumes and in the postvoid residual volumes after implantation. Urodynamic evaluation of the patients revealed almost complete normalization of voided volumes, flow rates, and residual volumes. The mean length of follow-up was 15.17 months (22). The exact mechanism of action is not known; however, in patients with retention, neuromodulation may assist in relaxing the pelvic floor and initiating micturition.

Behavior Modification

Patients with urinary retention can use a number of simple techniques to decrease the likelihood of elevated residual urine volume. The patient should be instructed to void in the sitting position, not in the squatting position, because this posture does not facilitate adequate relaxation of the pelvic floor. Patients should be educated about normal voiding mechanisms and instructed to relax the muscles of the pelvic floor. Because constipation can lead to bladder dysfunction, every attempt should be made to prevent this. Finally, the double-voiding technique, which requires two episodes of micturition a few minutes apart, can be very helpful for patients with large postvoid residual urine volumes.

In patients with hypotonic bladders, timed voiding is a very useful maneuver to decrease the likelihood of incontinence. The patients are instructed to void on a preset schedule regardless of their bladder sensation. This schedule is usually every 2 to 3 hours, depending on their frequency of incontinent episodes. This concept of scheduled voiding can also be used in patients who have overflow incontinence due to decreased bladder compliance and low urethral pressure. With this technique, the bladder volume is never allowed to reach the volume at which bladder pressure exceeds urethral pressure, and thus incontinence is avoided.

Finally, in patients with detrusor areflexia, application of manual pressure over the bladder, with or without Valsalva maneuver, can facilitate bladder emptying. However, some clinicians do not advocate this technique because of the possibility of vesicoureteral reflux (21) with increased detrusor pressure.

Surgical Intervention

In cases of detrusor areflexia, there are two therapeutic options. Although still under study, reduction cystoplasty has been used in some patients with excessively large bladders. Urinary diversion has been used in patients with progressive upper tract disease, presumably resulting from vesicoureteral reflux.

Conversely, patients with detrusor hyperreflexia may be treated with a number of surgical procedures, such as peripheral bladder denervation, selected sacral nerve resection, and augmentation cystoplasty, if more conservative options have failed. These procedures have not been widely studied, however.

REFERENCES

1. Abrams P, Blaivas JG, Stanton SL, et al. The standardization of terminology of lower urinary tract function recommended by the International Continence Society. *Int Urogynecol J* 1990;1:45–58.
2. Richardson DA. Overflow incontinence and urinary retention. *Clin Obstet Gynecol* 1990;33:378–381.
3. Dwyer PL, Desmedt E. Impaired bladder emptying in women. *Aust N Z J Obstet Gynecol* 1994;34:73–78.
4. Urinary Incontinence Guideline Panel. *Urinary incontinence in adults.* Clinical Practice Guideline. Rockville, MD: U.S. Department of Health and Human Services. AHCPR Publication No. 92-0038. March 1992.
5. Bhatia NN, Bergman A. Use of preoperative uroflowmetry and simultaneous urethrocystometry for predicting risk of prolonged postoperative bladder drainage. *Urology* 1986;28:440–445.
6. Person DA, Kaufman RH, Gardner HL, et al. Herpes virus type 2 in genitourinary tract infections. *Am J Obstet Gynecol* 1973;116:993–995.
7. Patel BR, Rivner MH. Herpes zoster causing acute urinary retention. *South Med J* 1988;81:929–930.
8. Nitti VW. Evaluation of the female with neurogenic voiding dysfunction. *Int Urogynecol J* 1999;10:119–129.
9. Muram D, Jerkins GR. Urinary retention secondary to a Gartner's duct cyst. *Obstet Gynecol* 1988;72:510–511.
10. Diokno AC, Hollander JB, Bennett CJ. Bladder neck obstruction in women: a real entity. *J Urol* 1984;132:294–298.
11. Nelson MS. Acute urinary retention secondary to an incarcerated gravid uterus. *Am J Emerg Med* 1986;4:321–322.
12. Rosenzweig BA, Soffici AR, Thomas S, et al. Urodynamic evaluation of voiding in women with cystoceles. *J Reprod Med* 1992;37:162–166.
13. Gardy M, Kozminski M, DeLancy J, et al. Stress incontinence and cystoceles. *J Urol* 1991;145:1211–1213.
14. Theofrastous JP, Swift SE. The clinical evaluation of pelvic floor dysfunction. *Obstet Gynecol Clin* 1998;25:783–804.
15. Steele AC, Kohli N, Mallipeddi P, et al. Pharmacologic causes of female incontinence. *Int Urogynecol J* 1999;10:106–110.
16. McGuire EJ. Editorial: bladder compliance. *J Urol* 1994;151:965–966.
17. Nyman MA, Schwenk NM, Silverstein MD. Management of urinary retention: rapid versus gradual decompression and risk of complications. *Mayo Clin Proc* 1997;72:951–956.
18. Wein AJ. Pharmacologic treatment of incontinence. *J Am Geriatr Soc* 1990;38:317–325.
19. Finkbeiner AE. Is bethanechol chloride clinically effective in promoting bladder emptying? A literature review. *J Urol* 1985;134:443–449.
20. Tammela T. Prevention of prolonged voiding problems after unexpected postoperative urinary retention: a comparison of phenoxybenzamine and carbachol. *J Urol* 1986;136:1254–1257.
21. Madersbacher H. The various types of neurogenic bladder dysfunction: an update of current therapeutic concepts. *Paraplegia* 1990;28:217–229.
22. Shaker H, Hassouna MM. Sacral root neuromodulation in the treatment of various voiding and storage problems. *Int Urogynecol J* 1999;10:336–343.

Ostergard's Urogynecology and Pelvic Floor Dysfunction, Fifth Edition. edited by A.E. Bent, et al.
Lippincott Williams & Wilkins, Philadelphia © 2003.

20

Management of Overactive Bladder

Joseph M. Montella

*Department of Obstetrics and Gynecology, Jefferson Medical College,
Jefferson University Hospital, Philadelphia, Pennsylvania*

DEFINITION

Overactive bladder (OAB) is a term coined by the International Continence Society to define the condition whereby a patient has symptoms of urgency and frequency with or without urge incontinence. It is a symptomatic diagnosis and therefore does not require the performance of urodynamic testing or cystometry for confirmation. Urgency is defined as the feeling that the patient must void immediately for fear of losing urine, and frequency is defined as greater than 10 micturitions in a 24-hour period. Urge incontinence describes involuntary loss of urine associated with an urgent, strong desire to void. The term detrusor instability (DI) (unstable bladder) is more restrictive and describes an OAB caused by detrusor contractions documented by cystometrogram. DI occurs when the bladder contracts spontaneously, or on provocation, during bladder filling while the patient is attempting to inhibit micturition. DI is diagnosed during provocative cystometry when one of the following conditions occurs: a true detrusor pressure rise of 15 cm H_2O (motor urge incontinence) or a true detrusor pressure rise of less than 15 cm H_2O in the presence of urgency or urge incontinence (sensory urge incontinence) (1). Subthreshold detrusor contractions of less than 15 cm H_2O may have clinical significance and have been shown to cause urinary incontinence in 10% and urgency in 85% of patients (2). Additionally, urodynamic diagnosis associated with the symptom of urge incontinence in a frail elderly patient is detrusor hyperactivity with impaired contractility (DHIC). These patients have involuntary detrusor contractions causing incontinence but are unable to empty their bladders completely, leaving a large postvoid residual (3). A pressure rise during filling may represent decreased bladder compliance or insufficient time to accommodate the increase in volume because cystometry is time dependent (4), and this would not be considered as DI in this context. Detrusor hyperreflexia is DI secondary to a known neurologic abnormality (1). The term neurogenic bladder is reserved for spinal cord injuries and other similar defects and their impact on bladder function.

Incorrect synonyms that have been applied to OAB include bladder dyssynergia and vesical instability. These terms should no longer be used.

INCIDENCE

The incidence of OAB is not well documented, but it is estimated to affect more than 17 million Americans, or 1 of 11 adults (5), with impact on quality of life equal to that of urinary incontinence. The occurrence of involuntary detrusor contractions in infancy is a normal state for bladder emptying and is later controlled by the development of cortical inhibition of reflex bladder activity.

Farrar and colleagues (6) described the prevalence of OAB as 8% to 50%, depending on age distribution. In more than 2,000 women studied by Abrams (7), OAB occurred in 38% of those 65 years of age or older and in 27% of those younger than 65 years of age. In institutionalized women, the incidence urinary incontinence secondary to OAB is greater than 80% (8). Thus, the prevalence of OAB is greatest at the extremes of life; OAB has a 5% to 10% occurrence in premenopausal patients, increasing to as much as 38% in elderly patients and perhaps to more than 80% in institutionalized incontinent elderly patients.

CLINICAL PRESENTATION

The symptoms of OAB include urgency, frequency (greater than 10 micturitions in a 24-hour period), urge incontinence, and nocturia (greater than or equal to two times). There can also be a history of childhood nocturnal enuresis in some patients (9). OAB may coexist with genuine stress incontinence, and stressful activity may trigger a detrusor contraction causing urge incontinence. In 100 women with the urodynamic diagnosis of DI, Wiskind and associates (10) reported that although 86% of patients had symptoms of urge incontinence, 76% also complained of stress incontinence. Sand and co-workers (11) reported on 188 incontinent women, and of those reporting only stress incontinence, 34.9% had DI. Only 32.6% of patients reporting both urge and stress incontinence had DI.

DIFFERENTIAL DIAGNOSIS

Because the symptoms of OAB overlap with those of other lower urinary tract conditions, a number of other diagnoses must be entertained. Table 20.1 lists the differential diagnosis for these symptoms. A special word must be written about urethral instability, which tends to be rather poorly defined.

TABLE 20.1. *Differential diagnosis of overactive bladder*

Severe genuine stress incontinence
Uninhibited urethral relaxation
Urethral diverticulum
Urinary tract fistula
Cystitis
Bladder foreign body (stone, suture, etc.)
Bladder tumor
Urethritis

Wise and associates (12) investigated the prevalence and significance of urethral instability in a group of women with OAB. This occurred in 42% of patients with OAB and was strongly associated with the sequence of relaxation of the urethra before unprovoked detrusor contraction. Women with OAB and a stable urethra exhibited primary contraction of the detrusor, whereas the symptom of stress incontinence was more common in women with urethral instability. The investigators postulated that women with OAB should be divided into two groups: those with and those without urethral instability, the latter group possibly benefiting from α-agonist therapy. In addition, Petros and Ulmsten (13) found that provocative urethrocystometry revealed a rise in detrusor pressure followed by a fall in urethral pressure, both preceded by urge symptoms. They concluded that urethral instability, OAB, and urge incontinence were different manifestations of a prematurely activated micturition reflex. Urethral instability may not be a separate entity but a part of urine loss associated with urge.

ETIOLOGY

Table 20.2 lists the etiologies of OAB. Neurologic diseases (multiple sclerosis, cerebrovascular disease, parkinsonism, Alzheimer's disease), local bladder and urethral irritants (cystitis, foreign bodies, tumors), outflow obstruction (severe cystocele or vaginal vault prolapse), and medications (parasympath-

TABLE 20.2. *Etiologies of overactive bladder*

Neurologic disease
Multiple sclerosis
Cerebrovascular disease
Parkinsonism
Alzheimer's disease
Local bladder or urethral irritation
Cystitis
Foreign bodies (stones, suture material)
Outflow obstruction
Tumors
Genitourinary prolapse (cystocele, vaginal vault
    prolapse)
Previous anti-incontinence surgery
Medication (parasympathomimetics)
Idiopathic
Disorder of bladder ganglia
Disorder of pacemaker cells
Generalized smooth muscle disorders
Increased sensory nerve density
Prostacyclin deficiency

omimetics) must be considered as etiologies. Most cases, however, apart from those in very young or elderly patients, are idiopathic in nature. Del Carro and colleagues (14) compared women with idiopathic OAB with age-matched controls using subtracted cystometry and anal sphincter electromyography sacral reflex analysis along with other neurologic tests using evoked potentials. All patients had normal neurophysiologic tests, and there was no significant difference between patients and controls.Because women with OAB do not appear to have either clinical or subclinical damage of central sensory or motor pathways, other investigators have put forth their theories regarding intrinsic bladder abnormalities. These include disorders of the bladder ganglia, disorder of pacemaker cells, generalized smooth muscle disorders, increased density of sensory nerves, and deficiency in prostacyclin production.

Disorders of the Bladder Ganglia

During the past few years, the role of neuropeptides as neurotransmitters at the various levels of the peripheral and central micturition reflex arc has been evaluated (15).

The sacral parasympathomimetics that originate from S-2 to S-4 are the major excitatory input to the urinary bladder. The corresponding ganglia lie within the bladder itself. Vasoactive intestinal polypeptide (VIP), a neuropeptide, has been found to be present in a certain proportion of cholinergic ganglion cells and functions as an inhibitory agent in this parasympathomimetic pathway. Furthermore, VIP is noted to be in reduced concentrations in detrusor muscles of patients with OAB (15).

Enkephalins may also be released from certain bladder ganglia and function as inhibitory agents in central and peripheral efferents controlling bladder capacity and stability. Exogenous enkephalins have been shown to depress the release of acetylcholine from the preganglionic nerve and thus inhibit transmission in bladder parasympathomimetic ganglia. This effect is demonstrated with the administration of opiate epidural drugs. This produces urinary retention in a significant number of patients and has been demonstrated urodynamically to reduce the magnitude of detrusor contractions and increase bladder capacity (16).

Disorder of Pacemaker Cells

The bladder is never really in a complete resting state. Rather, *in vitro* and *in vivo* studies show that it is in continuous activity, with rhythmic contractions that wax and wane (17,18). Van Duyl (19) suggested that small regional contractions from possible pacemaker cells might be the origin of large bladder contractions. In childhood, involuntary spontaneous and rhythmic contractions occur, but these are eventually suppressed with the maturation of cortical control. The persistence or reappearance of such uncontrolled contractions is possibly related to an aberrant control mechanism of pacemaker cells. *In vitro* studies by Kinder and Mundy (17) showed that muscles from bladders with OAB, regardless of the etiology, spontaneously contract more often and with a greater amplitude than muscles from urodynamically normal bladders. This suggests a disorder of the intrinsic neuromodulatory mechanism leading to OAB.

Generalized Smooth Muscle Disorder

A significant proportion of patients with irritable bowel syndrome have urinary complaints, including urgency and nocturia. Whorwell and colleagues (20) studied such patients urodynamically and found that 50% of these patients have OAB. They suggested that this high incidence of OAB is secondary to a diffuse disorder of smooth muscle or its innervation.

Increased Sensory Nerve Activity

Moore and co-workers (21) found that the density of subepithelial presumptive sensory nerves in the bladder wall was significantly greater in patients with OAB than in normal controls using bladder biopsy specimens stained for acetylcholinesterase activity. They suggested that a relative abundance of these nerves might serve to increase the appreciation of bladder filling, giving rise to the urgency and frequency of micturition characteristic of patients with OAB.

Deficiency of Prostacyclin Production

It is also postulated that women with OAB have a deficiency in the production of prostacyclin that was observed by *in vitro* studies using bladder biopsy specimens from women with OAB and from normal controls (22).

Local Bladder Irritation

Bladder or urethral irritation, especially in the proximal urethra and bladder trigone, aggravates and may possibly produce vesical instability through an increased sensory input that overfacilitates the detrusor reflex and results in loss of volitional control.

Outflow Obstruction and Antiincontinence Surgery

It has been thought that outflow obstruction in the male with prostatic hypertrophy is associated with OAB because the relief of this obstruction usually leads to the resolution of OAB. However, Abrams (7) has shown that OAB may be related to advanced age and that a postoperative decrease in instability may be due to interruption of sensory afferents. Obstruction with high outflow pressure in women is rare. Abrams studied more than 2,000 female patients and found that only 3.7% had outlet obstruction, defined by a maximum flow rate of less than 15 m/s. Additionally, there was no increased incidence of OAB in those patients with outflow obstruction.

It may be hypothesized that elevation of the vesical neck by surgical repair for stress incontinence leads to excessive urethral compression and could cause outflow obstruction, resulting in OAB. However, this is not correlated with changes in peak flow rates and maximum voiding pressures. Furthermore, patients with vaginal prolapse and preexisting OAB are not usually cured of their OAB by repairing the prolapse (23).

The incidence of *de novo* OAB in patients who preoperatively have only genuine stress urinary incontinence ranges from 5% to 18% (24,25). Cardozo and associates (24) postulated that repeat surgeries at the vesical neck interfere with the autonomic nerve supply of the bladder and result in OAB. In a review of six studies of patients who had a Burch colposuspension performed for stress incontinence, Vierhout and Mulder (26) found a prevalence of between 5% and 27%, with 68 of 396 patients developing *de novo* OAB.

Psychological Causes

Various methods of behavioral modification have been used with success in treating patients with OAB. These methods include bladder drills, biofeedback, and hypnotherapy (15–17). This lends evidence to a psychosomatic etiology for OAB in a certain number of patients.

DIAGNOSIS

All patients with OAB symptoms should undergo a basic evaluation as outlined in the guidelines proposed by the Agency on Health Care Policy and Research (27) that includes a history, physical examination, measurement of postvoid residual volume, and urinalysis. Any risk factors that are associated with urinary incontinence should be identified and attempts made to modify them.

The classic history of OAB is that of a strong urge to void or a voiding frequency of greater than 10 micturitions in a 24-hour period that can be associated with sudden urine loss. The history should also include the following elements:

1. A focused medical, neurologic, and genitourinary history that includes an assessment of risk factors and a review of medications
2. A detailed exploration of the OAB symptoms, including duration
3. Quality-of-life assessment
4. Associated symptoms, such as stress incontinence and pelvic organ prolapse
5. Fluid intake pattern by using a 24- to 72-hour voiding diary
6. Number of pads used
7. Previous treatments and their success
8. Expectations for outcomes of treatment
9. Assessment of mobility, living environment, and social factors

The physical examination should include the following:

1. Neurologic evaluation of the lower sacral segments, including bulbocavernosus and anal wink reflexes
2. Mental status examination
3. Abdominal examination to evaluate for masses or fluid collections, which may influence intraabdominal pressure and detrusor physiology
4. Pelvic examination, which usually reveals normal support in patients with OAB; however, severe genitourinary prolapse, hypoestrogenism, and urethral diverticulum must be ruled out because these conditions may contribute to the OAB symptoms. A rectal examination can determine sphincter tone, fecal impaction, or rectal mass.
5. Cough stress test to determine the presence of stress incontinence. Although the presence of stress incontinence does not rule out OAB, it can affect the treatment outcomes.
6. Estimation of postvoid residual volume either by catheterization or pelvic ultrasound. Residuals of less than 50 mL are considered normal. Repetitive postvoid residuals ranging from 100 to 200 mL or higher are considered incomplete bladder emptying. Postvoid residual determination is important to document adequate detrusor function and rule out DHIC.

Urinalysis and culture are used to rule out hematuria (which may be indicative of a tumor or stone in the urinary tract), glucosuria (which may cause increased voiding frequency), pyuria, and bacteriuria.

After any correctable problems (e.g., hematuria, infection) are identified and solved, therapy can be directed toward treating the OAB.

Advanced Testing

Advanced testing for OAB can be employed in the following situations:

1. Failure of the patient to respond to an adequate therapeutic intervention
2. Hematuria without infection
3. Persistent voiding dysfunction
4. Symptomatic genitourinary prolapse
5. Uncertain diagnosis from the basic evaluation

Uroflowmetry may reveal obstructive void-ing patterns secondary to severe genitouri-nary prolapse or tumor.

If urodynamic testing is to be employed, it is also important to duplicate closely the circum-stances surrounding urine loss, which would include provocative maneuvers such as cough-ing, positional changes, running water, hand washing, rapid filling, and temperature change of the filling medium. These can increase the sensitivity of the test (Fig. 20.1). Without provocation, DI will go undiagnosed in 30% to 40% of patients (10). In cases in which tradi-tional cystometry fails to produce a diagnosis, alternative methods may be used. One such method is extramural ambulatory urodynamic monitoring. McInerney and co-workers (28) and Webb and associates (29), in two separate studies, pronounced ambulatory monitoring as more sensitive in the diagnosis of DI than con-ventional cystometry. Porru and Usai (30) used this technique in 46 patients with urinary in-continence, 16 of whom had urge incontinence symptoms. Conventional cystometry identified detrusor contractions in only 50% of these pa-tients, whereas ambulatory monitoring identi-fied detrusor contractions in 93%. Another technique involves diuresis cystometry, in which a patient is given a diuretic to fill the bladder to approximate more closely the an-terograde filling phase. Van Venrooij and Boon (31) evaluated women with frequency and urge incontinence with a negative retrograde cys-tometrogram using diuresis cystometry and noted an increase in the detection of DI.

Finally, although multichannel standing cystometry is considered the gold standard for diagnosis, it may not always be possible to perform this test in patients with poor mobil-ity or in those who are unable to maintain a standing position. Simple cystometry at the bedside was found to have a specificity of 75% and a sensitivity of 88% compared with multichannel testing in the diagnosis of DI (32). This may be an excellent method of di-agnosing DI in frail elderly patients using a Toohey syringe attached to a Foley catheter (Fig. 20.2). The bladder is filled in incremen-tal fashion, and a rise in the meniscus repre-sents a detrusor contraction.

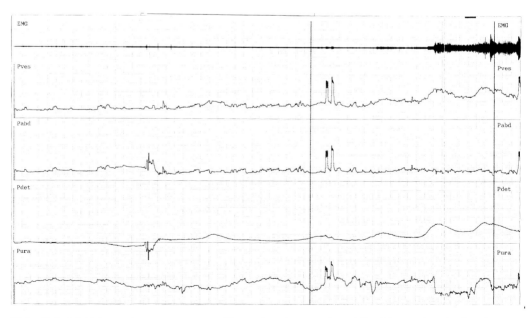

FIG. 20.1. Multichannel cystometrogram illustrating detrusor instability. The patient had a detrusor contraction after she washed her hands. Before provocation, she had no contraction.

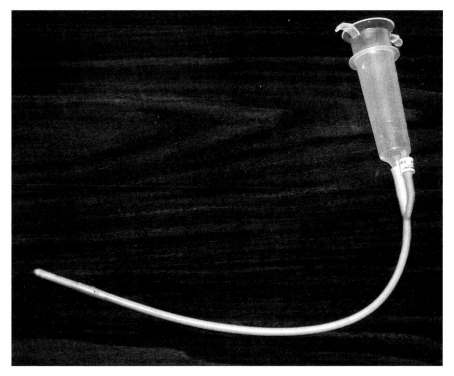

FIG. 20.2. Toohey syringe attached to catheter for bedside cystometrogram.

MANAGEMENT

Because OAB is a diagnosis based on symptoms, therapy may be instituted without performing any complex testing.

There are several methods of managing OAB, as listed in Table 20.3. Depending on the severity of the problem and its impact on the patient's quality of life and lifestyle, these treatments may be used separately or in tandem.

TABLE 20.3. *Management of overactive bladder*

Behavioral (timed voiding)
Electrical stimulation
Medical
Anticholinergics
Tricyclic antidepressants
Calcium-channel blockers
Surgical
Augmentation cystoplasty
Bladder denervation

Bladder Training (Timed Voiding)

There are three main components to bladder training: education, scheduled voiding with systematic delay of voiding, and positive reinforcement. The education portion combines written, visual, and verbal instruction that serves to familiarize patients with the anatomy and physiology of the lower urinary tract. Patients are then asked to resist or inhibit the sensation of urgency, to postpone voiding, and to urinate according to a timetable rather than according to the urge to void (33). Adjustment in fluid loads and delaying voiding to increase bladder volume may be used to augment this therapy (34). The patient is also asked to complete a daily diary as illustrated in Fig. 20.3.

Fantl and colleagues (35) conducted a controlled randomized study of 123 women with unstable detrusor function and sphincteric incompetence who received treatment in the form of behavioral strategies to decrease urge,

NAME _____   **DATE** _____

TIME	VOID	TIME	VOID	TIME	VOID
6 AM		2 PM		10 PM	
7 AM		3 PM		11 PM	
8 AM		4 PM		Midnight	
9 AM		5 PM		1 AM	
10 AM		6 PM		2 AM	
11 AM		7 PM		3 AM	
Noon		8 PM		4 AM	
1 PM		9 PM		5 AM	

Please place a check mark next to the time that you void.

FIG. 20.3. Timed voiding record.

patient education, and a schedule of voiding. Twelve percent became dry, and 75% had at least a 50% reduction in the number of incontinence episodes, with a greater effect in women with DI. Although primarily used for treatment of stress incontinence, pelvic floor muscle exercises may augment bladder training (36).

Behavioral Modification Protocol

An effective bladder training program that has produced good results consists of a 6-week outpatient voiding protocol (37). It is presented to the patient as a means of regaining cortical control over the detrusor and is offered as primary management for patients with OAB. Patients are assigned a voiding schedule based on their daily voiding interval; they are usually told to start by voiding every hour while awake for the first 2 weeks. Instructions to the patients include the following:

1. Empty your bladder at the scheduled time whether or not you feel the urge to void.
2. The important aspect is the voluntary initiation of voiding, not the amount voided.
3. Avoid going to the bathroom between scheduled times, and suppress the urge at other times.
4. Do not feel embarrassed if you leak.

The protocol requires follow-up every 2 weeks until the desired effect is obtained. Because this is a form of behavioral therapy, positive reinforcement is used. The voiding interval is increased by 15 to 30 minutes, depending on how well the patient did in the first 2 weeks. Combining this therapy with Kegel's exercises can increase the patient's ability to be continent because the increase in pelvic floor muscle tone will increase the patient's ability to hold urine. The treatment is considered successful if the patient achieves a voiding interval of 2.5 to 3 hours and is free of OAB symptoms.

Behavioral Modification in Elderly Patients

The overall incidence of OAB increases with age, and in older patients, OAB, cognitive deficits, and decreased mobility are more common causes of urinary incontinence. Hadley (38) described four scheduling regimens (Table 20.4) specifically tailored to the capabilities of the patient. They ranged from behavioral modification, used in cognitively intact ambulatory patients, to prompted voiding, used in patients with severe cognitive and mobility impairments. Hu and associates (39) used a randomized prospective protocol to study the efficacy of a prompted voiding regimen in 133 institutionalized women. Using nurses' aides to prompt and assist patients to void every hour for 14 hours of the day, they were able to reduce wet episodes by 0.6 per day, a reduction of 26% over baseline episodes. Ouslander and co-workers (40) designed a prospective study to look at the combined effects of a timed voiding schedule and oxybutynin chloride in 15 institutionalized patients with detrusor instability. In a longitudinal study design, timed voiding was implemented for the first 2 weeks alone. Oxybutynin was then added to the timed voiding regimen. Timed voiding significantly reduced the episodes of incontinence, and the addition of oxybutynin chloride did not confer any additional benefit. Fantl and colleagues (35) studied 123 community-dwelling women aged 50 years using a standard bladder training protocol. In this group of women they were able to reduce incontinence episodes by 57% and quantity of fluid loss by 54%.

Sacral Neuromodulation

Sacral neuromodulation has been confirmed as a valuable therapeutic tool in treating OAB. The current techniques of neuromodulation are anogenital electrical stimulation, transcutaneous electrical nerve stimulation (TENS), sacral nerve neuromodulation, percutaneous posterior tibial nerve stimulation (Stoler afferent nerve stimulation, SANS) and magnetic stimulation. It is unknown exactly how neuromodulation works, but at least two potential mechanisms are possible: (a) activation of efferent fibers to the striated urethral sphincter reflexively cause detrusor relaxation; and (b) activation of afferent fibers causes inhibition at a spinal or supraspinal level (41). Sacral neuromodulation is discussed more extensively in Chapter 22.

MEDICATION

See Table 20.5 for a list of medications used to treat OAB.

Anticholinergics

Anticholinergic agents are recommended as first-line medical therapy for OAB by working at the ganglionic receptor to block detrusor contractions in both the normal bladder and the OAB. These medications are contraindicated in patients with untreated narrow-angle glaucoma; however, few patients in the 21st century have this condition because they have been treated with laser surgery or with medications. If the physician is concerned about prescribing this class of medica-

TABLE 20.4. *Scheduling regimens for overactive bladder*

Regimen	Indication	Principle
Bladder training	Ambulatory, cognitive intact patient	Reestablishment of cortical inhibition of sacral reflexes
Habit training	Ambulatory, cognitive intact patient	Toileting schedule fitted to individual's voiding pattern
Timed voiding	Neurogenic bladder, minor cognitive impairment	Fixed voiding schedule to regularly empty bladder
Prompted voiding	Severe cognitive and mobility deficits	Attention focusing on need to void with assistance to void

TABLE 20.5. *Medications for overactive bladder*

Drug	Dosage forms	Dosage[a]
Tolterodine tartrate (Detrol, Detrol LA)	Tablets: 1, 2 mg	1–2 mg b.i.d.
	Timecaps: 2, 4 mg	2–4 mg q.d.
Oxybutynin chloride (Ditropan, Ditropan XL)	Tablets: 5, 10 mg	2.5–10 mg
	Syrup: 5 mg/5 mL	2.5–10 mg
	Timecaps: 5, 10, 15 mg	5–15 mg q.d.
Dicyclomine (Bentyl)	Tablets: 10, 20 mg	20 mg
	Syrup: 10 mg/5 mL	
Hyoscyamine (Levsin)	Tablets: 0.125 mg	0.125–0.25 mg
	Timecaps: 0.375 mg	0.375 mg b.i.d.
Propantheline (Pro-Banthīne)	Tablets: 7.5, 15 mg	7.5–15 mg + 30 mg q.h.s.
Flavoxate (Urispas)	Tablets: 100 mg	100–200 mg
Imipramine (Tofranil)	Tablets: 10, 25, 50 mg	25 mg

[a]Dosages are three to four times daily, unless otherwise noted.

tions in patients with narrow-angle glaucoma, consultation with the patient's ophthalmologist is recommended. The low dosage range is always initially used in elderly patients and titrated according to its effectiveness and side effects. Side effects of this class of medication involve atropine-like side effects, such as dry mouth and dry eyes, the severity of which are dose dependent; gastroparesis; constipation; gastroesophageal reflux; and somnolence. Less common side effects are headache, dizziness, and peripheral edema.

Based on the strength of scientific evidence through placebo controlled, double-blinded studies, there are two anticholinergic agents that are recommended as the starting point of medical therapy. In 1997, tolterodine tartrate was introduced to treat OAB. This is available in two forms: an immediate-release preparation and a timed-release preparation. Several placebo-controlled studies have documented the effectiveness of both forms of therapy in terms of significant reduction in urgency, frequency, and number of incontinence episodes (42,43). This medication is metabolized by the CYP2D6 isoform of the cytochrome P-450 system and must be used with caution in patients who are on any medications that competitively inhibit this enzyme, such as oral antifungals and macrolide antibiotics. The recommended dosage is 2 mg twice a day for the immediate-release preparation and 4 mg once a day for the timed-release preparation.

The second anticholinergic agent that has been considered highly effective in the treatment of OAB is oxybutynin chloride. This agent has both anticholinergic and smooth muscle relaxant properties. In five placebo-controlled studies in middle-aged outpatients, oxybutynin reduced incontinence frequency by 19% to 58% over placebo (44–48). Side effects were noted in all studies and included dry skin, blurred vision, nausea, constipation, and marked xerostomia. The severity of side effects increased with increasing dosages, with severe xerostomia occurring in 84% of patients receiving oxybutynin in a dose of 5 mg four times a day. The recommended dosage is 2.5 to 5 mg taken orally three or four times a day (44). Oxybutynin is also available in a timed-release formulation taken once a day in doses of 5, 10, or 15 mg. The side effects with the long-acting medication have been considerably reduced.

Propantheline is the prototype of anticholinergic agents used for urologic conditions because it best approximates atropine's effect on the bladder *in vitro,* although its central nervous system side effects are less marked. This is recommended as a second-line anticholinergic agent in doses of 7.5 to 30 mg three to five times per day and may need to be given in higher doses of 15 to 60 mg four times daily. Side effects include blurry vision, xerostomia, nausea, constipation, tachycardia, drowsiness, and confusion, the most common of which is xerostomia.

Two studies evaluated propantheline use in nursing home patients and found a 13% to 17% reduction of incontinence over placebo, which was statistically significant (49,50).

Dicyclomine hydrochloride is an anticholinergic agent with smooth muscle relaxant properties. Studies are limited, and those studies that were performed included small numbers of patients. No studies exist comparing this to other anticholinergics. However, clinical usefulness has been derived using 10 to 20 mg two to four times daily, and it may be a tolerable first-line approach in elderly patients.

Flavoxate is a tertiary amine that has smooth muscle relaxant properties *in vitro.* Four randomized controlled studies failed to demonstrate a significant benefit over placebo (46,51–53), and therefore, this medication is not recommended for the treatment of urge incontinence.

Hyoscyamine and other oral anticholinergics are known to be used for the treatment of OAB; however, there are no studies that adequately compare their effects to placebo. Dosage is 0.125 mg three to four times a day.

Tricyclic Antidepressants

The effects of tricyclic antidepressants on the lower urinary tract are twofold: anticholinergic properties as described previously, and α-adrenergic properties to increase tone of the urethra and bladder neck. Two randomized controlled studies revealed the effectiveness of doxepin and imipramine in reducing nocturnal incontinence in patients with OAB. Side effects noted in these studies included fatigue, xerostomia, dizziness, blurred vision, nausea, and insomnia (54,55). The usual oral dosages are 10 to 25 mg one to three times per day, with the daily total dose usually 25 to 100 mg.

Nonsteroidal Antiinflammatory Agents

Nonsteroidal antiinflammatory drugs are theorized to be effective for OAB because of their inhibition of prostaglandin synthetase, thereby interfering with prostaglandin-mediated bladder contractions. Limited research is available, and in general, the use of these medications has not been successful. Dosages that are effective in reducing bladder contractions produce extreme side effects of gastritis and ulceration.

Calcium-channel Blockers

Calcium-channel blockers stop the influx of extracellular calcium required for the contractile process of the detrusor and also prevent the mobilization from intracellular calcium stores with resultant inhibition of excitation contraction coupling (56). They are mainly used in the treatment of angina because of their ability to prevent intracellular movement of calcium through the slow channel in a membrane; however, investigators have used these drugs in the treatment of OAB because uninhibited bladder contractions have been shown to be dependent on calcium influx. No controlled studies for nifedipine, diltiazem, or verapamil have been performed, and their use for urge incontinence is not recommended at this time.

SURGERY

Surgery should be considered if behavioral or medical therapy has failed because this therapy is associated with advanced morbidity. As with any surgery for incontinence, the available surgical options vary in their invasiveness, efficacy, and durability. The three procedures most commonly performed are augmentation intestinocystoplasty, urinary diversion, and bladder denervation.

Augmentation Cystoplasty

Augmentation cystoplasty is recommended for patients with intractable severe OAB or for those with low-compliance bladders, the goal being to create a compliant and large-capacity urinary storage unit. The patient then employs clean intermittent self-catheterization to empty the reservoir; therefore, patients who are unable to catheterize themselves are not candidates for this surgery. Nearly all segments of the gastrointestinal tract, as well as the ureter, have been used for augmentation (57), but no single segment represents the ideal substitution because each has its own complications (58). The preoperative evaluation should include assessment of renal function (serum creatinine, 24-hour urine, serum electrolytes, and blood urea nitrogen), assessment of bowel function (sigmoidoscopy and barium enema), cystoscopy to rule out any intravesical abnormalities, and a urine culture. During surgery, the bladder is bivalved using a sagittal incision from 3 cm above the bladder neck to about 2 cm above the trigone. In the ileocystoplasty, a segment of terminal ileum about 20 to 40 cm long and at least 15 cm proximal to the ileocecal valve is chosen. The bowel is divided, and an end-to-end reanastomosis of the remaining intestine is done to restore intestinal continuity. The chosen ileal segment is then opened on its antimesenteric side and refashioned into a U or S shape, keeping its vascular supply intact. This is then anastomosed to the bladder. In the ileocecocystoplasty, a cecal pouch is created along with a segment of terminal ileum and anastomosed to the bladder. The goal of augmentation cystoplasty in patients with DI with lower motor neuron lesions or detrusor–sphincter dyssynergia is to induce urinary retention and allow the patient to empty using intermittent self-catheterization. Postoperative complications of augmentation intestinocystoplasty include urinary tract infections, stone formation, mucus production, metabolic acidosis, tumors, and perforation. The risks of this surgery include voiding difficulties, mucus or stone formation, and metabolic problems. Contraindications include renal insufficiency, bowel disease, and inability to perform self-catheterization. Mean cure rates were 77.2%; mean cure or improvement rates were 80.9% (59–62).

Urinary Diversion

Urinary diversion is usually considered the last option in patients who are not good candidates for reconstruction of the lower urinary tract and who are refractory to other forms of therapy. The two types of urinary diversion are the noncontinent and the continent urinary diversion, the former requiring an external collecting device. Bricker (63) established the ileal conduit as a method of noncontinent urinary diversion in 1950. Current technique involves the isolation of a 15- to 20-cm length of terminal ileum, 10 to 15 cm from the ileocecal anastomosis. The ureters are transected 3 to 4 cm from the bladder and anastomosed to either the antimesenteric border of the ileal loop or to the proximal end of the ileal loop. The remaining intestine is reanastomosed, and a stoma is created on the anterior abdominal wall using the ileal loop. Complications of this procedure include wound infection, ureteroileal leakage, intestinal obstruction, stomal stenosis, retraction, and hernia. Rare complications include urolithiasis involving the conduit and malignant transformation of the ileal loop.

The essential advantage of continent over incontinent urinary diversion is the elimination of the need for an external urine collection device. Several reservoirs designed from different combinations of the ileum, cecum, colon, sigmoid, and rectum have been used in which to divert the ureters. The ideal reservoir should have low intrinsic pressures as well as adequate capacity to preserve continence and prevent reflux. Usually, 40 cm of ileum or 20 cm of large bowel or a combination of these is needed to create a reservoir of adequate capacity. Like in noncontinent diversions, jejunum is unsuitable owing to its high intrinsic metabolic activity (64).

Bladder denervation can be accomplished by selective sacral rhizotomy, S-3 foramen injection, or paravaginal denervation. It is beyond the scope of this chapter to describe each procedure in detail. Complications include perineal hyperesthesia, wound infection, and intraoperative bleeding. Long-term follow-up revealed that 50% had persistent or recurrent incontinence, and an additional 20% were dry only with the addition of anticholinergic agents (65–67).

REFERENCES

1. Abrams P, Blaivas JG, Stanton SL, et al. The standardization of terminology of lower urinary tract function recommended by the International Continence Society. *Int Urogynecol J* 1990;1:45–58.

2. Coolsaet BLRA, Blok C, Van Venrooij GE, et al. Subthreshold detrusor instability. *Neurourol Urodyn* 1985; 4:309–311.

3. Resnick NM, Yalla SV, Laurino E. The pathophysiology of urinary incontinence among institutionalized elderly persons. *N Engl J Med* 1989;320:1–7.

4. Coolsaet BLRA. Bladder compliance and detrusor activity during the collection phase. *Neurourol Urodyn* 1985;4:263–265.

5. Payne CK. Advances in the nonsurgical treatment of urinary incontinence and overactive bladder. *Campbell's Urology Updates* 1999;1:1–20.

6. Farrar DJ, Whiteside G, Osborne J, et al. Urodynamic analysis of micturition symptoms in the female. *Surg Gynecol Obstet* 1975;141:875–877.

7. Abrams P. Detrusor instability and bladder outlet obstruction. *Neurourol Urodyn* 1985;4:317–319.

8. Starer P, Libow LS. The measurement of residual urine in the evaluation of incontinent nursing home residents. *Arch Gerontol Geriatr* 1988;7:75–81.

9. Fantl JA. Urinary incontinence due to detrusor instability. *Clin Obstet Gynecol* 1984;27:474–489.

10. Wiskind AK, Miller KF, Wall LL. One hundred unstable bladders. *Obstet Gynecol* 1994;83:108–112.

11. Sand PK, Hill RC, Ostergard DR. Incontinence history as a predictor of detrusor instability. *Obstet Gynecol* 1988;71:257–260.

12. Wise BG, Cardozo LD, Cutner A, et al. Prevalence and significance of urethral instability in women with detrusor instability. *Br J Urol* 1993;72:26–29.

13. Petros PE, Ulmsten U. Bladder instability in women: a premature activation of the micturition reflex. *Neurourol Urodyn* 1993;12:235–239.

14. Del Carro U, Riva D, Comi GC, et al. Neurophysiologic evaluation in detrusor instability. *Neurourol Urodyn* 1993;12:455–462.

15. de Groat WC, Kawatani M. Neural control of the urinary bladder: possible relationship between peptidergic inhibitory mechanisms and detrusor instability. *Neurourol Urodyn* 1985;4:285–288.

16. Rawal N, Mollefors K, Axelsson K, et al. An experimental study of urodynamic effects of epidural morphine and Naloxone reversal. *Anesth Analg* 1983;62: 641–647.

17. Kinder RB, Mundy AR. Pathophysiology of idiopathic detrusor instability and detrusor hyperreflexia: an in vitro study of human detrusor muscle. *Br J Urol* 1987; 60:509–515.

18. Kinder RB, Mundy AR. Inhibition of spontaneous contractile activity in isolated human detrusor muscle strips by vasoactive intestinal polypeptide. *Br J Urol* 1987;57: 20–23.

19. van Duyl WA. Spontaneous contractions in urinary bladder smooth muscle: preliminary results. *Neurourol Urodyn* 1985;4:301–304.

20. Whorwell PJ, Lupton EW, Erduran D, et al. Bladder smooth muscle dysfunction in patients with irritable bowel syndrome. *Gut* 1986;27:1014–1017.

21. Moore KH, Gilpin SA, Dixon JS, et al. Increase in presumptive sensory nerves of the urinary bladder in idiopathic detrusor instability. *Br J Urol* 1992;70:370–372.

22. Bergman A, Stanczyk FZ, Lobo RA. The role of prostaglandins in detrusor instability. *Am J Obstet Gynecol* 1991;165:1833–1836.

23. Stanton SL, Williams JE, Ritchie B. The colposuspension operation for urinary incontinence. *Br J Obstet Gynaecol* 1976;83:890–893.

24. Cardozo L, Stanton SL, Williams JE. Detrusor instability following surgery for genuine stress incontinence. *Br J Urol* 1979;51:204–206.

25. Langer R, Ron-el R, Newman M, et al. Detrusor instability following colposuspension for urinary stress incontinence. *Br J Obstet Gynaecol* 1988;95:607–610.

26. Vierhout ME, Mulder AF. De novo detrusor instability after Burch colposuspension. *Acta Obstet Gynecol Scand* 1992;71:414–416.

27. Clinical Practice Guidelines. *Urinary incontinence in adults: acute and chronic management.* Rockville, MD: Agency on Health Care Policy and Research, Number 2, 1996.

28. McInerney PD, Vainer TF, Harris SA, et al. Ambulatory urodynamics. *Br J Urol* 1991;67:272–274.

29. Webb RJ, Ramsden PD, Neal DE. Ambulatory monitoring and electronic measurement of urinary leakage in the diagnosis of detrusor instability and incontinence. *Br J Urol* 1991;68:148–152.

30. Porru D, Usai E. Standard and extramural ambulatory urodynamic investigation for the diagnosis of detrusor instability-correlated incontinence and micturition disorders. *Neurourol Urodyn* 1994;13:237–242.

31. van Venrooij GE, Boon TA. Extensive urodynamic investigation: interaction among diuresis, detrusor instability, urethral relaxation, incontinence and complaints in women with a history of urge incontinence. *J Urol* 1994;152:1535–1538.

32. Fonda D, Brimage PJ, D'Astoli M. Simple screening for urinary incontinence in the elderly: comparison of simple and multichannel cystometry. *Urology* 1993;42:536–540.

33. McCormick KA, Burgio K. Incontinence: an update on nursing care measures. *J Gerontol Nurs* 1984;10:16–23.

34. Frewen W. Role of bladder training in the treatment of the unstable bladder in the female. *Urol Clin North Am* 1979;6:273–277.

35. Fantl JA, Wymen JF, Harkins SW, et al. Efficacy of bladder training in older women with urinary incontinence. *JAMA* 1991;265:609–613.

36. Burton J, Pearce L, Burgio KL, et al. Behavioral training for urinary incontinence in elderly, ambulatory patients. *J Am Geriatr Soc* 1988;36:693–698.

37. Fantl JA, Hurt WG, Dunn LJ. Dysfunctional detrusor control. *Am J Obstet Gynecol* 1977;129:299–303.

38. Hadley EC. Bladder training and related therapies for urinary incontinence in older people. *JAMA* 1986;256: 372–379.

39. Hu T-W, Igou JF, Kaltreider DL, et al. A clinical trial of a behavioral therapy to reduce urinary incontinence in nursing homes. *JAMA* 1989;261:2656–2662.

40. Ouslander JG, Blaustein J, Connor A, et al. Habit training and oxybutynin for incontinence in nursing home patients: a placebo controlled trial. *J Am Geriatr Soc* 1988;36:40–46.

41. Groen J, Bsoch JLHR. Neuromodulation techniques in the treatment of the overactive bladder. *Br J Urol Int* 2001;87:723–731.

42. Van Kerrebroeck P, Kreder K, Jonas U, et al. Tolterodine once-daily: superior efficacy and tolerability in the treatment of the overactive bladder. *Urology* 2001;557: 414–421.

43. Appell RA, Abrams P, Drutz HP, et al. Treatment of overactive bladder: long-term tolerability and efficacy of tolterodine. *World J Urol* 2001;19:141–147.

44. Tapp AJ, Cardozo LD, Versi E, et al. The treatment of detrusor instability in postmenopausal women with oxybutinin chloride: a double-blind placebo controlled study. *Br J Obstet Gynaecol* 1990;97:521–526.

45. Holmes DM, Montz FJ, Stanton SL. Oxybutinin versus propantheline in the management of detrusor instability: a patient-regulated variable dose trial. *Br J Obstet Gynaecol* 1989;96:607–612.

46. Zeegers AGM, Kiesswetter H, Kramer AEJL, et al. Conservative therapy of frequency, urgency and urge incontinence: a double-blind clinical trial of flavoxate hydrochloride, oxybutinin chloride, emepronium bromide and placebo. *World J Urol* 1989;5:57–61.

47. Riva D, Casolati E. Oxybutinin chloride in the treatment of female idiopathic bladder instability. *Clin Exp Obstet Gynecol* 1984;11:37–42.

48. Moore KH, Hay DM, Imrie AE, et al. Oxybutinin hydrochloride (3 mg) in the treatment of women with idiopathic detrusor instability. *Br J Urol* 1990;66:479–485.

49. Dequeker J. Drug treatment of urinary incontinence in the elderly. Controlled trial with vasopressin and propantheline bromide. *Gerontol Clin* 1965;7:311–317.

50. Zorzitto ML, Jewett MAS, Fernie GR, et al. Effectiveness of propantheline bromide in the treatment of geriatric patients with detrusor instability. *Neurourol Urodyn* 1986;5:133–140.

51. Meyhoff HH, Gerstenberg TC, Nordling J. Placebo: the drug of choice in female motor urge incontinence? *Br J Urol* 1983;55:34–37.

52. Robinson JM, Brocklehurst JC. Emepronium bromide and flavoxate hydrochloride in the treatment of urinary incontinence associated with detrusor instability in elderly women. *Br J Urol* 1983;55:371–376.

53. Chapple CR, Parkhouse H, Gardener C, et al. Double-blind, placebo controlled, crossover study of flavoxate in the treatment of idiopathic detrusor instability. *Br J Urol* 1990;66:491–494.

54. Lose G, Jorgensen L, Thunedborg P. Doxepin in the treatment of female detrusor overactivity: a randomized double-blind crossover study. *J Urol* 1989;142:1024–1026.

55. Castleden CM, Duffin HM, Gulati RS. Double-blind study of imipramine and placebo for incontinence due to bladder instability. *Age Ageing* 1986;15:299–303.

56. Andersson KE, Sjogren C. Aspects on the physiology and pharmacology of the bladder and urethra. *Prog Neurobiol* 1982;19:71–89.

57. Hendron WH. Historical perspective in the use of bowel in urology. *Urol Clin North Am* 1997;24:703–713.

58. Duel BP, Gonzalez R, Barthold JS. Alternative techniques for augmentation cystoplasty. *J Urol* 1998;159: 989–1005.

59. Sidi AA, Becher EF, Reddy PK, et al. Augmentation enterocystoplasty for the management of voiding dysfunction in spinal cord injury patients. *J Urol* 1990;143:83.

60. George NK, Russel GL. Clam ileocystoplasty. *Br J Urol* 1991;68:487–489.

61. Strawbridge LR, Kramer SA, Castillo OA, et al. Augmentation cystoplasty and the artificial genitourinary sphincter. *J Urol* 1989;142:297–301.

62. Lockhart JL, Bejany D, Politano VA. Augmentation cystoplasty in the management of neurogenic bladder disease and urinary incontinence. *J Urol* 1986;135: 9069–9072.

63. Bricker EM. Bladder substitution after pelvic evisceration. *Surg Clin North Am* 1950;30:1511–1521.

64. Natarajan V, Singh G. Urinary diversion for incontinence in women. *Int Urogynecol J* 2000;11:180–187.

65. Opsomer RJ, Klarskov P, Holm-Bentzen M, et al. Long-term results of superselective sacral nerve resection for motor urge incontinence. *Scand J Urol Nephrol* 1984; 18:101–105.

66. Lucas MG, Thomas DG, Clarke S, et al. Long-term follow-up of selective sacral neurectomy. *Br J Urol* 1988; 61:218–220.

67. Hodgkinson CP, Drukker BH. Infravesical nerve resection for detrusor dyssynergia. *Acta Obstet Gynecol Scand* 1977;56:401–403.

Ostergard's Urogynecology and Pelvic Floor Dysfunction, Fifth Edition. edited by A.E. Bent, et al. Lippincott Williams & Wilkins, Philadelphia © 2003.

21

Interstitial Cystitis

Toby C. Chai

Division of Urology, University of Maryland Medical Center, Baltimore, Maryland

EPIDEMIOLOGY

Interstitial cystitis (IC) is best described as a chronic hypersensory bladder condition manifested by urinary frequency, urgency, and bladder pain without an identifiable etiology. This disease mainly afflicts women in their 30s and 40s (1). The female-to-male ratio is 10:1. Although the prevalence of IC in males is thought to be significantly underestimated, no formal epidemiologic studies have been conducted in the male population. Because females commonly have acute bacterial cystitis, the diagnosis of IC is often delayed. The primary care physician often treats IC with oral antibiotics because IC symptoms mimic acute bacterial cystitis and urine cultures are not typically sent before treatment of acute bacterial cystitis. The current estimated prevalence of IC in the United States is 66 per 100,000 population from the National Nurses Health Study (2). The estimation of the number of females afflicted with IC in the United States is between 450,000 and 700,000. It is thought that IC may be genetically inherited based on twin studies (3). This study found that there was a greater rate of concordance of IC among monozygotic twins than dizygotic twins. Future epidemiologic and genetic studies may help pinpoint etiologic mechanisms and also determine the natural history of this puzzling disease.

CLINICAL PRESENTATION

Because there are no proven etiologies for IC, there are no pathognomonic features of IC,

and therefore, there does not exist the ability to diagnose IC definitively. There are no classic physical examination findings, blood, histopathology, or radiologic tests for IC. Nevertheless, the clinical diagnosis of IC is currently made by a constellation of symptomatic features coupled with exclusionary criteria (namely, ruling out other defined diseases and conditions). The presentation of symptoms in IC is highly variable, and some have proposed that IC is a complex of diseases rather than just a single entity and, most likely, a combination of etiologies. Because bladder pain is a prominent symptom component of IC, some have included IC in the disease complex of chronic pelvic pain. When IC is better understood from the pathophysiologic standpoint, a more specific terminology may be developed.

Recently, a new International Classification of Diseases, 9th revision (ICD-9) (596.51), was created for the condition of overactive bladder. The symptoms of overactive bladder, such as urinary frequency and urgency, overlap with symptoms of IC. The etiology of overactive bladder is similarly enigmatic. The main difference between these conditions is that overactive bladder patients have no bladder or pelvic pain component. Nevertheless, there is overlap among these three conditions: IC, overactive bladder, and chronic pelvic pain. The Venn diagram (Fig. 21.1) depicts how patients diagnosed with any of these three conditions may actually have overlapping symptoms.

Patients who have IC with the prototypical symptom complex of urinary frequency, uri-

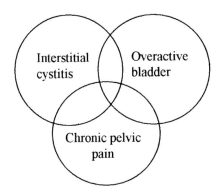

FIG. 21.1. Venn diagram showing how patients diagnosed with any of three conditions may actually have overlapping symptoms.

nary urgency, and bladder pain without a definable etiology have chronic symptoms that usually last longer than 6 months. The intensity of these symptoms typically waxes and wanes during the course of the disease. Because of the imprecise nature of these symptoms, IC patients are frequently thought to have recurrent urinary tract infection, urethritis, urethrotrigonitis, trigonitis, urethral pain syndrome, urethral stenosis, endometriosis, vulvodynia, vulvar vestibulitis, or pelvic congestion syndrome. A few studies have found associations between IC, vulvodynia, and chronic pelvic pain (4,5).

Recently, it has been speculated that IC may be a systemic disease because of its association with other conditions, such as irritable bowel disease, allergies, sensitive skin, inflammatory bowel disease, fibromyalgia, chronic fatigue syndrome, and systemic lupus erythematosus (6–9). Whether these associations represent common pathophysiologic mechanisms or spurious associations may relate to the relative nonspecific diagnostic criteria for all of these conditions and the potential for selection bias of cases and controls in these studies (10). Recently, a validated questionnaire for non–bladder-related symptoms was given to 35 IC patients (as defined by criteria detailed later) and 35 aged-matched controls, and it was found that IC patients did not have more nonbladder symptoms than controls (11).

Therefore, the diagnosis of IC remains primarily a process of exclusion and clinical sus-

picion. A list of exclusionary conditions has been set forth by the National Institutes of Health (NIH) and the National Institute of Diabetes and Digestive and Kidney Diseases (NIDDK) (12). The original intent of this criteria list was to ensure maximal objective standardization of patients enrolled into NIH-sponsored IC studies. These criteria were not designed as a diagnostic tool. Nevertheless, they can provide clinicians with a useful guide to other diseases and conditions that may cause symptoms similar to IC (Table 21.1).

The pain component of IC can be difficult for patients to describe. Because the bladder is autonomically innervated, it is classified as a visceral organ. From a neuroanatomic perspective, this simply means that there is an intervening synapse (ganglia) between the autonomic motor (preganglionic) neuron and the end effector organ (the bladder). However, from a sensory standpoint, patients often have difficulty localizing or describing visceral sensations. The pain may be referred to other areas of the pelvis. Besides the typical pain over the suprapubic (bladder) area, which may be relieved by voiding, IC patients may complain of

TABLE 21.1. *NIDDK criteria for NIH-sponsored IC studies*

NIDDK inclusion criteria for NIH-sponsored IC studies
1. Urinary frequency/urgency and pelvic pain of chronic duration (>9 mos)
2. Presence of glomerulations and/or Hunner's ulcers on cystoscopy and hydrodistention

NIDDK exclusion criteria for NIH-sponsored IC studies
1. Diagnosis of bacterial cystitis within a 3-month period
2. History of bladder calculi or current/active ureteral or urethral calculi
3. Genital herpes within past 12 wk
4. History of uterine, cervical, vaginal, or urethral cancer
5. Symptomatic urethral diverticulum
6. History of cyclophosphamide use, history of any type of chemical cystitis
7. History of tuberculous cystitis
8. History of pelvic irradiation
9. History of benign or malignant bladder tumors
10. Active vaginitis

NIDDK, National Institute of Diabetes and Digestive and Kidney Diseases; NIH, National Institutes of Health; IC, interstitial cystitis.

referred urethra-based pain, such as dysuria, stranguria, or constant burning. They may also complain of low back pain, vulvar pain, rectal pain, and dyspareunia. Quantitation of the severity of pain is quite difficult because of the waxing-waning presentation of symptoms, and there are no formal quantitative objective measures of bladder or pelvic pain.

Urinary urgency is another symptomatic component of IC that can be difficult to separate from pain in some patients. IC patients may describe a constant strong urge to void, despite low bladder volumes, that when severe, is described as pain. Urinary frequency is a manifestation of the actual act of voiding, but IC patients have been known not to void because they realize that frequent voiding does not necessarily lead to relief of pain and urge sensations. From the standpoint of quantification of IC symptoms, measurement of voiding frequency may be the best objective parameter.

In summary, the clinical presentation of IC is characterized by chronic urinary frequency, urgency, and pelvic pain in the absence of precise identifiable etiologic features. These symptoms do not necessarily follow a set pattern and may be quite different from one patient to another. IC patients may have one symptomatic component that predominates over the others. Finally, IC symptoms typically wax and wane, which further complicates the evaluation and treatment of this condition. The key is to rule out identifiable and potentially reversible causes of the bladder symptoms.

SYMPTOM QUANTITATION

Because IC symptoms are variable, it becomes important to quantitate these symptoms as objectively as possible. This is especially important for clinical researchers examining treatment options for IC. Two sets of validated instruments have been described in the literature. One questionnaire instrument was developed by O'Leary and colleagues in 1997 specifically to assess IC patients; this was then validated in a group of 45 IC patients and 67 controls (13). The questionnaire had two components: symptoms and quality-of-life quantification. This instrument is presented in Table 21.2.

TABLE 21.2. *Interstitial cystitis (IC) symptoms quantitation*

IC Symptom Index (ICSI)

1. During the past month, how often have you felt the strong urge to urinate with little or no warning?
   - 0_____not at all
   - 1_____less than 1 time in 5
   - 2_____less than half the time
   - 3_____about half the time
   - 4_____more than half the time
   - 5_____almost always
2. During the past month, have you had to urinate less than 2 hours after you finished urinating?
   - 0_____not at all
   - 1_____less than 1 time in 5
   - 2_____less than half the time
   - 3_____about half the time
   - 4_____more than half the time
   - 5_____almost always
3. During the past month, how often did you most typically get up at night to urinate?
   - 0_____not at all
   - 1_____less than 1 time in 5
   - 2_____less than half the time
   - 3_____about half the time
   - 4_____more than half the time
   - 5_____almost always
4. During the past month, have you experienced pain or burning in your bladder?
   - 0_____not at all
   - 1_____less than 1 time in 5
   - 2_____less than half the time
   - 3_____about half the time
   - 4_____more than half the time
   - 5_____almost always

IC Problem Index (ICPI)

During the past month, how much has each of the following been a problem for you?
1. Frequent urination during the day
   - 0_____no problem
   - 1_____very small problem
   - 2_____small problem
   - 3_____medium problem
   - 4_____big problem
2. Getting up at night to urinate
   - 0_____no problem
   - 1_____very small problem
   - 2_____small problem
   - 3_____medium problem
   - 4_____big problem
3. Need to urinate with little warning
   - 0_____no problem
   - 1_____very small problem
   - 2_____small problem
   - 3_____medium problem
   - 4_____big problem
4. Burning pain, discomfort, or pressure in your bladder
   - 0_____no problem
   - 1_____very small problem
   - 2_____small problem
   - 3_____medium problem
   - 4_____big problem

The interstitial cystitis symptom index (ICSI) and interstitial cystitis problem index (ICPI) were administered to a group of women with chronic pelvic pain before undergoing laparoscopy and cystoscopy with hydrodistention to determine whether these instruments can detect IC in this patient population. Using positive findings from cystoscopy and hydrodistention as objective criteria for IC (see Diagnosis), these investigators determined that the sensitivity, specificity, positive predictive value, and negative predictive value of these indices were 94%, 50%, 53%, and 93%, respectively (5). Furthermore, they found that 38% of these patients with chronic pelvic pain had IC.

A second symptom measurement instrument, the University of Wisconsin IC Scale (UW-ICS) has also been developed and validated (14,15). The UW-ICS is a 7-point, 0 to 6 rating scale with each item anchored between the extremes of 0 (not at all) and 6 (a lot) (Fig. 21.2). The scale is completed by the patient within the context of reporting the symptoms as, "How much have you experienced the following symptoms today?" Seven items are defined to characterize the IC patient, with a summary score being the sum of the seven individual items. This summated UW-ICS score will have a value ranging from 0 to 42.

Any of these validated instruments should be administered to the patients with IC to quantitate their symptoms during the course of evaluation and treatment. It is important to use these standardized instruments so that changes in patients' symptoms and quality of life can be followed as objectively as possible.

DIAGNOSIS

Cystoscopy with Hydrodistention

Cystoscopy with hydrodistention of the bladder under anesthesia is the standard method for the objective diagnosis of IC. The conventional wisdom is that IC bladders have the appearance of glomerulations (or petechiae) after bladder hydrodistention (nonulcerative form of IC). The appearance of Hunner's ulcers is uncommon in IC, although it has been suggested that the appearance of Hunner's ulcers is a more specific sign for IC (ulcerative form of IC). Hunner's ulcers may also be treated at the time of cystoscopy by laser fulguration (16). Anesthetic bladder capacity of IC patients may also be reduced, although typically, IC patients have normal anesthetic capacity. The presumed diagnostic specificity of appearance of post-distention bladder glomerulations or Hunner's ulcers resulted in the NIH using this as the only objective criterion in classifying a patient as having IC. Although this single criterion is not uniformly accepted by all clinicians, its main purpose is to standardize IC patients enrolled in NIH-sponsored stud-

How much have you experienced the following symptom today?	0 (not at all)	1	2	3	4	5	6 (a lot)
1. bladder pain							
2. bladder discomfort							
3. getting up at night to go to the bathroom							
4. going to the bathroom frequently in the day							
5. urgency to urinate							
6. difficulty sleeping because of bladder problems							
7. burning sensation in the bladder							

FIG. 21.2. The University of Wisconsin Interstitial Cystitis scale.

ies. It is unclear how to classify those patients who meet all criteria for IC except for the presence of glomerulations or Hunner's ulcers.

Whether individuals without symptoms have bladder glomerulations after hydrodistention is subject to debate. It has been thought that normal subjects do not have these findings. One study analyzed postdistention images in control women (those who had no bladder or voiding symptoms) undergoing anesthesia for tubal ligation (17). These investigators found that there were no differences in the incidence of pos-distention glomerulations between these controls and IC patients. Additionally, based on a visual severity scale of the cystoscopic images, the intensity of postdistention glomerulations was not different. Therefore, the diagnostic specificity of appearance of postdistention bladder was questioned.

The other potential utility of bladder hydrodistention is for IC symptom relief. Anecdotally, patients have had reduction in pain, urinary frequency, and urgency after anesthetic hydrodistention of the bladder, although there have also been patients who have fared worse for a period of time after hydrodistention. The mechanism underlying improvement may be a placebo effect because there have been no randomized trials comparing sham cystoscopy (without hydrodistention) to hydrodistention. Results from a recent study suggested possible beneficial effect of hydrodistention based on normalization of urine growth factor abnormalities associated with IC (18) (these urine growth factors produced by the bladder urothelium are described later under Role of Urinary Markers). The bladder, being a dynamic organ, may need to respond to repeated stretch to maintain physiologic homeostasis. In patients with IC, because the bladder is chronically understretched, the normal stretch stimulus is diminished, and this may be reflected by abnormal expression of growth factors by the IC bladder. Abnormalities in these growth factors may prevent normal growth and regeneration of the bladder urothelium, thereby causing IC symptoms.

Description of Hydrodistention

Hydrodistention is performed with the patient under general or regional anesthesia. A full cystoscopic examination of the bladder is performed first. Patients with IC have a completely normal-appearing bladder without evidence of uroepithelial lesions. Cystoscopic irrigant, water or saline, is then infused at a pressure of 80 to 100 cm H_2O into the bladder until filling stops (pressure cutoff). The bladder is distended for 2 to 5 minutes before all the irrigant is released from the bladder. Terminal bloody efflux of irrigant suggests the diagnosis of IC. The bladder epithelium is reexamined with the cystoscope during repeat filling. Glomerulations (petechiae) or Hunner's ulcers, appearing as fissures or cracks in the epithelium, is consistent with IC. The cystoscopic appearances of the bladder before and after distention are diagnostic (Fig. 21.3; See Color Plate 15 following page 204).

Potassium Sensitivity Test

The potassium sensitivity test (PST) was developed and popularized by Lowell Parsons (19) as a method to diagnose IC in a relatively noninvasive manner (as compared with cystoscopy and hydrodistention under anesthesia). The rationale of this test is based on the assertion that the bladder urothelium is "leaky" in IC patients because of a proposed deficiency in the glycosaminoglycan (GAG) layer (a proteoglycan or glycoprotein) on the luminal surface of the bladder uroepithelium. This theory was derived from several observations. First, in animal models, application of protamine sulfate, which purportedly "strips" the GAG layer, increased bladder permeability in rabbit bladder urothelium (20). Furthermore, the protamine-induced increased permeability was reversed by the addition of sodium pentosan

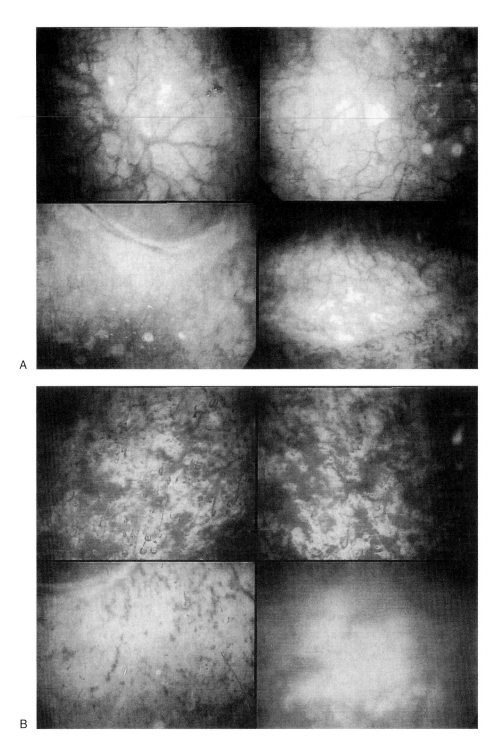

FIG. 21.3. A: Interstitial cystitis (IC) before hydrodistention. The initial filling of the bladder appears normal. **B:** IC after hydrodistention in same patient. Numerous petechiae and glomerulations appear after the bladder has been distended and emptied, then refilled, indicating a diagnosis of interstitial cystitis. Eventually, enough blood accumulates to cloud the picture in bottom right of figure. (See Color Plate 15 following page 204.)

polysulfate (Elmiron). Second, protamine placed into normal human volunteers induced pain, urinary frequency, urinary urgency, and increased bladder permeability to urea (21). Third, there was the finding of increased urea uptake by the IC bladders (when exogenous urea was introduced intravesically) compared with control bladders (22), suggesting increased bladder permeability IC. Finally, there was clinical evidence that sodium pentosan polysulfate alleviates some of the symptoms of IC (23,24). If urothelial leak were the pathophysiologic mechanism in IC, urinary potassium in the urine would cross the leaky IC urothelial barrier to activate (depolarize) the sensory nerve endings in the suburothelium.

The patient is awake and without anesthesia for the PST. The test is performed by infusing 40 mL of solution 1 (sterile water) into the bladder over 2 to 3 minutes. After 5 minutes, the patient rates her pain and urgency using a visual scale from 0 to 5, with 5 being worst. She voids the contents of her bladder. Next, 40 mL of solution 2 [0.4 molar potassium chloride (KCl)] is instilled into the bladder and left for 5 minutes. The patient rates her pain and urgency and voids the solution. A score of ≥2 in either pain or urgency is considered a positive PST, provided the patient does not respond to solution 1. It was shown in this same study that 75% of patients with IC have a positive PST, as compared with 4% of controls. Neither IC nor control subjects had a positive test with 40 mL of water infusion. Parsons observed that there was an 85% positive test when the KCl was administered to gynecologic patients with chronic pelvic pain (25), leading him to conclude that most gynecologic patients with chronic pelvic pain have IC. This is compared with a rate of 38% as determined by cystoscopy and hydrodistention in patients with chronic pelvic pain (5).

In addition to its diagnostic capability, the PST may also have a prognostic capacity. Recently, Teichman found that a positive PST predicted better response to oral sodium pentosan polysulfate than occurs in patients with a negative PST (26). In this study, the complete NIH criteria were not used for the diagnosis of IC. Specifically, not all patients received cystoscopy and hydrodistention to look for glomerulations or Hunner's ulcers. Therefore, most patients had an IC diagnosis based solely on symptoms and exclusionary criteria. Interestingly, the IC patient population in this study had a 34% negative PST rate. The investigators gave sodium pentosan polysulfate to all patients regardless of whether their PST was positive or negative. Those who had a positive PST fared better than those who had a negative PST. However, the predictive value of a positive PST was not consistent across all improvement categories (i.e., greater than 25% improvement, greater than 50% improvement).

There is still active debate about whether there is increased permeability of the IC bladder and whether this is directly related to GAG layer deficiency. Even the notion that a GAG layer exists on the luminal uroepithelial surface of a normal bladder is controversial. Part of the difficulty is that GAG localization techniques are not uniform or well defined, and different techniques suggest different findings. It is beyond the scope of this review to address these controversies adequately, but the assertion that the IC bladders have a "deficient" GAG layer must take this debate into account. Several studies have found no difference in the GAG layer between IC and control bladders (27–29).

The GAG layer is theorized to protect the bladder against both bacteria and urinary toxins (such as KCl) (30,31). However, it has been shown from ultrastructural studies that bacteria such as *Escherichia coli* invade the bladder uroepithelium by binding (through *E. coli* type 1 pili) to the uroplakin glycoproteins present on the apical surface of luminal epithelial cells (32,33). Attachment of bacteria to the urothelium is through the specific binding of type 1 pili to a specific structural pore in uroplakins Ia and Ib. These uroplakins are arranged in the apical urothelial membrane in a hexagonal array readily detected by electron microscopy. No GAG layer was visualized in these ultrastructural studies, but this may reflect processing techniques that removed the GAG. Nevertheless, it is clear from these studies that the interaction between the type 1 pili and the uroplakins is crucial for the invasion of the bacteria into the bladder urothelial cells. Whether GAG prevents this invasion from occurring is unknown.

The other theorized function of the GAG layer is to prevent "absorption" of substances from the urine; furthermore, the IC bladder is more permeable because of the decreased GAG layer. Direct measurements of bladder permeability with diethylenetriaminepentaacetic acid revealed no evidence of increased IC permeability (34). The observation that permeability of the bladder can be affected by protamine (20), solely by diminishing the GAG layer without injuring the urothelial cells, may be overly simplistic. Other studies have shown that protamine induces multiple changes in the urothelium and results in loss of the urothelial layer (35,36). Physiologic doses of intravesical potassium mimicking concentrations found in urine, which are significantly lower than the 0.4 M KCl used in the PST, significantly decreased the yield of the PST in the diagnosis of IC (37), diminishing the role of KCl

in the pathophysiology of IC. Additionally, because sodium pentosan polysulfate is poorly excreted in the urine (3% of ingested dose excreted in urine), it is expected that direct intravesical application of sodium pentosan polysulfate should revolutionize the therapeutic efficacy of sodium pentosan polysulfate, which is not the case. Finally, when the PST was compared with cystoscopy and hydrodistention as a diagnostic test, it fared no better in terms of positive predictive value (59% and 66%, respectively) in a population who had symptoms suggestive of IC (38). These investigators concluded that the general use of the PST is not validated and that we must continue to depend on cystoscopy and hydrodistention for the diagnosis of IC.

In conclusion, both "objective" diagnostic tests, hydrodistention under anesthesia and PST, have advantages and disadvantages (Table 21.3). Hydrodistention has been traditionally used to categorize patients in NIH-funded studies. The anesthetic capacity of the bladder can be measured, and other potential anatomic abnormalities of the bladder can be cystoscopically assessed. Some patients may symptomatically benefit from hydrodistention, although some also have a temporary worsening of symptoms. PST is a noninvasive test meant to induce temporary pain in IC patients. It might also help to pre-

TABLE 21.3. *Objective diagnostic tests*

Diagnostic test	Pros	Cons
Cystoscopy/hydrodistention	May be therapeutic Determine anesthetic bladder capacity Ability to treat Hunner's ulcers Ability to obtain bladder biopsy specimens Ability to rule out other intraluminal bladder pathologies	Invasive Requires anesthesia May not be specific
Potassium sensitivity test	Noninvasive May prognosticate sodium pentosan polysulfate (Elmiron) response	Nontherapeutic Does not result in higher diagnostic yield, may not be specific Painful to patients who have interstitial cystitis

dict those who will respond to sodium pentosan polysulfate. Taken in whole, the utility of these two tests requires further investigation. It also shows that until the pathophysiology of IC can be proved, a better diagnostic test (such as urine markers, discussed subsequently) awaits.

Role of Urinary Markers

Because of the dilemma that exists in the diagnosis of IC, many investigators have sought urine markers that might serve as noninvasive diagnostic surrogates. Finding a highly sensitive and specific urine marker will also serve to provide insights into the pathophysiologic mechanisms that may eventually lead to specific targeted treatments. Many urinary substances have been described as increased or decreased in patients with IC compared with controls. These substances, such as histamine, interleukins, GAGs, hyaluronic acid, epithelial growth factors, nerve growth factor, and others, were selected based on theorized etiologies for IC. One of the major problems in using many of these substances as a diagnostic marker is that, although the levels may be statistically significantly higher or lower in the IC population when averaged, there is significant overlap of values among control and IC subjects. The reasons for this may be that IC is multifactorial in etiology and that subgroups of IC patients exist depending on the cause. A more extensive review of urine markers has been recently published (39).

Two markers that have shown particular potential in diagnostic capability are glycoprotein-51 (GP-51) and antiproliferative factor (APF). GP-51 levels in urine were examined in controls and those who met NIDDK criteria for IC (40). There was no overlap in urinary GP-51 concentration between those control and IC individuals. APF is a low-molecular-weight protein present in IC urine that is able to inhibit the ability of cultured normal bladder urothelial cells to incorporate ^{3}H-thymidine (41). Because the structure of APF is not elucidated, the determination of the level of APF is an indirect assay based on inhibition of ^{3}H-thymidine incorporation. The levels of APF activity in patients who meet NIDDK criteria for IC and in control urine specimens do not overlap (42). Both of these markers were based on the gold-standard NIDDK objective criteria of presence of glomerulations on cystoscopy or hydrodistention, which may not be a specific finding. It is unknown how these urinary markers are altered in patients with painful bladder symptoms, overactive bladder, and other conditions that do not fulfill the NIDDK criteria for IC. Nevertheless, these two markers provide the foundation for elucidation of the pathophysiologic mechanisms involved in IC and may ultimately serve to be a diagnostic marker for IC.

Urodynamics

The use of urodynamics in the management of IC is also debated. The IC Database Study Group analyzed urodynamic data and compared them to data collected from voiding diaries (43). It was not surprising that urodynamic data closely correlated the findings of the voiding diaries. Patients with low-volume, high frequency voiding as recorded in a voiding diary had decreased cystometric capacity and decreased volume of first sensation. Therefore, it has been suggested that urodynamics are unnecessary in the evaluation of IC because the voiding diary, which is noninvasive, would capture the necessary information. However, some believe that urodynamics will allow discrimination between those patients with IC that have bladder symptoms and those with nonbladder symptoms (44). Patients who show motor instability on urodynamics are considered not to have IC and are treated with antimuscarinics. Additionally, urodynamic testing may be considered, especially when a patient will undergo catheterization for a PST (Fig. 21.4).

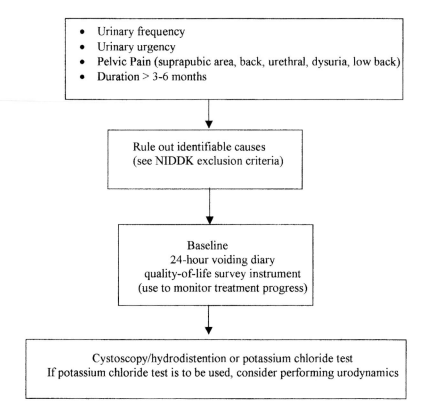

FIG. 21.4. Diagnostic algorithm.

TREATMENT OF SYMPTOMS

After the diagnosis of IC has been made, a cornucopia of therapies exists. Unfortunately, many of these therapies have not been tested in a rigorous, randomized, blinded fashion using standardized data collection techniques and standardized questionnaire instruments. Part of the difficulty with treatment studies relates to the subjective nature of this condition without an objective, proven clinical measure, such as a blood test or urine test. Additionally, the typical waxing–waning course of IC makes assessment of treatment modalities more difficult. Finally, because of the lack of understanding of the precise etiology of IC, there does not exist a highly effective treatment, and currently, there is no cure for this disease. These reasons make it imperative to assess the outcomes of the available treatments scientifically, so that clinicians can counsel patients on the best form of therapy.

The NIH, in its commitment to understanding the pathophysiology and treatment of IC, is currently conducting multicenter clinical trials examining outcomes of different IC treatments in a prospective, randomized manner that addresses all these problematic issues. These nine clinical centers across the United States compose the NIH Interstitial Cystitis Clinical Trials Group (ICCTG). The ICCTG recently completed a four-arm blinded, prospective, randomized study comparing sodium pentosan polysulfate plus placebo, hydroxyzine plus placebo, sodium pentosan polysulfate plus hydroxyzine, and placebo plus placebo. Results from these studies are pending. A second clinical trial is underway studying the effectiveness of intravesical bacille Calmette Guérin (BCG). It is

TABLE 21.4. *Interstitial cystitis therapies*

"Standard" oral therapies	"Standard" intravesical therapies
Sodium pentosan polysulfate (Elmiron)	Dimethyl sulfoxide (DMSO)
Amitriptyline (Elavil)	Steroids (methylprednisolone)
Hydroxyzine (Atarax)	Heparin
Gabapentin (Neurontin)	Local anesthetics (Lidocaine, Marcaine)
Antimuscarinics (Detrol, Ditropan)	Sodium pentosan polysulfate (Elmiron)
α-Blockers (Hytrin)	Astringents (Clorpactin, Silver Nitrate)

expected that findings from these randomized trials will be published over the next few years. However, until precise pathophysiologic mechanisms are identified, IC treatments will continue to be empiric (Table 21.4).

Oral-based Therapies

Oral pharmacologic treatments remain a mainstay of therapy. Each of the following agents has been used with a specific targeted pathway in mind, and most are used in other diagnoses besides IC. The rationale for these oral agents are presented.

1. Sodium pentosan polysulfate (Elmiron). This medication was developed as a specific treatment for IC based on the theory that IC is due to a leaky urothelium because of the deficiency of the GAG layer in the bladder. Sodium pentosan polysulfate, a weak heparinoid, supposedly replenishes the GAG layer and thus makes the urothelium less leaky. This is the first oral medication for IC that has undergone randomized, placebo-controlled clinical trials (24,45). These studies have shown that sodium pentosan polysulfate can significantly decrease certain IC symptoms. Several caveats should be discussed. First, there seemed to be a period of time (3 to 6 months) before maximal beneficial effect was seen, and this was found in an open-label continuation of the initial clinical trials (23). Second, differences between control and treated patients in the early trials, although statistically significant, were not dramatically different from a clinical standpoint [28% of sodium pentosan polysulfate treated patients had

more than 25% improvement versus 13% of placebo treated patients (24)]. If IC is truly due to only a GAG deficiency that is readily reversible with sodium pentosan polysulfate, a high concentration of sodium pentosan polysulfate introduced intravesically should ameliorate all the symptoms of IC (because only 3% of the oral dose is excreted into the urinary tract). Empirically, this is not the case. These points notwithstanding, this medication is well tolerated and simple to give, and long-term efficacy studies have shown continued benefit for those that respond initially to the therapy (23).

2. Amitriptyline (Elavil). This tricyclic antidepressant has been used to decrease the chronic pain associated with IC. This medication is given once daily at about 6:00 p.m. and may also have a beneficial effect on sleep disturbances and decrease nocturia. The medication is titrated to effect until the side effects are intolerable (starting at 10 to 25 mg daily). Its use in patients with IC has not been studied in a randomized, prospective manner, but is based on empiric observations and anecdotal references (46,47).

3. Hydroxyzine (Atarax). One of the theories for IC involves degranulation of mast cells with release of neuroactive and vasoactive chemicals. To prevent mast cell degranulation, antihistamines, such as hydroxyzine, have been suggested (48). Hydroxyzine also has a central nervous system effect, giving this medication sedative as well as anxiolytic effects. This medication was dosed at 25 mg given at bedtime and titrated up to 75 mg total (50

mg during the day and 25 mg at bed-time). Again, no large-scale, prospective, placebo-controlled randomized study had been performed for this medication until the ICCTG conducted its first clinical trial, which was closed in 2001. The possible synergy between hydroxyzine and sodium pentosan polysulfate should also be determined from this clinical trial.

4. Gabapentin (Neurontin). This is an antiepileptic medication that has gained popularity in the treatment of chronic pain disorders. Gabapentin is a neuronal stabilizer and thus can possibly hyperpolarize those neurons involved in pain transduction and increase sensory thresholds. Because chronic pelvic pain is a major component of IC symptoms, this medication is also being used clinically in IC patients (49). Because IC has a waxing–waning course and there are no objective markers for IC-related pain, studies on the efficacy of gabapentin in IC can prove to be difficult.

5. Antimuscarinics (oxybutynin, tolterodine). These agents have been developed as the primary agents to treat overactive bladder. Because the symptoms of overactive bladder overlap with IC, the use of these agents in IC is understandable. Antimuscarinics work by blocking the effect of acetylcholine at the neuromuscular junction in the detrusor smooth muscle. The efficacy of these medications is somewhat limited because both IC and overactive bladder are primarily hypersensory conditions of the bladder. Blocking the motor end of the pathway does not prevent the afferent signal (bladder pain, urinary urgency) from being relayed to the higher neural centers, such as the brain.

6. α-Blockers (terazosin). This agent has been used in the treatment of bladder symptoms, such as frequency, urgency, nocturia, and weak urinary stream in males with benign prostatic hyperplasia. The effect of the α-blocker was theorized to relax the smooth muscle within the prostatic capsule and thus decrease the resistance to outflow of urine out the bladder. However, several studies suggest that α-blockers also work by blocking micturition reflexes within the spinal cord (50–52). Because the central effects of α-blockers is in suppressing micturition reflexes, it has been suggested that terazosin be used in IC patients.

Intravesical Therapy

Intravesical therapy allows the introduction of medications directly into the bladder. There are potentially fewer side effects with intravesical administration primarily because of the lack of systemic absorption if the dwell time of the intravesical agent used is kept short. If the pathophysiology of IC is related directly to urothelial abnormalities, intravesical therapy makes more sense because these agents can directly target the urothelium. Intravesical therapy typically involves the mixture of multiple medications (as a "cocktail"). Again, as for the oral agents, no large prospective, randomized, and blinded trial has been performed for any of these agents, either singly or as a mixture. The following list includes the most commonly used agents.

1. Dimethyl sulfoxide (DMSO). This agent is probably the most used intravesical agent in the treatment of IC. The mechanism of action is thought to be antiinflammatory. Another described mechanism is depletion of sensory neuropeptides from afferent nerves over a period of time, which leads to a salutary response of decreased pain, voiding frequency, and urgency. The initial release of sensory neuropeptides may help explain the pain that DMSO causes during initial intravesical administration. Another potential mechanism of DMSO is mast cell inhibition. The dose of DMSO used intravesically is 50 mL of a 50% solution.

2. Steroids (methylprednisolone). Steroids can also be given intravesically. From 500 mg to 1 g of methylprednisolone can be reconstituted in a small volume (10 to 15

mL) and mixed with DMSO. The rationale for using this agent relates to its antiinflammatory actions.

3. Heparin. One of the etiologies of IC is theorized to be a decrease in the GAG layer of the uroepithelium. Heparin, which is a GAG derivative, is thought to help replenish this diminished layer. Typically 10,000 to 20,000 U of heparin in 2 to 5 mL of solution is used intravesically.

4. Local anesthetic. Lidocaine (1%) or bupivacaine (Marcaine) (0.5%) may be used. Usually, 20 to 30 mL of local anesthetic is sufficient.

These agents are mixed as a cocktail, infused into the bladder through a urethral catheter, and left to dwell for 30 to 60 minutes (or as long as patients can tolerate). Patients usually undergo one treatment per week for a 6-week period. The selection of this regimen is purely empiric. Some patients have more durable responses when a maintenance schedule of intravesical treatment is given (such as a biweekly or monthly treatment after the initial 6-week treatment).

Other agents that have been used intravesically include silver nitrate and Clorpactin. Both work as bladder astringents. Essentially, these agents coagulate the surface proteins on the urothelium and induce a regenerative reaction of the urothelium. Because of the nature of these agents, they cause pain when infused and thus are typically given under anesthesia in the operating room. These agents have fallen out of favor, not because of clinical data, but because they cause intense pain when infused and require anesthesia to administer.

Other intravesical therapies that are being studied and contemplated include several new agents. One is resiniferatoxin (RTX), a suprapotent analogue of the hot-pepper derivative, capsaicin. RTX works by releasing sensory neuropeptides, such as substance P and calcitonin gene-related peptide (CGRP). Over extended time, RTX should desensitize the sensory nerve of the bladder. An initial study in very few IC patients revealed that RTX was effective (53). Along these same lines (e.g., modulating the bladder sensory response), some have theorized that the phenotype and function of the sensory nerves can be modulated with gene therapy by introducing a vector through intravesical injection of a herpes simplex type 1 virus. This concept has been proved possible because a gene product (nerve growth factor) has been delivered to and expressed by the dorsal root ganglia (DRG) neurons (sensory neurons) from intravesical injection of the herpes simplex virus carrying the *NGF* gene (54). Therefore, the theory is that the virus can be engineered to carry a destructive gene that will knock out the sensory function of the DRG neurons and thus render the bladder asensate and that this could be used to treat the hypersensory disorder such as IC.

A current study by the ICCTG involves intravesical BCG bacilli. BCG is currently approved by the U.S. Food and Drug Administration (FDA) for treating bladder cancer (carcinoma *in situ*). Recently, in a small prospective, randomized, blinded, placebo-controlled trial, intravesical BCG has shown efficacy in reducing IC symptoms (55). However, these results were not replicable by another group of investigators (56). Therefore, the ICCTG is replicating this study using a multi-institutional prospective, randomized, placebo-controlled trial to enroll patients for a sufficiently statistically powered study. The mechanism of BCG's effect is unknown. BCG, when introduced intravesically, can modulate the immune response in the host. Perhaps, if IC is related to immune dysregulation, BCG can modulate the abnormality in immune response, thus decreasing IC symptoms.

Surgical Therapies to Reduce Symptoms

Major surgical intervention is not the mainstay in treatment of IC symptoms. Nevertheless, cystectomy or bladder augmentation has been described to treat IC (57–60). The uses of these aggressive interventions are typically reserved for those patients with a small contracted bladder as measured during cystoscopy and hydrodistention under general anesthesia. One would think that cystectomy with urinary diversion would alleviate these patients' symptoms, but there are anecdotal reports that symptoms persist despite urinary diversion. Although all these studies examining major surgical intervention in IC report excellent outcomes, these studies suffer the same methodologic flaws as all studies on IC, namely, too few patients with no standardized outcome parameters. Clearly, aggressive approaches to treating IC must be applied to carefully selected patients with clearly documented small, contracted bladders during cystoscopy under anesthesia.

Less invasive surgical approaches to treat IC include chronic sacral neuromodulation (InterStim, Medtronic Corporation, Minneapolis, MN). This therapy involves chronic electrical stimulation (by an implanted pulse generator) of the S-3 nerve root through an implanted lead placed through the S-3 foramen. The FDA has approved use of sacral neuromodulation for treatment of idiopathic urge incontinence, frequency–urgency syndrome, and idiopathic urinary retention (61–63). Symptoms of IC are similar to those of the frequency–urgency syndrome. The mechanisms by which sacral neuromodulation works are unknown. Perhaps, micturition and storage neural reflexes are altered in all patients with voiding dysfunction, be it IC or other conditions. S-3 neuromodulation, by virtue of stimulating the S-3 nerve roots, which innervate the bladder, bladder outlet, and pelvic floor, "corrects" or "balances" the abnormalities occurring in these reflexes. Because sacral neuromodulation can be tested through percutaneous test stimulation of the S-3 nerves, patients do not necessarily undergo implantation unless they have a positive response to the test stimulation. This therapy has been applied to IC patients in two small studies (64,65) with promising results.

The use of neodymium: YAG laser to fulgurate Hunner's ulcers to alleviate IC symptoms has also been described (16). Twenty-four patients underwent this procedure and had a mean follow-up time of 23 months. There was documented effectiveness in decreasing IC symptoms, but about half of the patients required one to four retreatments with repeat laser fulgurations during the mean 23 months of follow-up. Although this is a relatively noninvasive technique, most IC patients do not have Hunner's ulcers (66), which makes this therapy not widely applicable. Finally, as in most IC therapies, there has not been a randomized trial comparing outcomes of laser fulguration and cystoscopy alone.

FUTURE DIRECTIONS

It is obvious that the major goal in IC is to understand the pathophysiology of this disease. Many theories have been proposed, each based on some supporting experimental data. However, a consistent theme is that IC is a result of bladder urothelial abnormalities. Increased permeability of the bladder urothelium due to a deficient GAG layer was one of the early hypotheses that ultimately led to the use of sodium pentosan polysulfate for treatment and to the development of the PST for diagnosis of IC. It is unclear whether this is the final pathway in the development for IC because there is much debate about whether the IC bladder is truly more permeable and whether sodium pentosan polysulfate is uniformly effective (intravesically or orally) for IC patients.

Altered peptide growth factor production by the urothelial cells is another pathogenic hypothesis that is gaining acceptance. Studying biochemical alterations in IC urothelial cells will prove to be valuable for understanding the pathophysiology of IC and is hoped to lead to a noninvasive diagnostic test with high sensitivity and specificity. The growth factors that seem the most promising are heparin-binding epidermal growth factor (HB-EGF) and APF (41,67). It has been shown that the IC urothelium produces APF, which inhibits the growth of normal bladder urothelium and thus may inhibit the IC urothelium from regenerating properly, either in the course of normal bladder homeostasis or in response to some insult such as acute bacterial cystitis.

APF, furthermore, inhibits the production of other growth factors required for epithelial growth, such as HB-EGF. The abnormalities of these growth factors is providing the basis to develop a urinary test that can be performed in an office setting to diagnose IC. Additionally, another theory is that reversal of these growth factor abnormalities might ameliorate IC symptoms or even cure IC.

Recently, the bladder urothelium has been determined to have a sensory role in bladder function from experimental animal models (36,68–70), which represents a new paradigm for bladder urothelial function. Traditionally, the urothelium has been thought to serve only a protective function for the bladder, but several intriguing laboratory findings have suggested that the bladder urothelium may be crucial in relaying the sensation of bladder fullness to the brain. When the bladder urothelial cells are stretched during bladder filling, they release adenosine triphosphate, which then acts as a sensory neurotransmitter by binding to sensory nerve terminals located histologically just below the bladder urothelium. It has been shown that this process is augmented in IC, thus possibly explaining the hypersensory defect in IC (71). Vanillyoid receptor-1 has been detected in the bladder urothelial cells and, when activated, causes a release of nitric oxide (36,72), which can activate suburothelial nerves. These data taken together strongly suggest that the urothelium may serve as a sensory transducer for the bladder in addition to providing a barrier function. Currently, no medications are available to increase sensory thresholds of the bladder. Development of a bladder-specific analgesic agent could provide an effective treatment for IC. As discussed previously, the concept of gene therapy using a gene product delivered by a virus introduced into the bladder is also being actively studied (54). The goal of gene therapy would be to deliver a gene to the dorsal root ganglia cells or possibly the bladder uroepithelial cells that would interfere with the sensory function of the bladder or reverse the pathophysiologic defect identified (Table 21.5).

TABLE 21.5. *Potential future therapies (symptoms relief or cure)*

Gene therapy delivered intravesically
Sensory modulators (e.g., resiniferatoxin) Botulinum toxin
Growth factor regulators
Sacral neuromodulation

SUMMARY

IC is a disease complex with a core problem that involves the bladder. The epidemiology, genetics, diagnosis, and treatment of IC are still undergoing evolution. The key to IC undoubtedly is determining the etiology. It is probable that IC is multifactorial and therefore has different etiologies in different patients. However, our current diagnostic abilities cannot separate IC patients into different subcategories, except for perhaps ulcerative (Hunner's ulcer) versus nonulcerative IC. There is no cure for this debilitating problem, and current treatments only alleviate symptoms. To understand this disease will require a new paradigm in which sequential advances that characterize study of other diseases will not apply to IC. Advances in IC will occur in parallel in different arenas, including epidemiology, genetics, diagnosis, and treatment, which should all converge on the etiologies of this enigmatic disease.

REFERENCES

1. Simon LJ, Landis JR, Erickson DR, et al. The Interstitial Cystitis Data Base Study: concepts and preliminary baseline descriptive statistics. *Urology* 1997;49[Suppl 5A]:64–75.
2. Curhan GC, Speizer FE, Hunter DJ, et al. Epidemiology of interstitial cystitis: a population based study. *J Urol* 1999;161(2):549–552.
3. Warren JW, Keay SK, Meyers D, et al. Concordance of interstitial cystitis in monozygotic and dizygotic twin pairs. *Urology* 2001;57[6 Suppl 1]:22–25.
4. Gunter J, Clark M, Weigel J. Is there an association between vulvodynia and interstitial cystitis? *Obstet Gynecol* 2000;95[4 Suppl 1]:S4.
5. Clemons J, Arya LA, Myers DL. Diagnosing interstitial cystitis in women with chronic pelvic pain. *Obstet Gynecol* 2001;97(4):S7.
6. Pang X, Boucher W, Triadafilopoulos G, et al. Mast cell and substance P-positive nerve involvement in a patient with both irritable bowel syndrome and interstitial cystitis. *Urology* 1996;47(3):436–438.

7. Alagiri M, Chottiner S, Ratner V, et al. Interstitial cystitis: unexplained associations with other chronic disease and pain syndromes. *Urology* 1997;49[Suppl 5A]: 52–57.

8. Clauw DJ. The pathogenesis of chronic pain and fatigue syndromes, with special reference to fibromyalgia. *Med Hypoth* 1995;44(5):369–378.

9. Monga AK, Marrero JM, Stanton SL, et al. Is there an irritable bladder in the irritable bowel syndrome? *Br J Obstet Gynaecol* 1997;104(12):1409–1412.

10. Aaron LA, Buchwald D. A review of the evidence for overlap among unexplained clinical conditions [Review] [79 refs]. *Ann Intern Med* 2001;134(9 Pt 2):868–881.

11. Erickson DR, Morgan KC, Ordille S, et al. Nonbladder related symptoms in patients with interstitial cystitis. *J Urol* 2001;166(2):557–561; discussion, 561–562.

12. Gillenwater JY, Wein AJ. Summary of the National Institute of Arthritis, Diabetes, Digestive and Kidney Diseases Workshop on Interstitial Cystitis, National Institutes of Health, Bethesda, Maryland, August 28–29, 1987. *J Urol* 1988;140(1):203–206.

13. O'Leary MP, Sant GR, Fowler FJ, et al. The interstitial cystitis symptom index and problem index. *Urology* 1997;49[Suppl 5A]:58–63.

14. Goin JE, Olaleye D, Peters KM, et al. Psychometric analysis of the University of Wisconsin Interstitial Cystitis Scale: implications for use in randomized clinical trials. *J Urol* 1998;159(3):1085–1090.

15. Keller ML, McCarthy DO, Neider RS. Measurement of symptoms of interstitial cystitis: a pilot study. *Urol Clin North Am* 1994;21(1):67–71.

16. Rofeim O, Hom D, Freid RM, et al. Use of the neodymium: YAG laser for interstitial cystitis. A prospective study. *J Urol* 2001;166(1):134–136.

17. Waxman JA, Sulak PJ, Kuehl TJ. Cystoscopic findings consistent with interstitial cystitis in normal women undergoing tubal ligation. *J Urol* 1998;160(5):1663–1667.

18. Chai TC, Zhang C, Shoenfelt JL, et al. Bladder stretch alters urinary heparin-binding epidermal growth factor and antiproliferative factor in patients with interstitial cystitis. *J Urol* 2000;163(5):1440–1444.

19. Parsons CL, Greenberger M, Gabal L, et al. The role of urinary potassium in the pathogenesis and diagnosis of interstitial cystitis. *J Urol* 1998;159(6):1862–1866; discussion, 1866–1867.

20. Parsons CL, Boychuk D, Jones S, et al. Bladder surface glycosaminoglycans: an epithelial permeability barrier. *J Urol* 1990;143(1):139–142.

21. Lilly JD, Parsons CL. Bladder surface glycosaminoglycans is a human epithelial permeability barrier. *Surg Gynecol Obstet* 1990;171(6):493–496.

22. Parsons CL, Lilly JD, Stein P. Epithelial dysfunction in nonbacterial cystitis (interstitial cystitis). *J Urol* 1991; 145(4):732–735.

23. Hanno PM. Analysis of long-term Elmiron therapy for interstitial cystitis. *Urology* 1997;49[Suppl 5A]:93–99.

24. Mulholland SG, Hanno P, Parsons CL, et al. Pentosan polysulfate sodium for therapy of interstitial cystitis: a double-blind placebo-controlled clinical study. *Urology* 1990;35(6):552–58.

25. Parsons CL, Bullen M, Kahn BS, et al. Gynecologic presentation of interstitial cystitis as detected by intravesical potassium sensitivity. *Obstet Gynecol* 2001; 98(1):127–132.

26. Teichman JM, Nielsen-Omeis BJ. Potassium leak test predicts outcome in interstitial cystitis. *J Urol* 1999; 161(6):1791–1794; discussion, 1794–1796.

27. Dixon JS, Holm-Bentzen M, Gilpin CJ, et al. Electron microscopic investigation of the bladder urothelium and glycocalyx in patients with interstitial cystitis. *J Urol* 1986;135(3):621–625.

28. Nickel JC, Emerson L, Cornish J. The bladder mucus (glycosaminoglycan) layer in interstitial cystitis. *J Urol* 1993;149(4):716–718.

29. Anderstrom CR, Fall M, Johansson SL. Scanning electron microscopic findings in interstitial cystitis. *Br J Urol* 1989;63(3):270–275.

30. Parsons CL, Stauffer C, Schmidt JD. Bladder-surface glycosaminoglycans: an efficient mechanism of environmental adaptation. *Science*. 1980;208(4444):605–607.

31. Shrom SH, Parsons CL, Mulholland SG. Role of urothelial surface mucoprotein in intrinsic bladder defense. *Urology* 1977;9(5):526–533.

32. Wu XR, Sun TT, Medina JJ. In vitro binding of type 1-fimbriated Escherichia coli to uroplakins Ia and Ib: relation to urinary tract infections. *Proc Natl Acad Sci U S A* 1996;93(18):9630–9635.

33. Mulvey MA, Lopez-Boado YS, Wilson CL, et al. Induction and evasion of host defenses by type 1-piliated uropathogenic Escherichia coli [erratum appears in *Science* 1995;283(5403):795]. *Science* 1998;282(5393): 1494–1497.

34. Chelsky MJ, Rosen SI, Knight LC, et al. Bladder permeability in interstitial cystitis is similar to that of normal volunteers: direct measurement by transvesical absorption of 99mtechnetium-diethylenetriaminepentaacetic acid. *J Urol* 1994;151(2):346–349.

35. Eichel L, Scheidweiler K, Kost J, et al. Assessment of murine bladder permeability with fluorescein: validation with cyclophosphamide and protamine. *Urology* 2001;58(1):113–118.

36. Birder LA, Kanai AJ, de Groat WC, et al. Vanilloid receptor expression suggests a sensory role for urinary bladder epithelial cells. *Proc Natl Acad Sci U S A* 2001;98(23):13396–13401.

37. Payne CK, Sirinian E, Azevedo K. Effect of physiologic levels of urinary potassium on interstitial cystitis symptoms. *Urology* 2001;57[6 Suppl 1]:124.

38. Chambers GK, Fenster HN, Cripps S, et al. An assessment of the use of intravesical potassium in the diagnosis of interstitial cystitis. *J Urol* 1999;162(3 Pt 1): 699–701.

39. Erickson DR. Urine markers of interstitial cystitis. *Urology* 2001;57(6A):15–21.

40. Byrne DS, Sedor JF, Estojak J, et al. The urinary glycoprotein GP51 as a clinical marker for interstitial cystitis. *J Urol* 1999;161(6):1786–1790.

41. Keay S, Zhang CO, Trifillis AL, et al. Decreased 3H-thymidine incorporation by human bladder epithelial cells following exposure to urine from interstitial cystitis patients. *J Urol* 1996;156(6):2073–2078.

42. Keay SK, Zhang C, Shoenfelt J, et al. Sensitivity and specificity of antiproliferative factor, heparin-binding epidermal growth factor-like growth factor and epidermal growth factor as urine markers for interstitial cystitis. *Urology* 2001;57(6A):9–14.

43. Kirkemo A, Peabody M, Diokno AC, et al. Associations among urodynamic findings and symptoms in women enrolled in the Interstitial Cystitis Data Base (ICDB) Study. *Urology* 1997;49[Suppl 5A]:76–80.

44. Teichman JM, Nielsen-Omeis BJ, McIver BD. Modified urodynamics for interstitial cystitis. *Techniques Urol* 1997;3(2):65–68.

45. Parsons CL, Mulholland SG. Successful therapy of interstitial cystitis with pentosanpolysulfate. *J Urol* 1987; 138(3):513–516.

46. Hanno PM, Buehler J, Wein AJ. Use of amitriptyline in the treatment of interstitial cystitis. *J Urol* 1989;141(4): 846–848.

47. Renshaw DC. Desipramine for interstitial cystitis. *JAMA* 1988;260(3):341.

48. Theoharides TC. Hydroxyzine for interstitial cystitis. *J Allergy Clin Immunol* 1993;91(2):686–687.

49. Sasaki K, Smith CP, Chuang YC, et al. Oral gabapentin (neurontin) treatment of refractory genitourinary tract pain. *Techniques Urol* 2001;7(1):47–49.

50. Swierzewski SJ, Gormley EA, Belville WD, et al. The effect of terazosin on bladder function in the spinal cord injured patient. *J Urol* 1994;151(4):951–954.

51. Ishizuka O, Mattiasson A, Steers WD, et al. Effects of spinal alpha 1-adrenoceptor antagonism on bladder activity induced by apomorphine in conscious rats with and without bladder outlet obstruction. *Neurourol Urodyn* 1997;16(3):191–200.

52. Ishizuka O, Pandita RK, Mattiasson A, et al. Stimulation of bladder activity by volume, L-dopa and capsaicin in normal conscious rats: effects of spinal alpha 1-adrenoceptor blockade. *Naunyn-Schmiedebergs Arch Pharmacol* 1997;355(6):787–793.

53. Lazzeri M, Beneforti P, Spinelli M, et al. Intravesical resiniferatoxin for the treatment of hypersensitive disorder: a randomized placebo controlled study. *J Urol* 2000;164(3 Pt 1):676–679.

54. Goins WF, Yoshimura N, Phelan MW, et al. Herpes simplex virus mediated nerve growth factor expression in bladder and afferent neurons: potential treatment for diabetic bladder dysfunction. *J Urol* 2000; 165(5):1748–1754.

55. Peters K, Diokno A, Steinert B, et al. The efficacy of intravesical Tice strain bacillus Calmette-Guérin in the treatment of interstitial cystitis: a double-blind, prospective, placebo controlled trial. *J Urol* 1997;157(6): 2090–2094.

56. Peeker R, Haghsheno MA, Holmang S, et al. Intravesical bacillus Calmette-Guérin and dimethylsulfoxide for treatment of classic and nonulcer interstitial cystitis: a prospective, randomized double-blind study. *J Urol* 2000;164(6):1912–1915.

57. Peeker R, Aldenborg F, Fall M. The treatment of interstitial cystitis with supratrigonal cystectomy and ileocystoplasty: difference in outcome between classic and nonulcer disease. *J Urol* 1998;159(5):1479–1482.

58. Christmas TJ, Holmes SA, Hendry WF. Bladder replacement by ileocystoplasty: the final treatment for interstitial cystitis. *Br J Urol* 1996;78(1):69–73.

59. Linn JF, Hohenfellner M, Roth S, et al. Treatment of interstitial cystitis: comparison of subtrigonal and supratrigonal cystectomy combined with orthotopic bladder substitution. *J Urol* 1998;159(3):774–778.

60. Flood HD, Malhotra SJ, O'Connell HE, et al. Long-term results and complications using augmentation cystoplasty in reconstructive urology. *Neurourol Urodyn* 1995;14(4):297–309.

61. Hassouna MM, Siegel SW, Nyeholt AA, et al. Sacral neuromodulation in the treatment of urgency-frequency symptoms: a multi-center study on efficacy and safety. *J Urol* 2000;163(6):1849–1854.

62. Jonas U, Fowler CJ, Chancellor MB, et al. Efficacy of sacral nerve stimulation for urinary retention: results 18 months after implantation. *J Urol* 2001;165(1):15–19.

63. Schmidt RA, Jonas U, Oleson KA, et al. Sacral nerve stimulation for treatment of refractory urinary urge incontinence. Sacral Nerve Stimulation Study Group. *J Urol* 1999;162(2):352–357.

64. Chai TC, Zhang C, Warren JW, et al. Percutaneous sacral third nerve root neurostimulation improves symptoms and normalizes urinary HB-EGF levels and antiproliferative activity in patients with interstitial cystitis. *Urology* 2000;55(5):643–646.

65. Maher CF, Carey MP, Dwyer PL, et al. Percutaneous sacral nerve root neuromodulation for intractable interstitial cystitis. *J Urol* 2001;165(3):884–886.

66. Nigro DA, Wein AJ, Foy M, et al. Associations among cystoscopic and urodynamic findings for women enrolled in the Interstitial Cystitis Data Base (ICDB) Study. *Urology* 1997;49[Suppl 5A]:86–92.

67. Keay S, Zhang CO, Kagen DI, et al. Concentrations of specific epithelial growth factors in the urine of interstitial cystitis patients and controls. *J Urol* 1997;158(5): 1983–1988.

68. Cook SP, McCleskey EW. ATP, pain and a full bladder. *Nature* 2000;407(6807):951–952.

69. Cockayne DA, Hamilton SG, Zhu QM, et al. Urinary bladder hyporeflexia and reduced pain-related behavior in P2X3-deficient mice. *Nature* 2000;407(6807):1011–1015.

70. Vlaskovska M, Kasakov L, Rong W, et al. P2X3 knockout mice reveal a major sensory role for urothelially released ATP. *J Neurosci* 2001;21(15):5670–5677.

71. Sun Y, Keay S, De Deyne PG, et al. Augmented stretch activated adenosine triphosphate release from bladder uroepithelial cells in patients with interstitial cystitis. *J Urol* 2001;166:1951–1956.

72. Birder LA, Apodaca G, De Groat WC, et al. Adrenergic- and capsaicin-evoked nitric oxide release from urothelium and afferent nerves in urinary bladder. *Am J Physiol* 1998;275(2 Pt 2):F226–229.

Ostergard's Urogynecology and Pelvic Floor Dysfunction, Fifth Edition. edited by A.E. Bent, et al. Lippincott Williams & Wilkins, Philadelphia © 2003.

22

Sacral Neuromodulation

Mary T. McLennan

Department of Obstetrics, Gynecology, and Women's Health, St. Louis University, St. Louis University Hospital, St. Louis, Missouri

INDICATIONS

Tanagho and Schmidt introduced sacral neuromodulation in 1981 (1). Medtronic (Minneapolis, Minnesota) received initial approval to market InterStim therapy for the treatment of urge incontinence in 1997. The indications were expanded in 1999 to include frequency–urgency syndromes and nonobstructive urinary retention.

Most insurance companies do not approve this as first-line therapy. The latest Medicare recommendations include the following criteria:

1. Symptoms must be present for at least 12 months and have resulted in significant disability (i.e., limiting ability to work or participate in activities outside the home).
2. Other methods of conservative therapy have failed.
3. Conservative therapy must be documented.
   - Pharmacologic (two different medications)
   - Behavioral (pelvic floor exercises, behavioral modification, biofeedback, time voids, fluid management)
4. Successful test stimulation, defined as a 50% reduction in symptoms during a 3- to 5-day percutaneous test stimulation and symptom return when the stimulation is removed

PATHOPHYSIOLOGY

The mechanism of action is uncertain, but the effect appears to be by modulating afferent fibers. In the case of frequency–urgency–urge incontinence syndromes, stimulation of afferent input to S-3 activates spinal inhibitory pathways (2,3). Stimulation of sensory afferents from the pelvic floor can also inhibit the detrusor either at the spinal level or through neural pathways.

Idiopathic urinary retention is thought to be secondary to increased pelvic floor muscle activity (4). Continuous contraction of the pelvic floor is believed to cause detrusor inhibition. Based on the cat model, overactivity of the urethral sphincter results in detrusor hypotonia and suppression of bladder sensation. Fowler and colleagues described the so-called Fowler syndrome, in which the patient has an atonic detrusor and absent sensation of fullness (5). The same group later reported that successful neuromodulation resulted in a return of bladder perception, normal detrusor contraction presumably secondary to interfering with the increased afferent activity of the urethral sphincter (6). More recently, this same group was able to demonstrate that this effect does appear to be the result of an afferent mediated response (7).

In patients with chronic pain, for example, interstitial cystitis, it is thought that abnormal nonmyelinated C-afferent fibers are the basis for pain (8). Sacral neuromodulation acts by the afferent system once again and may be effective by modulating the C-afferent fibers. Other investigators have suggested that proximal activation of afferent fibers and peripheral nerves can lead to effective pain relief by exerting an inhibitory effect on the dorsal root (9).

EVALUATION

The patient should undergo the standard urogynecologic evaluation. This should include a detailed history focusing on medical and neurologic risk factors because certain conditions are relative contraindications to implantation (i.e., known neurologic disease). Aggravating factors (e.g., fluid intake, medications, and mobility) need to be assessed. Symptoms need to be detailed, including duration, pad use, degree of disruption to activities of daily living, and amount of frequency, urgency, and urge incontinent episodes. In the case of urinary retention, the amount voided and the amount obtained by self-catheterization need to be documented. Previous failed therapies, including duration of the trial, must be noted. Standard examination, including directed neurologic examination, postvoid residual, and urinalysis, is performed. Further studies may be performed as indicated (e.g., uncertain diagnosis, hematuria without infection, increased postvoid residual or symptoms of incomplete emptying, risk factors for bladder cancer). Urodynamics is not an absolute necessity.

Most centers do not perform electrodiagnosis before implantation. Tom Benson's group from Indianapolis recently presented initial work on the electrodiagnostic features of responders and nonresponders (10). An increased bladder–anal and clitoral–anal reflex sensory threshold correlated with improved outcome.

A baseline-voiding diary for a minimum of 3 days is required to assess eligibility. This provides the basis on which the 50% improvement during test stimulation is assessed. Medtronic provides a standardized diary, which is worthwhile to use because results can then be compared between centers.

TEST STIMULATION PHASE

The test stimulation phase is generally an office procedure but can be performed in an outpatient center if fluoroscopy is desired. No preparation by the patient is required. She is placed in the prone position with pillows under the abdomen to flatten the back and under the knees to elevate the lower limbs. The Medtronic kit contains all the supplies with the exception of lidocaine (Xylocaine) and bicarbonate. The lumbosacral area is prepared with povidone-iodine (Betadine), and the patient is draped in a sterile fashion. The bony landmarks are palpated and marked with a sterile marker. There are various ways to locate S-3. Most commonly, the greater sciatic notch is marked. S-3 is located at this level about 1 fingerbreadth lateral to the midline. Alternatively, the dropoff of the coccyx can be palpated, with S-3 about 3 fingerbreadths above and 1 fingerbreadth lateral to this.

The skin and subcutaneous tissue and periosteum are infiltrated with lidocaine or a lidocaine-bicarbonate solution (1% lidocaine with 8.4% bicarbonate in a ratio of 10:1). The addition of bicarbonate decreases stinging and burning from the highly acidic lidocaine. For the average-sized patient, a 3-inch 22-gauge spinal needle is inserted into the S-3 foramen. The operator needs to be aware of the sacral anatomy. The orientation of S-4 to the skin surface is about 90 degrees, but that of S-3 is only 60 degrees (Fig. 22.1). The spinal needle probes the bone and then drops into the foramen, a movement that has a distinct feel. The insulated spinal needle is connected to the temporary stimulator (Fig. 22.2). The parameters are preset at a stimulation frequency of 10 Hz, pulse duration of 210 ms, and current of 0.5 to 20 mA.

An appropriate S-3 response is plantar flexion of the ipsilateral great toe and contraction of the levator ani causing deepening of the groove between the buttocks—the so-called bellows response (11). Toe flexion is not requisite. S-4 stimulation results in appropriate sensation for the patient but no motor response. The patient typically reports a pulling sensation in the vagina or rectum or a vibrating or tingling sensation in the vagina or rectum. An S-2 response would involve plantar flexion and an eversion of the foot and a withdrawal-type clamping of the rectum.

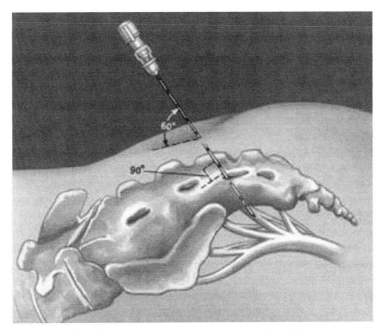

FIG. 22.1. Needle orientation for test stimulation.

When an appropriate response is obtained, a 3057 test electrode wire is threaded through the sheath of the spinal needle. This is the newer of the two electrodes. The original wire (041830-002) had a high rate of lead migration (30%) (Table 22.1). In a recent study comparing both leads, the mean range of lead migration with a new lead on radiograph was 4 mm (2 to 12 mm), compared with 12 mm (10 to 45 mm) for the old prototype, which was a significant difference (12). The reported clinical failure rate for the new lead in that study was 17%, half of previous reports. It is hoped that this new lead with coiled strands as opposed to straight wire will reduce the number of negative test stimulations thought to be secondary to lead migration.

The electrode is secured to the skin with a breathable elastic tape. It is important for the patient to avoid bending, and she should slide off the table rather than sit up and move. The lead is attached to the temporary stimulation device (Fig. 22.3). Some investigators obtain anteroposterior and lateral radiographs to document the position. The patient adjusts the voltage of the stimulation by turning a simple dial. She should feel the response at all times, but it should be comfortable. The patient should be made aware that the intensity may vary and have to be adjusted accordingly depending on her position and activity. She

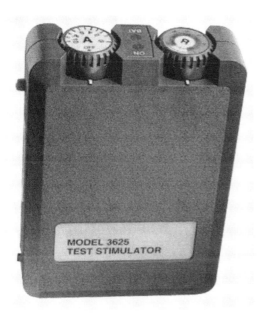

FIG. 22.2. Temporary stimulator.

TABLE 22.1. *Success rates with test stimulation phase*

Lead author	Study type	Diagnosis	N	Patients with >50% improvement (%)	Criteria
Dijkema (13)	Observational	UI, frequency, urge, pain	100	28	Diary
Koldewijn (14)	Observational	DI, UI, retention	100	47	Diary
Bosch (15)	Observational	UI	31	58	Diary
Weil (16)	Observational	DI, UI, retention	100	36	Diary
Bosch (17)	Observational	UI	70	57	Diary
Edlund (18)	Observational	UI	30	33	Diary
Weil (20)	Randomized	UI	123	75	Diary
Swinn (6)	Observational	Retention	38	68	Diary
Bosch (19)	Observational	UI	85	53	Diary
Carey (12)	Observational	UI	12	83	Diary

UI, urge incontinence; DI, detrusor instability.

should avoid strenuous activity, particularly bending, which may dislodge the lead. A minimum of 3 days of the voiding diary must be completed during the test stimulation phase. Direct comparison is made between these diaries and the one performed before stimulation to determine whether there has been at least a 50% improvement in symptoms to qualify for permanent implantation.

Successful response for the test stimulation phase is reported at a mean of 55% (range, 28% to 83%) (6,12–20) (Table 22.1). These success rates are with the old lead (average, 52%; range, 28% to 75%). Carey and associates reported 83% success with the new type (12).

Incorrect placement is an additional reason for failure. Janknegt and co-workers surgically implanted 10 nonresponders and noted that 8 of these subjects obtained a positive response (21). It appears that inappropriate positioning was the reason for failure. In an attempt to reduce this nonresponse rate, Benson reported on the addition of electrodiagnostic techniques (22). A ring electrode located on a Foley catheter is placed in the urethra. The muscle re-

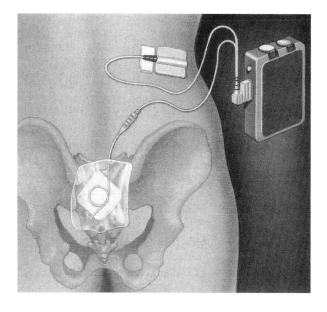

FIG. 22.3. Test stimulation phase.

sponse from the urethral sphincter is recorded. Benson reported a positive response rate of 80%. Of the responders, 46% did not have a bellows response, 74% had no toe response, and 46% had no vaginal sensation response, the responses typically looked for when relying on perineal and extremity visualization. A randomized prospective study is underway to determine whether such testing can increase efficacy as this initial report suggests.

PERMANENT IMPLANTATION

After induction of anesthesia and intubation on the stretcher, the patient is moved directly onto the operating room table and into the prone position. It is important to notify the anesthesiologist that long-acting muscle relaxants cannot be used because this abolishes the motor response needed to confirm correct placement. Prophylactic antibiotics (e.g., third-generation cephalosporins) are routinely used. If using adjunctive electromyography, a urethral lead is placed over the Foley catheter and the latter inserted (22). The patient must

be adequately supported with chest rolls, arm supports, and pillows under the knees. The feet must be exposed to determine a toe or foot response. The buttocks are taped to the table to expose the anus. The landmarks of the obturator notch and the coccyx dropoff are marked with the skin pen, and the patient is prepared and draped.

A spinal needle is placed in a similar manner to the test stimulation to confirm the response at the site of implantation. An 8- to 10-cm midline incision over the spinous process is made down to the lumbodorsal fascia. The fatty tissue is dissected off this layer for 1.5 to 2 cm to allow adequate exposure. The medial insertion of the gluteus maximus muscle can be visualized, which is the approximate line for the incision for the implant. A 1- to 1.5-cm incision is made in the muscle. Cautery is the preferred method but cannot be used if the spinal needle is in close proximity. The paraspinous muscle is then bluntly or sharply split longitudinally, and the sacrum can be visualized (Fig. 22.4). Scott's ring retractor may be helpful in a thin patient, but Weitlaner's re-

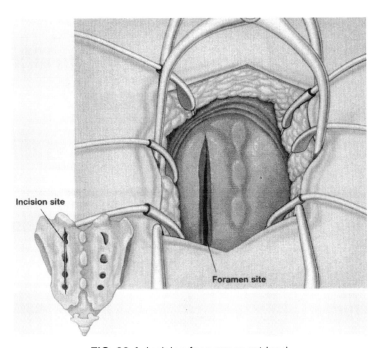

FIG. 22.4. Incision for permanent lead.

tractor is more useful for a larger patient because of the deeper blades. If the spinal needle is present, the foramen can easily be identified. Often, it can be palpated as a small indentation. A lacrimal duct probe is then used to dilate the fascial covering over the foramen. The initial recommendation was to insert the permanent lead, aiming inferolaterally toward the greater trochanter. However, Swinn and colleagues reported a series of patients with sciatica-like pain in the ipsilateral leg (23). Cadaver dissections showed that the more lateral in the foramen the lead is placed, the more intimate the association to the S-3 nerve route. In patients with leg pain, the lead may have impinged on dorsal rami. To avoid this, the current recommendation is to place the lead as far medially as possible so that the bend in the lead is directed medially. The length of the lead from the active electrode tip to the fixation cup is 3.5 cm. The lead is manipulated until muscle responses (anal or urethral) are obtained in at least two electrodes. The four electrodes are numbered 0, 1, 2, and 3, with 0 being the most distal. Each electrode is connected to the test stimulation control panel, and a bellows response of the perineum and flexion of the great toe is sought (Fig. 22.5). Full flexion of the foot (S-2) response should be avoided. The threshold for response should be 0.5 to 2 mA because lower thresholds may indicate the lead is too close to the nerve, which can cause postoperative pain.

After placement is confirmed to be ideal, the lead is secured to the periosteum. The recommendation is to place permanent sutures in the periosteum at three fixation points on the lead. It is often difficult to obtain a good purchase on the periosteum, and miniature bone anchors are useful as an alternative. The attached suture is placed around the lead and through the fixation points as would normally occur.

A transverse incision over the buttock is made for the generator [implantable pulse generator (IPG)] before closing the lead site. The lead is then tunneled to the proposed site of the IPG. The site is usually determined by the dexterity of the patient (i.e., which hand can more easily use the telemetry unit). Dissection of the fat is performed with cautery. It is important to leave at least a 1-cm fat layer over the muscle and a similar amount under the skin to decrease the risk for pain at the IPG site. The plastic sleeve "boot" is placed over the end of the extension lead, which is then connected to the IPG. The boot is manip-

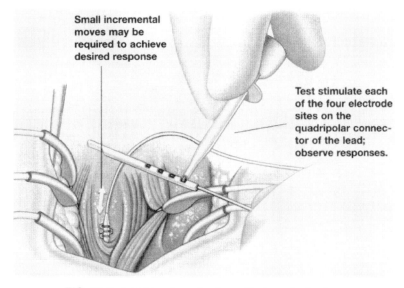

FIG. 22.5. Lead in place, testing with four electrodes.

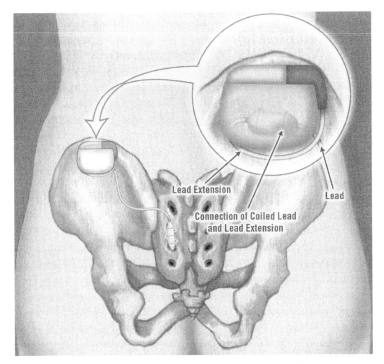

FIG. 22.6. Implantable pulse generator and lead in place.

ulated to cover the connection to ensure that liquid does not have access to the connection and is secured with two permanent sutures (Fig. 22.6). The IPG is placed in the pocket with the lettering uppermost. Extra wire can be placed around the perimeter of the IPG. A laparoscopic camera cover can be placed over the head of the telemetry unit to ensure sterility and the impedance of each electrode checked. It should be less than 2,000 Ω. Once all parameters appear functional, the fascia overlying the lead is closed for additional security. The fatty tissue over the lead and IPG is closed with absorbable suture to eliminate the dead space to reduce the risk for a seroma. A subcuticular suture is used for the skin incisions. If irrigation is desired, nonconductive sterile water is necessary.

POSTOPERATIVE CARE

Patients are typically hospitalized overnight (23-hour observation) for pain relief and additional doses of antibiotics as deemed necessary by the surgeon. Typically, the device is activated on the first postoperative day. With the new telemetry units, the patient may adjust the device at home after it is activated (Fig. 22.7). Patients need to be informed that the stimulation may need to be increased or decreased over the next several weeks depending on the amount of edema and trauma to the area. They should

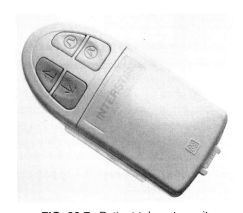

FIG. 22.7. Patient telemetry unit.

avoid twisting or bending and lifting for 4 to 6 weeks to minimize the risk for lead movement.

RESULTS

Frequency, Urgency, and Urge Incontinence

There are three randomized control trials evaluating Interstim in patients with frequency, urgency, or incontinence. Schmidt and colleagues randomized 34 patients with urge incontinence to immediate implantation and 42 patients to delayed implantation (24). At 6 months, 47% of the implanted group were dry, and 29% had a greater than 50% improvement. There was a significant reduction in leaks per day and pad usage. After stimulation was deactivated, the number of incontinent episodes increased back to baseline.

Hassouna and associates randomized 51 patients with frequency or urgency—25 patients to immediate implantation and 26 patients to delayed implantation (3). After 6 months, there was a statistically significant reduction in number of voids per day (16.9 ± 9.7 to 9.3 ± 5.1), volume per void (118 ± 74 mL to 226 ± 124 mL) and degree of urgency (rank, 2.2 ± 0.6 to 1.6 ± 0.9). Efficacy was sustained at 12 and 24 months.

European data confirm these results. Weil and co-workers randomized 21 patients to immediate implantation and 23 to continuation of conservative therapy (20). After 6 months, the control group was eligible to cross over; 56% of subjects were dry, and 75% had greater than a 90% improvement. Implanted patients exhibited improved quality-of-life measures, including physical function and emotional role, compared with controls.

These studies suffer from a number of epidemiologic problems, most notably patient dropout. Schmidt and colleagues initially implanted 86 patients, but 6-month data were reported on 58 patients (67%) (24). Similarly, Weil and associates randomized 21 patients to immediate implantation, but 16 patients were evaluable at 6 months (20). Long-term, the dropout numbers are even greater, with 36% of the original patients evaluable at 18 months (24). This raises the concern about the potential of significant bias because it is possible that those lost patients represented a disproportionate number of treatment failures.

Observational trials have produced similar results. It is important to note that all patients in observational studies were required to have successful test stimulation with greater than 50% improvement as documented by objective voiding diaries. These are the same criteria used in the randomized control trials. Cure rates have ranged from 50% to 68%, with greater than 50% improvement in 12% to 83% and greater than 90% improvement in 40% to 70% (1,3,13,15,16,19,24–30) (Table 22.2).

These studies did not include patients with known neurologic disorders or patients older than 70 years of age. It is difficult to know whether efficacy would be the same in the older patient population. However, after analysis of available data, Medicare on June 29, 2001 considered the scientific and clinical evidence sufficient to support coverage of this technology for Medicare beneficiaries nationwide.

Retention

There are a small number of studies on the use of sacral neuromodulation in urinary retention. In the only randomized control trial, Jonas and co-workers enrolled 177 patients with urinary retention refractory to standard therapy (31). Sixty-eight patients had successful peripheral nerve evaluations; 37 of these patients were randomly assigned to immediate implantation and 31 to delayed implantation. Results were reported on 29 of the implanted patients and 22 controls. Of the remaining 17 patients, 6 had not yet been enrolled, 3 were lost to follow-up, and 8 did not complete the voiding diary. At 6 months, 69% of those treated were voiding normally without catheterization, and 14% had greater than a 50% reduction in postvoid residual. Results were sustained at 18 months. These data have been supported by the observational data with reported cure rates of 50% to 71% (26,27, 30–32) (Table 22.3).

TABLE 22.2. *Success rate for treatment of urge incontinence (UI), frequency, and urgency*

Lead author	Study type	Diagnosis	N	No. of voids/day	No. of leaks/day	Pads	Degree of urgency	Patients with >90% improvement (%)	Patients with >50% improvement (%)	Cure (%)	Criteria	Follow-up (mo)
Elabbady (26)	Observational	Frequency, urge, pain	9	Improved by 37%	Improved by >50%	Improved by >50%			100		Diary	3–52
Schmidt (24)	Randomized	UI	34 Rx 42 delayed Rx		9.7/2.6 9.3/11.3	6.2/1.1 5.0/6.3			29	47	Diary	6
Bosch (15)	Observational	UI	18					61	83	50	Diary	×29
Thon (25)	Observational	UI	20						85		Not stated	Min, 12
Shaker (27)	Observational	UI	18		6.49/1.98				22	44	Diary, UDS	3–83
Weil (16)	Observational	UI	24	13.7/8.7	4.9/1.1	6.6/2.3		66	12		Diary, UDS	6
Dijkema (13)	Observational	UI, frequency, urge, pain	23		7.4/1.5	4.5/1.8		60	83		Diary	Mean, 12
Edlund (18)	Observational	UI	9		5.9/2.8	3/1.9					Diary	8–39
Weil (20)	Randomized	UI	44					75	33	56	Diary, UDS	6
Bosch (17)	Observational	UI	30	14.1/10.3	7.8/3.3	6.6/2.4					Diary, UDS	6–68
Tanagho (1)	Observational	UI	97							68	Not stated	Not stated
Hassouna (3)	Randomized	Urgency, frequency	25 Rx 26 delayed	16.9/9.3			2.2/1.6				Diary	24
Bosch (19)	Observational	UI	45		7.1/1.3	5.4/1.2		40	20		Diary, UDS	
Spinelli (30)	Observational	UI	86		5.4/1.1					57 65 55 59 43	Diary Diary Diary Diary Diary	3 6 9 12 18
Chartier-Kastler (29)	Observational	UI	9	16.1/8.2					100	56	Diary, UDS	7–72
Everaert (28)	Observational	UI, retention, pain	53						28	57	Diary	13–39

Rx, immediate treatment; delayed (Rx), delayed treatment; UDS, urodynamic studies.

TABLE 22.3. *Success rates with urinary retention*

Lead author	Study type	N	Self-catherization (preop/postop)	Cure (%)	Patients with >50% reduction in PVR (%)	Criteria	Follow-up (mo)
Elabbady (26)	Observational	8	4.2/1.3			Diary	3–52
Shaker (27)	Observational	20				Diary	1–18
Vapnek (32)	Observational	7		71		Subjective	2–48
Jonas (31)	Randomized	37 Rx 31 control		69	14	Diary	18
Spinelli (30)	Observational	45		67	13, cath 1/d	Diary	6
				50	33, cath 1/d		12

PVR, postvoid residual.

Interstitial Cystitis

Interstitial cystitis is currently not an approved indication for implantation. A small number of reports with small numbers of patients have been published. Zermann and coworkers reported a case of a patient with a 5-year history of interstitial cystitis who, 6 months after implantation, was pain free and had marked improvement in voiding (nocturia decreased from 4 to 2 and frequency from 21 to 10) (33). Chai and collaborators reported a small series of six patients undergoing test stimulation (34). Voiding frequency decreased from 23.1 ± 4.6 to 10.6 ± 4.0 and pain from 7.0 ± 1.6 to 2.3 ± 3.2 on a standard pain scale.

More recently, Maher and associates reported their results from 15 test stimulations. Bladder pain decreased from 8.9 to 2.4 on a standardized pain scale, frequency from 20 to 11, and nocturia from 6 to 2 (35). Quality-of-life variables also improved. Currently, this group of patients can be treated with Interstim if they have significant symptoms of frequency and urgency that meet the criteria.

URODYNAMIC CHANGES

There appears to be a general consensus in the literature that there is an increase in first sensation to void and maximum cystometric capacity for those with frequency, urgency, and

TABLE 22.4. *Urodynamic changes with Interstim*

Lead author	Indication	N	First sensation Pre/post (mL)	Maximum capacity Pre/post (mL)	Vol. at first contraction Pre/post (mL)	Peak flow rate Pre/post (mL/s)
Dijkema (13)	Retention, freq, pain	23		135/227[c]	80/167[c]	
Elabbady (26)	Retention, freq, pain	17		465/595		7.8/18
Bosch (15)	UI	18	204/318[a]	318/402	206/258[b]	
Shaker (27)	UI	18	133/203[c]	291/336[c]	80/124[c]	
Bosch (17)	UI	24/30	213/291[a]	306/380		
Shaker (36)	Retention	20	204/167	384/381		0/14[a]
Weil (20)	UI	21	93/167	266/370[a]	115/370[a]	
Groen (37)	UI	26		285/313		
Walsh (38)	UI	74	109/167[a]	345/404[a]		

[a]Significant with $p < 0.05$.
[b]8 of 10 patients had no contractions after stimulation.
[c]Significance not reported.

urge incontinence. Unfortunately, most studies published do not state whether this was a statistically significant change (Table 22.4) (13, 15,17,20,26,27,36–38). Of the two urodynamic reports on retention, there appears to be an increase in peak flow rate after implantation. Shaker's group (36) showed statistical significance, but Elabbady and colleagues (26) did not. This may be because in the former group, no patient voided preoperatively, but in the latter group, incomplete voiders were included.

Therefore, if a symptom diary shows significant reduction in frequency, urgency, and incontinence, and voiding is improved in the case of retention, the patient is eligible for implantation irrespective of urodynamic changes.

COMPLICATIONS

Tables 22.5 and 22.6 summarize the adverse events with test stimulation and perma-

nent implantation, respectively (13,24,3,6,20, 24,28,30). Revision rates range from 10% to 33%. Common complications are pain at the implant site (4% to 34%) followed by lead migration (4% to 17%). The high prevalence of pain is partially accounted for by the fact that the initial implantation devices (IPGs) were placed in the lower abdomen. It is currently standard practice to place these over the buttock; however, Everaert recently reported pain equally at all sites (28). Patients need to be informed of the relatively high rate of reoperation.

Recently, there have been reports of decreased efficacy or cessation of response with time. Weil and associates noted over a 6- to 36-month follow-up that 8 of 34 subjects (24%) had deterioration in primary outcome measures (20). On logistic regression analysis, they noted no predictors for these treatment failures. Everaert and colleagues re-

TABLE 22.5. *Incidence of complications with test stimulation*

Complication	Multicenter pooled data	Dijkema (13)	Schmidt (24)
Lead migration	9.90%	8.60%	
Lead/test stimulator disconnection	2.60%		
Stimulator defect		4.30%	
Temporary pain	2.60%	21.70%	2.9%
Change bowel habit	0.60%		
Infection or skin irritation	0.60%		5.70%

TABLE 22.6. *Complications with permanent implantation*

Lead author	Weil (20)	Schmidt (24)	Hassouna (3)	Spinelli (30)	Everaert (28)	Swinn (6)
No. of patients	21	34	219	103	53	38
Complication (%)						
Pain at IPG	29	19.1	15.3	3.9	34	
Lead migration	17	7	8.4		4	8
Lead pain			5.4			
Operative revision		32.5	33.3	9.7		24
Leg pain	17					8
New pain			9		17	
Leg stimulation	5				8	
Change in bowel function	5	2.9			6	
Urinary retention	2					
Vaginal cramps	2					
Anal pain	2					
Skin irritation	2	5.7				
Infection			6.1		2	
Wound problem				1.9		

IPG, implantable pulse generator.

ported 6 of 53 (11%) late device failures. Reoperation resulted in no improvement in 4 and a temporary response in 1, but the ultimate result was failure (28). The authors concluded that revision for late failures in patients with a good S-3 response is not successful. This has also been my experience.

PATIENT SATISFACTION

Few articles have specifically addressed patient satisfaction. This is particularly important in view of the fact that reoperation rates are high, which could be a potential deterrent for some patients. Despite the fact that 81% continued to use the device, Everaert and colleagues reported that 68% of patients were satisfied and 66% would repeat the procedure (28). They felt that the dissatisfaction with long-term success was explained by the occurrence of complications in all patients.

FUTURE DIRECTIONS

Future studies need to be directed at lowering the rate of negative responders to the initial test stimulation phase. Up to 50% of the patients are excluded from possible permanent implantation owing to a lack of response. The role of electrodiagnosis in reducing this number will be an important area of future research.

There are some centers now performing a staged implantation with direct surgical implantation of the initial lead into the foramen. There are two versions of the staged implantation. The first is a traditional implantation of the lead electrode under general anesthesia, with a connection of the implanted lead to an externalized lead extension. The second is a more minimally invasive technique involving a limited incision with fascial fixation of the lead electrode, and then externalization through a connection. Both have the advantage of allowing a longer period of time to assess the efficacy of therapy (2 to 4 weeks) and to reduce dramatically the potential for lead migration compared with the traditional test stimulation. This makes it a better option for certain groups, such as obese and pain patients. These approaches also eliminate the potential that the test stimulation would be successful but that the permanent implant would not feel the same or produce the same effect owing to a different lead placement because the trial and permanent lead placements are the same. Both techniques appear to reduce the false-negative and false-positive result rates compared with the traditional test stimulation, but this needs to be verified.

The less invasive technique is attractive because it can be done under conscious sedation and allows the patient to give sensory feedback during the permanent lead implantation. It also results in a much shorter, shallower incision and reduces the risk for wound complication from seroma or infection. It can be done on an outpatient basis, which provides cost savings. After both approaches, the final step is either to remove the permanent lead and extension if unsuccessful or to implant the IPG. Both can be accomplished in 2 to 4 weeks after the initial phase, which is particularly useful in pain patients who may take an extended period to determine whether there was an adequate enough response to warrant permanent implantation. Theoretically, the longer the interval, the greater the risk for infection. Studies on this particular staged implantation are still pending.

The other major research area should be directed toward lowering the reoperation rate. Despite these limitations, this therapy is the light at the end of the tunnel for a group of patients who are at the end of their therapeutic options.

CONCLUSIONS

Sacral neuromodulation is effective therapy for the treatment of frequency, urgency, urge incontinence, and idiopathic retention in patients with a history of poor response to other therapies. It is important to note that all studies have been done on patients who have failed conservative therapy and are considered to have recalcitrant disease. Until Interstim

(Medtronic Inc., Minneapolis, Minnesota), we had little else to offer such patients. Reported success rates of greater than 50% are therefore impressive in this group of patients. It is important, however, to counsel the patient that there is a high reoperation rate.

REFERENCES

1. Tanagho EA, Schmidt RA. Electrical stimulation in the clinical management of the neurogenic bladder. *J Urol* 1988;140:1331–1339.
2. Wheeler JS, Walter JS, Zaszczurynski PJ. Bladder inhibition by penile nerve stimulation in spinal cord injury patients. *J Urol* 1992;147:100–103.
3. Hassouna MM, Siegel SW, Lycklama À, et al. Sacral neuromodulation in the treatment of urgency-frequency symptoms: a multicenter study on efficacy and safety. *J Urol* 2000;163:1849–1854.
4. Goodwin RJ, Swinn MJ, Fowler CJ. The neurophysiology of urinary retention in young women and its treatment by neuromodulation. *World J Urol* 1998;16:305–307.
5. Fowler CJ, Christmas TJ, Chapple CR, et al. Abnormal electromyographic activity of the urethral sphincter, voiding dysfunction, and polycystic ovaries: a new syndrome? *BMJ* 1988;297:1436–1438.
6. Swinn MJ, Kitchen ND, Gooodwin RJ, et al. Sacral neuromodulation for women with Fowler's syndrome. *Eur Urol* 2000;38:439–443.
7. Fowler CJ, Swinn MJ, Goodwin RJ, et al. Studies of the latency of pelvic floor contraction during peripheral nerve evaluation show that the muscle response is reflexively mediated. *J Urol* 2000;163:881–883.
8. Barbanti G, Maggi CA, Beneforti P, et al. Relief of pain following intravesical capsaicin in patients with hypersensitivity disorders of the lower urinary tract. *Br J Urol* 1993;71:686–691.
9. Long DM. Electrical stimulation for the relief of pain from chronic nerve injury. *J Neurosurg* 1973;39:718–722.
10. Mastropietro M, Fuller E, Benson JT. Electrodiagnostic features of responders and non-responders to sacral neuromodulation test stimulation. *Int Urogynecol J Pelvic Floor Dysfunct* 2001;12[Suppl S1], paper 47.
11. Schmidt RA, Senn E, Tanagho EA. Functional evaluation of sacral nerve root integrity: report of a technique. *Urology* 1990;35:388–392.
12. Carey M, Fynes C, Murray C, et al. Sacral nerve root stimulation for lower urinary tract dysfunction: overcoming the problem of lead migration. *Br J Urol Int* 2001;87:15–18.
13. Dijkema HE, Weil EH, Mijs PT, et al. Neuromodulation of sacral nerves for incontinence and voiding dysfunctions. *Eur Urol* 1993;24:72–76.
14. Koldewijn EL, Rosier PF, Meuleman EJ, et al. Predictors of success with neuromodulation in lower urinary tract dysfunction: results of trial stimulation in 100 patients. *J Urol* 1994;152:2071–2075.
15. Bosch JL, Groen J. Sacral (S3) segmental nerve stimulation as a treatment for urge incontinence and detrusor instability: results of chronic electrical stimulation using an implantable neural prosthesis. *J Urol* 1995;154:504–507.
16. Weil EH, Ruiz-Cerda JL, Eerdmans PH, et al. Clinical results of sacral stimulation for chronic voiding dysfunction using unilateral sacral foramen electrodes. *World J Urol* 1998;16:313–321.
17. Bosch JL, Groen J. Neuromodulation: urodynamic effects of sacral (S3) spinal nerve stimulation in patients with detrusor instability or detrusor hyperflexia. *Behav Brain Res* 1998;92:141–150.
18. Edlund C, Hellstrom M, Peeker R, et al. First Scandinavian experience of electrical sacral nerve stimulation in the treatment of overactive bladder. *Scand J Urol Nephrol* 2000;34:366–376.
19. Bosch JL, Groen J. Sacral nerve neuromodulation in the treatment of patients with refractory motor urge incontinence: long-term results of a prospective longitudinal study. *J Urol* 2000;163:1219–1222.
20. Weil EH, Ruiz-Cerda JL, Eerdmans PH, et al. Sacral root neuromodulation in the treatment of refractory urinary urge incontinence: a prospective randomized clinical trial. *Eur Urol* 2000;37:161–171.
21. Janknegt RA, Weil EH, Eerdmans PH. Improving neuromodulation technique for refractory voiding dysfunction: two-stage implant. *Urology* 1997;49:358–362.
22. Benson JT. Sacral nerve stimulation results may be improved by electrodiagnostic techniques. *Int Urogynecol J Pelvic Floor Dysfunct* 2000;11:352–357.
23. Swinn MJ, Schott GD, Oliver SE, et al. Leg pain after sacral neuromodulation: anatomical considerations. *Br J Urol Int* 1999;84:1113–1115.
24. Schmidt RA, Jonas U, Oleson KA, et al. Sacral nerve stimulation for treatment of refractory urinary urge incontinence. *J Urol* 1999;162:352–357.
25. Thon WF, Baskin LS, Jonas U, et al. Neuromodulation of voiding dysfunction and pelvic pain. *World J Urol* 1991;9:138–141.
26. Elabbady AA, Hassouna MM, Elhilali MM. Neural stimulation for chronic voiding dysfunctions. *J Urol* 1994;152:2076–2080.
27. Shaker HS, Hassouna M. Sacral nerve root neuromodulation: an effective treatment for refractory urge incontinence. *J Urol* 1998;159:1516–1519.
28. Everaert K, De Ridder D, Baert L, et al. Patient satisfaction and complications following sacral nerve stimulation for urinary retention, urge incontinence and perineal pain: a multicenter evaluation. *Int Urogynecol J Pelvic Floor Dysfunct* 2000;11:231–236.
29. Chartier-Kastler EJ, Bosch JL, Perrigot M, et al. Long-term results of sacral nerve stimulation (S3) for the treatment of neurogenic refractory urge incontinence related to detrusor hyperreflexia. *J Urol* 2000;164:1476–1480.
30. Spinelli M, Bertapelle P, Cappellano F, et al. Chronic sacral neuromodulation in patients with lower urinary tract symptoms: results form a national register. *J Urol* 2001;166:541–545.
31. Jonas U, Fowler CJ, Chancellor MB, et al. Efficacy of sacral nerve stimulation for urinary retention: results 18 months after implantation. *J Urol* 2001;165:15–19.
32. Vapnek JM, Schmidt RA. Restoration of voiding in chronic urinary retention using neuroprosthesis. *World J Urol* 1991;9:142–144.
33. Zermann D-H, Weirich T, Wunderlich H, et al. Sacral nerve stimulation for pain relief in interstitial cystitis. *Urol Int* 2000;65:120–121.

34. Chai TC, Zhang C, Warren JW, et al. Percutaneous sacral third nerve neurostimulation improves symptoms and normalizes urinary BB-EGF levels and antiproliferative activity in patients with interstitial cystitis. *Urology* 2000;55:643–646.

35. Maher CF, Carey MP, Dwyer PL, et al. Percutaneous sacral nerve root neuromodulation for intractable interstitial cystitis. *J Urol* 2001;165:884–886.

36. Shaker HS, Hassouna M. Sacral root neuromodulation in idiopathic nonobstructive chronic urinary retention. *J Urol* 1998;159:1476–1478.

37. Groen J, van Mastrigt R, Bosch JL. Computerized assessment of detrusor instability in patients treated with sacral neuromodulation. *J Urol* 2001;165:169–173.

38. Walsh IK, Thompson T, Loughridge WG, et al. Non-invasive antidromic neurostimulation: a simple effective method for improving bladder storage. *Neurourol Urodyn* 2001;20:73–84.

PART B
Colorectal Disorders

Ostergard's Urogynecology and Pelvic Floor Dysfunction, Fifth Edition. edited by A.E. Bent, et al. Lippincott Williams & Wilkins, Philadelphia © 2003.

23

Fecal Incontinence

Mikio Albert Nihira* and Geoffrey W. Cundiff**

*Department of Obstetrics and Gynecology, Division of Urogynecology and Reproductive Pelvic Surgery, University of Texas Southwestern Medical Center, Dallas, Texas
** Department of Gynecology and Obstetrics, Johns Hopkins School of Medicine; and Department of Obstetrics and Gynecology, Johns Hopkins Bayview Medical Center, Baltimore, Maryland

EPIDEMIOLOGY

Defecation is a private function, and the inability to control bowel function often becomes an intense personal problem. Bowel control is learned in early childhood, and failure to control it may be associated with loss of independence resulting in lower self-esteem, social isolation, a sense of inadequacy or helplessness, and clinical depression.

Population-based postal surveys estimate the prevalence rates of fecal incontinence (FI) to be as high as 15% in women older than 50 years of age (1). Up to 3% of women who have delivered vaginally may develop FI. Less than half of women with FI seek professional help from their physicians (2). A fundamental limitation to the epidemiology of FI is that there is no standard definition. The prevalence varies according to the definition of FI used. Population-based surveys tend to underestimate the prevalence of FI owing to the embarrassing nature of the problem.

PATHOPHYSIOLOGY

The pathophysiology and the evaluation of FI have been reviewed in Chapter 15. Because multiple mechanisms are responsible for fecal continence, the pathophysiology is varied. Fecal continence requires normal anatomy and function of the anal sphincters and the pelvic floor muscles plus normal anorectal sensation. Other important variables include stool volume and consistency, intestinal transit time, and normal mentation. Table 23.1 lists the factors that maintain fecal continence.

The most common etiology of FI that an obstetrician-gynecologist encounters is the obstetric sphincter tear. Obstetric injury most often results in anterior disruption of the anal sphincters. Sultan and colleagues (3) observed that 35% of a group of primiparous women who clinically were thought to be intact had sphincter defects observed on endoanal ultrasound 6 weeks after delivery. More concerning was their observation that 13% of the primiparous women developed FI or fecal urgency after delivery. Faltin and associates (4) performed immediate postpartum endoanal ultrasound in 150 primiparous

TABLE 23.1. *Factors contributing to fecal continence*

Colonic factors
  Normal stool consistency and volume
Muscular factors
  Intact anal sphincters and normal resting anal tone
Neurologic factors
  Normal anorectal sensation (sampling)
  Intact innervation to the external anal sphincter
  Intact innervation to the puborectalis
  Intact anorectal reflexes
  Normal mentation to coordinate the process
Anorectal factors
  Intact anal seal of the vascular cushions
  Normal rectal capacity and compliance

TABLE 23.2. *Principal causes of fecal incontinence seen by an obstetrician-gynecologist*

Obstetric trauma
  Injury to the sphincter
  Injury to the levator ani
  Pudendal neuropathy (stretch injury)
  Levator ani neuropathy (compression injury)
Pelvic organ prolapse
  Descending perineum syndrome
Anorectal surgical trauma
  Sphincter disruption
  Sphincter stretch
Functional etiologies
  Fecal impaction
  Diarrhea

women. They identified clinically undetected anal sphincter tears in 42 of 150 women (28%). In a postal questionnaire 3 months postpartum or more, FI was reported by 22 women (15%). The odds ratio of those that had clinically undetected sphincter tears was 8.8 for the development of FI.

Vaginal delivery is associated with pudendal neuropathy, particularly during a prolonged or difficult second stage of delivery. A proposed mechanism of injury is that nerve damage results from traction or compression. This damage may develop into impaired rectal evacuation with the need to strain, perineal descent, and subsequent fecal and urinary incontinence. Other common conditions seen by an obstetrician-gynecologist that are associated with FI are presented in Table 23.2.

PREVENTION

Given that obstetrical trauma is the most common etiology of FI in women, efforts at prevention should be focused on the management of labor and delivery. There is an association between sphincter disruption and episiotomy (both midline and mediolateral). There is also a well-established association between operative delivery using forceps and anal sphincter trauma. Avoidance of episiotomy and use of vacuum-assisted vaginal delivery (as opposed to forceps) when operative delivery is indicated, as well as a low threshold for cesarean delivery, may be protective (3).

EVALUATION

Table 23.3 summarizes the differential diagnosis of FI. The goal of the diagnostic process is to understand the specific pathophysiology of FI in the individual and identify contributing treatable conditions so that appropriate therapy may be initiated. This usually requires imaging and ancillary testing before planning manage-

TABLE 23.3. *Differential diagnosis of fecal incontinence*

Anatomic derangements
  Developmental
    Congenital abnormalities
  Traumatic
    Obstetric trauma
    Surgery (hemorrhoidectomy, anal dilation or sphincterotomy)
    Fistula
    Anorectal trauma
  Functional
    Rectal prolapse
    Sequelae of anorectal infection, Crohn's disease
Neurologic disorders
  Central nervous system processes
    Dementia, sedation, mental retardation
    Stroke, brain tumor
    Spinal cord lesions
    Multiple sclerosis
    Tabes dorsalis
  Peripheral nervous system processes
    Cauda equina lesions
    Polyneuropathies
    Diabetes mellitus
    Shy-Drager syndrome
    Toxic neuropathy
  Traumatic neuropathy
    Obstetric trauma
    Perineal descent
    Idiopathic incontinence
  Altered rectal sensation (site of lesion not known)
    Fecal impaction
    Delayed sensation syndrome
    Skeletal muscle diseases
    Myasthenia gravis
    Myopathies, muscular dystrophy
Smooth muscle dysfunction
  Abnormal rectal compliance
    Proctitis due to inflammatory bowel disease, radiation
    Rectal ischemia
  Internal anal sphincter weakness
    Radiation proctitis
    Diabetes mellitus
    Childhood encopresis

From Johanson JF, Lafferty J. Epidemiology of fecal incontinence: the silent affliction. *Am J Gastroenterol* 1996;91:33–36, with permission.

ment. The basic evaluation of FI is discussed in Chapter 15, and the use of imaging in this evaluation is discussed in Chapter 14.

TREATMENT

FI treatments include behavioral therapy, medical therapy, biofeedback, and surgery. If the patient has other gastrointestinal conditions that may be contributing to the FI, it is prudent to maximize the treatment for that condition before initiating an extensive evaluation for other causes of incontinence. If FI persists, then other potential causes should be investigated. Table 23.4 is a summary of the principles of therapy for FI.

A significant challenge to the evaluation of the published literature is the lack of a consistent outcome measure. Success in some studies is based on a functional outcome but varies from a definition based on continence to gas, liquids, or solids. Other studies base success on subjective criteria, such as "improved" compared with the preoperative condition.

Nonsurgical Therapy

One approach to nonsurgical therapy is to maximize the continence mechanism through alteration of stool characteristics. Stool con-

TABLE 23.4. *Principles of therapy*

General principles
    Treat underlying disease, if possible
    Protective skin care
    Continence aids
    Psychological support
Medical therapy
    Stimulation of defecation at intervals
    Antidiarrheal (constipating) drugs
    Biofeedback training
Surgical therapy
    Sphincteroplasty
    Postanal repair
    Fecal diversion (ileostomy, colostomy)
Investigational interventions
    Sacral nerve root stimulator
    Dynamic graciloplasty
    Artificial anal sphincter

Adapted from Schiller LR. Constipation and fecal incontinence in the elderly. *Gastroenterol Clin North Am* 2001;30(2):497–515, with permission.

sistency and volume can be manipulated by dietary and pharmacologic means. The goal is to achieve passage of one or two well-formed stools per day. The rationale is that formed stool is easier to control than liquid stool. Predictable elimination of feces can be achieved by using the gastrocolic reflex, diet, and pharmacologic means.

Dietary Modifications

Increasing fiber consumption to the recommended 25 to 35 g/d can increase stool volume and density. Excessive fiber with an inadequate fluid intake may predispose elderly patients to fecal impaction. For some patients, avoidance of highly spiced foods or other dietary irritants, such as coffee, beer, diary products, or citrus fruits, that may precipitate diarrhea may also help.

Pharmacologic Agents

Constipating agents are helpful for patients who suffer from fecal frequency or urgency or who have chronic loose stools or diarrhea. Loperamide retards transit time and stimulates anal sphincter function. A 4-mg dose before meals has been demonstrated to increase anal tone and improve continence (5). The main side effect is constipation, which is usually better tolerated than FI. A balance between continence and constipation can usually be achieved with careful titration. Other useful constipating agents include codeine phosphate and diphenoxylate hydrochloride with atropine (Lomotil). Anticholinergic side effects include dry mouth, sleepiness, lightheadedness, and tachycardia.

Tobin and Brocklehurst (6) documented the effectiveness of pharmacologic treatment for FI in a geriatric population of 82 patients. Fifty-two subjects were randomly selected for pharmacologic therapy, whereas the other 30 served as controls. The study patients were separated into two therapeutic groups based on their history and physical examination. Those with FI secondary to fecal impaction were given a regimen of lactulose, 10 mL twice daily, and an enema once a week. Those diagnosed with neurogenic FI were constipated with codeine phosphate, 30 to 60 mg/d, and had two enemas a week three days apart to ensure that they would have only two bowel movements a week at predictable times. They reported that 60% of the study group members were continent, whereas another 4% had incontinence less than once a week. In the control group, 46% improved, although only 32% were continent.

α-Adrenergic agonists have theoretical utility as a means of improving the resting tone of the internal anal sphincter (IAS) (7), but there are no commercial preparations.

Bowel Regimens

Regimens of enemas or suppositories may be useful although potentially messy strategies to control incontinence. The goal is to leave the rectum empty between evacuations. The frequency of enemas must be titrated to the patient's baseline colonic activity but is usually once to twice daily. Cone-tip colostomy-irrigation catheters are useful for incontinent patients because they avoid the risk for rectal perforation and provide a dam to prevent efflux of the irrigating solutions (8). This approach is often used in patients who have failed other therapeutic modalities.

Biofeedback

Biofeedback can be an effective therapeutic modality provided patients are motivated and comprehend instructions. There are two proposed mechanisms through which biofeedback improves fecal continence:

Efferent training: voluntary contraction of the external anal sphincter (EAS) may be enhanced through training, allowing the patient to recruit more motor units and stimulate muscle hypertrophy.

Afferent training: impaired sensation in the anorectal canal may be improved through practice that recruits adjacent neurons to decrease the sensory threshold of volume stimulation.

Although there is little long-term data to support the efficacy of biofeedback for the treatment of FI, some investigators have observed success rates as high a 70% to 80% (9,10). Patients may be taught to contract the sphincters and the levators voluntarily in response to rectal distention. This strategy serves two purposes: one is to improve voluntary contraction of the puborectalis and the anal sphincters (efferent training); the other is to improve sensory discrimination for rectal filling (afferent training).

One of the most critical elements of biofeedback is patient education. An explanation of the influence of stool consistency or levator ani tone permits the patient to modify these parameters to improve continence. Similarly, an explanation of the physiology of the rectoanal inhibitory reflex can help patients with fecal urgency (7).

Norton and Kamm (11) reported the results of biofeedback in 100 patients with FI (84 of the 100 patients were women). The therapeutic goals were to isolate sphincter contraction from abdominal effort, increase maximal contraction, and improve rectal sensitivity. A manometric anal probe was employed to measure sphincter contractions. Treatments occurred weekly for a median duration of 5 weeks. Overall, 43% were symptomatically cured, and 24% improved. The patients with an intact EAS responded better to therapy than did those with EAS defects detected by endoanal ultrasound.

Despite the large number of patients who appear to have benefited from biofeedback, a critical examination of the evidence reveals significant methodologic weaknesses in the current literature. Norton and associates (12) scrutinized the published trials that involved biofeedback or anal sphincter exercises for the Cochrane Review. Only five studies met the standards of being adequately randomized controlled trials to evaluate the efficacy of this approach. They concluded that rectal volume discrimination training (afferent training) improves FI more than sham training. Further conclusions about the efficacy of biofeedback for FI were not possible based on the literature. They recommended that large, better-designed trials are needed to enable definitive conclusions about the efficacy of biofeedback therapy.

Surgical Therapy

The potential for surgical complications combined with less than perfect outcomes must be considered and discussed with patients when considering surgical therapy. A variety of surgical repairs have been advocated for FI. They generally compensate for different aspects of the faulty continence mechanism. For example, patients with complaints of postdefecatory fecal seepage in the context of a large rectocele with relatively intact anal sphincters and innervation often regain continence with a defect-directed rectocele repair (see Chapter 26). In this chapter, we highlight those procedures specifically described for FI and listed in Table 23.4.

Overlapping Sphincteroplasty

Sphincter repair is the procedure of choice for FI caused by a disrupted anal sphincter. Most authorities believe that an overlapping or flap-over technique is superior to an end-to-end repair, although direct comparisons are lacking in the literature. The rationale for the overlapping technique is that sutures should be less likely to tear through or pull out of scarred connective tissue than the sphincter muscle. The overlapping technique, therefore, preserves the scarred ends of the ruptured EAS for suture placement.

Technique

The procedure begins with wide mobilization of the ruptured EAS without excision of the scarred ends of the sphincter (Fig. 23.1). This is accomplished through an inverted semi-lunar perineal incision or a transverse incision at the posterior vaginal fourchette with infero-lateral extension in patients who have damage to the perineal body or rectovaginal septum. The latter incision facilitates repair of the perineal body and rectovaginal fascial attachments. Patients with EAS defects may have fibrous scar tissue intervening between the

viable muscular ends of sphincter, or they may have complete separation with scar tissue only present on the ruptured ends of the sphincter. In the latter case, the perineal body is usually compromised, and a complete reconstruction is indicated. A Pena muscle stimulator is invaluable to identify the distal ends of the EAS and to differentiate the viable muscle tissue from the scar tissue both before undertaking the dissection and during the dissection.

In dissecting out the EAS, care should be taken to avoid excessive lateral dissection around the EAS because the hemorrhoid branches of the pudendal nerve that serve the EAS enter at about the 3- and 9-o'clock positions. This can be a bloody dissection, and needlepoint cautery can maximize hemostasis. There is controversy about the importance of dissecting the EAS from the IAS before repair. This is accomplished by identifying the intersphincteric groove and keeping the dissection in this plane to avoid damage to either sphincter. If the IAS is also ruptured, its ends are identified before repair. This can be difficult because the IAS is intimately associated with the rectal mucosa but is facilitated by placing a finger in the anal canal.

The primary surgical goal is to repair at least 2 to 3 cm of the EAS to ensure that the anal canal is enclosed by an adequate bulk of muscular sphincter. Closure of the IAS and reconstruction of the perineal body and rectovaginal septum are also indicated to maximize the normal continence mechanism. A 3-0 delayed absorbable monofilament suture is used. Copious irrigation is used between layers. The EAS is overlapped with three or four stitches of 2-0 delayed absorbable suture placed through the distal scar tissue. The muscle ends are overlapped sufficiently to create snugness around an anal finger.

Finally, the perineal skin is closed with interrupted absorbable, monofilament suture. This frequently requires modification of the initial incision because of changes in the perineal architecture that result from repair of the sphincter. The most common approach is a Y closure of the incision.

Some surgeons recommend the overlapping repair regardless of whether the repair is a pri-

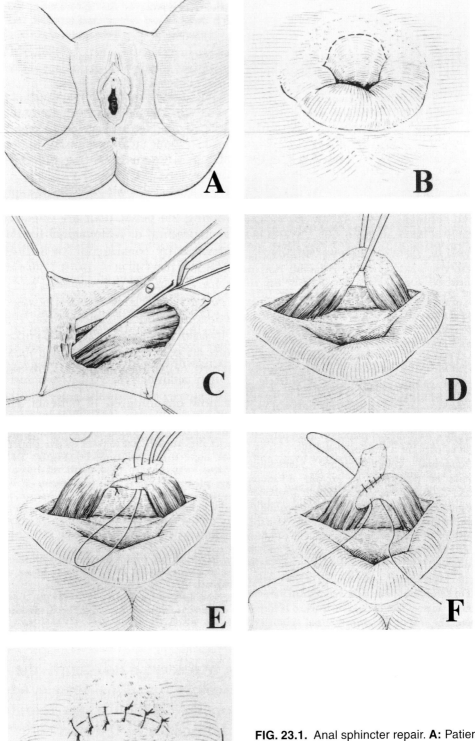

FIG. 23.1. Anal sphincter repair. **A:** Patient in lithotomy position for repair of anterior sphincter defect. **B:** Mucosa dissected off sphincter defect. **C:** The lateral components of the external anal sphincter are mobilized widely. **D:** The external anal sphincter is elevated and the scarred portion incised. **E, F:** A two-layer flap-over repair is performed. **G:** Completed repair.

mary repair, that is, immediately postpartum, or a secondary repair several years after an obstetric injury. Although the theoretical advantage of suture holding in the scar tissue does not apply to the primary repair, it does maximize surface area for scarification of the sphincter ends. In the case of secondary repairs, it is recommended to wait 3 to 6 months to permit all the postpartum inflammation to resolve.

Efficacy

One of the largest series with the longest reported follow-up was reported by Fang and colleagues (13). They examined the results of a 30-year experience with overlapping anal sphincteroplasty (OLAS). The mean duration of follow-up was 35 months. Of the 47 patients who underwent OLAS, 27 (57%) were continent to solid, liquid, and gas stool; another 17 (36%) had occasional incontinence of liquid stool. More recently, Malouf and colleagues (14) published a series that observed a similar rate of improvement after sphincteroplasty. They identified 55 patients who underwent OLAS at least 5 years previously. In all of these patients, sphincter damage was thought to be secondary to an obstetric trauma. The investigators observed that when compared with the results of a postoperative examination at 15 months, the symptomatic improvements were not maintained. The total follow-up consisted of 46 patients. In 8 of the 46 patients (17%), the sphincteroplasty failed, and those patients required further surgery that included colostomy. Of the 38 remaining patients, 27 (71%) reported improved bowel control, 5 (13%) were unimproved, and 6 (16%) were worse. No patient at the 5-year follow-up was fully continent (solids, liquids, and gas). Twenty-five of 38 (66%) patients complained that their current bowel control problems limited their lifestyle. Fifteen of the 25 (60%) patients reported this was "minor," but 10 reported it was "quite a lot" or "a great deal." Overall, the authors felt that at 5 years, 23 of the 46 (50%) patients had had a good outcome in terms of not requiring further surgery for continence and FI occurring less than once per month. Österberg and associates (15) found a similar result when they evaluated the performance of OLAS. After 1 year, 10 of 20 patients (50%) in the anterior sphincteroplasty group were continent of liquid and stool.

Some investigators have observed less success repairing patients with a sphincter defect complicated by pudendal neuropathy (16,17). They recommend concomitant postanal repair with the sphincter repair (18). Other investigators (15) have not observed this association and advise performance of sphincteroplasty alone, with patient counseling about the potential for less impressive results. Advanced patient age is also associated with reduced success of sphincteroplasty. Some researchers report lower success rates among patients older than 55 years of age (19,20), although others have found equivalent results regardless of age (21,22).

There is general consensus that a diverting colostomy does not usually improve the outcomes of the overlapping sphincteroplasty, and its routine use is discouraged. Some surgeons use diversion in women who are undergoing a second or third attempt at sphincter repair, although there is not evidence on which to base this decision (13).

Subsequent Deliveries

Bek and Laurberg (23) reported on 56 women that had sphincter lacerations after vaginal delivery and went on to have a second vaginal delivery. After the first delivery, 23 patients (41%) had transient FI. All but 4 recovered continence. Among the 23 that had transient FI after the delivery of their first child, an additional 4 women developed persistent FI after a subsequent delivery. As a result, the authors concluded that women should be counseled regarding the risk for FI with a subsequent vaginal delivery after an obstetric laceration of the anal sphincter.

Postanal Repair

Parks first described the postanal repair or posterior sphincter plication in 1975 (24). This procedure was originally designed to restore an acute anorectal angle and to elongate the functional length of the anal canal. It is indicated for patients with an intact EAS who have idiopathic or neurogenic FI and have failed conservative therapy. Postoperative defecography has demonstrated no change in the anorectal angle. It may improve continence by simply narrowing the lumen of the anal canal to increase passively the resistance to the passage of feces.

Technique

A curvilinear incision is made 3 cm inferior to the anal verge at the level of the coccyx. The EAS is dissected from the IAS, and the intersphincteric plane is opened. Waldeyer's fascia is incised transversely, and the rectum is mobilized off the sacrum. Interrupted sutures are then serially placed to plicate the medial limbs of the puborectalis and ileococcygeus muscles.

Efficacy

Parks initially reported a success rate of 81% in selected patients. Unfortunately, other surgeons have not been able to duplicate this success. Henry and Simpson (25) reported the results of postanal repair performed on 242 patients. The duration of follow-up ranged between 2 and 106 weeks, with mean of 46 weeks. Overall, 119 of the 204 patients (58%) had continence of liquid and solid stool. Seventy percent had incontinence of flatus. Most surgeons reserve this approach for a select group of patients with neurogenic FI who want to avoid diversion.

Diversion

The successful surgical repair of or compensation for a damaged fecal continence mechanism can be considerably more difficult to accomplish than the successful surgical repair of the damaged urinary continence mechanism. At the same time, salvage operations with diversion are considerably easier with FI than with urinary incontinence. Moreover, many patients achieve superior quality of life with a fecal diversion than with a less-than-successful repair. Although descriptions of techniques such as ileostomy and colostomy are beyond the scope of this book, the surgeon treating FI should keep these alternatives in mind for the difficult patient suffering from FI.

Novel and Investigational Procedures

Until recently, patients who were refractory to conservative therapy and sphincter repairs either had to live with FI or learn to live with a colostomy. Three new procedures—graciloplasty, artificial anal sphincters, and sacral nerve stimulation—offer hope when traditional approaches have failed or are inappropriate.

Graciloplasty

Adynamic graciloplasty (AGP) was first described in 1954 by Pickrell and colleagues. If repair of the EAS is not feasible because a large portion of the muscle is lost (because of trauma or because the muscle is too atrophied because of denervation), surgical reconstruction with a muscle flap should be considered.

Technique

A medial thigh incision is used to identify and mobilize the gracilis muscle (Fig. 23.2). The insertion onto the medial aspect of the tibia is divided. A transperineal tunnel is dissected around the anal canal. The gracilis muscle is then gently delivered through this tunnel, around the anus, to encircle the anal canal. The distal tendon of the gracilis is anchored to the ipsilateral ischial tuberosity. In patients with a large rectovaginal fistula or cloaca, the muscle flap can be mobilized with overlying skin and fat, and these can be sutured to help close the defect. Improvement in continence is due to passive increase of the resistance of the anal canal by the bulk of the encircling muscle.

Recent efforts to improve the effectiveness of this procedure have focused on developing resting tone in the transposed muscle through the use of an implanted neurostimulator. The

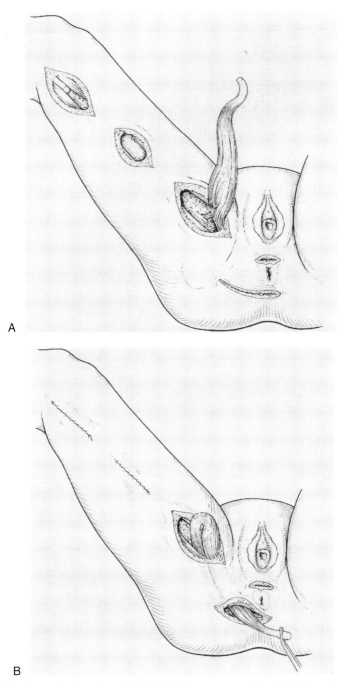

FIG. 23.2. Graciloplasty. **A:** A series of thigh incisions are used to identify and mobilize the gracilis muscle. Care must be taken proximally not to damage the neurovascular bundle, which enters the deep aspect of the muscle in the proximal third of the thigh. The tendon's insertion in the medial aspect of the tibia is divided. **B:** A tunnel is developed around the anal canal, and the tendon of the muscle is delivered around the anal canal to create a posterior sling. *(Continued on next page)*

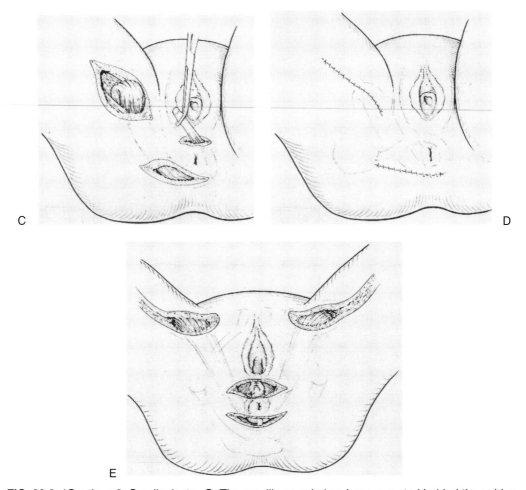

C   D

E

FIG. 23.2. (*Continued*) Graciloplasty. **C:** The gracilis muscle has been rerouted behind the sphincter. **D:** The tendon of the gracilis is sutured to the ischial tuberosity, and the skin has been closed. **E:** Double graciloplasty: both tendons are routed around the anus and sutured to each other.

intent of the stimulated graciloplasty is to convert the fast-twitch gracilis fibers into slow-twitch muscle fibers. The muscle is chronically stimulated for 2 months after surgery. The stimulation is adjusted to maintain tonic contraction around the anus. The patient interrupts the electric stimulation to defecate.

Efficacy of the Dynamic Graciloplasty

Niriella and Deen (26) performed an exhaustive review of the published literature. They identified 31 articles that included more than 200 patients. Cohorts were as large as 81

patients, but most were less than 20. The average reported rate of improved continence was 78%, and the average reported rate of failure was 28%. An international multicenter trial of dynamic graciloplasty has recently been published (27). A total of 123 adults received dynamic graciloplasty in this series. The success rates by different definitions of improved continence ranged between 55% and 66% in their patients. One hundred eighty-nine adverse events occurred in 91 patients (74%). Forty-nine patients (40%) required operative interventions to treat complications. The most significant complication was wound infection associated with failure of the dynamic graciloplasty.

Artificial Sphincter

The artificial sphincter is a modification of the device developed as an artificial urethral sphincter. It consists of three parts: (a) a Silastic inflatable cuff that encircles the anal canal, (b) a reservoir balloon, and (c) a patient-activated poppet valve that permits deflation of the cuff when the patient desires to defecate. The reservoir is placed in the retropubic space, and the poppet valve is placed in the labia majora. The sphincter cuff is placed through a perineal incision.

Efficacy

Experience with this device is limited to a few, highly specialized researchers. Presently, the literature consists only of pilot studies. Madoff (28) reported on the results of 28 patients who received artificial anal sphincters between 1997 and 1999. Seven artificial sphincters were removed (25%), six for infection. An additional six patients required surgical revision. One year after surgery, 9 of 12 patients were considered to have had a successful procedure as measured by reduced incontinence scores and improved quality-of-life scores.

Lehur and colleagues (29) described their implantation experience in 24 patients. At a median follow-up of 20 months, 20 patients had an activated implanted device. Incontinence scores improved drastically, and 75% of the patients had satisfactory results in terms of incontinence avoidance and ability to defecate.

Christiansen and co-workers (30) have the longest documented experience with the artificial anal sphincter. They have a cohort of patients 5 years or more (median, 7 years) after implantation. Originally, 17 patients were implanted. During the follow-up period, 2 died from unrelated conditions, 3 implants were removed secondary to infectious complications, and an additional 4 were removed secondary to malfunctions. Eight of the implants remained (47%). Four of these patients were continent of solid and liquid stool. The other four had "occasional" episodes of incontinence of liquid. Despite the challenges of postoperative infection and erosion that require device removal, the artificial sphincter appears to be relatively safe when under the care of an experienced specialist and offers the potential for good bowel control to a significant number of patients whose alternative may be fecal diversion.

Sacral Nerve Stimulation

Sacral nerve stimulation (SNS) has become an accepted form of treatment of urge urinary incontinence but has only been employed experimentally in the treatment of FI. The exact mechanism of action of SNS has not been fully elucidated. In the lower urinary tract, it appears to remodulate the sacral reflexes that influence urinary storage and micturition by balancing sympathetic and parasympathetic tone. Matzel and colleagues (31) published the first report of sacral nerve stimulation for the treatment of FI. Three patients experienced improved functional continence as well as increased closure pressure in the anal canal. Large populations and long-term data are presently lacking. The technique is described in Chapter 22.

Efficacy

The trials for this technique are very small. Malouf and associates (32) implanted SNS in five women with FI. All five had a 50% improvement over their baseline-voiding diary with percutaneous stimulation and proceeded to the permanent electrode. The continence scores on a validated instrument improved from a median of 16 (scale of 0 to 20) to 2 after surgery. The specific subgroup of patients for whom this modality is most effective has yet to be defined.

In an interesting report on two of these patients, the authors performed a double-blind trial in which the SNS pulse generator was turned off for a period of 2 weeks (33). The results were dramatic. There was a large reduction in the frequency of FI with the stimulator on. One patient had 10 episodes of incontinence with the unit off compared with 1 episode with the unit activated. The other patient had 30 episodes of incontinence with the unit off but only 2 episodes of liquid FI with the unit activated.

Treatment Summary

FI is a complex problem with a multitude of treatments. Lack of standard definitions and outcomes limits comparisons of different therapeutic approaches. Presently, care must be individualized to patients according to available resources. A conservative approach is recommended initially. Disrupted sphincters are surgically repaired if the initial therapy has failed. If the anal sphincters are intact, medical therapy and biofeedback are recommended. Continued research is necessary before it becomes clear which salvage procedure is best for patients who have failed this approach.

FUTURE AREAS OF RESEARCH

FI is not a homogeneous condition. It is imperative that standard definitions of FI that include important clinical subtypes are developed and employed in treatment trials so that optimal treatment strategies may be identified for women with different conditions. Another critical issue is the lack of standard outcome measurements.

REFERENCES

1. Roberts RO. Prevalence of combined fecal and urinary incontinence: a community-based study. *J Am Geriatr Soc* 1999;47:837–841.
2. Johanson JF, Lafferty J. Epidemiology of fecal incontinence: the silent affliction. 1996;91:33–37.
3. Sultan AH, Kamm MA, Hudson CN, et al. Anal-sphincter disruption during vaginal delivery. *N Engl J Med* 1993;329:1906–1911.
4. Faltin DL, Boulvain M, Irion O, et al. Diagnosis of anal sphincter tears by postpartum endosonography to predict fecal incontinence. *Obstet Gynecol* 2000;95(5):643–647.
5. Read M. Effects of loperamide on anal sphincter function in patients complaining of chronic diarrhea with fecal incontinence and urgency. *Dig Dis Sci* 1982;27(9):807–814.
6. Tobin GW, Brocklehurst JC. Faecal incontinence in res-

idential homes for the elderly: prevalence, aetiology and management. *Age Ageing* 1986;15:41–46.
7. Cundiff GW, Nygaard I, Bland DR, et al. Proceedings of the American Urogynecologic Society multidisciplinary symposium on defecatory disorders. *Am J Obstet Gynecol* 2000;182:1–15.
8. Madoff RD, Williams JG, Caushaj PF. Fecal incontinence. *N Engl J Med* 1992;326:1002–1007.
9. Rieger NA, Wattchow DA, Sarre RG, et al. Prospective trial of pelvic floor retraining in patients with fecal incontinence. *Dis Colon Rectum* 1997;40:821–826.
10. Patankar SK, Ferrara A, Levy JR, et al. Biofeedback in colorectal practice. *Dis Colon Rectum* 1997;40:827–831.
11. Norton C, Kamm MA. Outcome of biofeedback for faecal incontinence. *Br J Surg* 1999;86:1159–1163.
12. Norton C, Hosker G, Brazzelli M. Biofeedback and/or sphincter exercises for the treatment of faecal incontinence in adults (Cochrane Review). In: *The Cochrane library,* Vol. 2. Oxford: Update Software, 2001.
13. Fang DT, Nivatvongs S, Vermeulen FD, et al. Overlapping sphincteroplasty for acquired anal incontinence. *Dis Colon Rectum* 1984;27:720–722.
14. Malouf AJ, Norton CS, Engel AF, et al. Long-term results of overlapping anterior anal-sphincter repair for obstetric trauma. *Lancet* 2000;355:260–265.
15. Österberg A, Edebol Eeg-Olofsson K, Graf W. Results of surgical treatment for faecal incontinence. *Br J Surg* 2000;87:1546–1552.
16. Laurberg S, Swash M, Henry MM. Delayed external sphincter repair for obstetric tear. *Br J Surg* 1988;75:786–788.
17. Sitzler PJ, Thomson JP. Overlap repair of damaged anal sphincter: a single surgeon's series. *Dis Colon Rectum* 1996;39:1356–1360.
18. Keighley MRB, Williams NS. Faecal incontinence. In: Keighley MRB, Williams NS, eds. *Surgery of the anus rectum and colon.* London: WB Saunders, 1993:574.
19. Ctercteko GC, Fazio VW, Jagelman DG, et al. Anal sphincter repair: a report of 60 cases and a review of the literature. *Aust N Z J Surg* 1988;58:703–710.
20. Nikiteas N, Korsgen S, Kumar E, et al. Audit of sphincter repair: factors associated with poor outcome. *Dis Colon Rectum* 1996;39:1164–1170.
21. Young CJ, Mathur MD, Eyers AA, et al. Successful overlapping anal sphincter repair: relationship to patient age, neuropathy, and colostomy formation. *Dis Colon Rectum* 1998;41:344–349.
22. Simmang C, Birnbaum EH, Kodner IJ, et al. Anal sphincter reconstruction in the elderly: does advancing age affect outcome? *Dis Colon Rectum* 1994;37:1065–1069.
23. Bek KM, Laurberg S. Risks of anal incontinence from subsequent vaginal delivery after a complete obstetric anal sphincter tear. *Br J Obstet Gynaecol* 1992;99:724–726.
24. Soffer EE, Hull T. Fecal incontinence: a practical approach to evaluation and treatment. *Am J Gastroenterol* 2000;95:1873–1880.
25. Henry MM, Simpson JNL. Results of postanal repair: a retrospective study. *Br J Surg* 1985;72[Suppl]:S17–S19.
26. Niriella DA, Deen KI. Neosphincters in the management of faecal incontinence. *Br J Surg* 2000;87:1617–1628.
27. Baeten CG, Bailey HR, Bakka A, et al. Safety and efficacy of dynamic gracioplasty for fecal incontinence: report of a prospective, multicenter trial. Dynamic Gracioplasty Therapy Study Group. *Dis Colon Rectum* 2000;43:743–751.

28. Madoff RD. *Advances in the management of anorectal incontinence.* Presented at the 18th annual Houston Everett Memorial Course in Urogynecology. Baltimore, February 24, 2001.

29. Lehur PA, Roig JV, Duinslaeger M. Artificial anal sphincter: prospective clinical and manometric evaluation. *Dis Colon Rectum* 2000;43:1100–1106.

30. Christiansen J, Rasmussen Ø, Lindorff-Larsen. Long-term results of artificial anal sphincter implantation for severe anal incontinence. *Ann Surg* 1999;230:45–48.

31. Matzel KE, Stadelmaier U, Hohenfellner M, et al. Electrical stimulation of sacral spinal nerves for treatment of faecal incontinence. *Lancet* 1995;346: 1124–1127.

32. Malouf AJ, Vaizey CJ, Nicholls RJ, et al. Permanent sacral nerve stimulation for fecal incontinence. *Ann Surg* 2000;232:143–148.

33. Vaizey CJ, Kamm MA, Roy AJ, et al. Double-blind crossover study of sacral nerve stimulation for fecal incontinence. *Dis Colon Rectum* 2000;43:298–302.

Ostergard's Urogynecology and Pelvic Floor Dysfunction, Fifth Edition. edited by A.E. Bent, et al. Lippincott Williams & Wilkins, Philadelphia © 2003.

24

Defecatory Dysfunction

R. Mark Ellerkmann* and Howard Kaufman**

* Department of Gynecology, Johns Hopkins Medicine; and Division of Urogynecology, Greater Baltimore Medical Center, Baltimore, Maryland
**Department of Surgery, Johns Hopkins Medicine, Baltimore, Maryland

Defecatory dysfunction is a broad term that refers to any difficulty with defecation. Although the prevalence of this condition is difficult to ascertain, the incidence and prevalence of the individual conditions associated with defecatory dysfunction are better defined. Obstructive disorders may result from mechanical causes, such as neoplasia, benign strictures (Crohn's disease, low pelvic anastomosis, postirradiation), Hirschsprung's disease, rectal prolapse, prolapsing hemorrhoids, pelvic organ prolapse (POP), fecal impaction, or pelvic floor dyssynergia. Systemic diseases, such as diabetes mellitus, thyroid dysfunction, and multiple sclerosis may be associated with defecatory dysfunction. Functional disorders include irritable bowel syndrome (IBS), colonic inertia, and idiopathic constipation. Diet, lifestyle, and medications may also contribute to alteration in bowel habits. Finally, psychiatric causes, such as depression, eating disorders, and dementia, may lead to altered patterns of defecation.

CONSTIPATION

Epidemiology

Constipation remains one of the most common gastrointestinal disorders in America, with an estimated prevalence of 2% to 4% (1,2). Because it is a symptom, its presence and severity are often based on patient perception. Therefore, the frequency of self-reported constipation may be overestimated because epidemiologic studies have relied primarily on subjective survey by questionnaire. Constipation appears to be more commonly reported in women and with increasing age. The number of office visits for this complaint rises significantly after the age of 65 years (3). It has been correlated with lower economic status, fewer years of education (4), and sedentary lifestyle. Nonwhites are more frequently affected (5).

Differential Diagnosis

Although diet and stool bulk play an important role in the transit time of fecal material, constipation may be thought of as a disorder of gastrointestinal motility. Any number of etiologies can affect the motor function of the large intestine or its outlet from the pelvic floor (Table 24.1). These conditions range from underlying systemic diseases that directly impair bowel motor and sensory activity to secondary metabolic, endocrine, and neurologic disorders that affect motility and absorption. Functional disorders, such as IBS, ileus, and colonic inertia, may contribute to symptoms of constipation. In contrast, mechanical obstruction with POP, rectal prolapse, and neoplasm can lead to constipation

TABLE 24.1. *Differential diagnosis of constipation*

Systemic diseases
  Diabetes mellitus
  Thyroid disease
  Pregnancy
Collagen, vascular, muscular disorders
  Systemic sclerosis
  Amyloidosis
  Dermatomyositis
  Myotonic muscular dystrophy
Metabolic
  Hypercalcemia
  Hypokalemia
Endocrine
  Porphyria
  Panhypopituitarism
  Pheochromocytoma
  Glucagonoma
Neurologic
  Central
    Trauma, spinal cord lesions
    Sacral cauda equina lesions
    Meningomyelocele
    Multiple sclerosis
    Parkinson's disease
    Shy-Drager syndrome
  Peripheral
    Acquired
      Chaga's disease
      Paraneoplastic neuropathy
    Congenital
      Hirschsprung's disease
      Colonic aganglionosis
      Hyperganglionosis (neuronal dysplasia)
      Intestinal pseudoobstruction
      Sphincter achalasia
Functional causes
  Irritable bowel syndrome
  Ileus
  Colonic inertia
Idiopathic constipation
Outlet obstruction
  Neuromuscular
    Dyssynergic defecation
  Mechanical
    Pelvic organ prolapse
    Rectal prolapse
    Perineal descent
    Volvulus or intussusception
    Neoplasm
Other
  Cognition-dementia
  Mobility limited physical ability
  Nutrition
  Medication (see Table 24.2)
  Psychological causes

TABLE 24.2. *Drugs associated with constipation*

Analgesics
Anticholinergics
  Antispasmodics
  Antidepressants
  Antipsychotics
  Antiparkinsonian drugs
Neutrally active agents
  Opiates
  Antihypertensives
  Ganglionic blockers
  Vinca alkaloids
  Anticonvulsants
  Calcium-channel blockers
  Diuretics
Cation-containing agents
  Iron supplements
  Aluminum (antacids, sucralfate)
  Calcium (antacids, supplements)
  Barium sulfate
  Metallic intoxication (arsenic, lead, mercury)
Other
  5-HT$_3$ antagonists
    Granisetron
    Ondansetron

From Wald A. Approach to the patient with constipation. In: Yamada T, Alpers DH, Owyang C, et al., eds. *Textbook of gastroenterology*, 3rd ed. Philadelphia: Lippincott Williams & Wilkins, 1999;911, with permission.

from obstructed defecation. Dementia and limitations in a patient's physical ability to get to a bathroom can play a role in the pathogenesis of constipation and fecal impaction. Poor nutrition and certain medications can also lead to constipation (Table 24.2).

Systemic, Endocrine, and Neurologic Disorders

Diabetes mellitus, thyroid disease, and pregnancy are the most common underlying systemic causes of constipation. Symptoms tend to improve and become less severe after diabetic control is achieved or thyroid disease is corrected. Constipation in pregnancy has a reported prevalence of 11% to 38% (6). Etiologies include reduction in colonic motility and gut transit times because of the muscle-relaxing effects of progesterone, increased colonic water absorption related to increased aldosterone levels (7), and mechanical obstruction by the uterus. Less common but equally important systemic diseases known to cause constipation include collagen, vascular, and muscle disorders, such as systemic sclerosis, amyloidosis, dermatomyositis, and myotonic dystrophy. Metabolic disorders leading to electrolyte imbalances, such as hypercalcemia and hypokalemia, may also promote constipation, as may endocrinopathies such as porphyria, panhypopituitarism, pheochromocytoma, and glucagonoma.

Neural control of intestinal function is coordinated by the interrelationship of the enteric, sympathetic, and parasympathetic systems. Central nervous system lesions or injury involving the sacral nerves or spinal cord can compromise parasympathetic innervation of the bowel. Examples include trauma to the pelvic floor, lesions of the sacral cauda equina, injury to the lumbosacral spine, and meningomyelocele (8,9). Constipation can be associated with central neuropathies, such as multiple sclerosis, Parkinson's disease, and Shy-Drager syndrome. Multiple sclerosis, for example, has been shown to compromise bowel motility both directly (prolonged transit time, possible rectosphincteric dyssynergia) and indirectly (physical inactivity, medication side effects) (10). High spinal cord lesions may also be associated with constipation, even though lower colonic reflexes remain intact.

Peripheral neuropathies responsible for constipation may be either acquired or congenital. Patients who acquire Chagas' disease commonly present with progressively worsening symptoms of constipation and abdominal distention caused by segmental megacolon secondary to enteric neuronal degeneration. Nongastrointestinal neoplasms, such as carcinoid tumors and small cell carcinoma of the lung, have been associated with paraneoplastic visceral neuropathy, which can result in chronic constipation. The pathogenesis of this disorder is not entirely clear but may be related to either myenteric plexus inflammation or neuronal degeneration.

Congenital neuropathies may lead to functional obstruction and chronic constipation.

Hirschsprung's disease, the most well known of these disorders, is characterized by a congenital absence of intramural ganglion cell of both the submucosal and myenteric plexuses. The variability of clinical symptoms and poor correlation between symptoms and aganglionic segment length may result in delayed diagnosis in adulthood (11). Hallmark findings in adults include absence of the rectosphincteric inhibitory reflex, failure of the internal anal sphincter to relax after manometric distention, and absence of neurons on rectal wall biopsy (12). Other disorders of the enteric nervous system can include abnormally functioning or diminished concentration of enteric neurons (zonal colonic aganglionosis) (13) or loss or malfunction of inhibitory motor neurons, which serves as the pathophysiologic basis for disinhibitory motor disease (intestinal pseudoobstruction and sphincteric achalasia) (14).

Functional Constipation

Constipation has been traditionally defined as three or fewer bowel movements per week. However, patients may refer to other symptoms of defecatory dysfunction, including dyschezia, excessive straining, digital manipulation to facilitate defecation, abnormal variations in stool consistency, or sensations of incomplete emptying. In one study, only one third of patients complaining of constipation related this complaint to infrequent defecation. More common complaints included the inability to defecate when desired (34%), the passage of hard stools (44%), and straining associated with defecation (52%) (5). The Rome II criteria for functional constipation have been recommended to provide an operational definition in addition to one based solely on defecatory frequency, as follows:

Diagnostic Criteria

At least 12 weeks, which need not be consecutive, in the preceding 12 months, of two or more of the following:

1. Straining in more than 25% of defecations
2. Lumpy or hard stools in more than 25% of defecations
3. Sensation of incomplete evacuation in more than 25% of defecations
4. Sensation of anorectal obstruction or blockade in more than 25% of defecations
5. Manual maneuvers to facilitate more than 25% of defecations (e.g., digital evacuation, support of the pelvic floor)
6. Fewer than 3 defecations per week.

Loose stools are not present, and there are insufficient criteria for IBS.

Idiopathic Constipation

In approaching the differential diagnosis of constipation, it is necessary to consider and exclude conditions that could contribute to the symptom. When concurrent disease processes, diet, medications, and psychological factors cannot be identified, attempts to classify constipation as idiopathic may be based on age of presentation, colonic transit times, or anorectal sensory and motor dysfunction. Commonly, colonic transit times are used based on the presumption that there is some underlying colonic or anorectal motor dysfunction responsible for the disorder. To characterize constipation on this basis, four subtypes have been classified: (a) normal colonic and rectal transit time; (b) slow colonic transit time only; (c) slow rectal transit time only; (d) slow colonic and rectal transit times (3) (Table 24.3).

TABLE 24.3. *Diagnostic algorithm for idiopathic constipation*

Pathogenesis

Normal bowel motility depends on the action and combination of three distinct contraction patterns. Segmental contraction patterns result in mixing; propagating contractions result in the short-distance propulsion of colonic contents in either direction; and high-amplitude contractions result in the long-distance propulsion of stool boluses distally (3). Abnormalities in these contraction patterns, whether related to increased or decreased motor activity or lack of coordination, can result in colonic dysfunction.

The underlying physiologic abnormality is related to either diminished colonic motility (colonic inertia) or some type of pelvic outlet obstruction or abnormal rectal sensation (15). The pathogenesis is likely multifactorial, including underlying neurologic compromise, anorectal dysfunction, and any number of environmental factors. The most extensively studied has been the neural regulation of the enteric nervous system. Studies have demonstrated a neuronal deficit both in terms of actual neuronal loss (16,17) of the myenteric plexus supplying the colon and of diminished concentrations of vasoactive intestinal peptide, an inhibitory neurotransmitter (18). Anorectal dysfunction characterized by abnormal electromyographic and manometric studies showing paradoxical pelvic floor muscle contractions with defecation has also been documented in a subset of individuals with idiopathic chronic constipation (19).

Because the prevalence of idiopathic constipation changes with age, sex, social class, race, and culture, the role of environmental factors has been examined. Of these, diet has been most extensively studied. The efficacy of fiber in treating and preventing chronic constipation is a subject of ongoing debate (5,20). Other environmental risk factors include exposure to neurologic endotoxins (neurotoxic medications, laxative abuse) (21,22) and infectious agents (herpes simplex virus, herpes zoster virus, and cytomegalovirus) (5,23,24), which may adversely affect the myenteric plexus, as well as direct trauma to the pelvic nerves secondary to childbirth or pelvic surgery (20).

Age and Constipation

In children, chronic constipation may involve both physiologic and psychological factors. Children may present with symptoms of abdominal pain and distention when constipation is associated with fecal impaction with or without rectal (megarectum) and sigmoid (megacolon) dilation. Affected children may report the absence of a defecatory urge. Alternatively, they may demonstrate a conscious inhibitory or withholding reflex (learned response) related to previous experiences with dyschezia (possibly related to anal fissures or attempts to evacuate large stools) (12). Although decreased transit times localized to the distal colon and rectum have been demonstrated in many children with chronic constipation (25), manometric thresholds for rectal sensation and resting anal sphincter pressures are often normal (26,27). With the exception of children with Hirschsprung's disease, manometry usually demonstrates normal relaxation of the internal anal sphincter. Conversely, studies suggest that roughly two thirds of constipated children with encopresis suffer from anismus or rectosphincteric dyssynergia [failure to relax the puborectalis and external anal sphincter (EAS)] (12,28) (Fig. 24.1). The role of dietary fiber appears to be important; several studies have demonstrated that fiber alone is independently negatively correlated with chronic constipation and that an inadequate daily intake of fiber is a risk factor for chronic constipation in children (29,30).

Idiopathic constipation is twice as common in females than males in the young to middle-aged population (5). Of the patients who remain refractory to therapeutic intervention, 30% have normal colonic transit studies (31). Several studies have suggested that this subset of individuals has more psychopathology, including depression, than those individuals with delayed transit times (32,33), but there appears to be little efficacy in using psychological factors to characterize subtypes of idiopathic constipation (34).

There is an exponential increased prevalence of constipation after the age of 65 years (5). Although it is generally accepted that age does

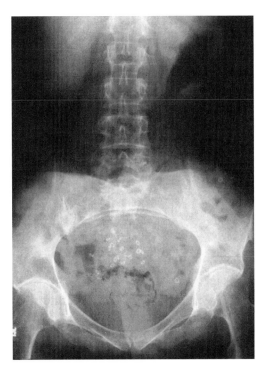

FIG. 24.1. Colonic transit study of a patient with rectosphincteric dyssynergia or colonic stricture on day 5 after ingestion of one Sitzmark capsule. The progression of markers to the rectum was normal.

not significantly affect colonic motor function in healthy individuals, this increase in prevalence could result from chronic stress to the enteric nervous system resulting in denervation and neuronal loss. This may be secondary to underlying systemic or colonic disorders or side effects from medications (12). Conditions affecting elderly patients, such as changes in mental status (dementia, Alzheimer's disease, confusion) and factors associated with mobility and bathroom access, may contribute to delayed defecation, which, in turn, may contribute to fecal impaction, a significant problem in elderly patients (35). Longstanding dilation of the rectum and rectosigmoid may contribute to denervation, diminished sensation, and worsening constipation.

Evaluation

The evaluation of the constipated patient begins with a careful history, with special consideration to the age of onset and duration of symptoms. Symptoms present since birth or childhood suggest an underlying congenital etiology. In contrast, constipation occurring later in life tends to be an acquired disorder. A sudden or recent change in bowel habits suggests an underlying organic lesion, whereas chronic symptoms usually represent a functional bowel disorder. A review of symptoms with respect to defecatory dysfunction must include questions regarding frequency and consistency of bowel movements, the presence of melena or hematochezia, the time required for a bowel movement, and the need to strain or digitally facilitate evacuation. Associated symptoms of dyschezia, obstipation, encopresis, incomplete defecation, anismus, fecal incontinence, abdominopelvic pain, or bloating must also be reviewed.

Medications (prescription, nonprescription, and alternative) should be reviewed in detail because many have constipating side effects (Table 24.2). Chronic laxative use or abuse is a common precipitating factor contributing to chronic constipation. Stimulant laxatives, such as the anthraquinones (aloe, senna, cascara), bisacodyl/castor oil, and the polyphenolic derivatives can cause degeneration of Meissner's and Auerbach's plexuses through neurotoxicity (5,36).

Patients should be questioned regarding a family history of both benign and malignant intestinal disorders. Psychosocial issues must also be addressed to detect any concurrent psychological diagnoses, history of emotional disorders, physical or sexual abuse, familial dysfunction, and other life stressors. A careful review of past medical, surgical, gynecologic, and obstetric history is essential.

Physical examination should include a focused abdominal, pelvic, and neurologic evaluation to rule out extraintestinal causes of constipation. Abdominal examination should include an assessment of previous incision sites and a search for ventral and inguinal hernias. Distention, tympany, and the presence of masses or hepatosplenomegaly should be documented. The presence of bowel sounds and any abdominal discomfort should be quantified and the location and quality described.

Rectal and pelvic examinations are essential. Typically performed in the dorsal or semi-Fowler's lithotomy position, a careful systematic evaluation of pelvic organ support is undertaken using the Pelvic Organ Prolapse Quantitation (POPQ) method (see Chapter 9). An overall stage of prolapse and compartment-specific stages are assigned. If present, attempts should be made to qualify and describe site-specific defects, especially with respect to anterior and posterior compartments. The degree of perineal descent and presence and type of rectal prolapse should be documented. Perineal examination should also look for any deformity, presence of surgical or traumatic scarring, ongoing sepsis, dovetail sign or flattening of the bilateral gluteal creases, or atrophy of the gluteal or perineal muscles. Rectal examination may reveal a stricture from previous anorectal surgery or trauma or may detect a neoplasm. The texture and amount of stool in the rectal vault should be noted. A large, hard mass of feces suggests impaction. Sphincter tone and symmetry should be assessed. With the patient straining, the presence of a paradoxical contraction of the puborectalis may indicate rectosphincteric dyssynergia. Neurologic examination should include an assessment of autonomic function and reflexes, including lower extremity deep tendon reflexes as well as pelvic and perineal sensation and bulbocavernosus and clitoral–anal reflexes.

In the patient with acute complaints of altered bowel habits, with a family history of colorectal cancer, or in the age group appropriate for colorectal cancer screening, colonoscopy, double-contrast barium enema, or computed tomographic colonography should be performed. If there is no evidence suggesting an underlying systemic or organic etiology, conservative therapy may be pursued (see later). For patients failing to respond to initial therapy, a 1- to 2-week bowel diary combined with a measurement of colonic transit time with either radiopaque markers or scintigraphic techniques is the most useful diagnostic study (37). Further testing and diagnostic studies should be tailored to the specific complaint (Table 24.3; also, see Chapter 15).

Treatment

Most patients presenting with uncomplicated idiopathic constipation may be treated conservatively with modifications in diet and toileting behavior, fiber supplementation, and laxatives. If fecal impaction was diagnosed on initial evaluation, the patient must first be disimpacted. Twice-daily enemas or oral polyethylene glycol may be used to facilitate this. For severe constipation, biofeedback and other pharmacologic agents may be used. If symptoms persist after failure of escalating medical therapy, diagnostic studies evaluating colonic and anorectal function should be undertaken.

Conservative Behavioral Therapy

Conservative therapy begins with patient education. Most patients require reassurance that their condition is not life threatening and can be successfully managed. Regular toileting strategies to prevent impaction are often used with children as well as with patients suffering from dementia, physical handicaps, and neurogenic constipation. Postprandial colonic motility can be enhanced, with behavior modification aimed at encouraging morning and postprandial defecation. Other initial recommendations include reducing excessive use of laxatives or cathartics, increasing daily fluid and fiber intake, and behavioral modification including daily exercise. Biofeedback using visible or audible signal recordings from rectal manometric or electromyographic monitoring may be useful in treating chronic constipation related to pelvic floor dyssynergia (38).

Fiber

Fiber is a bulking agent that increases fecal volume and density. Fiber consists of insoluble and soluble components that vary depending on the source. The cell wall in fiber resists digestion and contributes to the physical bulking property. It may also serve as a substrate for bacterial proliferation and gas production, which may stimulate colonic motility. It is hypothesized that the therapeutic effect of fiber on large bowel function is multifactorial. First, through enhancing bacterial metabolism and fermentation, fiber may enhance the absorption of bacterial metabolites, such as secondary bile acids. Second, gas production leads to colonic distention and increases in intraluminal pressures, which triggers peristaltic activity. Third, the presence of fiber promotes intraluminal water absorption, increasing fecal bulk and consistency (39).

Burkitt and colleagues first advocated the efficacy of dietary fiber in the early 1970s (40). Bowel frequency, stool weight, and intestinal transit times were compared between African and British cohorts. The authors concluded that the high prevalence of constipation in Western societies was associated with a diminished intake of dietary fiber. The role of fiber in the pathogenesis and prevention of constipation has been difficult to ascertain. Several studies have failed to detect a difference in dietary fiber intake in constipated patients versus healthy controls (20,41,42). Most studies demonstrate a beneficial effect of bran in treating constipation in patients with IBS (43–45) and diverticular disease (46–48). A meta-analysis of 27 studies investigating the relationship between dietary fiber and bowel function found that constipated patients continued to have lower stool weights and longer transit times despite being maintained on high-fiber diets (49). In another meta-analysis of 36 separate trials evaluating laxative and fiber therapy for the treatment of chronic constipation, Tramonte and co-workers found improved stool consistency, decreased abdominal pain, and an increase in weekly bowel movement frequency in patients treated with both daily fiber supplements and laxatives (50). The data could not determine, however, whether fiber was superior to laxatives or whether one type of laxative was better than another.

The accurate assessment of fiber intake is often difficult. Although the recommended daily intake of fiber is 25 to 35 g, or 10 to 13 g per 1,000 kcal (51), the average American typically consumes only 14 to 15 g daily. Fiber therapy may be recommended for patients who have constipation without evidence of impaction, megacolon or megarectum, or obstructing gastrointestinal lesions (Table 24.4). Patients may be started on a high-fiber cereal and should be

TABLE 24.4. *Fiber content*

Cereals	Amount of fiber (g)
All Bran-Extra Fiber ($1/2$ c)	15
Fiber One ($1/2$ c)	14
Bran Buds ($1/2$ c)	10
100% Bran ($1/3$ c)	9
Raisin Bran ($1/2$ c)	7
All Bran ($1/2$ c)	6
Fruit & Fiber ($2/3$ c)	5
Frosted Mini Wheats ($1/2$ c)	3
Frosted Flakes (1 oz)	1
Breads	
Whole wheat (1 slice)	2.0
White bread (1 slice)	0.5
Bagel (1)	1.0
Fiber supplements	
Konsyl (1 tsp)	6.0
Perdiem (1 tsp)	4.0
Konsyl D (1 tsp)	3.4
Maalox w/fiber (1 tbs)	3.4
Mylanta w/fiber (1 tsp)	3.4
Metamucil (1 tsp)	3.4
Citrucel (1 tbs)	2.0
Vegetables	
Lettuce (1 c)	1.4
Celery (1)	0.5
Tomato, raw (1)	1.0

encouraged to continue daily fiber consumption, increasing the amount to 25 to 35 g/d. Six to eight 8-oz glasses of water per day is recommended with this fiber load. Bloating can be a side effect that typically resolves over weeks. If bloating persists, a different type of fiber supplement or type of cereal may be substituted.

Laxatives

The use of laxatives is widespread in Western society, especially in the elderly population (4). Laxatives may be classified by their mechanism of action and content (Table 24.5).

Bulk-forming laxatives include both natural (psyllium) and synthetic (methylcellulose, polycarbophil) components, which increase the water content and bulk volume of stool. The mechanism of action is similar to that of fiber, and the net effect of bulk-forming laxatives is demonstrated by decreased colonic transit times, increased stool mass and density, and improved stool consistency (3).

TABLE 24.5. *Laxatives: mechanism of action and content*

Type of laxative	Adult dose	Onset of action	Side effects
Bulk-forming laxatives			
Natural (psyllium)	7 g PO	12–72 h	Impaction above strictures
Synthetic (methylcellulose)	4–6 g PO	12–72 h	Fluid overload
Emollient laxatives			
Ducusate salts	50–500 mg PO	24–72 h	Skin rashes
Mineral oil	15–45 mL PO	6–8 h	Decreased vitamin absorp
			Lipid pneumonia
Hyperosmolar laxatives			
Polyethylene glycol	3–22 L PO	1 h	Abdominal bloating
Lactulose	15–60 mL PO	24–48 h	Abdominal bloating
Sorbitol	120 mL 25% sol. PO	24–48 h	Abdominal bloating
Glycerine	3 g suppository	15–60 min	Rectal irritation
	5–15 mL enema	15–30 min	Rectal irritation
Saline laxatives			
Magnesium sulfate	15 g PO	0.5–3 h	Magnesium toxicity
Magnesium phosphate	10 g PO	0.5–3 h	
Magnesium citrate	200 mL PO	0.5–3 h	
Stimulant laxatives			
Castor oil	15–60 mL PO	2–6 h	Nutrient malabsorption
Diphenylmethanes			
Phenolphthalein	60–100 mg PO	6–8 h	Skin rashes
Bisacodyl	30 mg PO	6–10 h	Gastric irritation
	10 mg PR	0.25–1 h	Rectal stimulation
Anthraquinones			
Cascara sagrada	1 mL PO	6–12 h	Melanosis coli
Senna	2 mL PO	6–12 h	Degeneration of Meissner and Auerbach plexuses
Aloe (casanthrol)	250 mg PO	6–12 h	
Danthron	75–150 mg PO	6–12 h	Hepatotoxicity (w/docusate)

From Wald A. Approach to the patient with constipation. In: Yamada T, Alpers DH, Owyang C, et al., eds. *Textbook of gastroenterlogy*, 3rd ed. Philadelphia: Lippincot Williams & Wilkins, 1999; 921, with permission.

Emollient laxatives include docusate salts and mineral oil. The anionic action of docusate salts decreases stool surface tension, thereby enhancing the penetration and absorption of intestinal fluids, which results in softened stools. Docusate salts may also alter intestinal mucosal permeability, promoting absorption of other laxatives. Their overall efficacy in the treatment of chronic idiopathic constipation has been questioned because studies have failed to demonstrate objective improvement in defecatory frequency, colonic transit times, and stool weights (12). Mineral oil, administered orally or rectally as an enema, also works as an emollient to penetrate and soften stool.

Hyperosmolar laxatives include nonabsorbable sugars, such as lactulose and sorbitol, as well as glycerine and polyethylene glycol (GoLYTELY). These agents work by increasing intracolonic osmolarity, which promotes water absorption by stool with subsequent softening. Sorbitol and lactulose are poorly absorbed and are ultimately hydrolyzed by colonic coliform bacteria. Through hydrolysis, lactic, acetic, and formic acids are created and increase intracolonic osmolarity. Side effects include abdominal bloating and flatulence. Polyethylene glycol is not hydrolyzed and is typically associated with fewer symptoms of bloating and flatulence. Polyethylene glycol is usually used for preoperative bowel preparation; however, it may also be used in cases of severe constipation (3).

Saline laxatives include magnesium-containing solutions such as magnesium sulfate, phosphate, and citrate. Saline laxatives increase colonic osmolarity, which, in turn, results in increased water absorption and subsequent stool softening. Administered by enema or suppository, saline laxatives can give rise to mineral and metabolic imbalances and, in patients with renal insufficiency, magnesium toxicity (3).

Stimulant laxatives are typically indicated if bulk or osmotic laxatives are not effective. They include castor oil, the diphenylmethanes (phenolphthaleins, bisacodyl), and the anthraquinones (senna, aloe, cascara sagrada, and danthron). Castor oil, after intestinal conversion to ricinoleic acid, stimulates intestinal secretion and motility. The diphenylmethanes act directly to stimulate colonic motility and small intestine water absorption. The anthraquinones, in contrast, are catalyzed by intestinal microorganisms and promote colonic peristalsis by altering intraluminal fluid and electrolyte composition (12). Stimulant laxatives may be abused, and chronic daily use may lead to diarrhea, electrolyte abnormalities, and dehydration. However, use up to 2 to 3 times per week may be undertaken for longer periods.

Prokinetic agents include drugs that directly stimulate gastrointestinal motor activity. The efficacy of metoclopramide, cisapride, cholinergic agonists such as bethanechol, cholinesterase inhibitors such as neostigmine, and serotonin agonists in the treatment of chronic idiopathic constipation is questionable. Metoclopramide, for example, appears to be more effective in treating upper gastrointestinal motor disorders, whereas studies addressing the efficacy of cisapride report conflicting results. Current research is examining the facilitatory role of serotonin agonists on enteric cholinergic transmission and opioid receptor antagonist therapy in the treatment of chronic constipation (12).

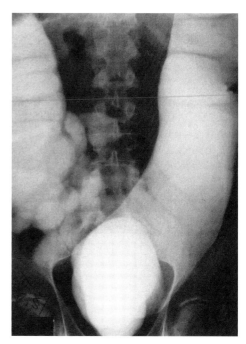

FIG. 24.2. Contrast enema showing megacolon above an anastomotic stricture.

sibilities include meningomyelocele and other lumbosacral spinal cord lesions. Secondary megacolon or megarectum is an acquired disease state usually found in children and elderly people. It may follow bowel surgery resulting in an anastomotic stricture (Fig. 24.1) and is usually associated with constipation or defecatory dysfunction. Diagnostic criteria are based on radiographic (Fig. 24.2) and manometric findings, including increased rectal compliance and elasticity, decreased rectal sensation, increased sensory thresholds, and diminished internal anal sphincter relaxation (52).

MOTILITY DISORDERS

Megacolon and Megarectum

Megacolon and megarectum may occur separately or together and may be divided into either primary or secondary entities (12). Primary megacolon or megarectum is usually present from birth and is associated with an underlying neurologic pathology. Although Hirschsprung's disease is the most classic example, other pos-

Irritable Bowel Syndrome and Functional Constipation

Diagnostic Criteria

Attempts to characterize IBS date back to 1820 when Powell first described a triad of pain, bowel dysfunction, and flatulence (53). It was not until 1962 that the syndrome was described in more detail (54), with the first classification of all the functional gastrointestinal disorders (FGIDs) appearing in 1979 (55). The Manning criteria (56) and the Kruis criteria (57) formed the basis for the first internationally recognized classification system for IBS, the Rome criteria. Since their introduction in 1988, the Rome criteria have become the gold standard for the diagnosis of FGIDs (58). Rome I criteria recommended that the diagnosis of IBS be based on the presence of abdominal pain or discomfort associated with a chronic change in bowel habit *and* two or more supporting criteria. Rome II criteria recommend that the diagnosis of IBS be based on the presence of two of the three main diagnostic criteria alone and provides consensus statements for each of the 25 FGIDs located throughout five anatomic regions (59).

The category of functional bowel disorders includes symptoms related to the middle and lower gastrointestinal tract. This group is further subclassified by Rome II into the following categories:

1. IBS
2. Functional abdominal bloating
3. Functional constipation
4. Functional diarrhea
5. Unspecified functional bowel disorders.

By definition, these diagnoses presume the absence of biochemical or structural etiologies, and symptoms must be present for at least 12 weeks (consecutive *or* nonconsecutive) within the past 12 months.

IBS is characterized by abdominal pain or discomfort associated with defecation or a change in bowel habit. Often having a chronic, relapsing course, symptoms of IBS often overlap with those of other FGIDs, and the diagnostic criteria are as follows (60):

Diagnostic Criteria

At least 12 weeks, which need not be consecutive, in the preceding 12 months, of abdominal discomfort or pain that has two of the following three features:

1. Is relieved with defecation
2. Has onset associated with a change in frequency of stool
3. Has onset associated with a change in form (appearance) of stool

Supporting symptoms may help to classify patients further into diarrhea- or constipation-predominant IBS and include the following (60):

1. Fewer than three bowel movements per week
2. Greater than three bowel movements per day
3. Hard or lumpy stools
4. Loose (mushy) or watery stools
5. Straining during a bowel movement
6. Urgency (having to rush to have a bowel movement)
7. Feeling of incomplete bowel movement
8. Passing mucus (white material) during a bowel movement
9. Abdominal fullness, bloating, or swelling

Diarrhea-predominant IBS

1 or more of 2, 4, or 6 and none of 1, 3, or 5

Constipation-predominant IBS

1 or more of 1, 3, or 5 and none of 2, 4, or 6

Functional abdominal bloating is characterized by feelings of abdominal fullness and bloating, which are typically less severe in the morning and tends to worsen as the day progresses. Symptoms suggestive of other functional bowel disorders, however, are lacking. Diagnostic criteria for functional abdominal bloating are as follows (60):

Diagnostic Criteria

At least 12 weeks, which need not be consecutive, in the preceding 12 months, of the following:

1. Feeling of abdominal fullness, bloating, or visible distension
2. Insufficient criteria for a diagnosis of IBS or other functional disorders

Functional constipation is characterized by symptoms of abnormal defecation, with respect to either frequency of bowel movements or the act of defecation itself. The diagnostic criteria are as follows (60):

Diagnostic Criteria

At least 12 weeks, which need not be consecutive, in the preceding 12 months, of two or more of the following:

1. Straining in more than 25% of defecations
2. Lumpy or hard stools in more than 25% of defecations
3. Sensation of incomplete evacuation in more than 25% of defecations
4. Sensation of anorectal obstruction or blockade in more than 25% of defecations
5. Manual maneuvers to facilitate more than 25% of defecations (e.g., digital evacuation, support of the pelvic floor)
6. Less than three defecations per week

Loose stools are not present, and there are insufficient criteria for IBS.

Functional diarrhea is characterized by the recurrent or continuous painless passage of watery or loose stools. The diagnosis depends on the exclusion of other diagnoses, such as pseudo diarrhea (defecation of solid stools associated with symptoms of urgency and frequency) and underlying organic disease. The diagnostic criteria for functional diarrhea are as follows:

Diagnostic Criteria

At least 12 weeks, which need not be consecutive, in the preceding 12 months, of the following (60):
1. Liquid (mushy) or watery stools
2. Present more than three fourths of the time
3. No abdominal pain

Unspecified functional bowel disorders are characterized by functional bowel symptoms that do not meet the criteria for the previously defined categories.

In summary, the Rome criteria currently serve as a standardized classification system for FGIDs. However, the ability of the Rome criteria to discriminate between functional and organic disease has not yet been validated.

Irritable Bowel Syndrome

IBS is a poorly understood, chronic disorder characterized by episodic abdominal pain and changes in bowel habits. In addition to gastrointestinal and defecatory dysfunction, individuals with IBS may also suffer from sleep disturbances, sexual and lower urinary tract dysfunction, and other nongastrointestinal pain syndromes (61). About 60% of patients report abdominal pain or discomfort as their primary complaint. Symptoms characterizing defecatory dysfunction appear to be equally divided between diarrhea-predominant IBS, constipation-predominant IBS, and a variation of the two (62).

Epidemiologic studies estimate that between 8% and 19% of adults worldwide experience symptoms consistent with IBS (63). In the United States, women are roughly twice as likely to be diagnosed with IBS than men (14 versus 7.7%). IBS symptoms are more prevalent in younger individuals (relative to those aged 45 years or older) and individuals with lower household income (2). Physician visits and prescriptions for IBS approximate $3.5 million and $2.2 million per year, respectively (64). Absenteeism from work is 2 to 3 times more likely in patients diagnosed with IBS (65).

Similar to other chronic functional syndromes, a conceptual model involving the interplay of cognitive, behavioral, psychological, genetic, infectious, dietary, and physiologic components has been developed to serve as a framework for understanding the multiple possible factors that may contribute to IBS symptoms. Because there is no single biochemical, physiologic, neurologic, or psychological marker for IBS, researchers have stressed the interrelationship of these multiple components.

Cognitive factors, including abnormal coping mechanisms; misconceptions regarding disease, nutrition, and medications; and illness behavior are common in patients with IBS. Behavioral factors, such as traumatic or stressful events, are often correlated to the first onset of IBS symptoms and have been associated with changes in stool pattern, abdominal pain, and defecation frequency (66,67). IBS is diagnosed more frequently in patients with a history of prior psychological trauma or physical or sexual abuse, especially if incurred during childhood (68,69). Concurrent psychological disorders have been diagnosed in 42% to 61% of patients and include depression, anxiety, panic, and somatization disorders (61,70). Genetic factors may also play a role in the development of IBS because symptoms also appear to be more common in first-degree relatives (71). Infectious disease may in some way be responsible for triggering IBS because several studies have shown an increase risk for IBS symptoms after gastrointestinal infection (72, 73). Histologic and biochemical studies have demonstrated evidence of long-term, persis-tent mucosal inflammation and changes in mucosal permeability in predisposed individuals suffering from IBS symptoms following an initial infectious insult.

There is little evidence to support a causal relationship between specific diet and the development of IBS. Patients intolerant or allergic to specific foods do not necessarily experience improvement of IBS symptoms when these food types are removed from their diets (61,74).

Many symptoms of IBS are consistent with dysfunction of the sensory and motor function of the enteric nervous system. These include dysfunction of neuroenteric regulation resulting in altered intestinal motility, myoelectrical activity, tone and compliance, sensation, and fluid and electrolyte absorption. Unfortunately, correlations between these alterations and IBS symptoms remain weak, raising the question of clinical relevance.

Evaluation

Diagnosis is based on identifying symptoms and differentiating IBS from other organic disease (Table 24.6). Once underlying

TABLE 24.6. *Differential diagnosis of inflammatory bowel syndrome*

Colorectal carcinoma
Chronic intestinal idiopathic pseudoobstruction
Disorders
  Thyroid disease
  Diabetes
  Endocrine tumors
Gastrointestinal infections
  Viral enteritis
  Parasitic (*Giardia* species, *Entamoeba histolytica*)
  Bacterial (*Clostridium, Salmonella, Yersinia, Campylobacter* species)
Inflammatory bowel disease
Lactose intolerance
Malabsorption syndromes/endocrine
  Celiac sprue
  Pancreatic insufficiency
Medications (constipating diarrhea-provoking)
Microscopic colitis
Psychiatric disorders

From Wald A. Approach to the patient with constipation. In: Yamada T, Alpers DH, Owyang C, et al., eds. *Textbook of gastroenterlogy*, 3rd ed. Philadelphia: Lippincot Williams & Wilkins, 1999; 921, with permission.

organic diseases are excluded, the Rome criteria demonstrate a sensitivity of 63%, a specificity of 100%, a positive predictive value of 100%, and a negative predictive value of 76% (75). Longitudinal studies examining a diagnosis of IBS based on symptoms and minimal diagnostic testing have shown that over time, fewer than 5% of IBS patients have other diagnoses responsible for their symptoms (76).

A detailed history and physical examination can usually exclude most organic diseases. Warning signs, including fever, weight loss or gain, anorexia, early satiety, anemia, intestinal bleeding, and palpable masses, must be ruled out and a differential diagnosis (Table 24.6) considered. Attention to stool consistency, defecatory frequency, and relationship of pain and bloating to activity and defecation can help to classify IBS. A symptom diary may be helpful in characterizing symptoms. Additional consideration should be given to reviewing psychosocial issues, including the patient's concerns and fears, possible stressors, the role of family support or dysfunction, reason for the visit including possible hidden agenda (e.g., disability or narcotic seeking), screening for previous psychological trauma, physical or sexual abuse, and history of concurrent psychological diagnoses.

Laboratory evaluation and diagnostic procedures should be undertaken in the initial evaluation to exclude structural lesions and systemic disease. These include a complete blood count and erythrocyte sedimentation rate, serum chemistries and metabolic profile, urine analysis, thyroid panel, and stool evaluation for occult blood, ova, and parasites. Further diagnostic studies should be tailored to address the patient's predominate symptoms and may be considered for those patients who are older than 50 years of age, have a positive family history of colon cancer, present with sudden onset of symptoms, or have symptoms that appear overly severe or disabling.

Current Rome criteria differentiate subtypes of IBS based on predominate symptoms. Patients who present with complaints of infrequent bowel movements, hard and lumpy stools, sensation of incomplete rectal emptying, or needing to strain or splint to facilitate defecation are classified as having constipation-predominant IBS. These patients also tend to have a higher frequency of other specific symptoms, including sexual and sleep dysfunction, anorexia, depression, dyspepsia, and musculoskeletal complaints. Patients presenting with symptoms of increased defecatory frequency and urgency and with loose, watery stools are classified as having diarrhea-predominant IBS. Finally, patients may present with chief complaints of abdominal pain rather than with changes in bowel habits. In this pain-predominant IBS subcategory, pain is commonly accompanied by abdominal bloating, distention, and gas.

After a preliminary diagnosis of IBS is made, basic therapy should be initiated. If no improvement is seen within 2 to 3 weeks, further studies, including colonic transit times (colonic inertia), flexible sigmoidoscopy (functional rectal outlet obstruction, organic lesions), and evaluation of stool weight and composition (malabsorption syndromes, steatorrhea), osmotic gap, and pH (secretory or osmotic diarrhea), can be helpful (76).

Treatment

Therapy for IBS is divided into dietary, pharmacologic, psychological, and behavioral approaches that focus on predominant symptoms and cofactors. Diet should be considered first, although attempts to modify dietary intake may be met with resistance. Avoidance of symptom-provoking agents, such as caffeine, alcohol, sorbitol, and gas-producing foods, including beans, raisins, apricots, carrots, celery, and onions, should be stressed (77). Dietary fiber (20 to 30 g/d) has been widely recommended and may be beneficial in the treatment of constipation-predominant IBS. By promoting free water absorption into the large bowel, fiber acts as a stool-bulking agent that facilitates defecation. Fiber has been shown to decrease intestinal transit time and intracolonic pressure (78). Current literature and meta-analysis evaluating the role of dietary and supplemental fiber in treating IBS reveal significant controversy regarding its long-term efficacy and effectiveness in treating diarrhea-predominant or pain-predominant subtypes (79).

Pharmacologic therapy for IBS is tailored toward alleviating predominant symptoms (Table 24.7). Prokinetic agents, such as cisapride, that stimulate colonic smooth muscle may be helpful as adjuvant therapy in constipation-predominant IBS. Conversely, in patients with diarrhea-predominant IBS, loperamide is the drug of choice. Cholestyramine may also be added because bile acid malabsorption may contribute to the diarrhea. For predominant symptoms of pain and bloating, antispasmodics, anticholinergics, and antidepressants have commonly been prescribed. Unfortunately, well-designed clinical studies are lacking, and outcome studies evaluating the efficacy of various drugs in these classes have shown conflicting results. In the class of antispasmodics or smooth muscle relaxants, many are anticholinergic. Although Klein's (80) frequently sited 1988 meta-analysis offered no convincing evidence of antispasmodic efficacy, Poynard and colleagues (81) reported on five antispasmodics (mebeverine, trimebutine, cimetropium, primaverium bromide, octyl onium) that were superior to placebo in alleviating IBS symptoms. Dicyclomine and hyoscyamine are commonly prescribed in the United States, and newer agents in this class, including zamifenacin and darifenacin, both M3-receptor antagonists, are showing promise in the treatment of IBS (65). Research evaluating the efficacy of peppermint oil, a natural antispasmodic, remains inconclusive (82).

Historically, antidepressants were used to treat IBS because a large percentage of these patients were thought to be clinically depressed. The neuromodulatory, anticholinergic, and analgesic properties of selected psychotropics provided some alleviation of IBS symptoms. Tricyclic antidepressants were the first to be used, and numerous studies have since demonstrated their varying degrees of efficacy in treatment of diarrhea- and pain-predominant IBS. Amitriptyline, doxepin, and imipramine are commonly prescribed, albeit usually in doses lower than those typically used for depression (79). More recently, the role of serotonin reuptake inhibitors in the treatment of IBS is being investigated, and preliminary results are promising (83).

Newer agents, including the 5-HT$_3$ antagonists (granisetron, ondansetron, and alos-

TABLE 24.7. *Dosage guidelines for drugs commonly used to treat the irritable bowel syndrome*

Drug	Dose
Anticholinergic agents	
Dicyclomine hydrochloride	20 mg every 6 h; can be increased to 40 mg every 6 h if tolerated
Hyoscyamine sulfate	0.125–0.25 mg sublingually every 4 h (0.375 mg extended-relief tablets: 1–2 tablets every 12 h)
Antidiarrheal agents	
Loperamide	4 mg/d initially, with a maintenance dose of 4–8 mg/d, in a single or divided dose
Diphenoxylate (2.5 mg) plus atropine sulfate (0.025 mg)	2 tablets 4 times a day
Cholestyramine resin	1 packet (9 g) mixed with fluid and taken once or twice a day
Osmotic laxatives	
Lactulose	10 mg/15 mL of syrup; 15–30 mL/d (usual dose), up to 60 mL/d
Polyethylene glycol solution	17 g dissolved in 240 mL (8 oz) of water, taken daily
Tricyclic compounds	
Amitriptyline	25–75 mg/d
Nortriptyline	25–75 mg/d
Desipramine	25–75 mg/d

From Horwitz BJ, Fisher RS. The irritable bowel syndrome. *N Engl J Med* 2001;344(24):1846–1850, with permission. (Copyright © 2001, Massachusetts Medical Society. All rights reserved.)

etron) and 5-HT$_4$ agonists (prucalopride and tegaserod), that may have peripheral visceral antinociceptive actions have also shown promise in treating diarrhea- and pain-predominant IBS subtypes. Several studies have shown fewer pain episodes, firmer stools, and fewer episodes of defecatory urgency and frequency in patients treated with these agents (84). Other substances that influence sensation and sensory thresholds to colonic distention include opioid receptor agonists. These include the κ-opioid receptor agonist fedotozine, and trimebutine, a μ-, κ-, and δ-receptor agonist (85). Pinaverium bromide and octylonium are calcium-channel blockers that have been shown to blunt intestinal motor activity. In contrast, motilin agonists provoke colonic motor activity and thereby reduce gut transit times and promote gastric emptying (79).

Psychological and alternative intervention has also been used to varying degrees of success in treating patients with IBS. Psychotherapy, hypnotherapy, and behavioral and cognitive therapy, as well as therapeutic massage and acupuncture, have undergone study with lack of scientific rigor. Factors that appear to correspond with a favorable response after psychotherapy include diarrhea- and pain-predominant IBS symptoms, especially when associated with and exacerbated by stress. In a recent review (86) evaluating the efficacy of hypnotherapy, relaxation training, and stress management for IBS, the authors found all three modalities effective (reduction in symptom scores; improvement in anxiety, pain, and bowel function; and decrease in gastric acid production and colonic motility). Based on their findings, it would appear that hypnotherapy leads to significant improvement in patients with poorly controlled IBS and that this therapy should be offered to all patients who fail conventional medical therapy.

Colonic Inertia

In the absence of outlet obstruction and following confirmatory transit studies, constipation refractory to fiber and laxative therapy is often referred to as idiopathic slow-transit constipation (STC). The underlying pathophysiology of this condition, representing a disorder of colonic motor function or ineffective colonic propulsion, is poorly understood. Schouten and associates (87) documented diminished neurofilament concentration in enteric ganglia, and others have confirmed similar findings with respect to the myenteric plexus in patients with this disorder (88). Other research has focused on neuropeptide composition, transmission, and abnormal hormonal responses to gastrin and motilin secretion. The term colonic inertia has been used to describe the failure of a meal or colonic stimulant, such as bisacodyl or neostigmine, to increase colonic activity. The term cathartic colon has been used by radiologists to describe abnormal barium enema studies demonstrating significant colonic dilation and redundancy, absence of haustral folds, and incompetent ileocecal valves. It was initially proposed that these findings were secondary to chronic stimulant laxative that had led to myenteric plexus neuropathy (89). The etiology is now less clear, and this term has fallen out of favor.

Women appear to be commonly affected by STC, with symptoms often beginning in childhood (20). Characterized by infrequent bowel movements, STC is also associated with many symptoms that are similar to those of constipation-predominant IBS. These include abdominal bloating and discomfort, flatulence, and defecatory dysfunction characterized by dyschezia, splinting, incomplete emptying, and lumpy, hard stools. Typically, abdominal pain is not a prominent feature in STC. After organic causes and underlying systemic disorders are excluded, the diagnosis of STC can be based on colonic transit measurements by radiopaque markers (Fig. 24.3) or scintigraphic techniques. Both procedures demonstrate good correlation with each other and are sensitive in demonstrating both overall and regional colonic transit delay. Further testing may be required to rule out concurrent outlet obstruction (secondary to dyssynergic defecation or mechanical obstruction) or chronic intestinal pseudoobstruction, an entity typically characterized by more pro-

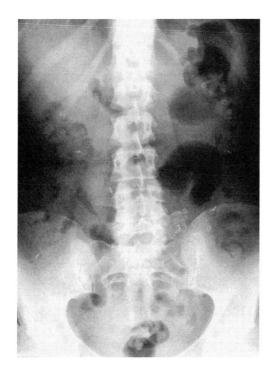

FIG. 24.3. Colonic transit study of a patient with slow transit constipation on day 5 after ingestion of one Sitzmark capsule.

nounced abdominal distress, including distention, pain, nausea, and vomiting.

Pharmacologic Treatment

After an empiric trial of fiber supplementation, patients with persistent STC may be treated with laxatives, usually beginning with bulk forming types such as psyllium and methylcellulose, followed by emollients or stimulant laxatives (Table 24.5). Caution should be used in prescribing laxatives for long-term use because some literature suggests that chronic stimulant laxative abuse may compromise myenteric plexus innervation, leading to further impairment of colonic motility (89). Enemas may also be used with caution to induce evacuation through colonic distention and mechanical lavage. Prokinetic agents such as the serotonin 5-HT$_4$ agonists, cisapride and metoclopramide, have not been proved effective in treating STC. In contrast, preliminary research involving prucalopride and tegaserod, both newer serotonin 5-HT$_4$ agonists, is encouraging. Both agents promote acceleration of colonic transit times (90). Investigational work involving selective recombinant human neurotrophic agents that enhance sensory neuronal growth and synaptic transmission may also lead to effective therapy for STC (91).

Surgical Treatment

Total abdominal colectomy with ileorectal anastomosis (IRA) may be curative for patients who have exhausted medical therapy. Before considering surgery, mechanical and other functional causes, such as Hirschsprung's disease, volvulus, rectal prolapse, tumors, anastomotic strictures, and pseudoobstruction, must be excluded. Additionally, concomitant extraintestinal and pelvic floor–related causes must be addressed. Wald proposes that at least four criteria be met before surgery: (a) chronic, disabling symptoms related to constipation refractory to medical therapy; (b) demonstration of slow proximal colonic transit; (c) no evidence or intestinal pseudoobstruction or mechanical obstruction; (d) normal anorectal function (3).

Lane was the first to publish his results on subtotal colectomy and to advocate this approach for the treatment of refractory constipation (92). Since then, subtotal colectomy with IRA has become the operation of choice for refractory STC, with success rates ranging from about 80% to 94%. Most authors contribute failures to preexisting or postoperative rectal dysfunction or to a more profound generalized intestinal motility disorder (93,94).

The largest series of long-term results of surgery for STC has been published by Nyam and colleagues from the Mayo Clinic (95). In this series, patients underwent extensive evaluation before surgical referral, and of 1,009 patients studied, only 53 with STC underwent colectomy with IRA. An additional 22 patients had STC with coexisting pelvic floor dysfunction and underwent pelvic floor retraining before IRA. At a mean follow-up of 56 months, all patients who underwent IRA were able to defecate spontaneously without the need of enemas, laxatives, or manual assistance. Of these patients, 97% were satisfied with surgery, and 90% reported an improvement in quality of life.

Other authors have reported similarly low operative rates after evaluation of patients for refractory constipation. Wexner and co-workers operated on only 16 of 163 patients initially evaluated for STC with a reported success rate of 94% (96). The importance of preoperative assessment and diagnosis was also emphasized by Sunderland and associates, who operated on only 18 of 228 patients evaluated for STC with an 88% success rate (97). Redmond and colleagues further categorized patients into those with colonic inertia alone and those with a more generalized intestinal dysmotility problem (94). After subtotal colectomy, the authors found improved success rates in those patients in the STC group (90%) compared with those with generalized intestinal dysmotility (13%).

In addition to abdominal colectomy with IRA, more and less aggressive procedures have been studied. Hosie and colleagues reported results of 13 patients with intractable constipation who underwent restorative proctocolectomy (ileal pouch–anal anastomosis), 8 of whom had previously failed colectomy with IRA (98). Despite a high complication rate, 85% of patients reported symptomatic improvement 20 months after surgery. Anorectal myectomy, an accepted procedure for short-segment Hirschsprung's disease, has also been used in patients with refractory idiopathic constipation. Although initial results were encouraging, long-term results are poor, with one study showing 70% of patients with no functional improvement at 30-months' follow-up (99). Finally, initially encouraging experience with the Malone antegrade continence enema (ACE) in the pediatric population has prompted some investigators to apply this option to adults with constipation and incontinence. In one study by Krogh and colleagues, time required for defecation was significantly reduced after ACE therapy, and 75% of patients reported overall satisfaction (100). Initially requiring an operative appendicostomy or exteriorization of other tubularized bowel, this procedure can be easily performed under fluoroscopic or colonoscopic guidance. Finally, a trapdoor cecostomy appliance (Fig. 24.4A,B)

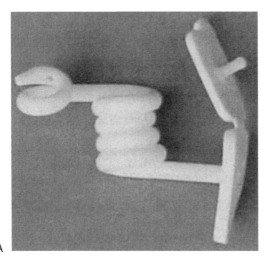

A

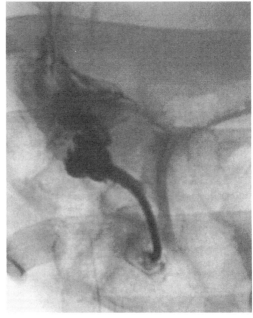

B

FIG. 24.4. A: Cecostomy button with trap door. **B:** Fluoroscopic confirmation of proper cecostomy placement.

allows for easy access to the proximal large intestine for antegrade colonic lavage.

OUTLET OBSTRUCTION

First described by Martelli and associates in 1978 (101), outlet obstruction has come to represent a subtype of slow-transit constipation in which there is normal passage of colonic transit Sitz markers until the level of rectum (Fig. 24.1). A number of functional (rectosphincteric dyssynergia, perineal descent, megarectum, mucosal intussusception, Hirschsprung's disease) or structural (rectocele or enterocele, hemorrhoids, anal fissure, anorectal neoplasia, rectal prolapse, fecal impaction) causes can lead to obstructive defecation. Numerous terms have been used to describe constipation associated with anorectal dysfunction. Anismus, for example, was first coined by Preston and Lennard-Jones to describe defecatory dysfunction related to paradoxic anal sphincter contraction (rectosphincteric dyssynergia) (102). Other terms, such as spastic floor syndrome, paradoxic puborectalis contraction syndrome, and pelvic floor dyssynergia, have been used to include the dysfunction of other muscles in the pelvic floor contributing to outlet obstruction. Currently, pelvic floor dyssynergia and resulting dyssynergic defecation are the preferred terms in the gastrointestinal literature (103, 104).

Dyssynergic Defecation

In normal defecation, cortical inhibition of the spinal reflex is required to allow relaxation of the EAS. In patients with rectosphincteric dyssynergia, there is a paradoxic contraction of the puborectalis and EAS at the time of desired defecation. This is analogous to detrusor–sphincter dyssynergia in patients with voiding dysfunction. The result is a narrowing of the anorectal angle and an increase in anal canal pressures leading to impaired evacuation. Rectosphincteric dyssynergia may be found in patients with both normal and decreased colonic transit times as well as in those with other causes for outlet obstruction (105). Although the etiology of dyssynergic defecation is unknown, psychosocial factors, including a history of sexual abuse, depression, eating disorders, obsessive-compulsive disorders, stress, and childhood constipation and dyschezia, appear to be important. Preliminary data in one survey by Rao and colleagues (106) suggest that dyssynergic defecation begins in childhood about one third of the time and is associated with a precipitating event in about 30% of individuals with this problem. The pathophysiology contributing to rectosphincteric dyssynergia (characterized by either paradoxic anal contractions or involuntary anal spasm during defecation) is likely multifactorial. The premise that this disorder is due only to the spasm of the EAS has been challenged by studies documenting minimal improvement after botulinum toxin injection or myectomy of the EAS (107,108). It seems more likely that multiple areas of rectoanal dysfunction are involved. In a study by Rao and co-workers (109), 35 patients with obstructive defecation were evaluated with anorectal manometry and rectal balloon expulsion. The authors found impaired rectal contraction in 61% and paradoxic anal contractions in 78%, whereas others demonstrated inadequate anal relaxation and impaired rectal sensation. Paradoxic muscle contraction is likely a learned acquired response because therapies using biofeedback and pelvic floor physical therapy have demonstrated improved defecation patterns (110,111).

The diagnosis is based on history, clinical findings, and diagnostic testing. Patients usually complain of impaired defecation associated with tenesmus and constipation. Other symptoms that may be present with any cause of outlet obstruction include the feeling of incomplete evacuation, anorectal pain or sensation of perianal heaviness, excessive straining with defecation, digital disimpaction, or vaginal splinting. In one survey evaluating symptoms associated with dyssynergic defecation, excessive straining was reported by 85% of patients, the need to facilitate defecation digitally by 66%, and the sensation of incomplete evacuation by 75% (106). Symptomatic criteria (Rome II) for the diagnosis of dyssynergic defecation have recently been published and are as follows (112):

Diagnostic Criteria for Pelvic Floor Dyssynergia

1. The patient must satisfy all criteria for functional constipation.
2. There must be manometric, electromyographic, or radiologic evidence of inappropriate contraction or failure of pelvic floor muscle relaxation during repeated attempts to defecate.
3. There must be evidence of adequate propulsive defecatory forces.
4. There must be evidence of incomplete evacuation.

Symptoms alone, however, are not helpful in differentiating between the different causes of outlet obstruction (113).

The diagnosis of a dyssynergic anorectal disorder is one of exclusion. Metabolic, systemic, and structural etiologies must first be ruled out with laboratory testing and sigmoidoscopy. The first clue to dyssynergic defecation may be perceived with a digital rectal examination in which there is a paradoxic contraction of the EAS. Rather than experiencing relaxation of the EAS, the clinician will appreciate a contraction of the puborectalis and EAS when the patient is asked to bear down to imitate a bowel movement. Confirmatory testing with anorectal manometry will demonstrate a heightened rather than diminished EAS pressure at the time of defecation that will coincide with increases in electromyographic recording activity from the puborectalis and EAS. Balloon expulsion testing and defecography have also been used diagnostically, with manometric correlation approximating 67% of cases (114). In addition to the symptom criteria listed previously, Rao has advocated using additional physiologic criteria based on manometry, balloon expulsion testing, and colon transit times to identify patients with dyssynergic defecation (115).

Treatment

Initial therapy should be aimed at addressing and alleviating constipation, a complaint usually always associated with this disorder. Standard therapies, including adequate fiber and fluid intake, avoidance of constipating medicines, scheduled toileting to maximize postprandial gastrocolonic and early morning waking responses, and laxative and prokinetic agents, should be tried first. In addition to addressing constipation, therapy must also be aimed at improving impaired rectal sensation and dyssynergic function of the abdominal, rectal, and anal sphincters that characterize this disorder. Biofeedback using manometry or electromyographic recording to provide visual or audible displays has been used in the treatment of dyssynergic defecatory dysfunction. Defecatory simulation with balloon expulsion and rectal sensory threshold conditioning are also used. Using the concept of operant conditioning, biofeedback enables patients to moderate motor and sensory function in response to desired visual displays representing ideal neuromuscular behavior. The efficacy of biofeedback in the treatment of dyssynergic defecation is difficult to access because randomized controlled trials are lacking and methodology including study design and treatment end points does not allow for good comparison or firm conclusions. In one meta-analysis by Ernst and Resch (116), the authors were unable to make any conclusions regarding the clinical effectiveness of biofeedback for the treatment of anismus, even though the results of subjective success rates in the 11 studies they reviewed ranged between 18% and 100%. Two other reviews (117, 118) have suggested cure rates ranging between 67% and 80%, with another suggesting 89% symptomatic improvement (119). Ho and colleagues reported on the results of biofeed-back in patients with dyssynergic defecation, both with and without measurable paradoxic puborectalis contractions. Clinical and anorec-tal physiologic parameters were evaluated, and subjective improvement was reported in 90% of patients after therapy (120).

For patients who fail to improve with bio-feedback, several other options exist. The use of botulinum toxin type A (BT) has been used with varying results in the treatment of spastic disorders of smooth muscle in the upper and lower gastrointestinal tract. Injection of BT into the EAS or puborectalis muscle has shown promising short-term results in the treatment of dyssynergic defecation (121). Surgical options as a last resort include sphincteric myectomy, obturator internus muscle auto transfer (122), sacral nerve modulation (off-label indication), and diverting colostomy.

ANATOMIC OBSTRUCTION

Chronic idiopathic constipation may be secondary to an underlying colonic motility disorder, an outlet obstructive disorder, or a combination of the two. In considering outlet obstruction, it is helpful to think in terms of either a mechanical etiology, such as POP, rectal prolapse, intussusception, or fecal im-paction, or a neuromuscular disorder, such as Hirschsprung's disease, dyssynergic defeca-tion, or anismus, as discussed previously. Constipation appears to be an important fac-tor in the pathogenesis of uterovaginal pro-lapse because a history of chronic straining has been shown to be an independent risk fac-tor for tissue attenuation and abnormal pu-dendal nerve function (123).

Pelvic Organ Prolapse

The true prevalence of POP has been diffi-cult to quantify, primarily because of difficul-ties related to data collection and, until re-cently, a universally accepted grading system. Samuelsson and colleagues (124) recently re-ported a 31% overall prevalence of prolapse in a Swedish population, with that number in-creasing to 56% in women aged 50 to 59 years. Swift described the distribution of POP stages in women seen for routine gynecologic care as representing a bell-shaped curve, with most women having stage 1 (43%) and stage II (48%) prolapse (125). Unfortunately, there is little published literature addressing symp-toms related to POP, especially when related to defecatory dysfunction.

Rectocele and Enterocele

It is commonly perceived that defecatory dysfunction related to outlet obstruction is secondary to posterior compartment defects. Rectoceles or herniations of the rectum through attenuated or site-specific breaks in the rectovaginal fascia are common forms of POP. Enteroceles are also common and may play some, as yet undefined, role in outlet ob-struction. Because the definition of an entero-cele is controversial and its diagnosis clini-cally challenging, the prevalence is difficult to quantify. It is estimated that enteroceles are found in 0.1% to 16% of women undergoing gynecologic surgery for POP (126).

Associated Symptoms

Rectoceles and enteroceles have commonly been associated with symptoms of bowel and defecatory dysfunction. This belief presum-ably stems from the direct involvement of the bowel and rectum in these defined areas of pelvic floor herniation. Symptoms usually at-tributed to rectocele and enterocele include pelvic pain and pressure, vaginal protrusion, constipation and splinting, sensation of in-complete evacuation, obstipation, fecal incon-tinence, and sexual dysfunction. However, a causal relationship between symptoms and posterior compartment prolapse has yet to be defined. Some researchers postulate that trauma to or intrinsic weakness of the recto-vaginal fascia leads to rectocele formation and subsequent defecatory dysfunction. In contrast, others believe that the primary insult is related to chronic colonic dysfunction (i.e., idiopathic constipation, dyssynergic defecation), which then leads to rectocele or enterocele formation.

Although symptoms related to defecatory dysfunction may coexist with POP, they have not been consistently correlated. Weber and coauthors (127) compared symptoms of bowel dysfunction with stage of posterior compartment prolapse and reported no clinically significant association. The authors did, however, find a weakly positive correlation between more advanced posterior vaginal prolapse and bowel dysfunction severity. Ellerkmann and associates (128) prospectively evaluated 273 patients and attempted to correlate symptoms with stage and location of POP. Although they found weak correlations between splinting and incomplete evacuation and worsening posterior compartment prolapse, they were not able to determine a specific stage of POP at which these symptoms became more pronounced. The use of proctography has also failed to show a correlation between rectocele size and defecatory symptoms (129,130).

Weidner and co-workers (131) attempted to characterize symptoms of defecatory dysfunction, including constipation and fecal incontinence, in 352 patients with urinary incontinence and POP and found that symptoms of constipation were more likely reported in patients with advanced stages of POP (stage III or IV). Interestingly, these authors also found a higher prevalence of fecal incontinence in patients with worsening stage of anterior and posterior vaginal wall prolapse. Jackson and colleagues (132) also reported significant correlations between POP and fecal incontinence. The effect of hormonal status on colorectal function is not clear. The effect of estrogen on the posterior compartment and concurrent fecal incontinence, for example, was examined by Donnelly and associates, who found improvement in anorectal physiologic parameters and improvement in quality of life after estrogen replacement therapy (133). In evaluating enteroceles and concurrent defecatory dysfunction, Chou and colleagues (126) found no association between symptoms of bowel function and the presence or absence of enterocele.

Treatment

Pessary

Treatment for POP may be thought of in terms of either surgical or nonsurgical approaches. Dating back to antiquity, pessaries have remained the mainstay of nonsurgical intervention for POP. Unfortunately, there is a paucity of literature regarding pessaries, with much being anecdotal and controversial. It has traditionally been advocated that pessaries should be used as a second-line therapy, reserved for those patients who either decline or have contraindications to surgery (134,135). In a recent survey of the American Urogynecologic Society, Cundiff and colleagues (136) confirmed this sentiment among gynecologic surgeons who had greater than 20 years of experience. In contrast, the same survey found that younger gynecologists reported using pessaries more frequently as a first-line therapy for POP. The reason for this difference in inclination toward pessary use is not known. The choice of pessary and its relative indications and contraindications are based primarily on subjective opinion rather than level I or II data. With the exception of one prospective study (137), which attempted to establish clinical parameters associated with successful pessary use, the large number of different pessaries and absence of uniform guidelines or recommendation have led to a lack of consensus regarding their use. With respect to posterior compartment defects, the efficacy of conservative pessary treatment is debated (138,139). Unfortunately, there are no studies that address the efficacy of pessaries in alleviating symptoms of pelvic floor herniation or defecatory dysfunction.

Posterior Colporrhaphy

The surgical repair of rectocele evolved in the 19th century, with the first procedures attempting to correct perineal tears by way of simple perineal closure. More aggressive approaches were soon undertaken to address prolapse, specifically elytrorrhaphy of the posterior compartment, which denuded the posterior vaginal mucosa, followed by closure and narrowing of the vaginal caliber. The traditional posterior colporrhaphy, advocated by Heidelberg and Simon in 1867, attempted to reduce rectoceles and uterovaginal prolapse by plicating the levator ani muscles and the inferior aspect of the vagina. This served to create a rigid inferior shelf that reduced herniations of the posterior compartment and prevented apical and uterine descensus. In 1870, Hegar introduced the concept of the colpoperineorrhaphy, which, by creating a tight introital band, sought to address all types of POP (140). The traditional posterior colporrhaphy has a reported success rate of 76% to 96% (141,142) for reducing actual rectocele herniation. Unfortunately, this approach appears to be less successful at alleviating defecatory dysfunction and may, in fact, exacerbate symptoms and contribute to *de novo* sexual dysfunction. Francis and Jeffcoate were the first to publish a significant correlation between posterior colporrhaphy and sexual dysfunction. In their series of 243 women, they reported postoperative dyspareunia in 50% of their patients (143). In a retrospective study by Kahn and Stanton, dyspareunia and defecatory dysfunction, including fecal incontinence, constipation, and incomplete evacuation, all increased postoperatively after posterior colporrhaphy (142). In one prospective study of posterior colporrhaphy, Mellgran and associates found a 48% prevalence of postoperative constipation in 25 patients 1 year after surgery (141). In this study, abnormal preoperative transit studies and dyssynergic defecation were risk factors for persistent postoperative constipation.

Transanal Repair

Colorectal surgeons traditionally approach rectocele repair through a transanal approach. The technique, first popularized by Sullivan and colleagues (144), includes plication of the rectal muscularis and attachment of this plicated tissue to the levator ani fascia bilaterally. Although this approach appears to alleviate constipation in 22% to 85% of patients

(145,146), it makes it difficult to address concurrently perineal descent, high rectocele, or enterocele. In one comparative study reviewing transanal and transvaginal approaches, Arnold and colleagues found no difference in surgical outcome with respect to fecal incontinence, constipation, or dyspareunia (147). Similar findings have also been published by Kahn and associates, who prospectively evaluated both approaches and found few differences with respect to postoperative defecatory dysfunction (148).

Defect-directed Repair

In the 1970s, Richardson popularized the concept of discrete fascial breaks rather than tissue attenuation as the primary cause of POP (149). With attention to the posterior compartment, he described five sites at which the rectovaginal fascia could be broken and advocated a site-specific repair for rectocele reduction. This concept allowed for a deviation from the traditional nonanatomic repair while still maintaining the basic principle of hernia repair. The site-specific repair does not attempt to plicate the levator ani fascia and, as such, may be associated with a lower incidence of postoperative morbidity. Cundiff and colleagues reported on their series of 69 women who underwent defect-directed repair for symptomatic rectocele (150). After this surgical approach, they reported resolution of several symptoms thought to be associated with rectocele, including constipation in 84%, splinting in 55%, and dyspareunia in 66%. The improved symptom outcome in this series was attributed to the defect-directed repair, which reestablished the normal integrity and anatomy of the rectovaginal fascia. Other authors have supported this premise. Porter and co-workers (151) and Glavind and Madsen (152) noted significant improvement in bowel symptoms after site-specific posterior colporrhaphy, and Kenton and associates (153) reported similar findings in patients undergoing rectovaginal fascia reattachment.

These reports suggest that the discrete site-specific repair may be preferable to the traditional posterior colporrhaphy incorporating levator plication in preventing postoperative dyspareunia and alleviating symptoms related to defecatory dysfunction.

Posterior Fascial Replacement

Attempts to augment rectocele repair with synthetic or allogenic material have met with varying results. Most initial reports involving permanent synthetic mesh have focused on anterior compartment support. Julian reported on his experience with Marlex mesh in the repair of recurrent anterior compartment prolapse. Although he reported no recurrence, the follow-up was relatively short, and the mesh erosion rate of 25% proved unacceptable (154). Numerous authors have confirmed the high erosion and infection rates with permanent types of mesh used in this application. As a result, others have attempted to use absorbable synthetic mesh material to prevent recurrent prolapse. Sand and associates recently published their results from a prospective randomized trial using polyglactin 910 (Vicryl) mesh in cystocele and rectocele repair (155). Although they found that the addition of mesh reduced the rate of recurrent central cystocele, there was no significant effect on the incidence of recurrent rectocele. Additionally, they reported no postoperative mesh erosions. Others have attempted to bolster attenuated rectovaginal fascia with natural materials, including autologous and allograft fascia lata, allogenic dermal grafts, and extracellular matrix xenografts. One of the first reports was by Oster and Astrup in 1981, in which the authors reported on their experience with dermal graft augmentation in rectocele repair in 15 patients (156). With a follow-up period of 1 to 4 years, they reported no recurrent prolapse and alleviation of most symptoms related to defecatory dysfunction, although five patients experienced persistent constipation. Other authors have reported using dermal allografts successfully in augmenting rectovaginal fistula (157). Two promising alternatives to synthetic materials for use in augmentation include Alloderm (Lifecell Corp., Branchburg, NJ), an acellular allogenic dermal matrix, and SurgiSIS (Cook

Ob/Gyn, Indianapolis, MN), an extracellular matrix derived from the submucosa of porcine small intestine. Alloderm grafts have been used extensively in plastic and periodontal surgery since 1994, whereas SurgiSIS has been used primarily in urologic and gynecologic applications. Although preliminary unpublished results suggest that these biomaterials are safe in vaginal applications, there are no data supporting that they add any additional strength or durability to the repair. It is doubtful whether the use of these materials will independently affect defecatory symptoms.

Although recent literature suggests that the defect-directed repair has better symptom-based outcomes than the traditional posterior colporrhaphy, controversy remains regarding the actual diagnosis of site-specific defects and the longevity of these repairs. The proponents of posterior fascia replacement augmentation maintain that these materials will add further durability to the repair with no increase in morbidity. Prospective randomized studies comparing these various approaches to posterior compartment prolapse are currently underway in an effort to establish which repair provides better symptom relief and durable surgical results.

PERINEAL DESCENT

Sir Allan Parks and colleagues first described the syndrome of the descending perineum in 1966 (158). The anatomic derangements that produce characteristic bulging of the pelvic floor with anterior displacement of the urethral axis and posterior displacement of the anal canal coexist with a variety of physiologic disturbances in the anorectum, vagina, and distal urinary tract. Associated clinical conditions may include symptomatic constipation, obstructed defecation, fecal incontinence, urinary incontinence, and anatomic abnormalities with single or multicompartmental POP (159,160). Because the endopelvic fascial support is often attenuated and significant pudendal neuropathy may coexist with descent, many surgeons consider perineal descent to be a nonoperative condition despite often disabling sequelae. This problem is compounded by the association of this syndrome with poor outcomes following other reconstructive anorectal procedures (161,162).

Biofeedback and behavioral modification with pelvic floor retraining have been the most common forms of nonoperative therapy for perineal descent and should be exhausted before pursuing operative repair. The avoidance of straining is of paramount importance, and early improvement in up to 64% of patients has been reported after intensive pelvic floor retraining (163). Unfortunately, the results are usually not durable, and defecatory disorders recur with behavioral relapse to chronic straining. With recurrence, the progression of symptoms may include obstructed defecation, fecal and urinary incontinence, POP, and rectal prolapse, leading to a very poor quality of life in severely affected women.

Early results presented by several groups may offer surgical alternatives for the management of perineal descent. Cundiff and colleagues modified the abdominal sacral colpopexy (164) (for apical prolapse) by extending the mesh support down to the perineal body in association with rectocele repair in patients with rectocele and perineal descent (165). The intent of this procedure, the abdominal sacral colpoperineopexy, is to restore and replace disrupted central perineal body support from the rectovaginal fascia and uterosacral-cardinal ligaments. The initial results of 19 patients who underwent abdominal sacral colpoperineopexy with Mersilene mesh have been reported. Postoperative stage of prolapse was significantly reduced, with no patient having greater than stage II prolapse on postoperative POPQ examination. Bowel symptoms improved in 8 of 11 women. Despite these encouraging early results, erosion of Mersilene mesh into the posterior vaginal wall occurred in up to 40% of patients (166). Alternatively, mesh erosion into the vault had only been reported in 3% of patients who underwent more apical mesh placement for abdominal sacral colpopexy (164).

Total pelvic mesh repair (TPMR) has been described by Sullivan and colleagues for the treatment of advanced POP (167). A trapezoidal sheet of Marlex mesh is attached to the perineal body through an abdominal approach, brought to the left of the rectum, and secured to the sacral periosteum at S-1 to S-2 (Fig. 24.5). A 2-cm strut of Marlex is secured from each side of the trapezoid to Cooper's ligament. A fourth strut is placed between the two anterior struts to support the bladder and vagina in patients with anterior prolapse.

The long-term follow-up on 236 patients operated on by TPMR from 1990 to 1999 has been reported (167). Indications included patients with previously failed conventional techniques of prolapse surgery and those with

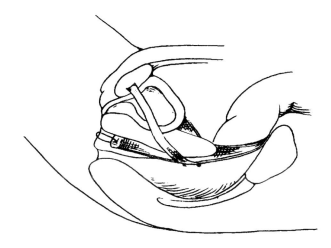

FIG. 24.5. Position of the trapezoidal and anterolateral mesh struts in the total pelvic mesh repair (TPMR). (From Sullivan ES, Longaker CJ, Lee PY. Total pelvic mesh repair: a ten-year experience. *Dis Colon Rectum* 2001;44:857–863, with permission.)

combined rectal and genitourinary prolapse. Rectal prolapse was common (74%) and included women with mucosal to full-thickness disease. Perineal descent was present in 64% of patients. There were no cases of recurrent stage IV vaginal vault prolapse or full-thickness rectal prolapse. Data were not reported on recurrence of perineal descent. Marlex erosion into the rectum or vagina occurred in 5% of patients. Additional procedures were subsequently performed for persistent urinary symptoms in 36% and anorectal symptoms in 28% of patients at a median interval of 197 days from the TPMR. Overall satisfaction was reported at 74% in patients followed more than 6 years.

The recto vaginopexy with polytetrafluoroethylene (PTFE, Gore-Tex has been proposed for the treatment of constipation and fecal incontinence with concomitant apical or posterior POP (Fig. 24.6). Although perineal descent was not specifically addressed by the authors, the attachments of the synthetic support may serve a similar purpose. The midpoint of a 20- × 1-cm strip of PTFE is sutured to the sacral promontory with the legs of this graft attached to the lateral rectum and uterosacral ligaments. Despite the absence of a separate rectocele or enterocele repair, these defects decreased from 74% and 33% preoperatively to 30% and 0%, respectively. There were no reports of PTFE erosion into pelvic viscera. Improvement in constipation was 76% at 1 year ($p = 0.0015$) and 71% at 4 years ($p = 0.005$). At 1 year, incontinence improved by 87% ($p = 0.0015$), which decreased to 53% at 4 years ($p = 0.09$).

Given the high rate of mesh erosion into the vagina when a transvaginal rectocele repair is performed in association with abdominal sacral colpoperineopexy, autologous fascia and other biomaterials have been used for attachment of the perineal body to the sacrum. Kaufman and colleagues used Alloderm as a graft in 11 women who did not desire autologous fascial harvest (168). Coexisting full-thickness or internal rectal prolapse or poor mesorectal fixation was documented by dynamic magnetic resonance imaging or cystocolpoproctography (169) in these patients with coexisting defecatory dysfunction. Simultaneous rectopexy (with or without sigmoid resection) was performed in association with abdominal sacral coloperineopexy in these patients for severe perineal descent with defecatory dysfunction (Fig. 24.7).

Highlights of this procedure include two teams beginning simultaneously, with the perineal surgeon performing a transvaginal rectocele repair (defect-directed or posterior colporrhaphy) and the abdominopelvic team beginning with sigmoid resection (if indicated) and rectal mobilization. The mesorectal plane is developed down to the pelvic floor

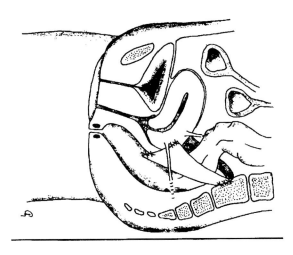

FIG. 24.6. Position of the polytetrafluoroethylene (PTFE) strip in the rectovaginopexy. The midpoint of the PTFE strip is sutured to the sacral promontory with the legs attached to the anterolateral aspects of the rectum and uterosacral ligaments. (From Silvis R, Goosen HG, van Essen A, et al. Abdominal rectovaginopexy: modified technique to treat constipation. *Dis Colon Rectum* 1999;42(1):82–88, with permission.)

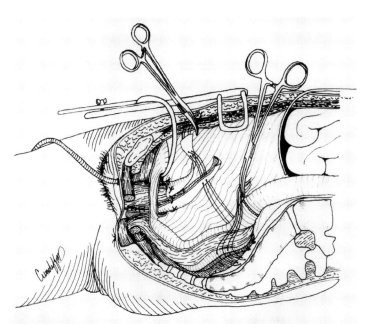

FIG. 24.7. Abdominal sacral colpoperineopexy with sigmoid resection and suture rectopexy. This sagittal view shows the posterior Alloderm graft sutured to the rectovaginal fascia and perineal body after defect-directed rectocele repair. The anterior sheet of Alloderm is sutured to the pubocervical fascia. Both sheets will be secured to the sacral periosteum to the right of the rectum. Rectopexy sutures (*left*) have not yet been tied and secured. (Courtesy of Geoffrey W. Cundiff, M.D.)

posteriorly, with care taken to identify and preserve the hypogastric nerves. The more distal autonomic pelvic plexus is preserved by avoiding lateral dissection and lateral ligament division. Sutures are placed from the fascia propria of the rectum to the sacral periosteum at S-1 to S-3 for the rectopexy. These sutures are not tied until the coloproctostomy is completed if the sigmoid has been resected. A 4- × 16-cm strip of nonmeshed Alloderm is sutured to the perineal body overlying the rectocele repair and passed into the pelvis through a defect made in the cul-de-sac. The proximal portion of this graft is secured to the sacrum by the right-sided rectopexy sutures along with a smaller anterior graft attached distally to the pubocervical fascia.

In early follow-up (12.5 ± 7.7 months), 9 of 11 patients (82%) remained free of perineal descent, whereas 2 patients had recurrences (168). Significant symptomatic improvement was noted in constipation, incomplete evacu-

ation, and need for assisted evacuation. Overall, 8 of 11 patients reported an improvement in their quality of life. In longer follow-up (unpublished data), there have been no cases of erosion of Alloderm through the vaginal mucosa or into the rectum or bladder. Furthermore, there have been no cases of erosion of the supporting sutures used to secure the Alloderm to the perineal body, rectovaginal fascia, or pubocervical fascia.

RECTAL PROLAPSE

Rectal prolapse results when the full thickness of the rectum intussuscepts through the anal canal. In adults, this syndrome most often affects elderly people, with the earliest onset usually occurring during the fifth decade. The female-to-male ratio is 5:1. Numerous congenital and acquired conditions have been implicated in the etiology of rectal prolapse and include chronic constipation, neurologic disease (congenital anomaly, spinal cord trauma, cauda equina lesion, dementia), weak anal sphincter (due to injury, denervation), and previous surgery (fistulotomy, sphincterotomy, hemorrhoidectomy, coloanal anastomosis). Anatomic findings associated with this process include a deep pouch of Douglas, patulous anus, redundant rectosigmoid, levator ani diastasis, and poor mesorectal fixation to the presacral tissues and pelvic sidewalls. A rectosigmoid lesion may also serve as a lead point for intussusception.

Patients usually present with a chief complaint of protrusion of the rectum, most often with attempts at defecation or with the Valsalva maneuver. With progression of disease, prolapse may occur without increases in intraabdominal pressure. Constipation has been reported in 25% to 50% of patients (170), and up to 75% of patients report fecal incontinence (171). Incontinence usually improves after surgical management of prolapse without any intervention directed at the anal sphincter. On physical examination, the surgeon must differentiate between full-thickness rectal prolapse, mucosal prolapse, and prolapsing hemorrhoids. Except for the most profound cases, patients often can only demonstrate rectal prolapse by sitting on a commode and straining to stool. A pelvic examination should be performed to rule out other POP.

More than 100 surgical procedures have been described to treat full-thickness rectal prolapse. These procedures may be broadly classified into those performed through the abdominal route and those performed through a perineal approach. Some surgeons prefer a perineal approach for nearly all patients; however, given overall lower recurrence rates after abdominal procedures, perineal procedures have classically been reserved for more debilitated patients.

Ripstein described the modern anterior sling rectopexy in 1965 (172). Although Ripstein anecdotally reported a very low recurrence rate, the details of his personal series of more than 1,500 patients were never published. Unfortunately, a relatively high constipation rate has been found in long-term follow-up of these

patients. Erosion of mesh and obstructed defecation secondary to a complete anterior wrap have been the major morbidities associated with this procedure. Subsequent modification to a two-thirds posterolateral wrap have led to improvements in postoperative defecatory dysfunction. Tjandra and colleagues reported the results of 142 Ripstein procedures performed over a 27-year period (173). The recurrence rate of complete prolapse was 8% and within the range reported from other series (5% to 10%) (172,173). Recurrence rates of 0% to 2% have been reported by others, but with shorter postoperative follow-up (174). Other related suspensions and fixation procedures include the Wells procedure, direct suture rectopexy, posterior Ivalon sponge rectopexy, and resection rectopexy (Frykman-Goldberg procedure) (171,175). Most series of prolapse surgery are retrospective, and there have been no data to suggest that the addition of a foreign sling provides any advantage to simple suture fixation alone. Debate continues about the value and extent of resection when combined with rectopexy (176).

Perineal operations for rectal prolapse have usually been reserved for more infirm and unfit patients who cannot tolerate an abdominal approach. Although easily tolerated, perianal encirclement procedures such as the Thiersch wire have largely been abandoned owing to poor success rates and high rates of recurrence and fecal impaction. Alternatively, the Altemeier procedure (Fig. 24.8A–C), a full-thickness rectosigmoidectomy with or without levator plasty, can be performed with minimal morbidity in this patient population. Although the incidence of recurrent rectal prolapse varies widely (3% to 60%) (177) after the Altemeier procedure, this operation can be easily repeated if necessary.

The Delorme procedure (Fig. 24.9), first described by a French army surgeon in 1900, entails mucosal stripping of the prolapsed rectum with subsequent recto mucosectomy and plication of the distal rectal wall (178). There was little interest in Delorme's procedure until the 1970s when several small series were reported. Senapati and colleagues published the results

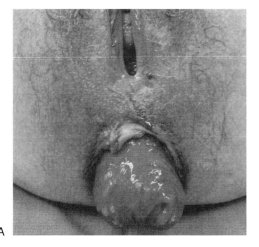

A

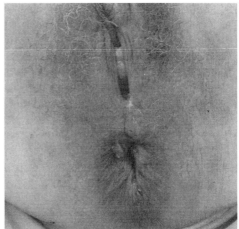

C

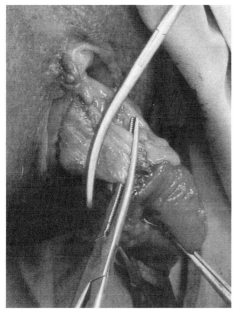

B

FIG. 24.8. Altemeier procedure (perineal rectosigmoidectomy). **A:** Preoperative appearance revealing full-thickness rectal prolapse. **B:** Mesorectal division and ligation. **C:** Postoperative view after end-to-end coloanal anastomosis.

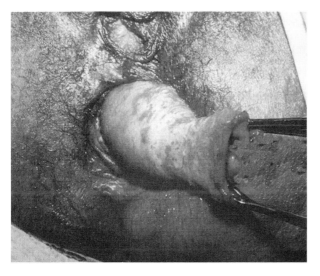

FIG. 24.9. Delorme's procedure. After mucosal stripping to the full extent of the prolapse, the circular smooth muscle of the rectum is plicated. A mucosa-to-mucosa anastomosis is then performed.

of this procedure in 32 patients (179). There was no mortality. At a mean follow-up of 24 months, 12.5% of patients developed a recurrence. Incontinence improved in 46%, and constipation improved in 50%. Oliver and coauthors reported their experience of 41 patients who underwent Delorme's procedure over a 10-year period (180). Twenty-two percent of patients developed a recurrence. Thirty-two patients (68%) claimed that their continence was enhanced after this procedure.

In conclusion, rectal prolapse is a multifactorial disease affecting mostly elderly people. For younger and fit patients, abdominal approaches offer low recurrence rates. Recently, laparoscopic approaches to suture rectopexy, sling rectopexy, and resection rectopexy have been described with satisfactory results (181). Regardless of the abdominal technique, continence is usually improved after repair. Elderly and debilitated patients, as well as younger patients with multiple medical problems, are best served by a perineal procedure.

CONCLUSIONS

In summary, defecatory dysfunction encompasses many disorders that are manifested by gastrointestinal symptoms, including but not limited to difficulty with evacuation. Epidemiologic studies attempting to characterize the prevalence of defecatory dysfunction have been difficult to perform because of the all-encompassing nature of the term and the lack of defining criteria. In approaching this subject, it is helpful to consider general etiologic factors. As we have seen, these include lifestyle issues such as the following: the effect of diet, exercise, medications, and patient mobility; systemic diseases, including underlying diabetes mellitus, thyroid dysfunction, and neuromuscular disorders such as multiple sclerosis and Hirschsprung's disease; functional disorders, such as IBS, colonic inertia, and idiopathic constipation; obstructive disorders resulting from either mechanical causes such as malignancy, POP, and impaction or from pelvic floor dyssynergia; and finally, psychiatric causes, such as depression, eating disorders, and dementia. Although considerable overlap exists within the subcategories of defecatory dysfunction, constipation is a common denominator.

Further research is needed to address many aspects of defecatory dysfunction. Most important is the need for a validated, disease-specific quality-of-life instrument to assist in clarifying the potential interrelationships between symptoms and their etiologies and respective therapies. Equally important are the development and standardization of normative data regarding normal physiologic defecation stratified by age, gender, and parity. Once established, these normal ranges will assist in defining diagnostic criteria and etiologies for various aspects of pelvic floor dysfunction, including important subcategories such as pelvic floor dyssynergia. Further advances in gastrointestinal diagnostic testing techniques and pelvic floor imaging will enhance our understanding of underlying pathology as it relates to both sensorimotor and pelvic support dysfunction. Further research is needed, for example, in defining the indications for and the utility of magnetic imaging in the evaluation and management of patients with POP. Advances in surgical innovation and biomaterial availability may ultimately enhance the longevity of surgical procedures addressing POP.

In the field of FGIDs, a better understanding of the enteric nervous system is needed. Factors influencing neural regulation and modulation are currently being defined that will clarify relationships between symptoms subgroups. This information will also shed light on the natural history of sensorimotor dysfunction and its respective relationship to the evolution of respective FGID symptoms. This, along with further research in genetics, will hopefully explain why there is such a broad range and overlap in FGID symptoms and their severity. New advances in pharmacologic research have led to the development of drugs that modulate visceral sensitivity, an important aspect of IBS therapy. Further research is needed to elucidate visceral afferent pathways, their respective neurotransmitters, and the gut–brain connection. The psychosocial aspects of the FGIDs also warrant further investigation, and validated instruments controlling for gender, sociocultural factors, and clinical settings are needed to assess psychosocial traits and bowel symptoms. Once these are established, the impact of psychological intervention and other similar treatment modalities (such as biofeedback) can be critically analyzed.

REFERENCES

1. Sonnenberg A, Koch TR. Epidemiology of constipation in the U.S. *Dis Colon Rectum* 1989;32:1–8.
2. Drossman DA, Li Z, Andruzzi E, et al. U.S. household survey of functional gastrointestinal disorders: prevalence, sociodemography and health impact. *Dig Dis Sci* 1993;38:1569–1580.
3. Wald A. Advances in gastroenterology. *Med Clin North Am* 2000;84(5):1231–1246.
4. Everhart JE, Go VLW, Johannes RS, et al. A longitudinal survey of self-reported bowel habits in the United States. *Dig Dis Sci* 1989;34:1153–1162.
5. Johanson JF, Sonnenberg A, Koch TR. Clinical epidemiology of chronic constipation. *J Clin Gastroenterol* 1989;11:525–536.
6. Jewell DJ, Younge G. Interventions for treating constipation in pregnancy (Cochrane review). In: *The Cochrane library*, Issue 2. Oxford: Update Software, 2001.
7. Perry E, Shields R, Turnball AC. The effect of pregnancy on the colonic absorption of sodium, potassium and water. *J Obstet Gynecol Br Commonw* 1970;77:900.
8. Devroede G, Lamarche J. Functional importance of extrinsic parasympathetic innervation to the distal colon and rectum in man. *Gastroenterology* 1974;66:273–281.
9. Devroede G, Arhan P, Duguay C, et al. Traumatic constipation. *Gastroenterology* 1979;77:1258.
10. Weber J, Grise P, Roquebert M, et al. Radiopaque markers transit and anorectal manometry in 16 patients with multiple sclerosis and urinary bladder dysfunction. *Dis Colon Rectum* 1987;30:95.
11. Metzger PP, Alvear DT, Arnold GC, et al. Hirschsprung's disease in adults: report of a case and review of the literature. *Dis Colon Rectum* 1978;21:113.
12. Wald A. Approach to the patient with constipation. In: Yamada T, Alpers DH, Owyand C, et al, eds. *Textbook of gastroenterology,* 3rd ed. Philadelphia: Lippincott Williams & Wilkins, 1999.
13. MacIver AG, Whitehead R. Zonal colonic aganglionosis: a variant of Hirschsprung's disease. *Arch Dis Child* 1972;47:233.
14. Wood JD, Alpers DH, Andrews PLR. Fundamentals of neurogastroenterology. *Gut* 1999;45[Suppl II]:6–16.
15. Shoulder P, Keighley MRB. Changes in colorectal function in severe idiopathic chronic constipation. *Gastroenterology* 1986;90:414.
16. Krishnamurthy S, Schuffler MD, Rohrmann CA, et al. Severe idiopathic constipation is associated with a distinctive abnormality of the colonic myenteric plexus. *Gastroenterology* 1985;88:26.
17. Dyer NH, Dawson AM, Smith BF, et al. Obstruction of the bowel due to a lesion in the myenteric plexus. *Br Med J* 1969;1:686.
18. Koch TR, Carney JA, Go L, et al. Idiopathic chronic constipation is associated with decreased colonic vasoactive intestinal peptide. *Gastroenterology* 1988;94:300–310.
19. Kuiipers HC, Bleijenberg G. The spastic pelvic floor syndrome. *Dis Colon Rectum* 1985;28:669–672.
20. Preston DM, Lennard-Jones JE. Severe chronic constipation of young women: idiopathic slow transit constipation. *Gut* 1986;27:41–48.
21. Odenthal KP, Ziegler D. In vitro effects of anthraquinones on rat intestine and uterus. *Pharmacology* 1988;36[Suppl 1]:57–65.
22. Schwarcz R, Foster AC, French ED, et al. Excitotoxic models for neurodegenerative disorders. *Life Sci* 1984;35:19–32.
23. Caccese WJ, Bronzo RL, Wadler G, et al. Oglivie's syndrome associated with herpes zoster infection. *J Clin Gastroenterol* 1985;7:309–313.
24. Walsch TN, Lane D. Pseudo-obstruction intestinale et infection a cyomegalovirus des plexus myenteriques. *Arch Fr Pediatr* 1985;42:713–715.
25. Corazzari E, Cucchiara S, Staiano A, et al. Gastrointestinal transit time, frequency of defecation, and anorectal manometry in healthy and constipated children. *J Pediatr* 1985;106:379.
26. Molnar D, Taitz LS, Urwin OM, et al. Anorectal manometry results in defecation disorders. *Arch Dis Child* 1983;58:257.
27. Loening-Baucke VA, Younoszai MK. Effect of treatment on rectal and sigmoid motility in chronically constipated children. *Pediatrics* 1983;71:774.
28. Loening-Baucke VA, Cruikshank B, Savage C. Defecation dynamics and behavior profiles in encopretic children. *Pediatrics* 1987;80:672.
29. Roma E, Adamidis D, Nikolara R, et al. Diet and chronic constipation in children: the role of fiber. *J Pediatr Gastroenterol Nutr* 1999;29(4):487.
30. Moarais MB, Vitolo MR, Aguiire AN, et al. Measurement of low dietary fiber intake as a risk factor for chronic constipation in children. *J Pediatr Gastroenterol Nutr* 1999;29(2):132.
31. Wald A. Colonic transit and anorectal manometry in chronic idiopathic constipation. *Arch Intern Med* 1986;146:1713.
32. Wald A, Hinds JP, Caruana BJ. Psychological and physiological characteristics of patients with severe idiopathic constipation. *Gastroenterology* 1989;97:932–937.
33. Wald A, Burgio K, Holeva K, et al. Psychological evaluation of patients with severe idiopathic constipation: which instrument to use. *Am J Gastroenterol* 1992;87:977–980.
34. Grotz RL, Pemberton JH, Talley NJ, et al. Discriminant value of psychological distress, symptom profiles, and segmental colonic dysfunction in outpatients with severe idiopathic constipation. *Gut* 1994;35:798–802.
35. Wald A. Constipation and fecal incontinence in the elderly. *Gastroenterol Clin North Am* 1990;19:405.

36. Odenthal KP, Ziegler D. In vitro effects of anthraquinones on rat intestine and uterus. *Pharmacology* 1988;36[Suppl 1]:57–65.

37. Ashraf W, Park F, Lof J, et al. An examination of the reliability of reported stool frequency in the diagnosis of idiopathic constipation. *Am J Gastroenterol* 1996;1:26.

38. Koutsomanis D, Lennard-Jones JE, Roy AJ, et al. Controlled randomized trial of visual biofeedback versus muscle training without a visual display for intractable constipation. *Gut* 1995;37:95–99.

39. Davies GJ, Crowder M, Reid B, et al. Bowel function measurements of individuals with different eating patterns. *Gut* 1974;27:1068–1074.

40. Burkitt DP, Walker ARP, Painter NS. Effect of dietary fiber on stools and transit-times and its role in the causation of disease. *Lancet* 1972;ii:1408–1411.

41. Watier A, Devroed G, Duranceau A, et al. Constipation with colonic inertia: a manifestation of systemic disease? *Dig Dis Sci* 1983;28:1025.

42. Lee AJ, Evans CJ, Hau CM, et al. Fiber intake, constipation, and risk of varicose veins in the general population: Edinburgh vein study. *J Clin Epidemiol* 2001; 54(4):423–429.

43. Manning AP, Heaton KW, Harvey RF, et al. Wheat fibre and irritable bowel syndrome: a controlled trial. *Lancet* 1977;2:417–418.

44. Arffmann S, Andersen JR, Hegnhay J, et al. The effect of coarse bran in the irritable bowel syndrome: a double blind cross-over study. *Scand J Gastroenterol* 1985;20:295.

45. Cann PA, Read NW, Holdsworth CD. What is the benefit of coarse wheat bran in patients with irritable bowel syndrome? *Gut* 1984;25:168.

46. Findlay JM, Smith AN, Michell WD, et al. Effects of unprocessed bran on colon function in normal subjects and in diverticular disease. *Lancet* 1974;1:146–149.

47. Brodribb AJM. Treatment of symptomatic diverticular disease with a high-fibre diet. *Lancet* 1977;2:664–666.

48. Ornstein MH, Littlewood ER, McLean Baird I, et al. Are fibre supplements really necessary in diverticular disease of the colon? A controlled clinical trial. *Br Med J* 1981;282:1353–1356.

49. Müller-Lissner S. Effect of wheat bran on weight of stool and gastrointestinal transit time: a meta analysis. *Br Med J* 1988;296:615–617.

50. Tramonte SM, Brand MB, Mulrow CD, et al. The treatment of chronic constipation in adults: a systematic review. *J Gen Intern Med* 1997;12(1):15–24.

51. Slavin JL. Implementation of dietary modifications. *Am J Med* 1999;106:46S–49S.

52. Verduron A, Devroede G, Bouchoucha M, et al. Megarectum. *Dig Dis Sci* 1985;30:1164.

53. Powell R. On certain painful affections of the intestinal canal. *Med Trans Coll Physicians* 1820;114:841.

54. Chaudhury NA, Truelove SC. The irritable colon syndrome. *Q J Med* 1962;32:307.

55. Thompson WG. *The irritable gut.* Baltimore: University Park Press, 1979.

56. Manning AP, Thompson WD, Heaton KW, et al. Towards positive diagnosis in the irritable bowel syndrome. *BMJ* 1978;2:653–654.

57. Kruis W, Thieme CH, Weinzierl M, et al. A diagnostic score for the irritable bowel syndrome: its value in the exclusion of organic disease. *Gastroenterology* 1984; 87:1–7.

58. Drossman DA, Richter JE, Talley NJ, et al, eds. *The functional gastrointestinal disorders: diagnosis, pathophysiology and treatment,* 1st ed. McLean, VA: Degnon Associates, 1994.

59. Drossman D, Corazziari E, Talley NJ, et al., eds. *Rome II: the functional gastrointestinal disorders,* 2nd ed. McLean, VA: Degnon Associates, 2000.

60. Thompson WG, Longstreth GF, Drossman DA, et al. Functional bowel disorders and functional abdominal pain [Review]. *Gut* 1999;45[Suppl 2]:43–47.

61. Mayer EA. Emerging disease model for functional gastrointestinal disorders. *Am J Med* 1999;107(5A):12S.

62. Talley NJ, Zinsmeister AR, Melton LJ. Irritable bowel syndrome in a community: symptom subgroups, risk factors, and health care utilization. *Am J Epidemiol* 1995;142:76–83.

63. Heaton KW. Symptoms of irritable bowel syndrome in a British urban community: consulters and nonconsulters. *Gastroenterology* 1992;102:1962–1967.

64. Gralnek IM. Health care utilization and economic issues in irritable bowel syndrome. *Eur J Surg* 1998; 583[Suppl]:73.

65. Rothstein RD. Irritable bowel syndrome. *Med Clin North Am* 2000;84:1247–1257.

66. Drossman DA, Sandler RS, McKee DC. Bowel patterns among subjects not seeking health care. *Gastroenterology* 1982;83:529–534.

67. Whitehead WE, Crowell MD, Robinson JC, et al. Effects of stressful life events on bowel symptoms: subjects with irritable bowel syndrome compared with subjects without bowel dysfunction. *Gut* 1992;33:825–830.

68. Talley NJ, Fett SL, Zinsmeister AR, et al. Gastrointestinal tract symptoms and self-reported abuse: a population-based study. *Gastroenterology* 1994;107: 1040–1049.

69. Drossman DA, Leserman J, Nachmann G, et al. Sexual and physical abuse in women with functional or organic gastrointestinal disorders. *Ann Intern Med* 1990; 113:828–833.

70. Walker EA, Katon WJ, Jemelka RP, et al. Comorbidity of gastrointestinal complaints, depression and anxiety disorders in the epidemiologic catchment (ECA) area study. *Am J Med* 1992;92(1A):26S–30S.

71. Locke GR III, Talley NJ, Zinsmeister AR, et al. The irritable bowel syndrome and functional dyspepsia: familial disorders? *Gastroenterology* 1996;110:A26(abst).

72. Rodriguez LAG, Ruigomez A. Increased risk of irritable bowel syndrome after bacterial gastroenteritis: cohort study. *BMJ* 1999;318:565–566.

73. Gwee KA, Graham JC, McKendrick MW, et al. Psychometric scores and persistence of irritable bowel after infectious diarrhoea. *Lancet* 1996;347:150–153.

74. Zwetchkenbaum J, Burakoff R. The irritable bowel syndrome and food hypersensitivity. *Ann Allergy* 1988; 62:47–49.

75. Vanner S, Glenn D, Paterson W. Diagnosing irritable bowel syndrome: predictive values of Rome criteria. *Gastroenterology* 1997;112:A47(abst).

76. Schmulson MW, Chang L. Diagnostic approach to the patient with irritable bowel syndrome. *Am J Med* 1999;107(5A);20S–26S.

77. Almoundjed G, Drossman DA. Newer aspects of the irritable bowel syndrome. *Prim Care* 1996;23(3): 477–495.

78. Camilleri M. Clinical evidence to support current ther-

apies of irritable bowel syndrome [Review]. *Aliment Pharmacol Ther* 1999;13:48–53.

79. Camilleri M. Therapeutic approach to the patient with irritable bowel syndrome. *Am J Med* 1999;107(5A): 27S–32S.

80. Klein KB. Controlled treatment trials in the irritable bowel syndrome. *Gastroenterology* 1988;95:232–241.

81. Poynard T, Naveau S, Mory B, et al. Meta-analysis of smooth muscle relaxants in the treatment of irritable bowel syndrome. *Aliment Pharmacol Ther* 1994;8: 499–510.

82. Pittler MH, Ernst E. Peppermint oil for irritable bowel syndrome: a critical review and meta-analysis. *Am J Gastroenterol* 1998;93(7):1131–1135.

83. Clouse RE. Antidepressants for functional gastrointestinal syndromes. *Dig Dis Sci* 1994;39:2352–2363.

84. Gunput MD. Review article: clinical pharmacology of alosetron. *Aliment Pharm Ther* 1999;70;[Suppl 2]:70.

85. Corazziari E. Role of opioid ligands in the irritable bowel syndrome. *Can J Gastroenterol* 1999;13[Suppl A]:71A.

86. Vicker AJ. *Hypnotherapy for irritable bowel syndrome: a report commissioned by North East Thames Regional Health Authority.* London: Research Council for Complimentary Medicine, 1994.

87. Schouten W, ten Kate F, de Graaf E, et al. Visceral neuropathy in slow transit constipation: an immunohistochemical investigation with monoclonal antibodies against neurofilament. *Dis Colon Rectum* 1993;36: 1099–1101.

88. Krishnamurthy S, Schuffler M, Rohrmann C, et al. Severe idiopathic constipation is associated with a distinctive abnormality of the colonic myenteric plexus. *Gastroenterology* 1985;88:26–34.

89. Bharucha AE, Phillips SF. Slow transit constipation. *Gastroenterol Clin North Am* 2001;30(1):77–95.

90. Camilleri M, McKinzie S, Burton D, et al. Prucalopride accelerates small bowel and colonic transit in patients with chronic functional constipation or constipation-predominant irritable bowel syndrome. *Gastroenterology* 2000;118:A845.

91. Coulie B, Szarka LA, Camileri M, et al. Recombinant human neurotrophic factors accelerate colonic transit and relieve constipation in humans. *Gastroenterology* 2000;119(1):41–50.

92. Lane W. Remarks on the results of the operative treatment of chronic constipation. *BMJ* 1908;1:126–130.

93. Christiansen J, Rasmussen OO. Colectomy for severe slow-transit constipation in strictly selected patients. *Scand J Gastroenterol* 1996;31(8):770–773.

94. Redmond JM, Smith GW, Barofsky I, et al. Physiological tests to predict long-term outcome of total abdominal colectomy for intractable constipation. *Am J Gastroenterol* 1995;90:748–753.

95. Nyam DCNK, Pemberton JH, Ilstrup DM, et al. Long-term results of surgery for chronic constipation. *Dis Colon Rectum* 1997;40:273–279.

96. Wexner SD, Daniel N, Jagelman DG. Colectomy for constipation; physiologic investigation is the key to success. *Dis Colon Rectum* 1991;34:851–856.

97. Sunderland GT, Poor FW, Lauder J, et al. Video-proctography in selecting patients with constipation for colectomy. *Dis Colon Rectum* 1992;35:235–237.

98. Hosie KB, Kmiot WA, Keighley MR. Constipation: another indication for restorative proctocolectomy. *Br J Surg* 1990;77(7):801–802.

99. Pinho M, Yoshioka K, Keighley MRB. Long term results of anorectal myectomy for chronic constipation. *Br J Surg* 1989;76:1163–1164.

100. Krogh K, Laurberg S. Malone antegrade continence enema for faecal incontinence and constipation in adults. *Br J Surg* 1998;85:974–977.

101. Martelli H, Devroede G, Arhan P, et al. Mechanisms of idiopathic constipation: outlet obstruction. *Gastroenterology* 1978;75:623.

102. Preston DM, Lennard-Jones J. Anismus in chronic constipation. *Dig Dis Sci* 1985;30:413–418.

103. Whitehead WE, Wald A, Diamant N, et al. Functional disorders of the anorectum. In: Drossman DA, ed. *International Working Party consensus: Rome criteria II.* McLean, VA: Degnon, 2000:482–532.

104. Rao SSC. Dyssynergic defecation. *Gastroenterol Clin North Am* 2001;30(1):97.

105. Read NW, Timms JM. Defecation and the pathophysiology of constipation. *Clin Gastroenterol* 1986;15:937.

106. Rao SSC, Vellema T, Kempf J, et al. Symptoms, stool patterns and quality of life in patients with dyssynergic defecation. *Gastroenterology* 2000;118:A782.

107. Joo JS, Agachan F, Wolff B, et al. Initial North American experience with botulinum toxin type A for treatment of anismus. *Dis Colon Rectum* 1991;35: 145–150.

108. Pinho M, Yoshioka K, Keighley MRB. Long term results of anorectal myectomy for chronic constipation. *Br J Surg* 1989;76:1163–1164.

109. Rao SSC, Welcher K, Leistikow J. Obstructive defecation: a failure of rectoanal coordination. *Am J Gastroenterol* 1998;93:1042–1050.

110. Enck P. Biofeedback training in disordered defecation: a critical review. *Dig Dis Sci* 1993;38:1953.

111. Bleijenberg G, Kuiipers HC. Treatment of the spastic pelvic floor syndrome with biofeedback. *Dis Colon Rectum* 1987;30:108.

112. Whitehead WE, Wald A, Diamant NE, et al. Functional disorders of the anus and rectum. *Gut* 1999;45: 1143–1147.

113. Rao SSC. Dyssynergic defecation. *Gastroenterol Clin North Am* 2001;30(1):101.

114. Wald A, Cauana BJ, Friemanis MG, et al. Contributions of evacuation proctography and anorectal manometry to evaluation of adults with idiopathic constipation. *Dig Dis Sci* 1990;35:481.

115. Rao SSC. Dyssynergic defecation. *Gastroenterol Clin North Am* 2001;30(1):107.

116. Ernst E, Resch KL. A meta-analysis of biofeedback treatment for anismus. *Eur J Phys Med Rehabil* 1995, 5(5):157–159.

117. Enck P. Biofeedback training in disordered defecation: a critical review. *Dig Dis Sci* 1993;38:1953–1960.

118. Rao SSC, Loening-Baucke V, Enck P. Biofeedback therapy for defecation disorders. *Dig Dis Sci* 1997; 15[Suppl 1]:78–92.

119. Rao SSC. Dyssynergic defecation. *Gastroenterol Clin North Am* 2001;30(1):109.

120. Ho YH, Tan M, Goh HS. Clinical and physiologic effects of biofeedback in outlet obstruction constipation. *Dis Colon Rectum* 1996;39(5):520–524.

121. Joo JS, Agachan F, Wolff B, et al. Initial North American experience with botulinum toxin type A for treat-

ment of anismus. *Dis Colon Rectum* 1996;39(10): 1107–1111.

122. Farag A. Obturator internus muscle autotransfer: a new concept for the treatment of anismus. Clinical experience. *Eur Surg Res* 1997;29(1):42–51.

123. Spence-Jones C, Kamm MA, Henry MM, et al. Bowel dysfunction: a pathogenic factor in uterovaginal prolapse and urinary stress incontinence. *Br J Obstet Gynecol* 1994;101:147–152.

124. Samuelsson EC, Arne Victor FT, Tibblin G, et al. Signs of genital prolapse in a Swedish population of women 20-59 years of age and possible related factors. *Am J Obstet Gynecol* 1999;9:961–964.

125. Swift SE. The distribution of pelvic organ support in a population of female subjects seen for routine gynecologic health care. *Am J Obstet Gynecol* 2000;183: 277–285.

126. Chou Q, Weber AM, Piedmonte MR. Clinical presentation of enterocele. *Obstet Gynecol* 2000;96(4):599–603.

127. Weber AM, Walters MD, Ballard LA, et al. Posterior vaginal prolapse and bowel function. *Am J Obstet Gynecol* 1998;179(6 Pt 1):1446–1449.

128. Ellerkmann RM, Cundiff GW, Bent AE, et al. Correlation of symptoms with location and severity of pelvic organ prolapse. *Am J Obstet Gynecol* 2001;185(6): 1332–1337.

129. Goei R. Anorectal function in patients with defecatory disorders and asymptomatic subjects: evaluation with defecography. *Radiology* 1990;174:121–123.

130. Yoshioka K, Matsui Y, Yamada O, et al. Physiologic and anatomic assessment of patients with rectocele. *Dis Colon Rectum* 1991;34:704–708.

131. Weidner AC, Coates KW, Cundiff GW, et al. Dysfunctional bowel symptoms in women with urinary incontinence and pelvic organ prolapse. (Submitted for publication.)

132. Jackson SL, Weber AM, Hull TL, et al. Fecal incontinence in women with urinary incontinence and pelvic organ prolapse. *Obstet Gynecol* 1997;89(3):423–427.

133. Donnelly V, O'Connell PR, O'Herlihy C. The influence of oestrogen replacement on faecal incontinence in postmenopausal women. *Br J Obstet Gynaecol* 1997; 104(3):311–315.

134. Sulak PJ, Kuehl TJ, Shull BL. Vaginal pessaries and their use in pelvic relaxation. *J Reprod Med* 1993;38: 919–923.

135. Zeitlin MP, Lebherz TB. Pessaries in the geriatric patient. *J Am Geriatr Soc* 1992;40:635–639.

136. Cundiff GW, Weidner AC, Visco AG, et al. A survey of pessary use by members of the American urogynecology society. *Obstet Gynecol* 2000;95(6 Pt 1):931–935.

137. Wu V, Farrell SA, Baskett TF, et al. A simplified protocol for pessary management. *Obstet Gynecol* 1997; 90:990–994.

138. Davila GW. Vaginal prolapse. *Postgrad Med* 1996;99: 171–185.

139. Sulak PJ, Kuehl TJ, Shull BJ. Vaginal pessaries and their use in pelvic relaxation. *J Reprod Med* 1993;38: 919–923.

140. Jeffcoat TNA. Posterior colpoperineorrhaphy. *Am J Obstet Gynecol* 1959;77:490–502.

141. Mellgren A, Anzén B, Nilsson BY, et al. Results of rectocele repair: a prospective study. *Dis Colon Rectum* 1995;38:7–13.

142. Kahn MA, Stanton SL. Posterior colporrhaphy: its effects on bowel and sexual function. *Br J Obstet Gynaecol* 1997;104:882–886.

143. Francis WJA, Jeffcoate TNA. Dyspareunia following vaginal operations. *J Obstet Gynaecol Br Emp* 1961; 68:1–10.

144. Sullivan ES, Leaverton GH, Hardwick CE. Transrectal perineal repair: an adjunct to improved function after anorectal surgery. *Dis Colon Rectum* 1968;11:196–214.

145. Sehapayak S. Transrectal repair of rectocele: an extended armamentarium of colorectal surgeons. A report of 355 cases. *Dis Colon Rectum* 1985;28: 422–433.

146. Khubchandani AT, Clancy JP, Rosen L, et al. Endorectal repair of rectocele revisited. *Br J Surg* 1997; 84:89–91.

147. Arnold MW, Stewart WRC, Aguilar PS. Rectocele repair: four year's experiences. *Dis Colon Rectum* 1990; 33:684–687.

148. Kahn MA, Stanton SL, Kumar DA. *Randomized prospective trial of posterior colporrhaphy versus transanal repair of rectocele.* Presented at American Urogynecologic Society, September 1997.

149. Richardson AC, Lyon JB, Williams NL. A new look at pelvic relaxation. *Am J Obstet Gynecol* 1976;568: 568–573.

150. Cundiff GW, Weidner AC, Visco AG, et al. An anatomic and functional assessment of the discrete defect rectocele repair. *Am J Obstet Gynecol* 1998;179(6 Pt 1):1451–1456.

151. Porter WE, Steele A, Walsh P, et al. The anatomic and functional outcomes of defect-specific rectocele repairs. *Am J Obstet Gynecol* 1999;181(6):1353–1359.

152. Glavind K, Madsen H. A prospective study of the discrete fascial defect rectocele repair. *Acta Obstet Gynecol Scand* 2000;79(2):145–147.

153. Kenton K, Shott S, Brubaker L. Outcome after rectovaginal fascia reattachment for rectocele repair. *Am J Obstet Gynecol* 1999;181:1360.

154. Julian TM. The efficacy of Marlex mesh in the repair of severe, recurrent vaginal prolapse of the anterior midvaginal wall. *Am J Obstet Gynecol* 1996;175: 1472–1475.

155. Sand PK, Koduri S, Lobel RW, et al. Prospective randomized trial of polyglactin 910 mesh to prevent recurrence of cystoceles and rectoceles. *Am J Obstet Gynecol* 2001;184(7):1357–1362.

156. Oster S, Astrup A. A new vaginal operation for recurrent and large rectoceles using dermis transplants. *Acta Obstet Gynecol Scand* 1981;60(5):493–495.

157. Miklos JR, Kohli N. Rectovaginal fistula repair utilizing a cadaveric dermal allograft. *Int Urogynecol J Pelvic Floor Dysfunct* 1999;10(60):405–406.

158. Parks AG, Porter NH, Hardcastle J. The syndrome of the descending perineum. *Proc R Soc Med* 1966;59: 477–482.

159. Bartolo DC, Read NW, Jarett JA, et al. Differences in anal sphincter function and clinical presentation in patients with pelvic floor descent. *Gastroenterology* 1982;85:68–75.

160. Mackle EJ, Parks TG. Clinical features in patients with excessive perineal descent. *J R Coll Surg Edinb* 1989; 34:88–90.

161. Yoshioka K, Hyland G, Keighley MR. Anorectal func-

tion after abdominal rectopexy: parameters of predictive value in identifying return of continence. *Br J Surg* 1989;76:64–68.

162. Korsgen S, Deen KI, Keighley MR. Long-term results of total pelvic floor repair for postobstetric fecal incontinence. *Dis Colon Rectum* 1997;40:835–839.

163. Harewood GC, Coulie B, Camilleri M, et al. Descending perineum syndrome: audit of clinical and laboratory features and outcome of pelvic floor retraining. *Am J Gastroenterol* 1999;94:126–130.

164. Addison WA, Cundiff GW, Bump RC, et al. Sacral colpopexy is the preferred treatment for vaginal vault prolapse. *J Gynecol Tech* 1996;2:69–74.

165. Cundiff GW, Harris RL, Coates KW, et al. Abdominal sacral colpoperineopexy: a new approach for correction of posterior compartment defects and perineal descent associated with vaginal vault prolapse. *Am J Obstet Gynecol* 1997;177:1345–1355.

166. Visco AG, Wiedner AC, Barber MD, et al. *Vaginal erosion with abdominal sacral colpoperineopexy.* Presented at the 20th Annual Scientific Meeting of the American Urogynecologic Society, San Diego, October 1999.

167. Sullivan ES, Longaker CJ, Lee PY. Total pelvic mesh repair: a ten-year experience. *Dis Colon Rectum* 2001;44:857–863.

168. Kaufman H, Cundiff G, Thompson J, et al. Suture rectopexy and sacral colpoperineopexy with Alloderm® for perineal descent. *Dis Colon Rectum* 2000;43:A16.

169. Kaufman HS, Buller JL, Thompson JR, et al. Dynamic pelvic magnetic resonance imaging and cystocolpoproctography alter surgical management of pelvic floor disorders. *Dis Colon Rectum* 2001;44:1575–1584.

170. Jurgeleit HC, Corman ML, Coller JA, et al. Procidentia of the rectum: Teflon sling repair of rectal prolapse, Lahey Clinic experience. *Dis Colon Rectum* 1975;18:464.

171. Duthie GS, Bartolo DCC. Abdominal rectopexy for rectal prolapse: a comparison of techniques. *Br J Surg* 1992;79:107–113.

172. Ripstein CB. Surgical care of muscle rectal prolapse. *Dis Colon Rectum* 1965;8:34–38.

173. Tjandra JJ, Fazio VW, Church JM, et al. Ripstein procedure is an effective treatment for rectal prolapse without constipation. *Dis Colon Rectum* 1993;36: 501–507.

174. Gordon PH, Hoexter B. Complications of the Ripstein procedure. *Dis Colon Rectum* 1978;21:277–280.

175. Frykman HM, Goldberg SM. The surgical treatment of rectal procidentia. *Surg Gynecol Obstet* 1969;129: 1225–1230.

176. Kuijpers HC. Treatment of complete rectal prolapse: to narrow, to wrap, to suspend, to fix, to encircle, to plicate or to resect? *World J Surg* 1992;16:826–830.

177. Wassef R, Rothenberger D, Goldberg S. Rectal prolapse. *Curr Probl Surg* 1986;23:402.

178. Delorme R. Sue le traitement des prolapses du rectum totavx pour l'excision de la mucueuse rectele ou rectocolique. *Bull Mem Soc Chir Paris* 1900;26:498.

179. Senapati A, Nicholls RJ, Thomson JPS, et al. Results of Delorme's procedure for rectal prolapse. *Dis Colon Rectum* 1994;37:456–460.

180. Oliver GC, Vachon D, Eisenstat TE, et al. Delorme's procedure for complete rectal prolapse in severely debilitated patients. *Dis Colon Rectum* 1994;37:461–467.

181. Graf W, Stefansson T, Arvidssom D, et al. Laparoscopic suture rectopexy. *Dis Colon Rectum* 1995;38: 211–212.

182. Horwitz BJ, Fisher RS. The irritable bowel syndrome. *N Engl J Med* 2001;344(24):1846–1850.

183. Silvis R, Goosen HG, van Essen A, et al. Abdominal rectovaginopexy: modified technique to treat constipation. *Dis Colon Rectum* 1999;42(1):82–88.

PART C
Pelvic Organ Prolapse

Ostergard's Urogynecology and Pelvic Floor Dysfunction, Fifth Edition. edited by A.E. Bent, et al. Lippincott Williams & Wilkins, Philadelphia © 2003.

25

Nonsurgical Management of Pelvic Organ Prolapse

Scott A. Farrell

Department of Obstetrics and Gynecology, Dalhouse University, Halifax, Nova Scotia, Canada

The causes of pelvic organ prolapse include failure of support structures, deterioration of tissue integrity, and neuromuscular dysfunction. The etiology of these causes has only been partially elucidated. Conservative, nonsurgical management of pelvic organ prolapse has been pragmatic and based to a large extent on accepted wisdom. Scientific evidence for the efficacy of most nonsurgical interventions is limited, and their adoption into the clinical armamentarium of gynecologists is dependent to a large extent on clinical practices prevailing during their formal residency training. This chapter discusses the two most common nonsurgical treatments: pessaries and pelvic muscle exercises (PMEs).

HISTORICAL PERSPECTIVE

Pessaries

The problem of pelvic organ prolapse has prompted the development and use of many ingenious devices designed to restore and maintain the pelvic organs in their normal position within the pelvis. Although undoubtedly effective, the materials used for early pessaries, everything from pomegranates to wax balls, were often incompatible with long intravaginal retention (1). Gynecologic enthusiasm for pessaries peaked in the 19th century when most of the ills suffered by women were attributed to malposition and inflammation of the uterus (1). Pessaries were frequently used to address these problems. The advent of asepsis, improvements in anesthesia, and the development of surgical techniques to treat pelvic organ prolapse, which all occurred in the early 20th century, signaled the beginning of a declining interest in pessaries. The focus on surgical management of pelvic organ prolapse, which has come to dominate gynecologic thinking, prompted Emil Novak to lament in 1923: "Gynaecology has become so predominately a surgical specialty that one hesitates to undertake even a very much qualified defense of such a non-surgical implement as the pessary." He went on to say, "the young gynaecologist of today frequently has no conception of what the pessary is meant to do, and he is apt to be irritated at the suggestion that such an implement should be accorded at least a modest position in his armamentarium" (2). This loss of enthusiasm for pessaries happened during a time when refinements in synthetics were permitting the production of pessaries that were much less likely to produce unpleasant side effects such as vaginal discharge and bleeding. Most modern pessaries are made from silicone, a very inert, nonreactive, durable material, using precast molds. The result is that women find modern pessaries very comfortable, with a low incidence of troublesome symptoms.

PELVIC MUSCLE EXERCISES

PME was advocated for recovery and maintenance of pelvic health as early as 1861 (3).

Although a number of authorities advocated the use of PME in the early 1900s, it is Arnold Kegel who is credited with devising a standardized approach to the teaching of pelvic floor exercises (4). Kegel employed a simple balloon perineometer as a biofeedback device to enhance his patient's efforts to contract and strengthen their pelvic floor muscles. Over the course of a number of years, Kegel reported an overall cure rate in excess of 84% in more than five hundred patients (5). Greenhill, a contemporary of Kegel, advocated PME to prevent and treat urinary incontinence, as a treatment for pelvic floor prolapse, and to enhance sexual sensation (6). Much of the work done on pelvic floor exercises in the late 20th century has focused on their effectiveness as a conservative treatment for stress urinary incontinence (3). There is a paucity of research on the effectiveness of PME as a treatment for pelvic organ prolapse.

Before Training: Patient Evaluation

Most of the research examining factors that are predictive of successful use of PME have focused on the treatment of urinary incontinence. Before initiating a course of PME, clinical evaluation should be designed to assess the integrity of the pelvic floor muscles and their contractility (7,8). Questions the examiner should consider during the examination of the functional integrity of the pelvic muscles include the following:

1. Are the muscles morphologically symmetric?
2. Are there any defects in the muscles, such as hernias or tears from obstetric trauma?
3. Is there any scarring?
4. What is the volume of the muscles?
5. Is there voluntary symmetric contraction?
6. Does contraction elevate the bladder neck and anorectal angle?

The examiner uses both inspection and palpation to answer these questions. During inspection, when the levator ani muscle group is healthy, voluntary contraction of these muscles results in a puckering and in-drawing of the vaginal introitus, anal sphincter, and perineal body. Coughing should produce little or no descent of the perineum either in the supine or standing position. In the patient whose levator ani muscle function is compromised, voluntary contraction may produce minimal puckering or no movement at all. Coughing when levator muscle function is compromised produces perineal descent and gaping of the vaginal introitus with accompanying pelvic organ prolapse. The standing position may be necessary to demonstrate the full extent of prolapse and perineal descent.

During palpation, the examiner attempts to evaluate muscle bulk, resting tone, contractile strength, and reflex response to cough. Vaginal examination with a gloved index finger permits assessment of the resting bulk and symmetry of the levator ani muscles, primarily the pubococcygeus muscle (PCM) (Fig. 25.1). Normally, the PCM is felt as a distinct 1- to 2-cm band that surrounds the vaginal introitus and closes it. A weak or attenuated PCM may be indistinguishable from the surrounding tissues. During rectal examination, the intact external anal sphincter grasps the examining finger. The PCM swings around the anorectal junction, and at rest, it pulls the junction forward to create an acute angle between the anal canal and the rectal ampulla.

The voluntary function of the pelvic floor muscles can be assessed subjectively. A more sophisticated evaluation of pelvic floor function, known as PERFECT, involves assessment of the power (P), endurance (E), and the number of repetitions (R) that a subject is able to achieve. Every (E) contraction (C) is timed (T) to ensure that progress can be objectively demonstrated (8). Using this system, the power of the muscular contraction is graded from 0 (no movement) to 5 (strong contraction), based on the Oxford grading system. Both slow- and fast-twitch muscle fibers contribute to power. The endurance, measured in seconds, is the duration of time that a maximum vaginal contraction can be maintained and reflects the activity of slow-twitch fibers. Other aspects of pelvic muscle function that can be evaluated include coordination and re-

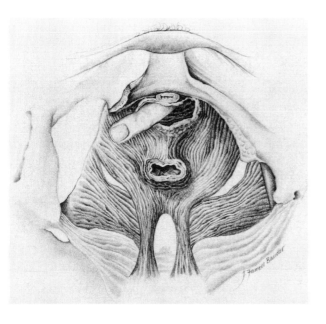

FIG. 25.1. Vaginal palpation of the pubococcygeus muscle. (Modified from Schüssler B, Laycock J, Norton P, et al, eds. *Pelvic floor re-education.* London: Springer-Verlag, 1994, with permission.)

flex response. A patient with a healthy functioning pelvic floor should be able to contract and relax the pelvic floor both quickly and slowly on command. An increase in intraabdominal pressure should result in a reflex contraction of the pelvic floor muscles that can be observed at the introitus and palpated digitally.

Although research into the factors predictive of successful use of PME for the treatment of urinary incontinence has had contradictory results, there is no research evidence concerning their usefulness to treat pelvic organ prolapse. Most authorities would agree that some ability to contract the pelvic floor muscles, a strong conviction concerning the efficacy of PMEs, and a commitment to conservative treatment are essential to success. Duration of therapy may extend up to 12 months, and continued practice is necessary to maintain the effect that has been achieved.

Techniques for Instruction

Although verbal and written forms of instruction have been the mainstay of teaching methods for PMEs, considerable evidence indicates that this approach is unsatisfactory for many women. Kegel observed that about 40% of his patients were unable to perform the exercises properly after simple verbal instructions (4). Bump and colleagues found that only 60% of women who received brief verbal instruction were able to perform a Kegel contraction sufficient to increase their urethral pressure profile area by more than 120% (9). Bø and associates focused on two basic principles of strength training for muscles: overload and specificity (10). Specificity means that the specific muscle group that requires strengthening can be isolated and contracted by the patient. Several studies have demonstrated that up to 30% of women are unable to perform pelvic floor muscle exercises at their first attempt (11,12). Common errors include the performance of a Valsalva maneuver or the contraction of other muscle groups, such as the abdominal, gluteal, or hip abductor muscles. Correct pelvic floor contractions are best achieved by instruction that involves feedback from digital palpation. In some cases, repeated evaluation may be necessary over several months to ensure that exercises are correctly performed.

Kegel stated that, "only the exceptional woman, however, will continue the exercise long enough to produce results on mere instruction to do this. Many women, in addition, have no 'awareness of function' and, unless provided with some way of knowing they are being successful, soon become discouraged or are unwilling to make even an initial attempt at exercise" (4). He indicated that the perineometer, because it provided accurate information concerning the power of pelvic floor contractions as well as visual feedback to the patient, was essential to continuity of practice. Recently, more sophisticated approaches to PME training have been developed.

The PERFECT system of evaluation of pelvic floor function has been used as the basis of an exercise prescription for patients (8). Power (P) is reflected by the grade of the contraction, the endurance (E) by the duration that the contraction can be held, and repetitions (R) by the number of contractions of that power and duration that can be performed consecutively. These figures provide a baseline for an exercise regimen that ensures that the patient performs enough exercises to "overload" and thus strengthen the muscle. Progress is assessed by regular repeat digital examinations and perineometry when visual feedback of progress is indicated.

Bø and associates studied an instruction program, which began with an introductory session that included personalized instruction concerning the anatomy and physiology of the pelvic muscles and digital and perineometric confirmation that exercises were performed properly (13). After the individual education session, participants attended weekly 45-minute group exercise sessions. Exercises were performed in a number of positions in which the legs were abducted so that extraneous muscle groups could not be contracted (Fig. 25.2). The intervention group performed intensive contractions, which involved holding a maximal pelvic muscle contraction for a duration of 6 to 8 seconds, after which 3 to 4 fast contractions were superimposed. At home, participants were encouraged to do 8 to 12 of these contractions three times a day and to keep a diary of their exercise sessions. The control group received the same instruction but performed their contractions "as

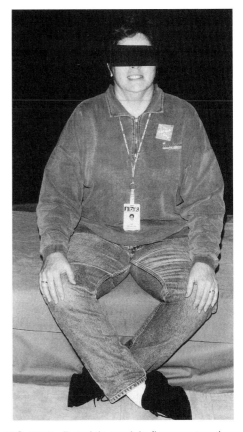

FIG. 25.2. Practicing pelvic floor contractions.

hard as possible." This study lasted for 6 months and demonstrated that the intensive exercise group showed greater objective pelvic strength and significantly better symptomatic improvement.

Although Kegel recommended performance of between 100 and 300 contractions daily, recent, more sophisticated work has suggested that exercise regimens using fewer numbers of contractions may be equally or perhaps more effective (13). He believed that the visual feedback of the perineometer provided a woman with a direct reflection of her progress. He noted that evidence of progress in muscle strength preceded clinical improvements in urinary incontinence. Kegel described four phases of the recovery of pelvic floor muscle function. It was not until the woman had reached the third phase or "period of regeneration" that changes in clinical symptoms could be expected to occur.

Other research has suggested that some form of biofeedback enhances the chances of successful therapy for urinary incontinence. Castleden and co-workers trained 19 incontinent women with pelvic floor exercises alone and subsequently using biofeedback with a perineometer (14). They found that although PCM strength was not increased by biofeedback, patients experienced greater clinical improvements. Burgio and associates conducted a study of two groups of women with urodynamically proven genuine stress incontinence (15). One group was taught muscle contraction by digital examination and verbal feedback. The other group had this teaching reinforced by bladder sphincter biofeedback. The biofeedback group experienced a 76% decrease in their incontinence, compared with a 51% decrease in the verbal feedback group. Peattie and colleagues trained 30 premenopausal women with stress incontinence using weighted vaginal cones (16). These cones provided biofeedback to the patient by slipping out if the pelvic floor muscles were not properly contracted. Seventy percent of the patients in their study reported a cure or significant improvement of their symptoms after 1 month of therapy. Despite these good results with biofeedback, a recent prospective randomized study comparing pelvic muscle training to vaginal electrical stimulation and vaginal cones found that the highest compliance to treatment was in the supervised exercise group (17). Although at 6 months, the mean pelvic floor muscle strength had improved significantly from baseline in all three treatment groups, this was highest at 75% in the exercise group. Using an objective stress pad test, 78% of the supervised exercise group had a significant decrease in their urine leakage, compared with 13% in the electrical stimulation group and 30% in the vaginal cone group.

Efficacy in Treating Prolapse

Although PMEs are clearly an effective treatment of stress urinary incontinence, their utility in the treatment of pelvic organ prolapse is unproved. It has been hypothesized that pelvic organ prolapse may begin when the ability of the pelvic floor muscles to support the pelvic organs is compromised. This compromise may occur as a result of mechanical injury to the muscles (a stretching or widening of the genital hiatus) or as a consequence of denervation and subsequent muscle atrophy. When pelvic muscle support is compromised, excessive stresses on the ligamentous and fascial support structures of the pelvic organs results in stretching and attenuation. If PMEs result in recovery of muscle function, the result may be a reversal of minor degrees of pelvic prolapse and prevention of progression to more severe degrees of pelvic prolapse. Prospective studies are needed to clarify the role of pelvic floor exercises in the treatment and prevention of pelvic floor prolapse.

PESSARIES

The demographic shifts that will occur in the North American population during the near future will mean that a greater number of women than ever before will be entering the postmenopausal age group, in which problems with urinary incontinence and pelvic prolapse become much more common. Both gynecologists and family physicians must be prepared to meet the growing demand for conservative options to manage both urinary incontinence and pelvic prolapse. Physician and patient reluctance to use a pessary for the management of pelvic prolapse arises from a lack of familiarity with this device. Before seeing a modern pessary, many patients imagine arcane instruments that may effectively treat pelvic prolapse but at the cost of ongoing discomfort. Physicians who have little experience with using pessaries (this is the case for most senior obstetrics and gynecology residents in North America) are daunted by the prospects of fumbling inefficiency and troublesome frequent follow-up visits. Recent evidence, however, suggests an increased interest and willingness among younger gynecologists to use pessaries (18). Current management information dispensed with each pessary by the manufacturer calls for frequent visits that are both inconvenient and costly to the health care system. A more relaxed approach to pessary management is described in this chapter.

Selection

A variety of pessary models are available, each with its purported indications (Fig. 25.3). In most cases, these indications are based on accepted wisdom rather than scientific data. A survey of members of the American Urogynecology Society (AUGS) found that from 60% to 89% selected a pessary based on the specific stage and location of prolapse (18). On the other hand, 22% preferred to use the same pessary model as a first-line treatment in all prolapse patients, resorting to other models when the preferred pessary model failed. The most common first choice was the ring pessary and the second, the Gellhorn pessary.

Choice of pessary model should be predicated on several factors. Although efficacy is paramount among these factors, acceptability to both patient and physician is arguably equally important. Pessaries that are difficult for the patient and physician to insert and remove and that require troublesome frequent follow-up visits are unlikely to be used. In a recent prospective study, the ring pessary was used as a first-line treatment for all locations and degrees of pelvic organ prolapse (19). When the ring pessary failed, second-line pessaries, including the Gellhorn, cube, and donut, were used. Of 110 women, 81 (79%) were successfully fitted with pessaries. Of the 81 successfully fitted women, 78 (96%) were fitted with ring pessaries. At the time of initial evaluation, a composite score representing the severity of pelvic organ prolapse was calculated (Table 25.1). The impact of the degree of pelvic prolapse on pessary fitting success was evaluated by determining the composite pelvic prolapse score of each patient. A higher composite score reflecting more severe degrees of support failure in all compartments did not predict failure of pessary fittings.

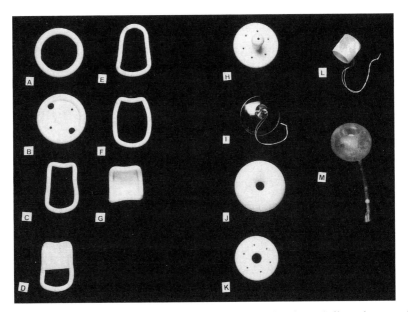

FIG. 25.3. Pessary types: support pessaries (columns 1 and 2 from *left*) and space-filling pessaries (columns 3 and 4 from *left*). (From Cundfiff GW, Weidner A, Visco AG, et al. A survey of pessary use by the members of the American Urogynecologic Society. *Obstet Gynecol* 2000;95:933, with permission.)

TABLE 25.1. *Composite score of pelvic prolapse and pessary fitting success*

Score[a]	No. of patients	No. of successful fittings	Successful fittings (%)
2	1	1	100
3	3	3	100
4	22	16	73
5	22	14	64
6	31	23	74
7	12	10	83
8	13	11	85
9	3	1	33
10	1	0	0

[a]Score calculated by adding point values equivalent to the grade of prolapse in the front, middle, and posterior pelvic compartments. Grading based on descent to following landmarks: grade 1, cystocele or rectocele—midvaginal axis; grade 1, uterine and vault—ischial spines; grade 2, prolapse in all compartments to the introitus; grade 3, prolapse in all compartments through the introitus. Procidentia was scored as 4.

The x^2 test for trend revealed no significant differences.

From Wu V, Farrell SA, Baskett TF, et al. A simplified protocol for pessary management. *Obstet Gynecol* 1997;90:990–994, with permission.

In a retrospective review of 101 women who had been successfully fitted with a Gellhorn pessary, the most common support defect was a grade 3 or 4 anterior vaginal wall prolapse, which was experienced by 58% of these women (20). Thirty-three women (33%) had grade 3 or 4 prolapse of the vaginal cuff or cervix. In the study by Wu and colleagues, although a history of previous surgery appeared to reduce the chances of a successful pessary fitting, this was not a statistically significant effect (19). Similarly, adequate perineal support as determined by the physician on pelvic examination did not influence pessary fitting success rates.

Urinary tract symptoms do influence the success of pessary fitting. Compared with the symptoms of urgency, frequency, and urgency incontinence, women with the symptom of stress incontinence were statistically less likely to consider the use of a pessary to be satisfactory (19). Sulak and associates found that among 19 women complaining of urinary incontinence at the time of pessary fitting, 6 reported a decrease or total relief of their urinary incontinence symptoms (20). Thirteen (68%) either discontinued pessary use or underwent surgery. Prior hysterectomy and current sexual activity have been considered contraindications to pessary use. The survey of the AUGS found that fewer than half of respondents considered these features to be contraindications to pessary use (18). Wu and colleagues found that prior hysterectomy did not influence pessary fitting success rates (19).

Recommended Pessaries for Prolapse

Most cases of prolapse can be managed with a limited pessary armamentarium. In order of utility, this armamentarium should include the ring with support, cube, and Gellhorn. It is our opinion that the donut, Gehrung, inflato-ball, and Schaatz pessaries will be used infrequently.

The ring pessary with or without a supportive membrane is the most versatile pessary model available. There are several reasons for this assertion:

1. The ring pessary is shaped like a diaphragm and designed to be folded in half for easy introduction through the vaginal introitus.
2. It is less likely to sequester vaginal secretions, which degenerate and produce odor.
3. It works for most patients who will be able to use a pessary successfully.
4. Patients are more likely to manage this type of pessary themselves.
5. The ring with support and knob can be used to treat concomitant prolapse and stress incontinence.

Most modern pessaries are manufactured from medical-grade silicone, which can be steam sterilized. It is most convenient to maintain a selection of pessary sizes readily available in your office. Experience with pessary fitting permits the selection of the correct pessary size in most fittings, but many fittings require several attempts with different sizes of pessaries. In their prospective study, Wu and colleagues found that 70% of successfully fitted patients used ring pessaries sizes 3, 4, or 5. Pessaries discarded during a fitting can be resterilized for reuse.

Patient Evaluation

Pelvic examination should include an assessment of the degree of estrogenization of the vaginal mucosa and quantification of the prolapse in the anterior, middle, and posterior compartments of the pelvis. A complete description of the evaluation of pelvic organ prolapse is provided in Chapter 9.

To determine pessary size, a vaginal examination is undertaken. The depth and width of the vaginal barrel will determine the size of the first pessary. The goals of the pessary fitting are: (a) correction of the symptoms attributed to prolapse; (b) a proper match of pessary size to vaginal caliber, which will avoid the morbidity associated with compression of the vaginal mucosa—abrasion, erosion, and bleeding; and (c) the patient should not feel the pessary (21).

Pessary Insertion

Inspection of the ring pessary with diaphragm shows that it has two larger and two smaller perforations. In addition to these markings, there is a slight indentation on the inner aspect of the ring next to the larger perforations (Fig. 25.4). The larger perforations

mark the point where the pessary flexes and can be folded in half.

Step 1

With both hands gloved, the pessary is held by the thumb and index finger of the dominant hand in the folded position. Lubricant is placed on the vaginal introitus and on the leading edge of the folded pessary. The hand holding the pessary should be dry (Fig. 25.5). The thumb and index finger of the left hand are used to keep the pessary folded as it slides into the vagina.

Step 2

With the labia minora held separated at the posterior introitus, the pessary, which is oriented at a 90-degree angle to the floor, is introduced into the vagina. Pressure is maintained in an inferior direction during introduction of the pessary (Fig. 25.6).

Step 3

An alternate method of introduction is very effective in seating the pessary in the posterior

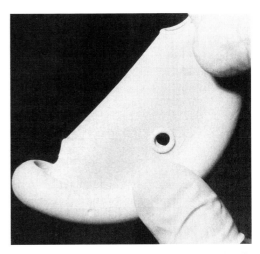

FIG. 25.5. The pessary is maintained in the folded condition by the dominant hand. (From Farrell SA. Practical advice for ring pessary fitting and management. *J SOGC* 1997;19:627, with permission.)

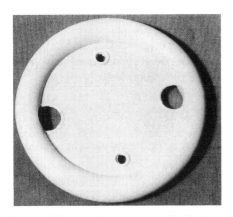

FIG. 25.4. Silicone ring pessary with diaphragm. (From Farrell SA. Practical advice for ring pessary fitting and management. *J SOGC* 1997;19:626, with permission.)

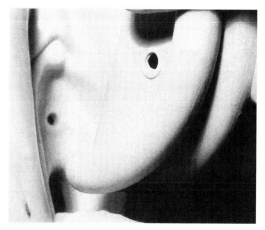

FIG. 25.6. Introduction of the pessary into the vaginal introitus. (From Farrell SA. Practical advice for ring pessary fitting and management. *J SOGC* 1997;19:627, with permission.)

vaginal fornix of patients who have a uterus. Once it has been folded, the pessary is held with the curved edge upward and introduced into the vagina by rotating it backward against the posterior vaginal wall (Fig. 25.7).

Step 4

Once the pessary has been introduced into the vagina, two maneuvers help to seat it

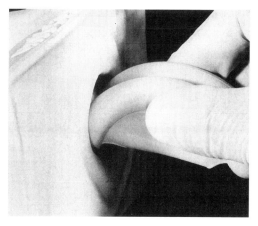

FIG. 25.7. Alternative position for backward rotational introduction of the pessary. (From Farrell SA. Practical advice for ring pessary fitting and management. *J SOGC* 1997;19:629, with permission.)

properly. First, the index finger of the right hand is directed into the posterior vaginal fornix to ensure that the cervix is resting above the pessary. It is possible to direct the leading edge of the pessary beneath the cervix to ensure that it is properly placed. Second, if difficulty is encountered in placing the pessary beneath the cervix, it is sometimes helpful to elevate the outer edge of the pessary behind the symphysis pubis, thus rotating the leading edge of the pessary posteriorly.

Step 5

When the pessary is properly placed, the cervix will be supported by the diaphragm with the ring of the pessary sitting in the posterior vaginal fornix (Fig. 25.8).

Step 6

It is important to assess how well the pessary fits. It should be possible to slide the ring of the pessary easily up and down along the vaginal sidewall. When the labia are separated, a well-supported pessary is not usually visible. When a ring pessary is in proper position, it lies parallel to the vaginal axis. It is not usual for it to sit behind the symphysis pubis. With the labia separated, the patient should be asked to perform a Valsalva maneuver and to cough. Some descent of the pessary with these maneuvers is to be expected, but the pessary should return to its normal position when these efforts are stopped. If the pessary descends to the introitus with these maneuvers, a larger size should be tried.

Once satisfactory support has been achieved in the supine position, the patient should be asked to stand. In the standing position, the patient should be asked to cough and to walk around the examining room. Examination of the patient in the standing position will confirm that the pessary is not slipping down to the introitus. Initial fitting is judged successful if the patient does not feel the pessary coming down, and examination confirms that it is staying in position.

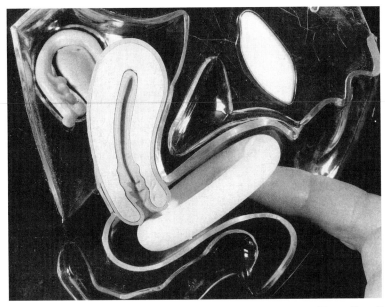

FIG. 25.8. Anterior rotation of the pessary to assist in proper placement. (From Farrell SA. Practical advice for ring pessary fitting and management. *J SOGC* 1997;19:629, with permission.)

Pessary Removal

Step 1

The index fingers of both hands are inserted into the vagina to hook the leading edge of the pessary ring from above and below. With these fingers, traction is applied along the vaginal axis to bring the pessary down toward the introitus.

Step 2

Once the pessary has been brought to the introitus, it can be grasped with the thumb and index finger of the dominant hand. The nondominant hand is held above the vaginal introitus, where the index finger and thumb can be used to compress the pessary as it is pulled through the introitus, thus facilitating pessary removal without patient discomfort. Once the pessary has been removed, it is washed with tap water and dried with a paper towel.

The vaginal walls are inspected using a speculum to look for evidence of abrasions or erosion caused by the pessary. If the vaginal mucosa is healthy and the pessary is still intact and flexing normally, it can be reinserted.

Patient Instructions

Before discharge from the clinic after a pessary fitting, the patient is given a set of instructions (Table 25.2). These instructions describe the management of commonly encountered problems. The patient is also given the manufacturer's booklet that accompanied the pessary. Hormone replacement is recommended for patients whose vaginal epithelium is thin.

Follow-up

Recommendations for pessary follow-up frequency and timing are included in the literature distributed by the manufacturer. These recommendations call for recheck visits at 4- to 6-week intervals, a schedule that is both inconvenient for the patient and costly to the health care system. A variety of recommendations are found in the literature, most based on the wisdom of recognized experts (1,6). A re-

TABLE 25.2. *Guidelines for pessary care*

Pessary type_____
size_____

1. After your initial pessary fitting is successful, you will be asked to return for a follow-up appointment in about 2 weeks. The purpose of this visit is to check the pessary and examine the vagina to ensure that it is healthy. Follow-up appointments will follow this schedule:
   1st year—every 3 to 6 months
   2nd year and beyond—every 6 months
   You may learn to care for the pessary yourself. For those patients who can remove and insert the pessary themselves, we recommend weekly overnight removal and cleansing of the pessary with soap and warm water. These patients should see the doctor at least once per year.
2. The following is a list of problems you may encounter with the pessary and our recommendations for the management.

Problem	Management
a. The pessary falls out.	Keep the pessary and notify your doctor's office. An appointment will be made. It may be possible that a change in the size or the type of pessary is needed.
b. You experience pelvic pain.	Notify your doctor's office. If the pessary has slipped and you can remove it, do so. Otherwise, have your doctor remove the pessary. A change in pessary size or type may be needed.
c. Vaginal discharge and odor.	You can douche with warm water and you may want to try using Trimosan vaginal gel 1–3 times a week.
d. Vaginal bleeding.	Vaginal bleeding may be a sign that the pessary is irritating the lining of the vagina. Call your doctor's office and arrange an appointment.
e. Leaking from the bladder.	Sometimes, the support provided by the pessary will cause leaking from the bladder. Notify your doctor and discuss this problem.

From Farrell SA. Practical advice for ring pessary fitting and management. *J SOGC* 1997;19:632, with permission.

cent survey of the members of AUGS found that recommended follow-up intervals ranged from 1 to 3 months (18).

The following timetable for pessary follow-up has been proved to be both safe and acceptable (19):

1. First visit after initial fitting—2 weeks.
2. Follow-up visits in the first year after successful pessary fitting—3 months.
3. Follow-up visits after first year of successful pessary use—6 months.

At each follow-up visit, the pessary is removed and inspected. The vagina is examined by speculum looking for any evidence of abrasions caused by the pessary. When the pessary becomes stiff or encrusted with secretions, it is replaced. Most of the silicone pessaries can be used for up to 2 years without replacement. If the vagina is healthy and the pessary is in good condition, it is reinserted. Patients can be taught to remove and insert the ring pessary themselves. This option is of-

fered to all patients. In a recent survey, 45% of physicians taught all of their patients to remove and insert their pessary (18), and 45% used this approach only for women using a support pessary (ring or lever pessary models). We recommend that women who are able should remove the pessary and leave it out overnight at least once a week. Women who manage their own pessaries can be seen at 6-month intervals (19).

Management of Pessary Problems

Pessary Falls Out with Valsalva Maneuvers

The first pessary may prove to be inadequate to provide support. This will be evident either immediately in the office or after several days of normal activity. Pessaries are particularly prone to be discharged at the time of straining associated with bowel movements. If the pessary falls out with a Valsalva maneuver, a larger size should be tried. Some accommodation of the vagina to a pessary may account for the need to increase the pessary size at the time of follow-up visits. If a larger-sized ring pessary is not effective, alternative pessaries should be tried. Because the patient can handle the Gellhorn pessary relatively easily, it should be tried as the second option. If the Gellhorn pessary fails, a cube pessary may be inserted. If perforations are made in the cube pessary, this does not diminish its efficacy but does permit vaginal secretions to drain, allowing the cube pessary to be left in place for longer intervals.

Patient Experiences Pelvic Pain

If the pessary is too large, the patient will be aware of its presence in the vagina and will complain of discomfort; the patient should not feel a properly fitted pessary. This is an indication for substituting a smaller-sized pessary. In most cases, a smaller pessary will still provide the necessary support without causing any pain.

Patients who are successfully fitted and comfortable with a pessary may subsequently return complaining of pain. In these cases, the position of the pessary should be ascertained. It may be that the pessary has rotated its position within the vagina or, because it was providing inadequate support, has descended to the introitus. In these cases, a larger pessary may be appropriate.

Vaginal Bleeding Occurs

If the chosen pessary is too large, it may compress or abrade the vaginal epithelium. Superficial abrasions, if the pessary is left in place, will progress to frank erosions of the vaginal epithelium. Vaginal bleeding is a warning sign that must not be ignored and should prompt immediate evaluation of the patient. If the pessary is too large, it can be removed and left out for several weeks while the vaginal epithelium heals. Subsequently, a trial with a smaller pessary is appropriate. Patients with thin vaginal epithelium should be given some form of local estrogen replacement, such as vaginal estrogen cream or an estrogen-releas-

ing ring, to help thicken the vaginal epithelium. The cube pessary is prone to producing vaginal abrasions and erosions. For that reason, it may have to be removed regularly for short intervals to allow the vaginal epithelium to heal.

Patient Complains of Urinary Incontinence

Significant degrees of pelvic prolapse may mask stress incontinence by kinking the urethrovesical junction. When the prolapse is reduced, either by surgery or a pessary, latent stress incontinence may by unmasked. The ring pessary with support and knob can be used effectively to treat both prolapse and stress urinary incontinence. Although the plain incontinence ring is effective at treating stress incontinence, it does not provide sufficient pelvic support to be used in cases of combined prolapse and stress incontinence.

Patient Complains of Vaginal Discharge or Odor

Vaginal discharge is often increased by the presence of a pessary. All pessaries tend to trap vaginal secretions and obstruct their normal drainage. These accumulated secretions break down and produce an odor. Strategies to deal with this problem of odor include the intravaginal insertion of Trimo-San gel (Milex Products Inc., Chicago, Illinois) once or twice weekly. This gel helps to reduce the bothersome odors that often accompany pessary use. Patients may also be encouraged to douche with warm water mixed with a small amount of vinegar to rinse out vaginal secretions. The problem of vaginal discharge and odor is usually not encountered by patients who learn to remove and insert the pessary themselves. Patients who are able to do this should be encouraged to remove the pessary on a weekly basis, and after washing it with warm water, leave it to dry overnight.

Factors Affecting Long-term Use of Pessaries

The most common reasons for pessary discontinuation after successful fitting include

TABLE 25.3. *Life-table analysis of pessary continuation[a]*

Time interval (mo)	Using pessary at beginning of time interval	Pessary discontinued during interval	Censored at time of analysis	Cumulative probability of continued pessary use
1–6	62	14 (13-S, 1-O)	4	0.767
6–12	44	6 (5-S, 1-O)	5	0.656
12–18	33	1 (1-O)	3	0.635
18–24	29	0	5	0.635
24–30	24	2 (1-S, 1-O)	6	0.575
30–36	16	1 (1-O)	5	0.532
36–42	10	0	3	0.532
42–48	7	0	3	0.532
48–54	4	0	3	0.532

S, opted for surgery; O, opted for observation.
[a]Data are presented as number of patients.
From Wu V, Farrell SA, Baskett TF, et al. A simplified protocol for pessary management. *Obstet Gynecol* 1997;90:990–994, with permission.

failure to sustain support of the prolapse, intolerable urinary incontinence, vaginal discharge, pelvic pain, and vaginal abrasions and erosions. Wu and colleagues found that women with stress incontinence were more likely to undergo surgery than were women without symptoms (19). They found that current hormone replacement did not predict successful pessary fitting. The risk for vaginal abrasions increased significantly as the vaginal epithelium became thinner, and there was no correlation between current hormone use and rates of vaginal abrasions. Vaginal erosions were strongly associated with cube pessary use as compared with ring pessary use. A number of women, despite taking systemic hormone replacement, were found to have thin vaginal epithelium. Some form of local hormone replacement is recommended for women with thin or atrophic vaginal epithelium.

Sulak and associates found that patients with more severe degrees of pelvic prolapse were more likely to continue using a pessary (20). In their study group, 47 women (46%) discontinued use of their pessary. Their reasons for discontinuation were as follows: 19 women (40%) complained of either inconvenience or inadequate relief of symptoms; 11 (23%) had difficultly removing the pessary; 6 (13%) experienced discomfort with the pessary; 6 (13%) chose to have surgery; in 3 (6%) the pessary fell out; and 2 (5%) were un-

able to urinate. Most discontinued pessary use within a few days to a few weeks of fitting. Wu and colleagues excluded patients who were not satisfied with their pessary at the initial 2-week follow-up visit. A life-table analysis of pessary use (Table 25.3) revealed that the highest rate of pessary discontinuation occurred in the first 12 months. The cumulative probability of continued use of a pessary after 24 months was 0.532 (19).

CONCLUSIONS

Pessaries represent an effective and appropriate alternative to surgery for pelvic organ prolapse. A limited armamentarium of pessaries can be used successfully to manage pelvic organ prolapse. Because there is no evidence that any one pessary is superior in specific circumstances, physician familiarity and patient comfort should guide the choice of pessary. Although surgery for pelvic organ prolapse is effective, there is a significant recurrence rate over time and a significant risk for complications associated with surgery. Novak concluded his discussion of pessaries by quoting Bantock, who wrote, "I am not aware that there is on record a single case in which a woman has lost her life through the use, or even the abuse, of a vaginal pessary" (2). Although cases of cervical and vaginal cancer have been reported in association with the use of pessaries, the mean interval between pessary insertion and cancer diagnosis was 18 years in one study (22). Unfortunately, in this report, the authors failed to determine whether appropriate pessary surveillance had been used. In most cases, when vaginal cancer has developed, the pessary was either neglected for many years or changed periodically without a speculum examination of the vagina (23). Neglected pessaries have also eroded into the bladder and become impacted in the vagina, necessitating surgical removal. It is likely that if appropriate follow-up protocols are used, including regular Papanicolaou smears, precancerous changes would be detected and neglected pessary problems avoided.

Although many patients who have pelvic prolapse opt for surgical correction of this problem, the vaginal pessary offers a management option that can be used over the short term to relieve symptoms during the preoperative waiting period or over the long term by patients who, either by personal preference or medical necessity, are not candidates for surgery. In the coming decades, a large cohort of North American women will be entering their postmenopausal years, a time when problems of pelvic support are most likely to occur. Despite high surgical success rates, gynecologists will find that the pessary is an indispensable part of their armamentarium—one that should be as familiar to the gynecologist as the compass is to the navigator.

AREAS OF FUTURE RESEARCH

Pelvic Floor Exercises

Pelvic floor exercises have proven efficacy in the treatment of stress urinary incontinence. Although the levator ani muscles' contribution to pelvic support is better understood today than it was at the time that Arnold Kegel conducted his original research, the effect on pelvic prolapse of strengthening these muscles has not been examined. Areas of research could include the efficacy of pelvic floor muscle exercises in the management of moderate pelvic prolapse and the contribution

of postoperative Kegel exercises to the long-term efficacy of surgery.

Pessaries

Although pessaries have been used for more than 1,000 years, the mechanism by which they affect support is disputed. Research should focus on elucidating the mechanisms of support enlisted by the pessary, protocols for insertion and removal that could enhance pessary acceptability to patients, effectiveness of pessary models designed to treat concomitant prolapse and incontinence, and the value of concomitant use of pessaries and pelvic floor exercises.

REFERENCES

1. Miller DS. Contemporary use of the pessary. In: Sciarra JJ, Droegemueller W, eds. *Gynecology and obstetrics.* Philadelphia: JB Lippincott, 1992;1(39):1–12.
2. Novak E. The vaginal pessary: its indications and limitations. *JAMA* 1923;80:1294–1298.
3. Wall LL, Davidson TG. The role of muscular re-education by physical therapy in the treatment of genuine stress incontinence. *Obstet Gynecol Surv* 1992;47:322–330.
4. Kegel AH. Progressive resistance exercises in the functional restoration of the perineal muscles. *Am J Obstet Gynecol* 1948;56:238–248.
5. Kegel AH. Stress incontinence of urine in women: physiologic treatment. *J Int Coll Surg* 1956;25:487.
6. Greenhill JP. The nonsurgical management of vaginal relaxation. *Clin Obstet Gynecol* 1972;15:1083–1097.
7. Schüssler B. Aims of pelvic floor evaluation. In: Schüssler B, Laycock J, Norton P, eds. *Pelvic floor re-education.* London: Springer-Verlag, 1994;39–41.
8. Laycock J. Clinical evaluation of the pelvic floor. In: Schüssler B, Laycock J, Norton P, et al, eds. *Pelvic floor re-education.* London: Springer-Verlag, 1994:42–48.
9. Bump RC, Hurt WG, Fantl A, et al. Assessment of Kegel pelvic exercise performance after brief verbal instruction. *Am J Obstet Gynecol* 1991;165:322–329.
10. Bø K, Larsen S, Kvarstein B, et al. Classification and characteristics of responders to pelvic floor muscle exercises for female stress urinary incontinence. *Neurourol Urodynam* 1990;9:395–397.
11. Benvenutti F, Caputo GM, Bandanelli S, et al. Re-educative treatment of female genuine stress incontinence. *Am J Phys Med* 1987;66:155–168.
12. Hesse U, Schüssler J, Frimberger N, et al. Effectiveness of three step pelvic floor re-education in the treatment of stress urinary incontinence: a clinical assessment. *Neurourol Urodyn* 1990;9:397–398.
13. Bø K, Hagen RH, Kvarstein B, et al. Pelvic floor muscle exercise for the treatment of female stress urinary incontinence: effects of two different degrees of pelvic floor muscle exercises. *Neurourol Urodyn* 1990;9: 489–502.

14. Castleden CM, Duffin HM, Mitchell EP. The effect of physiotherapy on stress incontinence. *Age Ageing* 1984; 13:235–237.

15. Burgio KL, Robinson JC, Engel BT. The role of biofeedback in Kegel exercise training for stress urinary incontinence. *Am J Obstet Gynecol* 1986;154:58–64.

16. Peattie A, Plevnik S, Stanton SL. Vaginal cones: a conservative method of treating genuine stress incontinence. *Br J Obstet Gynaecol* 1988;95:1049–1053.

17. Bø K, Talseth T, Holme I. Single-blind, randomized controlled trial of pelvic floor exercises, electrical stimulation, vaginal cones and no treatment in management of genuine stress incontinence in women. *BMJ* 1999; 318:487–493.

18. Cundiff GW, Weidner A, Visco AG, et al. A survey of pessary use by the membership of the American Urogynecology Society. *Obstet Gynecol* 2000;95:931–935.

19. Wu V, Farrell SA, Baskett TF, et al. A simplified protocol for pessary management. *Obstet Gynecol* 1997;90: 990–994.

20. Sulak PJ, Kuehl TJ, Shull BL. Vaginal pessaries and their use in pelvic relaxation. *J Reprod Med* 1993;38: 919–923.

21. Farrell SA. Practical advice for ring pessary fitting and management. *J SOGC* 1997;19:625–632.

22. Schraub S, Sun XS, Maingon PH, et al. Cervical and vaginal cancer associated with pessary use. *Cancer* 1992;69:2505–2509.

23. Russell JK. The dangerous vaginal pessary. *BMJ* 1961; 5:1595–1597.

Ostergard's Urogynecology and Pelvic Floor Dysfunction, Fifth Edition. edited by A.E. Bent, et al.
Lippincott Williams & Wilkins, Philadelphia © 2003.

26

Surgical Management of Pelvic Organ Prolapse

Julia B. Van Rooyen* and Geoffrey W. Cundiff**

* Department of Gynecology and Obstetrics, The Johns Hopkins School of Medicine, Baltimore, Maryland
** Department of Gynecology and Obstetrics, Johns Hopkins School of Medicine; and Department of Obstetrics and Gynecology, Johns Hopkins Bayview Medical Center, Baltimore, Maryland

CHOOSING A REPAIR

Virtually all parous women and many active nulliparous women can be demonstrated to have less than perfect pelvic support on careful examination. Many of these women, however, have few, if any, symptoms associated with their support defects, and only 10% to 15% ultimately undergo surgery for prolapse. Unfortunately, up to 30% of women who seek surgical repair return for a subsequent procedure (1). The conscientious surgeon, therefore, is obliged to recognize the limitations of surgical repairs.

The symptoms associated with specific support defects have not been well characterized and overlap from one type of support defect to another. Symptoms such as pelvic pressure and tissue bulging from the vagina can be associated with anterior, posterior, or apical support defects. Symptoms such as lower abdominal or back pain or pelvic pressure are even less specific and may be altogether unrelated to support defects. Our ability to distinguish clinically significant pelvic organ prolapse (POP) from normal variation in support is impaired by an absence of longitudinal studies that identify symptoms consistently associated with prolapse and a dearth of controlled interventional trials that establish cure rates for these symptoms.

SURGICAL LIMITATIONS

Support defects may result from damage to any of the pelvic floor structures, including connective tissues, muscles, or nerves. In recent years, we have made significant improvements in characterizing nerve injuries with neurodiagnostic testing, including pudendal and perineal nerve terminal motor latency testing, evaluation of the sacral nerve reflexes, and external anal sphincter electromyography. We are accumulating information on the adverse impact that neuropathy can have on surgical outcome, so that neurodiagnostic testing can be helpful in counseling patients regarding outcomes. Despite these advances, neurologic injury remains irreversible at present, and we are limited to surgical correction of connective tissue tears or breaks and rehabilitation of pelvic floor muscles.

SURGICAL GOALS

The goals of surgical correction are to alleviate the symptoms of pelvic floor support defects, to strive for normal anatomic relationships, and to maximize bladder, bowel, and coital function. Urinary symptoms can include incontinence, retention, and lower urinary tract symptoms such as frequency and urgency. Bowel symptoms can include

incontinence, constipation, incomplete emptying, urgency, and dyschezia. Other symptoms include pelvic pressure and tissue protrusion. In correcting any support defect,
care must be taken to avoid overcorrection,
which can lead to new support problems.
This has been well described, with the anterior deflection of retropubic urethropexies
predisposing to apical prolapse and enterocele formation and with the development of
anterior support defects associated with posterior deflection due to sacrospinous ligament fixation.

Successful correction of POP, therefore,
must balance the goals and limitations of
surgery and address support defects at all
levels. A systematic evaluation of the anterior, posterior, and apical compartments
must be made before surgery and any defects identified must be confirmed intraoperatively with careful evaluation at that time
as well.

SURGICAL APPROACH

Numerous surgical procedures have been
described for each type of support defect.
Pelvic reconstructive surgery can be accomplished through a vaginal approach, an open
abdominal approach, a laparoscopic abdominal approach, or some combination thereof.
Too often, the choice of procedure and route
of approach has been based on the surgeon's
biases or preferences rather than on anatomic
principles. Improved understanding of normal
and abnormal pelvic anatomy and function
now permits a more rational selection of the
procedure and route that can be tailored to the
individual patient.

Considerations that affect the choice of
procedure include the precise defects responsible for the POP, the etiology of the defects, whether the inciting and promoting
events are continuing processes, and the patient's desires and expectations. Table 26.1
includes a more complete list of the factors
that can contribute to POP and its recurrence
(see Chapter 3).

TABLE 26.1. *Factors contributing to pelvic organ prolapse*

Predisposing (congenital) factors
  Musculoskeletal
  Neurologic
  Connective tissue
  Racial
Inciting (acquired) factors
  Vaginal delivery
  Surgery
  Neurologic injury
Promoting factors
  Obesity
  Smoking
  Lung disease
  Constipation
  Recreational or occupational stressors
Decompensating factors
  Aging
  Menopause and hormonal deprivation
  Neuropathy or myopathy (progressive or acquired)
  Debilitation
  Medication

CATEGORIES OF SURGICAL REPAIRS

For the frail patient whose health status
precludes prolonged, extensive surgery, an
obliterative procedure such as vaginectomy or
colpocleisis affords symptom relief with minimal morbidity owing to shorter operative
time and more superficial dissection. Such a
procedure is obviously contraindicated, however, for any woman with a desire to maintain
vaginal function. For women with discrete defects in the fibromuscular layer of endopelvic
fascia, an anatomic vaginal repair that simply
corrects the defects of the indigenous tissues
may be sufficient. Such restorative repairs can
be accomplished from the vaginal approach.
This approach has the advantages of less
blood loss and a shorter recovery than procedures performed through a laparotomy.

There are circumstances such as ongoing occupational or recreational stressors or chronic
illness, however, that may compromise the
longevity of restorative repairs. Surgeries that
use native tissues depend on normal muscular
support and function to support the repaired tissue and might be at increased risk for failure in
the presence of neuromuscular compromise of

TABLE 26.2. *Surgical repairs for prolapse and indications*

Obliterative
 Medical indications for short operative time
 Medical indications for regional or local anesthesia
 No desire for future sexual intercourse
Restorative
 Adequate native pelvic fascia
 Adequate pelvic floor muscles
 Desire to maintain coital function
Compensatory
 Ongoing causes of prolapse
 Weak pelvic floor muscles
 Recurrent prolapse

the pelvic diaphragm. Extreme attenuation of native tissues may also compromise the success of these repairs. In addition, women with recurrent POP may require a stronger repair than is provided by a simple anatomic repair. Under these circumstances, a compensatory repair that provides an additional support mechanism is indicated (Table 26.2).

OBLITERATIVE REPAIRS

The primary advantage of obliterative procedures is the shorter operative time required, which decreases acute perioperative morbidity. Another advantage is the ease and safety of employing regional or local anesthesia with sedation in place of general anesthesia. These factors significantly decrease the overall risks of surgery for patients with chronic illnesses. Obliterative procedures also have the advantage of minimizing the uncommon but serious complications of hemorrhage or nerve injury associated with other reconstructive procedures because the dissection is carried out in a superficial plane away from large vessels and nerves. Blood loss tends to occur more gradually and is more easily controlled than the sudden blood loss that can occur with sacrospinous or sacral colpopexy procedures. Such gradual blood loss may be better tolerated than sudden fluid shifts by patients with chronic illnesses.

Although a short operating time is a goal of the obliterative techniques, obtaining optimal results still demands attention to critical support principles. It is important to provide preferential support to the urethrovesical junction and to reduce the enterocele component of the prolapse adequately during colpocleisis if stress incontinence and recurrent prolapse are to be avoided. Because obliterative procedures preclude subsequent evaluation of the cervix and uterine cavity, vaginal hysterectomy should be considered before colpocleisis. In cases in which this is not desired, preoperative evaluation should include a Papanicolaou smear, pelvic sonogram, and endometrial biopsy.

The fact that undergoing an obliterative procedure will preclude sexual intercourse must be discussed and must be acceptable to the patient. Many women with massive prolapse have ulcerations of the cervix or vaginal epithelium. An attempt can be made to heal these ulcers preoperatively by prescribing a course of topical estrogen. If there is any suspicion of malignancy, biopsies should be performed before surgery. For benign ulcers that do not heal with topical estrogens, the affected areas should be completely excised at the time of surgery.

Preoperative evaluation, including urodynamics, is useful for women with preexisting incontinence or evidence of urethral hypermobility. Specific surgical procedures for incontinence are discussed elsewhere in the book, but vaginal procedures such as one of the variations of a suburethral sling can be performed at the time of an obliterative procedure with minimal additional morbidity.

Obliterative procedures include partial or total colpocleisis and colpectomy. In the absence of a uterus, either complete colpocleisis or colpectomy can be performed, whereas the presence of the uterus necessitates partial colpocleisis, leaving lateral drainage channels for cervical secretions.

Techniques

The most commonly described technique for partial colpocleisis is a variation of the operation originally described by LeFort in 1877. Neugebauer, Langmade, Denehy and others have described modifications in the procedure (2–4). The prolapsed cervix is grasped with a tenaculum and brought out through the introitus. A surgical marking pen is used to outline the area of vaginal epithelium that is to be removed both anteriorly and posteriorly. The epithelium is incised sharply with a scalpel, and Strully or Metzenbaum scissors are then used to dissect sharply the underlying rectovaginal and pubocervical fascia off of the epithelium. The electrosurgical unit can also be used for the dissection and has the advantage of decreased blood loss. The dissection is continued until the entire area previously marked on both the anterior and posterior surfaces has been dissected free of underlying fascia. The epithelium is then excised (Fig. 26.1A).

Nonabsorbable sutures placed in an inverting Lembert fashion are then used to approximate the pubocervical fascia to the rectovaginal fascia on either side of the cervix. Progressive sutures are placed, creating a lateral channel on either side of the cervix for drainage of cervical secretions (Fig. 26.1B).

The cervix is then inverted, and a second layer of imbricating sutures is placed from the pubocervical fascia anteriorly to the rectovaginal fascia posteriorly in front of the cervix, permanently inverting it (Fig. 26.1C). Successive layers of plicating sutures are then placed in a caudad direction until the bulk of the prolapse has been reduced, obliterating the upper portion of the vagina (Fig. 26.1D). The vaginal epithelial edges are then reapproximated with absorbable suture.

The technique for total colpocleisis is similar, with the exception that it is not necessary

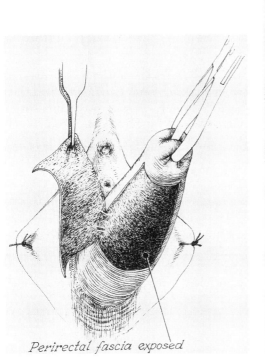

A   *Perirectal fascia exposed*

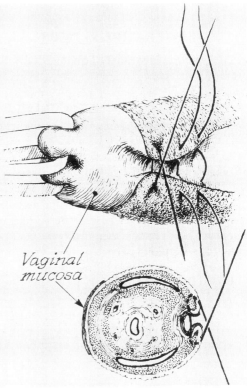

Vaginal mucosa

B

FIG. 26.1. A: The posterior vaginal epithelium is removed, exposing the rectovaginal fascia. **B:** The anterior and posterior epithelium has been excised. The pubocervical fascia is being attached to the rectovaginal fascia on either side, creating lateral drainage channels for cervical mucous.

to leave lateral drainage channels. A circumferential incision is made in the vaginal epithelium just cephalad to the hymenal ring. The epithelium is dissected sharply off of the underlying fascia and excised. The anterior and posterior fascia are then reapproximated either with sequential pursestring sutures or with interrupted sutures placed in an anterior-to-posterior fashion until the lumen of the vagina is obliterated. Plication of the levator ani muscles is frequently added to provide a firm site of attachment for colpectomy stitches. In either partial or total colpocleisis, once most of the prolapse has been reduced, appropriate bladder neck procedures can be performed as needed, before completing the colpocleisis. The fixation of the anterior wall

to the posterior is usually not carried out all the way to the hymenal ring because this artificially flattens the posterior vesical neck angle and predisposes to incontinence.

A colpectomy is performed in a similar manner, grasping the vaginal apex and everting it completely through the introitus. A circumferential incision is made in the vaginal epithelium, extending through the pubocervical fascia anteriorly and the rectovaginal fascia posteriorly. The vagina is then marked into four quadrants, and each is removed by sharp dissection. A series of pursestring permanent sutures is then placed. The vault of the soft tissue is then inverted, and the pursestring sutures are sequentially tied down, progressively inverting the soft tissue.

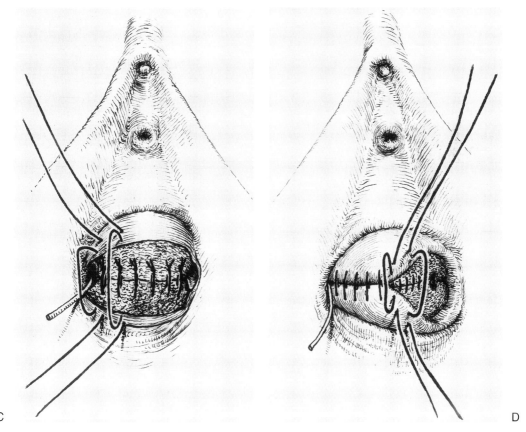

C   D

FIG. 26.1. (*Continued*) **C:** The cervix has been inverted, and the pubocervical and rectovaginal fascia are approximated in an anterior-to-posterior fashion in sequential layers. **D:** The anterior and posterior epithelium is reapproximated. (From Wheeless CR Jr. *Atlas of pelvic surgery.* Baltimore, MD: Williams & Wilkins, 1997:79, 81, with permission.)

Results

In the most recently published evaluation of total colpocleisis, DeLancy reported successful treatment in 32 of 33 women (5). One woman had a recurrence of her vault eversion at 1 year, and she was treated successfully with a repeat colpocleisis. Average length of follow-up was 35 months. No new cases of stress urinary incontinence (SUI) developed in this group. Earlier papers on the outcome of colpocleisis reported similar cure rates of 86% to 100%, although what constitutes a cure is generally not defined. In a series reported by Ridley, 50 of 58 patients (86%) had a "satisfactory" outcome a minimum of 1 year after the colpocleisis (6). In the same series, 6 of 58 women (10%) required subsequent surgery; 3 patients had surgery for recurrent prolapse, and 3 had surgery for SUI. Reported complications following colpocleisis are few, with the most common being development of SUI. Most series report postoperative incidences of SUI of 1% to 9%.

RESTORATIVE AND COMPENSATORY REPAIRS

In planning a reconstructive procedure designed to maintain vaginal function, it is essential to address defects of support at all levels during both anatomic (restorative) and compensatory procedures. Although most women require multiple steps for successful repair, for the sake of organization, we will address the vaginal apex, the anterior compartment, and the posterior compartment separately.

Apical Prolapse

Regardless of the anchoring site for the vaginal vault suspension, it is essential to reestablish continuity of the anterior and posterior vaginal fascia at the vaginal apex. Failure to approximate these fibromuscular planes can result in a vault enterocele where the small bowel herniates behind the thin vaginal epithelium lacking its myofascial layer.

Techniques

There are many techniques for suspending the vaginal apex. For the patient with good pelvic floor muscle strength as assessed by clinical examination and reasonably substantive endopelvic fascia, a vaginal approach using native tissues may be appropriate.

McCall Culdoplasty

McCall popularized a technique of uterosacral suspension of the vaginal vault commonly used in New Orleans, in conjunction with an extensive posterior culdoplasty (7). Following the opening of the vaginal apex, either after completion of a vaginal hysterectomy or after rectocele, cystocele, or enterocele repair, the uterosacral ligaments are identified and placed under tension. The uterosacral ligaments are then plicated with nonabsorbable sutures placed from one uterosacral ligament to the other, reefing the peritoneum of the posterior cul-de-sac in between (Fig. 26.2A). Two to three separate sutures are placed in a progressively cephalad fashion. These initial sutures, or internal stitches, are placed from within the peritoneal cavity. Additional sutures, the external stitches, are then placed from the vaginal side of the incision into the peritoneal cavity, incorporating the vaginal cuff and both uterosacral ligaments. When the stitches are tied down, the internal stitches plicate the uterosacral ligaments in the midline, whereas the external stitches suspend the cuff from the plicated uterosacral ligaments (Fig. 26.2B).

Uterosacral Suspension

Modifications of this procedure have been recommended over the years. We presently perform uterosacral ligament suspension that avoids plicating the uterosacral ligaments in the midline. Once the apex has been opened, the patient is placed in Trendelenburg position, and a 6-inch moistened Kerlix is used to pack the bowels up out of the sacral hollow. This greatly aids in visualization of the uterosacral ligaments. A headlamp is also useful to improve visualization.

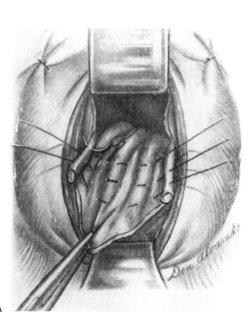

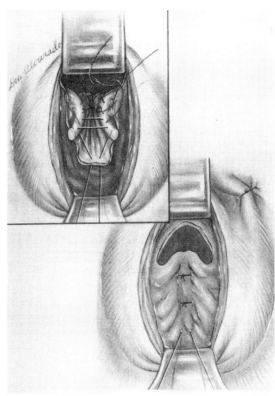

B

FIG. 26.2. A: The three internal stitches have been placed, from one uterosacral ligament to the other, incorporating peritoneum in between. **B:** In the upper frame, the internal stitches are tied down, plicating the uterosacral ligaments in the midline. In the lower frame, the external stitches are tied down, suspending the vaginal cuff to the uterosacral ligaments.

Buller and colleagues performed a cadaveric investigation aimed at describing the optimal location for suture placement in the uterosacral suspension (8). The surrounding vasculature and nerves in conjunction with suture pullout studies suggested the intermediate segment of the uterosacral ligament as the optimal compromise between strength and safety. The ischial spine was found to be a good marker of this intermediate segment.

They also noted that the proximity of the ureter to the anterior border of the fan-shaped uterosacral ligament varies along its length, being closest at the level of the cervix and farthest at the sacrum. Inappropriate suture placement can kink the ureter, causing obstruction. The potential for ureteral injury can be minimized by placing sutures at least 1 cm posterior to the anterior border of the uterosacral ligament. Placing the distal uterosacral ligament on tension demonstrates the anterior border of the ligament.

A single permanent suture of 2-0 Ti-Cron is then placed through the uterosacral ligament at about the level of the ischial spine, 1 cm posterior to the anterior border. One arm of this suture is brought out through the lateral aspect of the pubocervical fascia, whereas the other arm is brought out through the lateral aspect of the rectovaginal fascia. A second suture is placed through the contralateral uterosacral ligament and then attached as previously described to the pubocervical and rectovaginal fascia. Some authors describe placing additional sutures through each uterosacral ligament in a cephalad fashion and attaching them to progressively more medial aspects of the vaginal cuff.

A horizontal mattress stitch is used to close the intervening cuff medial to the lateral suspension stitches. This stitch reapproximates the anterior and posterior fascia, to prevent subsequent enterocele formation. Tying the uterosacral sutures closes the lateral aspects of the vaginal cuff and anchors them to the uterosacral ligaments in an anatomic configuration (Fig. 26.3). Finally, absorbable sutures are used to close the vaginal mucosa.

No attempt is made to plicate the uterosacral ligaments in the midline because this is not anatomic and can lead to narrowing of the upper vagina with resultant dyspareunia. It also increases the risk for ureteral obstruction. The ureter runs along the distal aspect of the anterior border of the uterosacral ligament and is frequently attached to it by a fibrous band. This leads to a risk for obstruction or injury to the ureter with all procedures that use the uterosacral as an anchorage. The rate of obstruction with uterosacral suspension has been reported to be as high as 11% (9). Should obstruction occur, simply releasing the suture may be sufficient to restore ureteral flow, although in other cases, reimplantation may be necessary. Regardless, postoperative cystoscopy is essential to a safe repair.

The uterosacral suspension can also be performed from an abdominal or laparoscopic approach. These approaches have the advantage of permitting uterine preservation in patients who wish to avoid hysterectomy. To perform a laparoscopic suspension, we place four ports in the abdomen: a 10/12-mm port at the umbilicus; a second 10/12-mm port just to the left of midline, about midway between the symphysis and the umbilicus; and two 5-mm ports in the left and right mid-lower quadrants (Fig. 26.4). Port site placement is crucial to the success of

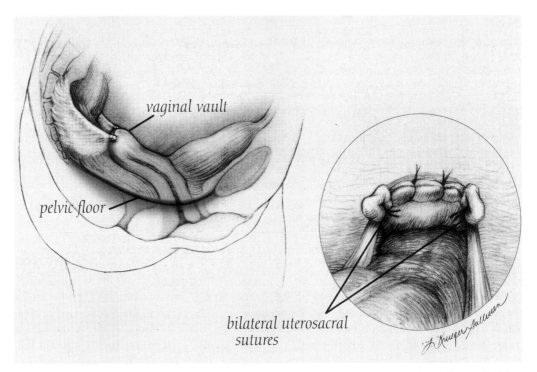

vaginal vault

pelvic floor

bilateral uterosacral sutures

FIG. 26.3. After one arm of each uterosacral suture has been passed through the pubocervical fascia and the other through the rectovaginal fascia on each side, they are tied down, anchoring the vaginal cuff to the uterosacrals. Additional sutures are placed in the midline, approximating the anterior and posterior fascia in the middle. The end result is a normal vaginal axis and length.

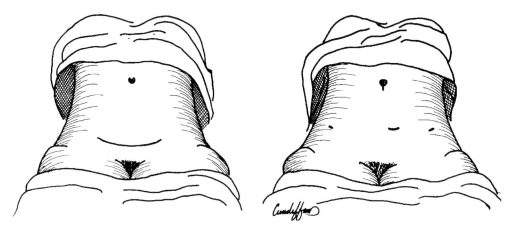

FIG. 26.4. The four laparoscopic port sites are placed (on *right*): a 10-mm port through the umbilicus; a second 10-mm port just to the left of midline, about midway from the umbilicus to the symphysis; a 5-mm port in the right lower quadrant; and a second 5-mm port in the left lower quadrant. The alternative is a laparotomy through a Pfannenstiel incision (on *left*).

a laparoscopic repair. The port placed just off midline must not be too low or it will not be useful to suture in the pelvis, whereas placement that is too high will interfere with good visualization from the camera through the umbilical port. The lateral ports must not be too low in the pelvis, or suturing will be prohibitively difficult.

After the ports are in place, the uterosacral suspension is performed using nonabsorbable 2-0 suture on a 5/8 circle curved needle. The ureter is identified, and the location of the ischial spine is palpated with a blunt probe. A single suture is placed through the uterosacral ligament at about the level of the ischial spine, 1 cm posterior to the anterior border. A second bite of tissue is then taken caudad to the first, incorporating mostly peritoneum, before finally passing the needle through the uterosacral as it inserts onto the posterior cervix (or through the uterosacral remnant on the posterior vaginal cuff). When the suture is tied down, the uterosacral ligament is effectively shortened. The procedure is repeated on the other side. No attempt is made to plicate the uterosacral ligaments in the midline (Fig. 26.5).

Ileococcygeus Suspension

In cases in which it is not possible to visualize the uterosacral ligaments or when they are extremely attenuated, the fascia of the iliococcygeus muscle, just anterior to ischial spine can be used to suspend the vaginal vault. The procedure is similar to the description of the uterosacral suspension but uses a different anchorage site. As described by Shull and coauthors, the fascia overlying the iliococcygeus muscle is identified lateral to the rectum and anterior to the ischial spine (10). The bowel is retracted medially, and a suture is placed just anterior to the spine beside the arcus tendineus fascia pelvis and brought out through the pubocervical fascia anteriorly and the rectovaginal fascia posteriorly on the ipsilateral side. Tying the sutures suspends the vagina bilaterally.

Sacrospinous Fixation

Finally, fixation of the apex to the sacrospinous ligament is a widely advocated and used option (11). Both anterior and posterior approaches to the pararectal space have been described. And although fixation is most commonly performed unilaterally, bilateral fixation has also been described (12). After the pararectal space has been entered, the spine is located and the sacrospinous ligament is identified over its course from the spine to the sacrum. The use of a Miya hook ligature carrier makes placement of the sacrospinous

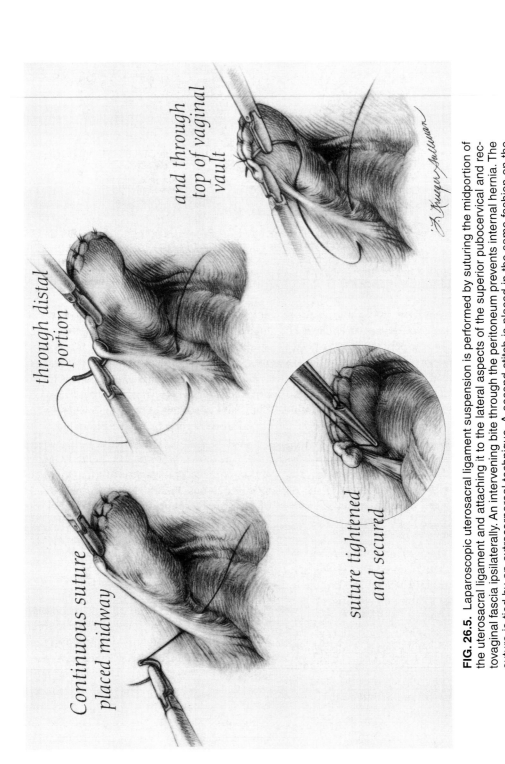

Continuous suture placed midway

through distal portion

and through top of vaginal vault

suture tightened and secured

FIG. 26.5. Laparoscopic uterosacral ligament suspension is performed by suturing the midportion of the uterosacral ligament and attaching it to the lateral aspects of the superior pubocervical and rectovaginal fascia ipsilaterally. An intervening bite through the peritoneum prevents internal hernia. The suture is tied by an extracorporeal technique. A second stitch is placed in the same fashion on the contralateral side.

sutures significantly easier. Two nonabsorbable sutures are placed through the ligament, the first about 2 cm medial and 1 cm cephalad to the spine and the second about 1 cm medial to the first. One arm of each suture is then brought through the posterior rectovaginal fascia, and the other is brought through the anterior pubocervical fascia. The sutures are then tied down, directly approximating the vagina to the sacrospinous ligament complex, without a suture bridge.

Each of these procedures for restorative repair of apical prolapse has advantages and disadvantages. The lateral and posterior deflection of the vagina with the typical unilateral sacrospinous ligament fixation is clearly not anatomic owing to posterior deflection of the vaginal axis (Fig. 26.6). This exposes the anterosuperior vaginal wall to increased force during increases in abdominal pressure. Numerous papers have reported an increase in the incidence of anterior wall prolapse after sacrospinous fixation, although a recent retrospective study challenges this assumption

(13). Although the iliococcygeus suspension maintains the normal alignment of the vaginal cylinder, the ischial spines are considerably inferior to the normal position of the vaginal apex, resulting in loss of vaginal length (Fig. 26.6). The origins of the uterosacral ligaments, if sufficiently strong on both sides, allow better vaginal depth with normal alignment (Fig. 26.6). When attenuation of the ligaments mandates plication at the level of the suspension, the resulting midline suspension is not anatomic.

Sacral Colpopexy

The woman with attenuated fascia, poor pelvic floor muscle strength, or severe ongoing physical stress is better served by a technique of vault suspension that provides compensatory support. Our preferred compensatory repair is the sacral colpopexy, which replaces the normal apical support with interposition of a suspensory bridge of either autologous fascia or synthetic material

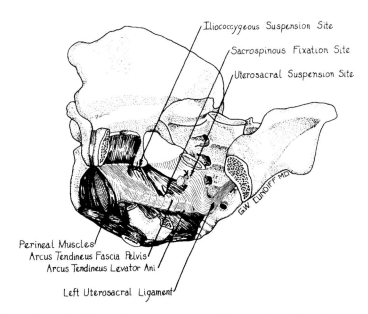

FIG. 26.6. Oblique view of pelvis to demonstrate three different sites of attachment for vaginal vault suspensions. A window is viewed in the vaginal vault to permit viewing of these anchorage sites. The iliococcygeous suspension is in the normal vaginal axis but falls short of the normal vaginal length. The sacrospinous ligament is deflected posteriorly. The uterosacral ligaments are in the normal vaginal axis and do not compromise vaginal length.

between the prolapsed vagina and the anterior sacrum. A variety of synthetic materials, including polyethylene terephthalate, polypropylene, and expanded polytetrafluoroethylene, can be used, as well as xenografts such as small intestine submucosa or allografts including cadaveric skin or fascia lata. Alternatively, native tissue can be harvested from the rectus fascia or fascia lata of the thigh. The material is then placed in the manner described subsequently.

If synthetic material is chosen, two straps of tissue measuring 5.5 cm at the base and extending 15 cm in length are cut into a rhomboid shape. Any defect in the rectovaginal or pubocervical fascia is repaired before attaching the graft. This is particularly important with rectocele repair to ensure continuity of support from the sacrum all the way down to the perineal body. A large obturator is placed in the vagina to assist in elevating the vaginal cuff. The bladder is dissected off of the vaginal cuff exposing the superior aspect of the pubocervical fascia to provide a sufficiently broad area to attach the graft. Similarly, the posterior peritoneum is opened at the vaginal apex, and the rectovaginal space is dissected until the superior edge of the rectovaginal fascia can be identified.

It is preferable to reestablish the integrity of the pubocervical ring by suturing the superior aspects of the pubocervical fascia and the rectovaginal fascia if they are not already attached. The two straps are attached separately, one anteriorly and the other posteriorly, taking care to attach the material over a wide surface area. Most failures occur as a result of avulsion of the mesh from the vagina. Attaching the graft over a wide surface area, which distributes the force that any one suture has to withstand, can minimize the risk for avulsion. It is also important to avoid bunching of graft material under the sutures and to avoid tying the sutures too tightly, which may predispose to necrosis and mesh erosion. After the straps have been attached anteriorly and posteriorly, they are sutured laterally to each other, creating a circumferential attachment around the vaginal cuff (Fig. 26.7A).

Many surgeons perform a culdoplasty before attaching the mesh to the sacrum, to prevent bowel from slipping behind the mesh. Nonabsorbable suture is used, incorporating the inferior edge of the posterior piece of mesh in the culdoplasty (Fig. 26.7A). Failure to obliterate the cul-de-sac has led to reports of enterocele formation behind the posterior mesh. After the culdoplasty, the peritoneum is closed over the mesh, until all mesh is covered.

The presacral space is entered by carefully grasping the overlying peritoneum, elevating it anteriorly, and then using the Bovie to incise the peritoneum and underlying loose areolar tissue. The goal of this dissection is to expose the anterior sacral ligament without injuring the hypogastric nerves or avulsing the middle sacral vessels. This is best accomplished by a combination of blunt and sharp dissection with the electrosurgical unit, with use of the Bovie directed away from the sacrum. The hypogastric nerves should be identified and avoided. After the anterior longitudinal sacral ligament has been cleared of loose connective tissue, two 2-0 nonabsorbable sutures are placed through it at the level of the S-2–S-3 junction. It is helpful to use a needle with a $5/8$ circle curve to place these sutures. We encircle the middle sacral vessels so that in the event of bleeding, the sutures can be tied, easily controlling the bleeding. Early reports of the procedure described attachment of the suspensory bridge to the sacrum at the S-3 to S-4 level. This site has been associated with an increased risk for hemorrhage, and the anterior ligament is thinner at this location (14). The area from the sacral promontory to the upper third of the sacrum appears to be a preferable site for attachment.

Each suture is passed through both the anterior and posterior pieces of mesh and then tied down, ensuring that neither strap is under undue tension (Fig. 26.7B). The anterior strap is left somewhat longer than the posterior strap to avoid over elevation of the anterior vaginal wall, which can increase the angle at the posterior urethrovesical junction and lead to incontinence.

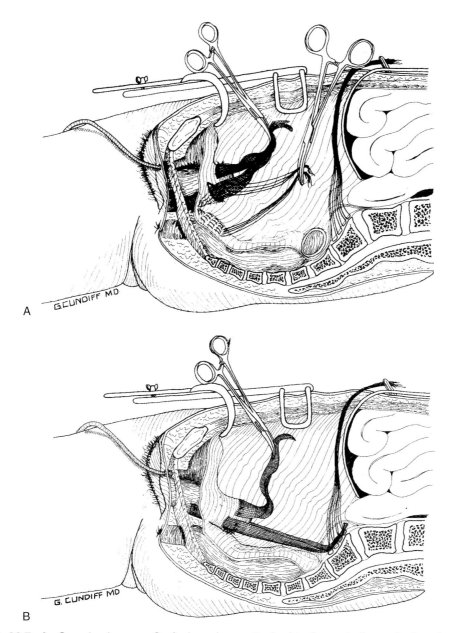

FIG. 26.7. A: Sacral colpopexy. Grafts have been attached to the posterior vaginal vault and anterior vaginal vault. Halban culdoplasty sutures are placed but untied. Sutures are placed in the longitudinal sacral ligament. **B:** Sacral colpopexy. The culdoplasty stitches are tied, and the posterior graft is anchored to the sacral stitches. The anterior and posterior graft are anchored separately to avoid overelevating the anterior wall, which predisposes to urinary incontinence.

Paraiso and colleagues have described an approach for laparoscopic sacral colpopexy (15). A minimum of four ports are placed as follows: a 10/12-mm infraumbilical port, two additional 10/12-mm ports, one in each lower quadrant, and a 5-mm port in the left midabdomen, lateral to the rectus muscles at the level of the umbilicus. An additional 5-mm port may be placed in the right midabdomen as needed for retraction.

The procedure itself is performed in a similar manner to that described for the open approach. The technique described employs a T-shaped piece of synthetic mesh of either polypropylene or Dacron. A large obturator is placed in the vagina and used to elevate the vaginal cuff, which assists in the dissection of the bladder off the vaginal cuff anteriorly to expose pubocervical fascia and in the opening of the rectovaginal space to identify the superior edge of the rectovaginal fascia.

The integrity of the pubocervical ring should be established by attaching the pubocervical fascia to the rectovaginal fascia, if they are not already attached. The T-shaped piece of mesh is then attached anteriorly first, using 0-0 nonabsorbable sutures to attach the mesh over a wide surface area and incorporating the full thickness of the vagina, but excluding the epithelium. The sutures are placed through the lower quadrant ports and the knots are tied extracorporeally. The ends of the T are then wrapped around the cuff and attached in a similar manner posteriorly. A Halban procedure or other culdoplasty is performed using 2-0 nonabsorbable sutures.

The sacral promontory is then identified and the presacral space is exposed. The use of a fan retractor may improve exposure, or the patient may be tilted to her left. The peritoneum overlying the sacrum is opened in a vertical manner, and the anterior longitudinal ligament is identified. Once again, care must be taken to identify and avoid the patient's right ureter, the presacral vessels, and the hypogastric nerves. The laparoscopic dissection may be accomplished with the assistance of a hydrodissector. The free end of the mesh is then attached to the longitudinal ligament of the sacrum in two rows of 2-0 nonabsorbable suture, avoiding undue tension. Alternatively, titanium tacks or hernia staples may be used to attach the mesh to the ligament. Excess mesh is trimmed and excised. The peritoneum is then closed over the mesh with 2-0 absorbable suture.

Results

There is a considerable difference of opinion among surgeons regarding the relative merit of vaginal and abdominal approaches to surgery for POP. Benson and colleagues reported the only prospective randomized study comparing vaginal and abdominal approaches for POP (16). This study compared outcomes for all vaginal segments and noted a significantly higher rate of reoperation for recurrent prolapse with surgery from a vaginal approach compared with surgery from an abdominal approach, 33% versus 16%. Although this is an appropriate study design for comparing two seemingly equivalent interventions, we believe these operations are appropriate for different subsets of patients and we would anticipate a higher failure rate with indiscriminate use of a restorative approach. Although the authors hypothesized that some of this difference was due to neuropathy caused by the vaginal dissection, some of the difference might also be explained by the use of the sacrospinous ligament suspension and needle urethropexies in the vaginal group. Most of the vaginal failures involved the anterior segment, and sacrospinous fixation has been shown to predispose to recurrent anterior wall prolapse, particularly when combined with needle bladder neck suspensions. Other complications described after sacrospinous fixation include vaginal shortening, sexual dysfunction, pain, and hemorrhage (11,12,14). The latter complications are related to the close proximity of pudendal nerves and vessels laterally and gluteal vessels and sacral nerve roots superiorly.

Although the technique of uterosacral suspension was described four decades ago, there are relatively little data regarding its efficacy. McCall reported no recurrent enteroceles during a 3-year follow-up (7), and Given reported a 5% failure rate with an average follow-up of 7 years (17). Elkins and associates compared high uterosacral suspension to sacrospinous ligament fixation and found a greater vaginal depth with the former, 10.2 versus 8.3 cm (18). Shull and colleagues reported on 289 patients with short-term follow-up after a vaginal uterosacral suspension (19). They reported that 87% had optimal anatomic outcomes, with a 1% transfusion rate and 1% ureteral injury rate. Their report was limited to anatomic results, but Barber and colleagues reported on 46 women followed for a mean of 15 months after a vaginal uterosacral suspension, noting that 90% had both resolution of prolapse symptoms and improvement in the stage of prolapse (9).

In distinction to the sacrospinous and uterosacral ligaments, the iliococcygeus fascia does not have critical structures, such as the pudendal nerve or ureter, immediately adjacent to it. Meeks and colleagues reported a 4% recurrence rate for anterior segment prolapse in 110 women after iliococcygeus suspension (20). This is better than the 19% failure rate in a study of 42 women undergoing iliococcygeal suspension reported by Shull and colleagues, although 10 women with recurrence had minimal anterior defects and only 5% had failure of apical support in this series (10).

Abdominal sacral colpopexy has a consistent cure rate of more than 90% (21). It is not without complications, including the risk for rare, but potentially life threatening, intraoperative hemorrhage and a 3% to 10% incidence of vaginal mesh erosion. Erosions can usually be managed with vaginal excision of all visible mesh followed by partial colpocleisis. A small subset of patients requires multiple extirpative surgeries for complete removal of eroded mesh. The cure rates and complication rates for apical prolapse corrected laparoscopically are consistent with those published for the open approach, although data are sparse.

Anterior Compartment Defects

Cystoceles have traditionally been repaired by plicating the pubocervical fascia in the midline with a series of horizontal mattress sutures, regardless of where breaks in the fascia are located. More recently, interest has turned to a more anatomic repair, the defect-directed repair, with careful preoperative as well as intraoperative evaluation of the precise defect in the fascia. Defects in the anterior segment can occur laterally, superiorly, and in the midline. Superior defects are addressed with closure of the cuff, establishing continuity of the anterior and posterior fascia and ensuring adequate apical support. The original description of the repair of lateral defects, the paravaginal repair, used the vaginal approach, but recently the approach is more commonly performed with an abdominal approach and has also been described through a laparoscopic approach. Defect-directed repairs are described subsequently.

Techniques

When performed vaginally, the epithelium is incised and dissected from the underlying endopelvic fascia from beneath the descending pubic rami to the lateral pelvic sidewalls. Placing the contralateral index finger on the ischial spine helps to identify the arcus tendineus fascia pelvis. The arcus tendineus fascia pelvis runs from the tip of the finger along the medial aspect of the finger to the proximal intraphalangeal joint. Lateral defects can be identified by attempting to swing the finger anteriorly and by the identification of retropubic space fat. If a lateral defect is present, permanent sutures are placed at 1-cm intervals into the arcus tendineus fascia pelvis from the spine to the pubic bone, while retracting the bladder medially. When all sutures are placed, they are then brought through the lateral aspect of the pubocervical fascia and tied down (Fig. 26.8A). Central defects are most easily accessible from the vaginal approach. The rent is identified by looking for the contrast between the ruddy red detrusor muscle and the white pubocervical fascia.

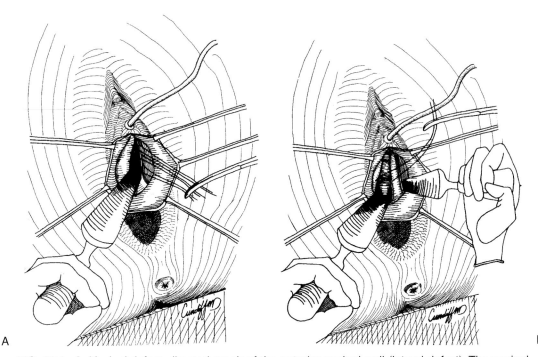

A

B

FIG. 26.8. A: Vaginal defect–directed repair of the anterior vaginal wall (lateral defect). The vaginal epithelium has been dissected from the underlying tissue, revealing a left paravaginal defect. Sutures have been placed through the arcus tendineus fascia pelvis (*white line*) and lateral aspect of the pubocervical fascia and are ready to be tied. **B:** Vaginal defect–directed repair of the anterior vaginal wall (midline defect). The vaginal epithelium has been dissected from the underlying tissue, revealing a midline longitudinal defect. A suture has been placed through both margins of the pubocervical fascia and is ready to be tied.

The detrusor muscle also bleeds more easily. The defect is closed in an interrupted fashion with permanent suture, and the vaginal epithelium is closed (Fig. 26.8B).

Abdominally, the retropubic space is dissected to expose several important landmarks, including the arcus tendineus fascia pelvis running between the posterior aspect of the pubis and the ischial spine and the more superior and lateral obturator neurovascular bundle. After landmarks are identified, the endopelvic fascia and lateral vaginal sulcus are sutured to the arcus with interrupted nonabsorbable sutures (Fig. 26.9).

This dissection can also be completed laparoscopically. Four laparoscopic ports are placed as described previously for laparoscopic apical support procedures, and the bladder is filled in a retrograde fashion to help delineate its boundaries. The peritoneum is grasped in the midline, anterior and superior to the bladder dome, and is sharply incised with endoshears. This incision is extended bilaterally until the lateral boundaries of the obliterated umbilical arteries are reached. A combination of blunt and sharp dissection is then used to expose Cooper's ligament. Once the ligament is identified, the dissection of the space of Retzius is continued bluntly posteriorly and inferiorly to the ischial spine, which can be palpated with a blunt probe. Interrupted sutures of 2-0 Prolene on a 5/8 circle curved needle are then placed, starting with the inferior-most stitch, near the spine, through the arcus, and then through the lateral vaginal sulcus until the defect is obliterated.

Access to the central defect from the abdominal approach is achieved by opening the

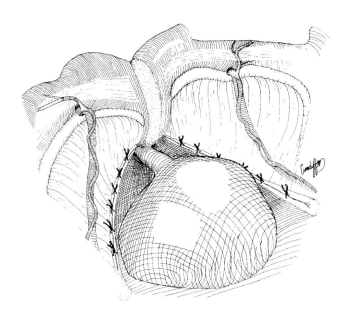

FIG. 26.9. Abdominal defect–directed repair of the anterior vaginal wall (lateral defect). The retropubic space has been dissected, revealing right and left paravaginal defects. Sutures have been placed through the arcus tendineus fascia pelvis (*white line*) and lateral aspect of the pubocervical fascia bilaterally and are tied.

vesicouterine peritoneal reflection and mobilizing the bladder after clamping and ligating the bladder pillars. Abdominal repair has been reported to be as efficacious as vaginal repair, although there may be an increased risk for bleeding with this approach. In addition, although repair of central defects is possible from this approach, we generally avoid it because of the neurologic injury that can occur with ligation of the bladder pillars, as can be seen after radical hysterectomy.

For the occasional patient whose endopelvic fascia is too attenuated to repair, a compensatory repair using a piece of synthetic mesh or heterologous fascia can be used for an anterior fascial replacement. An attempt is made to correct any obvious breaks in the fascia, and the graft is then placed over the fascia, in a manner that a patch would be placed. The graft is secured bilaterally to the arcus tendineus fascia pelvis along its entire course and superiorly to the vaginal cuff.

After the correction of all fascial defects, support procedures for the urethrovesical junction can be performed as needed for patients with genuine stress incontinence or potential incontinence.

Results

Although there are considerable data regarding the efficacy of the abdominal paravaginal defect repair for genuine stress incontinence (GSI), its efficacy for anterior POP is not as well documented. Richardson reported a cure rate of 95% (22). Shull and Baden also reported a 5% recurrence rate for cystocele but noted a 6% incidence of vault prolapse and a 5% incidence of enterocele (23). Young reported a 98% objective cure rate at 1-year follow-up, using a vaginal approach to paravaginal repair, but there are no studies reporting cure rates for the defect-directed approach with all anterior wall defects (24). There is also a paucity of information on the anterior fascial replacement. Julian reported a 66% cure rate for standard vaginal anterior colporrhaphy for recurrent anterior prolapse, compared with a 100% cure rate when Marlex mesh was used to substitute for the endopelvic fascia (25). There was, however, a 25% incidence of mesh-related complications. Others have reported a 25% recurrence rate of cystoceles at 1 year when mesh was used as part of the anterior repair, compared with a 43% recurrence rate with anterior repair alone (26).

Posterior Compartment Defects

Repair of rectoceles has traditionally been performed with plication of the levator muscles in the midline, creating a nonanatomic barrier between the vagina and rectum. This approach has been associated with dyspareunia and constipation postoperatively. As with cystocele repairs, recent investigations have advocated a defect-directed approach to repairing rectoceles.

Techniques

The epithelium is incised in a transverse manner, just outside the hymenal ring. This incision is carried cephalad to the cuff or until the defect has been exposed. The underlying rectovaginal fascia is dissected sharply off the underlying tissue out laterally to its lateral fascial attachments to the levator ani and obturator fascia. After the dissection is complete, the rent is identified. Displacing the anterior rectal wall with a finger in the rectum facilitates identification of discrete fascial tears (Fig. 26.10A). Careful attention to the attachment of the posterior fascia to the perineal body is essential to prevent recurrent rectocele and to help correct perineal descent (Fig. 26.10B). Superior defects are corrected by attachment of the rectovaginal fascia to the pubocervical fascia anteriorly as well as reestablishing apical support as previously described. Lateral breaks are corrected by reattaching the fascia to the lateral pelvic sidewall in a manner similar to that described previously for paravaginal repairs. Perineal reconstruction is performed before reattachment of the rectovaginal fascia to the perineal body

only if there are discreet breaks in the superficial perineal muscles. A perineorrhaphy that artificially enlarges the perineum and superficially constricts the genital hiatus creates abnormal anatomy with poor functional results.

For women with extremely attenuated fascia, posterior fascial replacement can be considered. It is performed in a manner similar to that described previously for anterior fascial replacement, attaching the graft to the arcus tendineus fascia rectovaginalis laterally, the uterosacral ligaments and pubocervical fascia anteriorly, and the perineal body inferiorly.

The abdominal sacral colpoperineopexy is an abdominal approach to the correction of posterior segment prolapse associated with severe perineal descent and vault prolapse (27). The procedure is similar to the sacral colpopexy, except that the posterior strap is taken all the way down to the perineal body, where it is attached with several interrupted permanent sutures (Fig. 26.11A). An assistant can perform a rectovaginal examination, elevating the perineal body for easier suture placement. An initial vaginal dissection as described previously is the only way to ensure attachment of the strap to the perineal body; however, the strap should be passed down from above and then sutured in place. Placement of a synthetic mesh strap vaginally, first attaching the strap to the perineal body and then pushing the strap cephalad, led to rejection and erosion rates reportedly as high as 40%, although we have not had rejection of allogenic or autologous straps (Fig. 26.11B).

Results

Although traditional posterior colporrhaphy effectively reduces the vaginal bulge in 76% to 96% of cases, relief of associated defecatory and sexual dysfunction symptoms has been much less satisfactory, with dyspareunia in 20% to 50% postoperatively and persistent splinting in 21% to 50% (28,29). One study documenting the cure rate for repair of discrete posterior fascial defects showed improvement in Pelvic Organ Prolapse Quantification (POPQ) stage at 6 weeks in 67 of 69

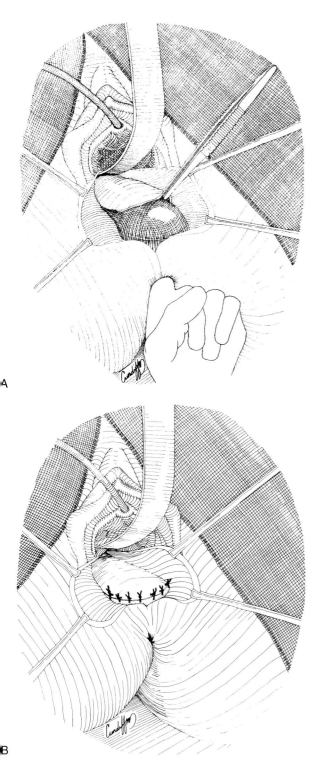

FIG. 26.10. A: Vaginal defect–directed repair of the posterior vaginal wall (inferior defect). The vaginal epithelium has been dissected from the underlying tissue, revealing a detachment of the rectovaginal septum from the perineal body. The defect is highlighted by the rectal finger. **B:** Vaginal defect–directed repair of the posterior vaginal wall (inferior defect). The detached rectovaginal septum has been reapproximated to the perineal body with interrupted stitches.

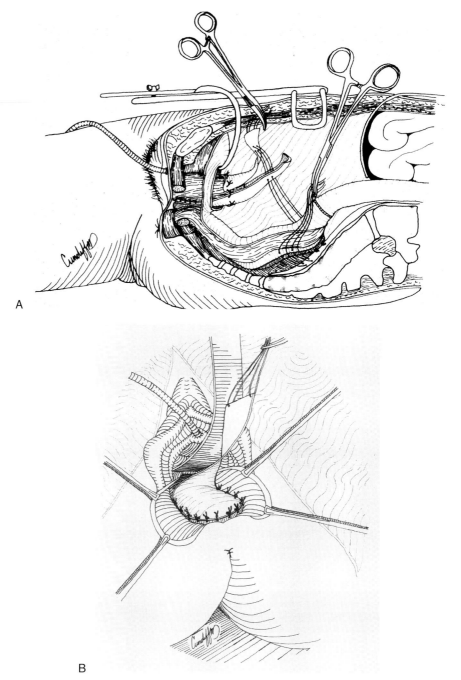

A

B

FIG. 26.11. A: Sacral colpoperineopexy. Grafts have been attached to the posterior vaginal vault and anterior vaginal vault. The posterior graft is attached to the perineal body and brought through the rectovaginal space into the abdominal field. On the patient's left, rectopexy sutures are placed through the longitudinal sacral ligament and the lateral ligaments of the rectum and are untied. On the patient's right, rectopexy sutures are placed through the longitudinal sacral ligament, the lateral ligaments of the rectum, and the anterior and posterior vaginal grafts and are untied. **B:** Sacral colpoperineopexy. The posterior graft is attached to the perineum through a vaginal approach and then brought through the rectovaginal space to the abdominal field.

women (29). 18% were found to have recurrent rectoceles at one year. Others have reported similar success rates in the range of 81% to 90% with similar follow-up (28). Statistically significant improvement in bowel symptoms, such as constipation, splinting, and incontinence, and in other symptoms such as dyspareunia has been documented. There are no studies to date evaluating the efficacy of posterior fascial replacement. Our early experience with abdominal sacral colpoperineopexy demonstrates correction of severe recurrent prolapse to stage 0 in 12 of 19 patients (63%), to stage I in 4 (21%), and to stage II in the remaining 3 (16%) (22). Only 1 (5%) had a recurrent rectocele, and two thirds of patients had resolution of chronic bowel symptoms (27).

FUTURE AREAS OF RESEARCH

At its most basic, future research regarding the surgical management of POP needs to be prospective, randomized, and outcomes based. In addition, functional outcomes are perhaps a more appropriate target than strictly structural ones. The consistent use of a standardized system for objective, reliable quantification of support defects performed both preoperatively and postoperatively is essential so that meaningful inferences can be made after surgical intervention. This will allow larger, multicentered trials to be performed and will also enable comparisons to be made between studies evaluating different procedures.

A significant area of weakness has been our inability to predict which patients will fail restorative approaches and might benefit from a compensatory approach. Knowing which patients are at increased risk for failure would allow improved preoperative counseling and more appropriate choice of surgical procedure. The increased use of neurophysiologic testing to evaluate the presence of neurologic injury or evaluation of individual connective tissue types are interesting possibilities that deserve further attention. Other parameters that may be identified preoperatively to predict the function of the pelvic diaphragm postoperatively include

imaging studies that evaluate muscle mass, perineal descent, and pelvic diaphragm axis may prove to be valuable as well.

REFERENCES

1. Olsen AL , Smith VJ, Bergestrom JO, et al. Epidemiology of surgically managed pelvic organ prolapse and urinary incontinence. *Obstet Gynecol* 1997;89:501–506.
2. Goldman J, Ovadia J, Feldverg D. The Neugebauer-Le Fort operation: a review of 118 partial colpocleises. *Eur J Obstet Gynecol Reprod Biol* 1981;12(1):31–35.
3. Langmade CF, Oliver JA. Partial colpocleisis. *Am J Obstet Gynecol* 1986;154(6):1200–1205.
4. Denehy TR, Choe JY, Gregori CA, et al. Modified Le Fort partial colpocleisis with Kelly urethral plication and posterior colpoperineoplasty in the medically compromised elderly: a comparison with vaginal hysterectomy, anterior colporrhaphy, and posterior colpoperineoplasty. *Am J Obstet Gynecol* 1995;173(6):1697–1702.
5. DeLancy JO, Morley GW. Total colpocleisis for vaginal eversion. *Am J Obstet Gynecol* 1997;176(6):1228–1232.
6. Ridley JH. Evaluation of the colpocleisis operation: a report of fifty-eight cases. *Am J Obstet Gynecol* 1972;113:1114–1119.
7. McCall ML. Posterior culdoplasty: surgical correction of enterocele during vaginal hysterectomy. A preliminary report. *Obstet Gynecol* 1957;10:595–602.
8. Buller JL, Thompson JR, Cundiff GW, et al. Uterosacral ligament: description of anatomic relationships to optimize surgical safety. *Obstet Gynecol* 2001;97:873–879.
9. Barber MD, Visco AG, Weidner AC, et al. Bilateral uterosacral ligament vaginal vault suspension with site-specific endopelvic fascia defect repair for treatment of pelvic organ prolapse. *Am J Obstet Gynecol* 2000;183:1402–1411.
10. Shull BL, Capen CV, Riggs MW, et al. Bilateral attachment of the vaginal cuff to iliococcygeus fascia: an effective method of cuff suspension. *Am J Obstet Gynecol* 1993;168:1764–1771.
11. Nichols DH. Sacrospinous fixation for massive eversion of the vagina. *Am J Obstet Gynecol* 1982;142:901–904.
12. Pohl JF, Frattarelli JL. Bilateral transvaginal sacrospinous colpopexy: preliminary experience. *Am J Obstet Gynecol* 1997;177(6):1356–1361.
13. Richter K, Albrich W. Long-term results following fixation of the vagina on the sacrospinal ligament by the vaginal route (vaginaefixatio sacrospinalis vaginalis). *Am J Obstet Gynecol* 1981;141:811–816.
14. Sutton GP, Addison WA, Livengood CH, et al. Life-threatening hemorrhage complicating sacral colpopexy. *Am J Obstet Gynecol* 1981;140:836–837.
15. Paraiso MF, Falcone T, Walters MD. Laparoscopic surgery for enterocele, vaginal apex prolapse and rectocele. *Int Urogynecol J* 1999;10:223–229.
16. Benson JT, Lucente V, McClellan E. Vaginal versus abdominal reconstructive surgery for the treatment of pelvic support defects: a prospective randomized study with long-term outcome evaluation. *Am J Obstet Gynecol* 1996;175:1418–1422.
17. Given FT. "Posterior culdoplasty": revisited. *Am J Obstet Gynecol* 1985;153:135–139.

18. Elkins TE, Hopper JB, Goodfellow K, et al. Initial report of anatomic and clinical comparison of the sacrospinous ligament fixation to the high McCall culdoplasty for vaginal fixation at hysterectomy for uterine prolapse. *J Pelvic Surg* 1995;1:12–17.

19. Shull BL, Bachofen C, Coates KW, et al. A transvaginal approach to repair of apical and other associated sites of pelvic organ prolapse with uterosacral ligaments. *Am J Obstet Gynecol* 2000;183:1365–1374.

20. Meeks GR, Washburne JF, McGehee RP, et al. Repair of vaginal vault prolapse by suspension of the vagina to iliococcygeus (prespinous) fascia. *Am J Obstet Gynecol* 1994;171:1444–1454.

21. Addison WA, Bump RC, Cundiff GW, et al. Sacral colpopexy is the preferred treatment for vaginal vault prolapse in selected patients. *J Gynecol Tech* 1996;2:69–74.

22. Richardson AC, Lyon JB, Williams NL. A new look at pelvic relaxation. *Am J Obstet Gynecol* 1976;568:568–573.

23. Shull BL, Baden WF. A six year experience with paravaginal defect repair for stress urinary incontinence. *Am J Obstet Gynecol* 1989;160:1432–1440.

24. Young SB, Daman JJ, Bony LG. Vaginal paravaginal repair: one-year outcome. *Am J Obstet Gynecol* 2001;185(6):1360–1366.

25. Julian TM. The efficacy of Marlex mesh in the repair of severe, recurrent vaginal prolapse of the anterior mid-vaginal wall. *Am J Obstet Gynecol* 1996;75:1472–1475.

26. Sand PK, Kodure S, Lobel RW, et al. Prospective randomized trial of polyglactin 910 mesh to prevent recurrence of cystoceles and rectoceles. *Am J Obstet Gynecol* 2001;184:1357–1364.

27. Cundiff GW, Harris RL, Coates KW, et al. Abdominal sacral colpoperineopexy: a new approach for correction of posterior compartment defects and perineal descent associated with vaginal vault prolapse. *Am J Obstet Gynecol* 1997;177(6):345–355.

28. Porter WE, Steele A, Walsh P, et al. The anatomic and functional outcomes of defect-specific rectocele repairs. *Am J Obstet Gynecol* 1999;181:1353–1359.

29. Cundiff GW, Weidner AC, Visco AG, et al. An anatomic and functional assessment of the discrete defect rectocele repair. *Am J Obstet Gynecol* 1998;1791451–1791457.

PART D
Urinary Incontinence

Ostergard's Urogynecology and Pelvic Floor Dysfunction, Fifth Edition. edited by A.E. Bent, et al.
Lippincott Williams & Wilkins, Philadelphia © 2003.

27

Vesicovaginal and Ureterovaginal Fistulae

W. Glenn Hurt

Department of Obstetrics and Gynecology, Virginia Commonwealth University, School of Medicine; and Department of Obstetrics and Gynecology, Medical College of Virginia Hospitals, Virginia Commonwealth University Health System, Richmond, Virginia

A genitourinary fistula can be a cause of great suffering and emotional distress for a woman. The constant leakage of urine interferes with her work, restricts her social life, and in many cases, results in rejection by the rest of society. Genitourinary fistulas are common in the developing countries, where the leading cause is childbirth; they are uncommon in the developed countries, where the leading cause is pelvic surgery (1).

In 1840, John Peter Mettauer, a surgeon in rural Virginia, reported the first successful cure of a vesicovaginal fistula in the United States (2). In 1852, James Marion Sims, a surgeon in Alabama, acknowledged the cures of Mettauer in Virginia and of Hayward in Massachusetts when he described his procedure for the treatment of vesicovaginal fistulas (3). The surgical cure of vesicovaginal fistulas was such an important event that even today it is credited with being the beginning of "modern" gynecologic surgery.

INCIDENCE

As a result of underreporting, the true incidence of genitourinary fistulas, especially in the developing countries, is unknown. However, with respect to developed countries, Finland has a nationwide report on the incidence of urinary tract injuries among 62,379 hysterectomies carried out from 1990 through 1995 (4). The total incidences of ureteral injury after all hysterectomies were 1.0 of 1,000 procedures: 13.9 of 1,000 after laparoscopic, 0.4 of 1,000 after total abdominal, 0.3 of 1,000 after supracervical abdominal, and 0.2 of 1,000 after vaginal hysterectomy procedures. The failure rates of primary repair of a ureteral injury were 5%, 12%, 0%, and 0%, respectively. The incidence of bladder injury was 1.3 of 1,000 procedures. Sixty-five percent of reported bladder injuries were vesicovaginal fistulas, giving an incidence of 0.8 of 1,000 procedures after all hysterectomies: 2.2 of 1,000 after laparoscopic, 1.0 of 1,000 after total abdominal, 0 of 1,000 after supracervical abdominal, and 0.2 of 1,000 vaginal hysterectomy procedures. The failure rates of primary repair of a simple bladder injury were 5%, 18%, 0%, and 0%, respectively; the failure rates of primary repair of a vesicovaginal fistula were 17%, 20%, 0%, and 0%, respectively.

ETIOLOGY

As noted, most vesicovaginal and vesicourethrovaginal fistulas in the developing countries of the world are due to childbirth—a combination of obstructed labors, poorly trained birth attendants, and inaccessible or deficient health care facilities. A few are the result of Gishiri cuts of the vagina and bladder, a traditional and regional custom of treating a variety of obstetric and gynecologic conditions.

In the developed countries of the world, genitourinary fistulas are uncommon. Access

TABLE 27.1. *Etiology of genitourinary fistulas*

Childbirth
    Obstructed labor
    Operative deliveries
Pelvic surgery
    Laparoscopy
    Hysterectomy
    Bladder neck suspensions
    Bladder surgery
    Bowel surgery
    Colporrhaphy
    Diverticulectomy
Pelvic radiation
Diseases
    Cancer
    Infections
    Stones
Instrumentation and support devices
    Dilations
    Catheterization
    Endoscopic trauma
    Pessaries
Miscellaneous
    Foreign bodies
    Accidental trauma
    Congenital

TABLE 27.2. *Surgical techniques for minimizing lower urinary tract injuries during gynecologic surgery*

1. Prepare, position, and drape to allow both abdominal and vaginal access.
2. Provide continuous bladder drainage.
3. Provide adequate exposure, lighting, and suctioning of the surgical field.
4. Restore anatomic relationships.
5. Identify the course of each ureter and keep them out of harm's way.
6. Perform sharp dissection along anatomic planes.
7. Dissect and develop the extraperitoneal spaces.
8. Secure hemostasis while avoiding frantic blind attempts to control bleeding.
9. Clamp, cut, and suture under direct vision while avoiding large tissue pedicles.
10. Perform intraoperative testing of the integrity of the lower urinary tract, with cystoscopy or cystotomy as indicated.

to modern health care facilities and trained birth attendants has made childbirth a rare cause of genitourinary fistulas. In these countries, pelvic surgery is the most common cause of genitourinary fistulas. The lower urinary tract and the genital tract are intimately related, both embryologically and anatomically. The diseases and conditions that affect one often affect the other. A pelvic disease process and its treatment (Table 27.1) create an opportunity to develop a genitourinary fistula. Unfortunately, in the United States, most genitourinary fistulas that are caused by pelvic surgery occur in women who had their surgery for a benign condition. Therefore, it is reasonable to believe that most genitourinary fistulas may be preventable.

PREVENTION

A number of steps can be taken at the time of surgery to help prevent lower urinary tract injuries that may result in the formation of a genitourinary fistula (Table 27.2).

Patients undergoing advanced or challenging gynecologic procedures should be positioned, prepared, and draped to allow access to both abdominal and vaginal approaches. This is facilitated by the use of the "universal" stirrups and the availability of disposable double-access (e.g., laparoscopic-abdominal-vaginal-hysterectomy, or LAVH) drapes. This technique allows manipulation of the vagina during complicated abdominal cases, abdominal and vaginal access during procedures for urinary incontinence, and access for a rectocele repair at the time of abdominal reconstructive procedures. It also helps in positioning a patient for transurethral cystoscopy.

Bladder drainage is usually accomplished by the placement of a two-way transurethral balloon catheter (14 or 16 French) connected to straight drainage. When the need for intraoperative bladder filling is anticipated, a three-way balloon catheter (14 or 16 French) may be placed and connected to a bag of sterile water or normal saline, with or without a dye such as indigo carmine. This enables the surgeon to fill and empty the bladder during the procedure to define the limits of the bladder, to test the bladder for partial or full-thickness injuries of its wall, or to fill the bladder to perform a cystotomy for a surgical procedure, suprapubic cystoscopy (i.e., teloscopy), or suprapubic bladder catheter placement. When operating vaginally on patients who have had prior cesarean sections or who have lower-segment uterine fibroids, it may be helpful to drain the bladder with a transurethral catheter, inject undiluted indigo carmine (5 mL) through the catheter into the bladder, and clamp the catheter in order to keep the dye within the bladder. Then, if the bladder is injured during the course of the operation, the presence of the dye will help the surgeon to determine the location and extent of the injury so that it can be repaired.

There has been a lot of discussion regarding preoperative intravenous urograms and the preoperative placement of ureteral catheters in an effort to prevent surgical injuries to the lower urinary tract. Intravenous urograms are useful in detecting congenital anomalies and in documenting the involvement of the lower urinary tract by pelvic tumors, pelvic inflammatory disease, endometriosis, and malignancies. However, routine urograms have not been shown to reduce the incidence of surgical injury to the ureters and bladder. Likewise, the preoperative placement of ureteral catheters is not always practical or desirable because most ureteral injuries occur in patients whose procedures are otherwise uncomplicated. They cannot be expected to reduce the incidence of ureteral injuries. In addition, ureteral catheters may cause mucosal injury or impart stiffness to a ureter that may predispose it to devascularization or laceration. If, at the time of surgery, it is found that ureteral catheterization is desirable, the catheters may be placed by transurethral cystoscopy or by a cystotomy placed in the extraperitoneal dome of the bladder.

Suspected injuries of the lower urinary tract should be evaluated at the time of surgery. The direct injection of indigo carmine into the lumen of a ureter above the site of possible injury is easily accomplished using a butterfly needle (22 or 23 gauge) and syringe. Leakage of dye from a damaged ureter suggests the need for stenting or repair of that ureter; passage of dye into the bladder is evidence of ureteral patency. The intravenous

administration of indigo carmine may demonstrate a damaged ureter but cannot be used to demonstrate bilateral ureteral patency unless cystoscopy or a cystotomy is performed and colored urine is seen to be coming from each ureteric orifice. As noted, ureteral catheters may be placed by transurethral cystoscopy or by abdominal cystotomy. These catheters may be used to demonstrate ureteric injury and to stent the ureter for repair, to drain urine from the kidney pelvis, or to prevent urine leakage and stenosis during the healing of minor crush injures.

When testing the bladder for possible injuries, it should be remembered that the injuries could involve a partial or full thickness of the bladder wall. To demonstrate injuries, the bladder should be distended with either dyed (e.g., indigo carmine or methylene blue) sterile water or saline or with sterile milk (e.g., infant's formula). Because vesicovaginal fistulas may follow partial- or full-thickness injuries of the bladder wall, both types of injuries should be repaired when they occur. Superior results are obtained when complete lacerations of the base or trigone of the bladder are covered with a layer of peritoneum or with a portion of omentum. The location and type of bladder injury dictates the need for postoperative bladder drainage.

Cystoscopy is frequently performed at the time of urogynecologic and reconstructive pelvic procedures. It should be performed whenever there is a question about the integrity of the lower urinary tract. Common distending media include sterile water, normal saline, and hypertonic glucose (i.e., 10% to 50%). The administration of 5 mL of intravenous indigo carmine or methylene blue (not preferred because of the formation of methemoglobin) should result, within 4 to 8 minutes, in bilateral excretion of blue urine from the ureters into the bladder. When hypertonic glucose is used as the distending medium, the blue urine from the ureters has a lower specific gravity than the hypertonic glucose in the bladder, and the stream of blue urine is more easily seen, especially in patients with some delay in kidney function. Transabdominal cystoscopy (i.e., teloscopy) should be performed through the extraperitoneal dome of the bladder because openings in this portion of the bladder are more likely to heal without complications. First, the bladder is distended with sterile water or normal saline using a transurethral catheter, and a pursestring suture is placed around the site selected for telescope placement. A stab incision is then made within the pursestring suture through which the telescope is inserted into the bladder. Usually, the balloon of the transurethral catheter will have to be displaced upward from the bladder neck or removed to see both ureteric orifices. Whenever cystoscopy is performed, it is always important to inspect the inside of the bladder for foreign bodies (e.g., misplaced sutures), injuries, or abnormalities of the bladder wall.

CLASSIFICATION

A simple classification of genitourinary fistulas is recommended (Table 27.3). Many classifications of genitourinary fistulas have been suggested, but none has international acceptance. Because classifications tend to obscure details, it is best to describe the physical findings in each case of genitourinary fistula and in each publication on genitourinary fistulas. This is the only way there can be a critical analysis of the world literature, especially when fistulas involve more than two organs and more than just the urethra, bladder, and ureters. In this chapter, attention is directed to the diagnosis and treatment of urethrovaginal, vesicovaginal, and ureterovaginal fistulas.

CLINICAL PRESENTATION AND EVALUATION

The evaluation of genitourinary fistulas should determine their cause, the organs involved, the presence of any infection, the condition of the tissues around the fistula, and the general condition and prognosis of the patient. The elements of such an evaluation are listed in Table 27.4.

Clinical Presentation

Women with genitourinary fistulas usually complain of the uncontrollable loss of urine from their vagina that may be continuous or intermittent. A large number of perineal pads, diapers, rags, or towels are needed to help control the resulting wetness and to prevent soilage of their clothes and everything around them. The unpleasant, ammonia odor of urine often accompanies them. In taking their history, an attempt should be made to determine the cause of their genitourinary fistula with specific questions about known etiologies (Table 27.1). It is also important to obtain prior medical records regarding diseases, conditions, or therapies that may have caused the development of the fistula as well as any treatments or procedures that may have been undertaken to cure the fistula.

Vaginal Examination

There usually is a wetness of the vulva and perineum accompanied by the odor of urine. There may be skin irritation that is the result of the constant presence of urine or the wearing of

TABLE 27.3. *Classification of genitourinary fistulas*

Simple
Vesicovaginal
Ureterovaginal
Urethrovaginal
Complex
Urethrovesicovaginal
Other genitourinary fistulas

TABLE 27.4. *Evaluation of genitourinary fistulas*

Clinical presentation
Vaginal examination
Diagnostic testing
Dye or milk
Water and air ("flat tire")
Imaging
Intravenous urography
Retrograde urography
Cystography
Computed tomography

absorbent pads or diapers. With the aid of a speculum, it is often easy to locate a genitourinary fistula that involves the bladder or urethra when the patient is examined in the lithotomy position. A Sims speculum is recommended for examining the walls of the vagina, and a small probe may be used to demonstrate a fistula between the urethra or bladder and the vagina. The collection of urine in the posterior fornix of the vagina is always an abnormal finding. How it gets there must be explained. Although a vaginal examination may locate the opening of a genitourinary fistula, and urinary leakage may be demonstrated, further evaluation of these findings is recommended.

Diagnostic Testing

Dye tests (e.g., indigo carmine or methylene blue in sterile water or normal saline) or milk (e.g., sterile infant's formula) may be used to fill the bladder through a transurethral catheter. When there is a vesicovaginal fistula, the dyed liquid or milk can usually be seen leaking into the vagina. When the fistula is small, it may be necessary to place a few cotton balls loosely throughout the vaginal canal and have the patient move around to cause leakage from the bladder into the vagina. When this occurs, there will be a wetness and discoloration of the cotton balls within the vagina.

Moir's cotton ball or tampon test (5) may be used to help detect a ureterovaginal fistula. After a vesicovaginal fistula has been ruled out and the bladder has been drained of all blue dye, cotton balls are loosely placed throughout the length of the vaginal canal, and indigo carmine (5 mL) is administered intravenously. The patient is then asked to walk around the room. After 10 to 15 minutes, the cotton balls are sequentially removed from the vagina; if the cotton balls in the lower vagina have not been colored by the blue dye and those in the vaginal apex are blue, one should suspect a ureterovaginal fistula.

Water and air (flat-tire) test can be used to detect vesicovaginal fistulas. With the patient in the knee–chest position, the vagina is filled with sterile water or normal saline, and air or carbon dioxide is placed into the bladder through a small transurethral catheter. The escape of gas through a fistula is demonstrated by bubbles passing though the liquid within the vagina. In this respect, it is much like testing an inner tube or flat tire for a puncture. The test is most helpful in diagnosing very small vesicovaginal fistulas.

Endoscopic Examination

Cystourethroscopy is an essential part of the preoperative evaluation of patients with genitourinary fistulas. It helps determine the exact anatomic location of the fistulas and the relationship of vesicovaginal fistulas to the openings of the ureters. Importantly, cystourethroscopy also permits the evaluation of the tissues surrounding the fistula. The condition of these tissues determines the timing of surgical repair. It is likely that cystourethroscopy will have to be repeated several times during the preoperative and intraoperative management of patients with genitourinary fistulas.

Imaging

Intravenous urography should be considered in women with genitourinary fistulas, especially when their fistulas are the result of a disease process, hysterectomy, or radiation therapy. A significant number of these women have a ureterovaginal fistula or ureteral obstruction.

Retrograde ureterography may be needed to evaluate ureteral involvement or to place ureteral catheters. Cystography or hysterosalpingography may be helpful to diagnose some complicated vesicouterine fistulas. Computed tomography scans may be done in place of intravenous urograms in women with genitourinary fistulas that are associated with pelvic neoplasms and ureteral obstruction

MANAGEMENT

Preoperative Care

It is important to help the patient cope with her urine loss and improve her general health. Those who are hypoestrogenic should be given estrogen replacement, unless there is a contraindication, to improve the integrity and resistance of their vaginal tissues. Urinary tract and vaginal infections must be eradicated before any surgical procedure. It is the patient's general health and the condition of the tissues around the fistula that determine the timing of surgery for genitourinary fistulas.

Nonsurgical Treatment

Some lower urinary tract injuries that could develop into genitourinary fistulas will heal spontaneously if urine is kept from the site of the injury (6). Recent publications have recommended immediate ureteral stenting once the diagnosis of ureterovaginal fistula has been made, and the stents should be left in place for 6 to 8 weeks. In one series (7), 82% of cases healed when the fistulas were less than 1 month old, and 33% healed when the fistulas were older.

Some vesicovaginal fistulas up to 3 mm in diameter can be cured by superficial electro-surgical coagulation (8) of the epithelium of the fistulous tract followed by prolonged bladder drainage. However, deeper coagulation is more likely to devitalize and enlarge the fistula.

Surgical Treatment

Historically, the surgical approach to repairing vesicovaginal fistulas has been divided among surgical specialties, with gynecologists preferring the vaginal approach and urologists preferring the abdominal approach. More recently, however, the vaginal approach has been favored for most vesicovaginal and urethrovesicovaginal fistulas (9–11). The abdominal approach is used in cases of ureterovaginal fistulas, genitourinary fistulas that involve other organs (e.g., uterus, bowel), recurrent pelvic malignancies, or prior extensive pelvic radiation therapy. A number of general principles that apply to the repair of genitourinary fistulas (Table 27.5). Adher-

TABLE 27.5. *Principles of repair of genitourinary fistulas*

1. Prescribe prophylactic perioperative antibiotics.
2. Optimize surgical exposure, lighting, and suction.
3. Widely mobilize tissue layers about fistula.
4. Maintain meticulous hemostasis.
5. Perform multilayered, tension-free closure.
6. Provide uninterrupted postoperative urinary drainage.

ence to these principles greatly improves the results of fistula surgery.

Vesicovaginal Fistulas

Latzko Procedure

The Latzko procedure (Fig. 27.1) is recommended for small apical vesicovaginal fistulas that develop as a result of a vaginal or abdominal hysterectomy usually performed for a benign condition (12). Such fistulas are located at, or just above, the interureteric ridge (Mercier's bar) and open into the vagina anterior to the vaginal cuff. Because the procedure is actually an apical colpocleisis and does not involve surgery on the fistula tract or bladder, it can often be done soon after the development of a vesicovaginal fistula. With the patient in the lithotomy position, four stay sutures are placed around the vaginal apex at the 12-, 3-, 6-, and 9-o'clock positions, at least 2 cm from the edge of the fistula. With traction on these stay sutures, a circle or an oval is drawn 2 cm in all directions from the edge of the fistulous opening, and this is roughly divided into four quadrants. Hydrodissection with saline or a dilute vasoconstrictive agent may be used to separate the vaginal epithelium within the circle from the underlying fibromuscular layer. All of the squamous epithelium is systematically removed from within the circumference of the circle. Often, the placement of a small balloon catheter through the fistula helps in mobilizing and exposing the vaginal apex. After all of the vaginal epithelium has been removed, the vagina is closed over the fistulous tract with a first layer of interrupted absorbable (e.g., 3-0 or 4-0 chromic) suture and then two layers of inter-

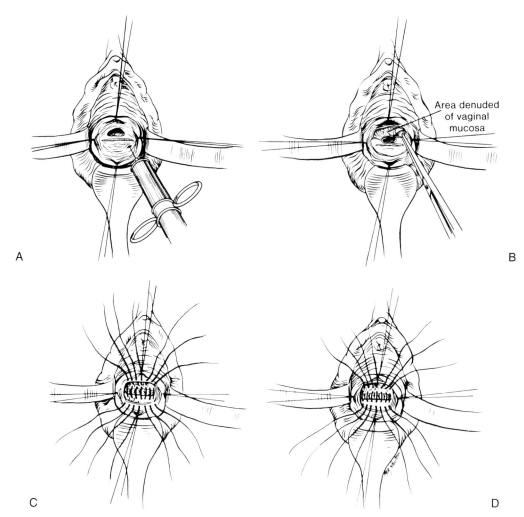

Area denuded
of vaginal
mucosa

A

B

C

D

FIG. 27.1. Latzko procedure for apical vesicovaginal fistula. **A:** Four stay sutures are placed about 2 to 3 cm from the vaginal opening of the fistula at 3, 6, 9, and 12 o'clock, and hydrodissection is used to separate the vaginal epithelium around the fistula from the underlying fibromuscular wall of the vagina. **B:** All of the vaginal epithelium is removed for a distance of 2 cm around the opening of the fistula. **C:** The fibromuscular wall of the vagina is closed in two layers using interrupted delayed-absorbable sutures. **D:** The vaginal epithelium is approximated using interrupted delayed-absorbable sutures.

rupted delayed-absorbable (e.g., 3-0 or 4-0 polyglactin or polyglycolic acid) suture. At this point, the closure is tested for watertightness by placing 250 to 300 mL of a sterile solution (e.g., indigo carmine dyed water or saline or milk) into the bladder. If there is any leakage, the site of the leakage is oversewn with additional interrupted delayed-absorbable sutures. Once the closure is watertight, the

vaginal epithelium is approximated with interrupted delayed-absorbable sutures.

Layered Vaginal Repair

Layered repairs (Figs. 27.2 through 27.4) are recommended for other genitourinary fistulas along the anterior vaginal wall. They may be urethrovaginal, vesicovaginal, or ure-

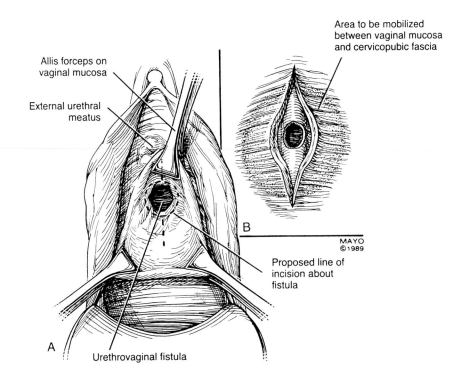

FIG. 27.2. Vaginal repair of anterior vaginal wall fistula. **A:** Proposed incision around fistulous opening. **B:** Area to be mobilized after excising scarred fistulous tract. (From Lee RA. *Atlas of gynecologic surgery.* Philadelphia: WB Saunders, 1992. By permission of Mayo Foundation.)

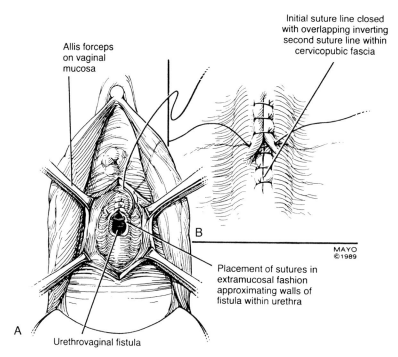

FIG. 27.3. Vaginal repair of anterior vaginal wall fistula (continued). **A:** Closure of fistula with placement of interrupted sutures in an extramucosal position. **B:** Second suture line reinforcing inverted original suture line. (From Lee RA. *Atlas of gynecologic surgery.* Philadelphia: WB Saunders, 1992. By permission of Mayo Foundation.)

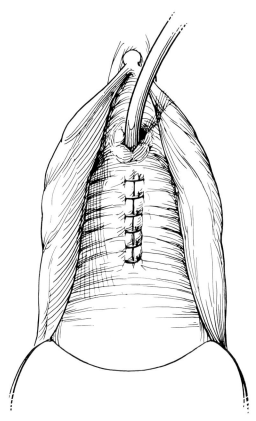

FIG. 27.4. Vaginal repair of anterior vaginal wall fistula (continued). Closed vaginal suture line with balloon catheter in place. (From Lee RA. *Atlas of gynecologic surgery.* Philadelphia: WB Saunders, 1992. By permission of Mayo Foundation.)

throvesicovaginal. Removal of the entire fistulous tract has a tendency to enlarge the fistulous opening into the bladder and may put the subsequent closure of the bladder under significant tension. It is often preferable to leave the fistulous opening into the bladder and to preserve its fibrotic ring. This minimizes tissue loss and bleeding. After widely mobilizing the tissues around the fistula, a first layer of interrupted absorbable (e.g., 3-0 or 4-0 chromic) sutures is placed in the submucosa of the bladder to close the fistula by inverting the bladder mucosa into the lumen of the bladder. After closure of the opening into the bladder, a layered closure of the bladder muscularis and subsequently of the fibro-

muscular wall of the vagina is performed using interrupted delayed-absorbable (e.g., 3-0 polyglactin or polyglycolic acid) sutures. At this point, the bladder is tested for watertightness, and any site of leakage is oversewn with interrupted delayed-absorbable sutures. Once the closure is watertight, the edges of the vaginal epithelium are approximated with more interrupted delayed-absorbable sutures. It is important to emphasize that all suture lines must be tension-free to promote healing.

Abdominal Repair

The abdominal approach is recommended for complex genitourinary fistulas involving the ureters or other pelvic organs (e.g., uterus, bowel) or those that may be associated with malignancies or are the result of radiation therapy. The vesicovaginal component of the fistula may be reached by a sagittal cystotomy to provide access to the site of the fistula (Fig. 27.5). The fistulous tract is excised, and the vesicovaginal space is widely dissected. The opening into the vagina is closed in two layers using delayed-absorbable (e.g., 3-0 polyglactin or polyglycolic acid) sutures, and the opening in the bladder is closed in three layers using absorbable (e.g., 3-0) suture to approximate the submucosa and two layers of delayed-absorbable (3-0 polyglactin or polyglycolic acid) suture to imbricate the adjacent muscularis (Fig. 27.6). It is recommended that omentum or peritoneum be placed to separate the vaginal and bladder repairs (Fig. 27.7). The involvement of adjacent organs must be individualized.

Ureterovaginal Fistulas

Historically, ureterovaginal fistulas associated with gynecologic disorders or surgery involve the distal 4 to 5 cm of the ureter. These are best treated by ureteroneocystotomy, most commonly performed using an abdominal approach. Ureterovaginal fistulas that involve the upper ureter and that are associated with a viable segment of distal ureter may be treated by ureteroureterostomy.

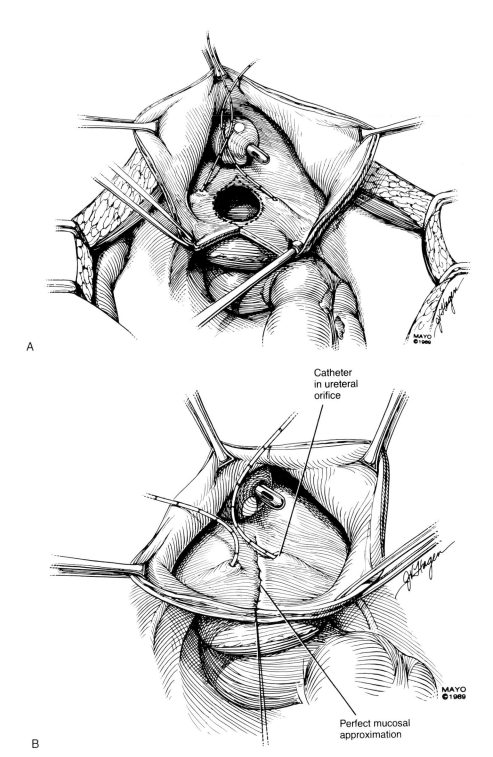

A

Catheter
in ureteral
orifice

Perfect mucosal
approximation

B

FIG 27.5. Abdominal repair of vesicovaginal fistula. **A:** Bladder opened with outline of area to be re-sected before placement of initial suture line. **B:** Extramucosal approximation by sutures resulting in approximation of bladder mucosa. (From Lee RA. *Atlas of gynecologic surgery.* Philadelphia: WB Saunders, 1992. By permission of Mayo Foundation.)

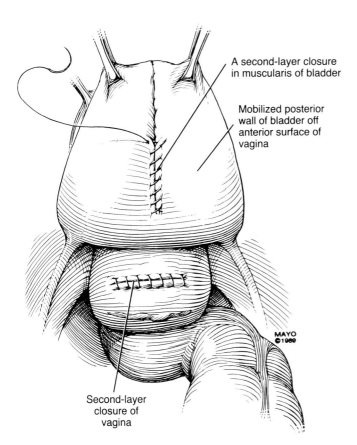

A second-layer closure
in muscularis of bladder

Mobilized posterior
wall of bladder off
anterior surface of
vagina

Second-layer
closure of
vagina

FIG. 27.6. Abdominal repair of vesicovaginal fistula (continued). Previously closed vagina suture line separated from second layer of inverting suture within wall of bladder. (From Lee RA. *Atlas of gynecologic surgery.* Philadelphia: WB Saunders, 1992. By permission of Mayo foundation.)

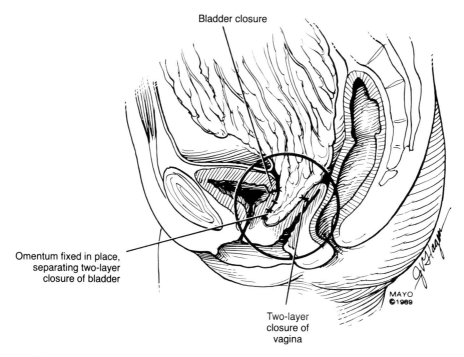

Bladder closure

Omentum fixed in place,
separating two-layer
closure of bladder

Two-layer
closure of
vagina

FIG. 27.7. Abdominal repair of vesicovaginal fistula (continued). Mobilized omentum sutured in place between closed bladder and vagina. (From Lee RA. *Atlas of gynecologic surgery.* Philadelphia: WB Saunders, 1992. By permission of Mayo foundation.)

Ureteroneocystostomy

Ureteroneocystostomy is most often done by an abdominal approach (Fig. 27.8). The distal segment of the ureter next to the bladder is ligated or oversewn with permanent suture material. The dome of the bladder is incised, and the fundus of the bladder is displaced toward the proximal end of the ureter that is to be implanted into the bladder. It is important that the anastomosis between the end of the ureter and the bladder be tension free. If there is any question about this, the bladder may be mobilized by dissecting the retropubic space and freeing the bladder from its retropubic attachments. The displacement of the bladder toward the end

of the ureter may be maintained by suturing the fundus of the bladder to the psoas muscle (e.g., psoas hitch) with permanent suture material. The female bladder is considered a low-pressure organ; therefore, it is usually satisfactory to perform a direct implantation of the end of the ureter into the bladder. After the end of the ureter is tagged with fine suture material, a tonsil clamp is passed through the wall for the bladder from inside the bladder toward the end of the ureter. The opening in the bladder is stretched to prevent stenosis. The ends of the suture tags are grasped, and the end of the ureter is brought into the bladder. The ends of the ureter are spatulated for a distance of about 0.5 cm on opposite sides of the ureter, and the

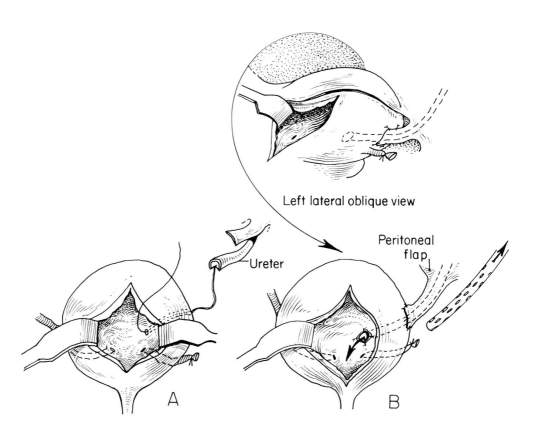

FIG. 27.8. Abdominal ureteroneocystostomy. **A:** Abdominal cystotomy in extraperitoneal dome of bladder with traction suture drawing ureter through wall of bladder; ligation of distal ureteral segment. **B:** Ureter sutured to bladder mucosa; peritoneal flap and adventitial sheath of ureter sutured to bladder muscularis at its site of entry into bladder. (From Symmonds RE. Ureteral injuries associated with gynecologic surgery: prevention and management. *Clin Obstet Gynecol* 1976;19: 623–644, with permission.)

resulting flaps are sutured to the inside of the bladder with absorbable (e.g. 3-0 or 4-0 chromic) sutures. The adventitial sheath of the ureter is then anchored to the outside of the bladder with delayed-absorbable (e.g., 3-0 or 4-0 polyglactin or polyglycolic acid) sutures. The incision in the dome of the bladder is closed by two layers of delayed-absorbable (e.g., 3-0 polyglactin or polyglycolic acid) sutures. Whenever there is concern about ureteral reflux, tunneling of the distal ureter within the wall of the bladder is protective of the kidneys. The site of anastomosis of the end of the ureter and the bladder should have a suction drain placed to evacuate any urine or serum that might jeopardize the repair.

Ureteroureterostomy

Ureteroureterostomy joins the two ends of a cut ureter. It is important to freshen the ends of any damaged tissue and to anastomose the ends without tension. The ends of the ureter are spatulated to protect the anastomosis from stricture, and the ends are sutured together over a stenting catheter using fine interrupted absorbable or delayed-absorbable suture. This anastomosis site should be drained with a suction drain to remove any urine or serum that may jeopardize the repair.

Complex Genitourinary Fistulas

In these cases, defects in the ureters, bladder, and urethra are repaired using the general principles of genitourinary fistula repair through either the vaginal or abdominal approach that has been described. The management of other organs that may be involved in the fistula has to be individualized. The surgeon is encouraged to use peritoneum or omentum to separate the layers of a repair that involves the urinary tract, vagina, and bowel.

Postoperative Complications and Care

Common postoperative complications may be grouped as occurring early or late (Table 27.6). It is important that all repairs be performed with attention to obtaining strict hemostasis and a watertight, tension-free approximation of tissues. The development of a hematoma or urinoma will jeopardize the results of a repair.

TABLE 27.6. *Postoperative complications*

Early
Bleeding
Bladder spasms
Wound infection
Wound dehiscence
Late
Stress incontinence
Vaginal stenosis
Small capacity bladder
Dyspareunia

After most genitourinary fistula repairs, it is important to provide adequate, uninterrupted urinary drainage. As for the bladder, this may be accomplished by a suprapubic or transurethral catheter. The catheter must be of large-enough caliber to allow for the passage of blood and some clots. Ureteroneocystostomies and ureteroureterostomies usually leave the operating room with ureteral and bladder catheters. The ureteral catheters drain the kidney and act as stents to help prevent stricture at the site of the anastomosis; the bladder catheters drain the bladder to protect the cystotomy site. There are those who use catheters in patients who have Latzko procedures and those who do not. It would be better to provide urine drainage rather than risk the disruption of a repair as a result of urinary retention. Surgery on the lower urinary tract and the presence of catheters can predispose to painful bladder spasms. When these occur, anticholinergic therapy should be considered.

Perioperative prophylactic antibiotics are recommended for genitourinary fistula repairs. Whether to continue the antibiotics during the immediate postoperative period is left up to the surgeon's discretion. Under any circumstances, if a urinary tract infection develops, the organism must be identified and treated with appropriate antibiotic therapy.

After the repair of a genitourinary fistula, it is recommended that the patient observe a period of "pelvic rest," refraining from using vaginal tampons, administering vaginal douches, or having vaginal intercourse. In most cases, the physician performing a digital or speculum examination of the vagina during the immediate postoperative period gains little. It is best to refrain from manipulation of the vagina for at least 8 to 12 weeks after the repair of most genitourinary fistulas.

Results

The two most controversial topics regarding surgical repair of genitourinary fistulas are the timing of surgery and the surgical approach, whether vaginal or abdominal. Recent reports support early repair after the inflammatory process around the fistula has subsided. However, patients who are considered poor surgical risks for other reasons and those whose fistulas are the result of radiation therapy or recurrent malignancies may benefit from a delay in their fistula repair. Also, the surgical literature now reflects the general opinion that genitourinary fistulas that involve the urethra, bladder, and vagina may be approached, at least initially, vaginally. Those that involve the ureter and adjacent organs and those caused by radiation therapy or recurrent malignancy may be approached abdominally.

Most sizeable series report the cure rate of vesicovaginal fistulas to be higher than 90% to 95% on the first attempt at repair.

REFERENCES

1. Flores-Carreras O, Cabrera JR, Galeano PA, et al. Fistulas of the urinary tract in gynecologic and obstetric surgery. *Int Urogynecol J* 2001;12:203–214.
2. Mettauer JP. Vesico-vaginal fistula. *Boston Med J* 1840; 22:154–155.
3. Sims JM. On the treatment of vesico-vaginal fistula. *Am J Med Sci* 1852;23:59–82.
4. Härkki-Sirén P, Sjöberg J, Tiitinen A. Urinary tract injuries after hysterectomy. *Obstet Gynecol* 1998;92:113–118.
5. Moir JC. Vesico-vaginal fistulae as seen in Britain. *J Obstet Gynaecol Br Commonw* 1973;80:598–601.
6. Waaldijk K. The immediate surgical management of fresh obstetrics fistulas with catheter and/or early closure. *Int J Gynaecol Obstet* 1994;45:11–16.
7. DeBaere T, Roche A, Lagrange C. Combined percutaneous antegrade and cystoscopic retrograde approach in the treatment of distal ureteral fistulae. *Cardiovasc Intervent Radiol* 1995;18:349–352.
8. Stovsky JD, Ignatoff JM, Blum MD, et al. Use of electrocoagulation in the treatment of vesicovaginal fistulas. *J Urol* 1994;152:1443–1444.
9. Blaivas JG, Heritz DM, Romanzi LJ. Early versus late repair of vesicovaginal fistulas: vaginal and abdominal approaches. *J Urol* 1995;153:1110–1113.
10. Blandy JP, Badenoch DF, Fowler CG, et al. Early repair of iatrogenic injury to the ureter or bladder after gynecological surgery. *J Urol* 1991;146:761–765.
11. Selzman AA, Spirnak JP, Kursh ED. The changing management of ureterovaginal fistulas. *J Urol* 1995;153: 626–628.
12. Latzko W. Postoperative vesicovaginal fistulas; genesis and therapy. *Am J Surg* 1942:58:211–228.

Ostergard's Urogynecology and Pelvic Floor Dysfunction, Fifth Edition. edited by A.E. Bent, et al. Lippincott Williams & Wilkins, Philadelphia © 2003.

28

Nonsurgical Treatment of Stress Urinary Incontinence

John James Klutke* and Arieh Bergman**

* Department of Obstetrics and Gynecology, USC-Keck School of Medicine, Los Angeles, California
** Department of Obstetrics and Gynecology, University of Southern California, School of Medicine, Los Angeles, California

Not all incontinent women are bothered enough to accept the risks of surgery. With 13 million incontinent women in the United States, the costs of surgery would exclude it from being a therapy of first choice in most. The magnitude of the problem of incontinence and its cost, more than $26 billion annually in the United States, has inspired interest in effective and relatively inexpensive nonsurgical alternatives for treating stress incontinence (1). Current recommendation of the Agency for Health Care Policy and Research is to advise nonsurgical therapy in nearly all patients with stress incontinence before surgery is attempted (2). Given the aging of the American population, the trend toward nonsurgical therapy can only be expected to increase.

Surgery has great success in correcting stress urinary incontinence but may limit future therapeutic options. After a failed anti-incontinence operation, a subsequent surgery will itself have a higher failure rate. Conservative estimates predict that nonsurgical therapy will cure 10% of patients with stress incontinence and substantially improve another 40% (3). When 50 women with stress incontinence were randomly treated with either surgery or exercises, almost half of the conservatively treated group were improved or cured (4). Those patients that failed the conservative treatment still had the option of surgery open to them in the future.

Many women are suited to nonsurgical therapy. They include frail elderly patients who face a prohibitive surgical risk and young patients who want to have children in the future. Younger women may not want to deal with a long convalescence after surgery. Surgery for stress incontinence remains an elective procedure in all cases.

PELVIC FLOOR MUSCLE REHABILITATION

The pelvic floor muscles contribute to continence by supporting the vagina and acting as a bladder sphincter (5). The striated muscle component contains two fiber types: slow-twitch or type I fibers, which use aerobic oxidative metabolism; and fast-twitch or type II fibers, which use anaerobic glycolytic metabolism for rapid forceful contractions in response to sudden increases in intraabdominal pressure.

Muscle fibers with greater aerobic oxidative capacity have less resistance to fatigue, and vice versa. The periurethral levator ani muscle is composed of 70% type I fibers and 30% type II fibers. The levator ani supports the pelvic organs and forms the scaffolding to which the pelvic ligaments attach (6). The striated urethral sphincter muscle contains almost exclusively type I or slow-twitch fibers and is important in intrinsic urethral function and passive continence (7).

The strength of muscular contraction depends on the muscle's cross-sectional area. Partial denervation of the pelvic floor muscles occurs with aging and childbirth (8). Delayed conduction of impulses to the pelvic floor muscles is present in women with stress urinary incontinence (9). Denervated muscle tissue atrophies, resulting in weaker muscular contractions and more rapid onset of fatigue. Both types of fibers, but especially the slow-twitch fibers, are capable of hypertrophy with appropriate training. Exercises that cause hypertrophy of the pelvic floor muscles improve the efficiency of their supportive and sphincteric actions.

Arnold Kegel posited that denervation injury occurs with childbearing and was the first to develop a method to rehabilitate the pelvic floor muscles (10). In Kegel's original publication, he recognized the importance of segregation, guidance, and progression in pelvic floor muscle training. These principles are often forgotten when pelvic floor exercises are prescribed. Indeed, because the appropriate muscles are anatomically hidden and not normally noticed in daily activity, inadequate instruction in their identification may result in exercises that are counterproductive to the control of incontinence. Patients frequently contract the rectus abdominis muscle, promoting loss of urine. Bump and colleagues (11) showed that more than half of a series of patients with stress incontinence contracted inappropriate muscles after brief verbal instruction in Kegel exercises.

Digital vaginal examination with one hand palpating the patient's abdomen should confirm contraction of the pubococcygeus and not the abdominal muscles. We instruct our patients to sit on the toilet seat at home to identify the pubococcygeus muscle by stopping the flow of urine without moving their legs. Once the appropriate muscle is isolated, patients are instructed to contract and hold for 10 seconds in groups of 10 contractions, three times daily. To train both fast- and slow-twitch fibers, sustained maximal contractions should be combined with "quick flicks," that is, brief forceful contractions. Patients should perform the contractions in different positions to limit Valsalva-type efforts. They need close follow-up and frequent positive reinforcement for the exercises to be optimally effective. The exercises are supervised by a dedicated physiotherapist, and, ideally, follow-up is twice weekly in the initial sessions. Patients who improve should note a change within 2 to 3 months.

A study assessed the effect of Kegel exercises in an objective manner. Fifty-six percent of stress incontinent women considered their problem substantially improved or cured when Kegel exercises were performed under optimal conditions (36 subjects studied) (12). Other researchers reported similar success rates of 47% to 67% in patients treated with Kegel exercises for stress incontinence (13–15).

Peattie and colleagues (16) used a novel and ingenious technique to strengthen the pelvic floor muscles. Patients used a weighted vaginal cone in the vagina, inserted tip down, and retained it for 15 minutes. Cones of increasing weights from 20 to 100 g were used progressively. The cone orients vertically in the vagina with the apex pointing downward, and lateral pressure from contraction of the pelvic floor muscles causes retention, whereas force directed at the cone's base (Valsalva) causes it to slip out. The tactile feedback of the cone slipping out of the vagina directs the patient to contract the pelvic floor muscles while she relaxes the muscles that cause a Valsalva. Seventy percent of women participating reported significant improvement after using these cones for 1 month. Similar results were reported by other groups (17–19).

BIOFEEDBACK

Filling and storage of urine requires accommodation of increasing volumes of urine without bladder contraction in the presence of a competent bladder outlet. Detrusor control and contraction of the striated muscle sphincter are learned processes, making incontinence a kind of behavioral deficit. Biofeedback, a behavioral therapy, effectively facilitates the learning of skills necessary to overcome this deficit.

Biofeedback is a therapeutic process that furnishes information on the state of a physiologic variable to enable the individual to gain voluntary control over the variable being monitored. The goal in applying biofeedback to stress incontinence is to increase the efficiency and magnitude of muscular contraction of the pelvic floor muscles. Its application to pelvic floor muscle exercises is not new and dates back to Kegel's original work (10). Kegel's technique involved monitoring the intravaginal pressure with a device called a perineometer. Patients were able to increase progressively the efficiency of their pelvic floor muscle exercises using the visual feedback of intravaginal pressure. Kegel reported a 90% improvement in 455 patients treated.

Another variable monitored for feedback is vaginal electrical activity. This can be detected in the pelvic floor with a surface electrode and furnished to the patient as an audi-tory or visual cue. Using electrical activity for biofeedback has the advantage of reflecting pelvic floor muscular activity only, independent of abdominal muscle contraction. An investigation of this technique in patients with stress urinary incontinence reported a 76% reduction in incontinence (20). Like pelvic floor muscular exercises, all forms of biofeedback require a highly motivated patient and the supervision of a trained therapist.

FUNCTIONAL ELECTRICAL STIMULATION

Functional electrical stimulation is based on the premise that contraction of the periurethral and paraurethral striated muscles reflexively causes inhibition and relaxation of the detrusor (Fig. 28.1). Electrical stimulation of the nerves supplying the pelvic floor initiates this process. The technique is passive in

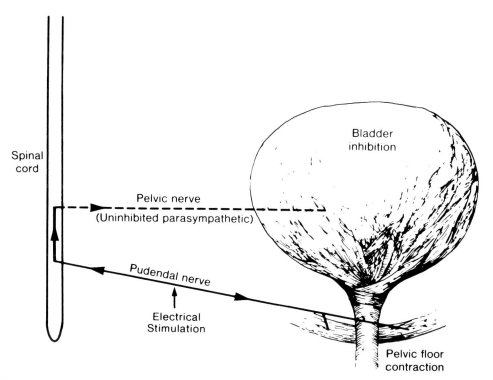

FIG. 28.1. Electrical stimulation. Pudendal nerve stimulation can cause a direct pelvic floor contraction, an increase in urethral pressure, and, through the spinal cord, a reflex pelvic nerve stimulation, which results in inhibition of bladder activity.

that it does not require the active participation of the patient. Functional electrical stimulation may be particularly suited to mixed incontinence because of the simultaneous detrusor inhibition. Like pelvic floor muscular exercise, however, at least partial innervation of the pelvic floor musculature must exist for the technique to be effective.

Bors (21) first described the effect of electrical stimulation on the bladder neck, and Caldwell and associates (22) demonstrated its effectiveness in the treatment of incontinence. Early attempts, although effective, were cumbersome technically. In the technique described by Caldwell and associates, electrodes were surgically implanted in the pelvic floor. Since then, sophisticated and reliable devices have evolved. Electrodes are removable, in the form of vaginal pessaries or vaginal and anal plugs. Treatment can be given in the office or with portable battery-operated devices that the patient takes home. To date, the effectiveness and the optimal parameters for treatment have not been established.

Electrical stimulation has been used widely in the area of muscle rehabilitation to improve the function of weak or atrophied muscles. Women with stress incontinence benefit by application of this therapy to the muscles of the pelvic floor. It is difficult to compare this therapy to other forms of muscle rehabilitation because the effects are more profound than those of a "passive Kegel." Besides contraction of the pelvic floor muscles, activation of an inhibitory reflex on the detrusor muscles occurs, achieving relaxation of the bladder detrusor. Chronic stimulation, moreover, is thought to induce changes in the composition of the striated sphincter muscles as the nervous control of the muscles is reprogrammed (23). Available modalities include direct stimulation of the sacral nerve roots and stimulation of the pudendal nerve with electrodes placed in the vagina or anus. Optimal patterns of stimulation have not been established. Sand and colleagues (24) achieved cure or significant improvement in 89% in women with stress incontinence treated with an insertable vaginal electrode,

the Innova device (Empi, Inc., St. Paul, Minnesota), for 12 weeks. Recommended parameters for stimulation with this device are a frequency of 50 Hz with current up to 100 mA as determined by the patient's comfort level. The device is used for 15 minutes twice a day, every other day. Frequency settings for stress incontinence are, in general, higher than for urge incontinence.

MEDICATIONS

Treating incontinence often falls within the much broader context of treating the menopausal woman. Estrogen-replacement therapy in deficient women has a well-established role in reducing atrophic changes and osteoporosis.

Menopause is associated with a general weakening of connective tissue owing to impaired synthesis and metabolism of collagen (25). The density of bone and dermal thickness, for example, decline in parallel after menopause (26). Collagen is the main constituent of these tissues and is also the key structural component in the support of the pelvic organs. Fibroblasts in the pelvic ligaments produce and secrete collagen and have estrogen receptors (27,28). Lack of estrogen, therefore, may explain an accelerated rate of pelvic organ prolapse in menopause. Defective anatomic support of the bladder neck is largely responsible for stress incontinence (29).

As a short-term remedy for stress incontinence, estrogen's role remains unproved. Only a small number of randomized clinical trials have adequately studied the effect of estrogen on genuine stress incontinence (30–35). None of these studies assessed estrogen's role as a preventative measure.

If estrogen has a theoretical basis in anatomic support, its effect on the urethra's intrinsic function is clear. Intrinsic urethral function describes the component of urinary continence not dependent on anatomic support of the urethra (36). The physiologic factors responsible for this function include the periurethral striated muscle, neurologic tone of the bladder neck, urethral vascularity, and mucosal surface tension. All of these factors depend on estrogen stimulation.

The lower urinary tract and vagina develop from a common primordial structure. The histochemical similarities between mature vaginal and urethral tissue include a high concentration of estrogen receptors (37). Estrogen stimulation causes maturation of the mucosa of the urethra, with improvement in lower urinary tract symptoms, such as incontinence (38,39). Estrogen replacement therapy in the patient with atrophic vaginitis improves blood flow to the pelvis, manifested as decreased dyspareunia and increased vaginal lubrication (40).

Estrogen potentiates α-adrenergic transmission in the urethra in animal tissue preparations (41–43). The combination of an α-adrenergic agonist with estrogen in women with stress incontinence improves estrogen's effectiveness both subjectively and in terms of specific urodynamic parameters. Beisland and co-workers (44) treated 18 postmenopausal women with stress incontinence in a prospective randomized crossover trial. Oral phenylpropanolamine and vaginal estriol were given separately and in combination. With combined treatment, 8 patients became completely continent, and 9 were considerably improved. Similar cure rates were reported in another prospective clinical trial using norepinephrine in combination with oral estradiol (45). Kinn and Lindskog (46) carried out a randomized crossover trial with 36 postmenopausal women with stress incontinence. Additive effects of combination treatment with oral estriol and phenylpropanolamine reduced the number and amount of leakage episodes by 40%. Finally, Ahlstrom and colleagues (47) studied 29 postmenopausal women with stress incontinence in a randomized double-blind trial. They showed that a combination treatment of phenylpropanolamine and oral estriol was more effective than estriol alone in treating the incontinence.

Medications with α-adrenergic properties are common constituents of over-the-counter diet suppressants (Table 28.1). We prescribe Ornade Spansules, one tablet orally twice a day. Imipramine and other tricyclic antidepressants have anticholinergic effects in addition to α-adrenergic effects. We prefer imipramine in patients with mixed incontinence. Patients may be given up to 150 mg daily. A trial of 8 weeks is allowed for these medications.

TABLE 28.1. *Currently available dietary suppressants containing phenylpropanolamine*

		Dosages	
Drug	How supplied	Phenylpropanolamine (mg)	Caffeine (mg)
Anorexin	C	25	100
Anorexin One-Span	C, SR	50	200
Appedrine	T	25	100[a]
Contac	C, SR	75	—[b]
Control	C, SR	75	—
Dexatrim Extra Strength	C, SR	75	200
Dexatrim	C, SR	75	—
Diet Gard	C, T	25	—
Dietac	C, SR	50	200
Dietac	T	25	—
Dietac	D	25	—
E-Z Trim	C, SR	75	—
Ornade	C, SR	75	—
Prolamine	C	37.5	140[b]
Super Odrinex	T	25	100

C, capsule; SR, sustained release; T, tablet; D, drops.
[a]Also contains vitamins.
[b]Also contains chlorpheniramine.

Until evidence disproves estrogen's role in stress urinary incontinence, we recommend its use in all estrogen-deficient women without contraindication to estrogen replacement therapy. We prefer to use conjugated equine estrogen cream, 2 g intravaginally every other day, with the dose reduced by half once a response is demonstrated. Ideally, patients are simultaneously prescribed α-sympathomimetic drugs. These latter medications, however, affect the vascular tone, and their contraindications should be observed carefully.

OBSTRUCTIVE DEVICES

Stress incontinence results when the bladder outlet no longer resists increases in intraabdominal pressure, and the aim of corrective surgery is to create increased urethral resistance. The effect of a successful operation is obstructive in the sense that leakage of urine occurs at higher abdominal pressures, if at all. Ideally, obstruction in the surgically cured patient is in effect during filling but not during voiding. The physiology that results in continence is complex, however, and it is not possible to separate filling from voiding. Feedback regulates the two states, and surgical intervention to increase urethral resistance during the filling state risks interfering with normal voiding. Although new surgical techniques are simpler and minimize perioperative morbidity, the risk for inducing voiding dysfunction will be present as long as the procedure has efficacy in correcting stress incontinence. Controllable obstructive devices are appealing in that the therapeutic effect is reversible, and obstruction can be overridden at the time of voiding.

These simple devices include small adhesive patches that occlude the urethra, urethral inserts, and vaginal prostheses that press on the anterior vaginal wall. Their use is office-based and can be terminated at any time by the patient.

Brubaker and co-workers (48) reported the results of a large multicenter study investigating the safety and efficacy of the Miniguard

(Advanced Surgical Innovations, San Clemente, California), an adhesive foam patch that sticks to the external urethral meatus and occludes it. The study was an uncontrolled trial and was supported by the manufacturer. It was limited to women with mild or moderate incontinence symptoms, and the examiners were not blinded for evaluation of the data. Three hundred forty-six women completed the 21-week trial and reported a significant decrease in the severity score of their leakage. Although efficacy was reported in subjective measures and pad testing, most of the patients did not attain complete control of their symptoms. This was attributed to the limited adhesive power of the device, and the authors surmised that it would be ineffective in women with severe incontinence. The device was well tolerated, and only three women discontinued the trial. There was a significant incidence of vulvar irritation (3.8%) and irritative voiding symptoms (6.1%) associated with use of the device. An average of four of the disposable devices were used each day, but the cost per device was not specified.

Although the Miniguard appeared to benefit the patients studied, no comparison was made in the study to other nonsurgical therapies. Kegel exercises will benefit many women with mild to moderate incontinence symptoms. It is impossible to determine from Brubaker's study whether the Miniguard is more effective than simple exercises.

FemAssist (Insight Medical, Boston, Massachusetts) is a small cup-shaped disk that adheres to the external urethral meatus by suction vacuum pressure. The device can, according to the manufacturer, be reused for up to 1 week. Although the expense of FemAssist is offset somewhat by its reusability, its efficacy is limited, and many patients discontinue use of the device because of discomfort. Moore and colleagues (49) enrolled 97 patients in a study of the FemAssist, of which only 57 (57%) completed the 1-month trial. Of the 57 women who completed 1 month of use, 27 (47%) were continent on pad testing.

Several intraurethral occlusive devices have been developed. They are held in place by a plate or knob at either end that lodges the plug between the bladder neck and the external urethral meatus. The device can be removed when the user wants to void. Because the base of the plug protrudes from the urethra, there is a risk for bacterial colonization and urinary tract infection.

Sand and associates (50) evaluated the Reliance device (Uromed, Norwood, Massachusetts), a small urethral insert with a balloon at its proximal end that the patient inflates to hold the device in place. The balloon rests above the bladder neck, obstructing the flow of urine. The balloon can be deflated by an attached string, allowing removal of the device and voiding. The device is disposable and is approved by the U.S. Food and Drug Administration. In the study by Sand and associates, urine loss was reduced or eliminated in 91% of 63 women who answered a validated questionnaire. Complications associated with the Reliance device include bacteriuria in 30% of users, gross hematuria in 24%, and mucosal irritation in 9% (51). The device costs $3 per insert, and, averaging four voids each day, use of the Reliance device would result in a yearly expense of $4,368.

Bladder neck support prostheses are worn in the vagina and press against the anterior vaginal wall and urethra. Although the mechanism of these devices in correcting incontinence is presumably by obstruction, the effect is apparently mild, and urine flow rates are unaffected during voiding (52). Support prostheses include the Conveen Continence Guard (Johnson & Johnson, New Brunswick, New Jersey) and the Introl device (Uromed, Norwood, Massachusetts). Of 69 women included in an open prospective study of one prosthesis, 4 (6%) could not be fitted, and 39 (56%) later withdrew from the study, mainly because of lack of efficacy and adverse events (52). Twenty of the remaining 26 patients (77%) achieved cure or social continence. Another study evaluated reuse of the Conveen Continence Guard, a device recommended by the manufacturer for single use only. Although harmful bacteriologic or biochemical changes in the vagina were not identified, the investi-gators also noted a decreased efficacy associated with reuse (53).

Conventional vaginal pessaries have also been used to prevent stress incontinence. Several pessaries, such as the Smith, Hodge, and Gellhorn types, provide support to the proximal urethra. These pessaries restore continence by stabilizing the bladder base and increasing functional urethral length (54). There are now specific ring and dish continence pessaries available with urethral support for women who need temporary relief during vigorous activity.

INDWELLING INTRAURETHRAL DEVICES

To date, little attempt has been made to develop a remotely controlled sphincter that is entirely intraurethral. This design would minimize bacterial colonization and allow long-term use. The challenge of this approach from a design standpoint would be to devise a non-reactive device that functions reliably in the body's hostile environment. It would need to stay in place in the urethra and have a fail-safe mechanism to prevent transmission of high pressures to the upper urinary tract. Expanding biomedical and material technology may make this challenge attainable.

Recently, an Israeli group reported the development of and early experience with a new intraurethral sphincter prosthesis containing a remote-controlled valve and pump (55). The device is made of silicone and is held in place at the bladder neck with soft, expandable silicone fins. Although initial experience with the device was encouraging, the experience of another group assessing the device was somewhat disappointing (56). Eighteen women with neurogenic voiding disorders and urinary retention were evaluated prospectively. Only 6 patients (33%) were satisfied with the device and continued to use it at 16 months of follow-up. Incontinence or urethral irritation led to removal of the device in 10 patients (55%), and 2 others (11%) were unable to use it properly. Twelve patients (67%) had bacteriuria while using the device, and 6 of these developed symptoms of urinary tract infection.

SUMMARY

The mainstay of therapy for stress incontinence since the 1900s has been to suspend the bladder neck by one of several surgical techniques that have significant morbidity. In 1995, the societal cost associated with incontinence in individuals 65 years of age and older was estimated at $3,565 per individual (1). With the aging of the American population, an inexpensive and effective treatment of incontinence is becoming increasingly important.

A trial of nonsurgical therapy is recommended in virtually all patients with stress incontinence. Up to 50% of patients treated in this conservative fashion may improve enough to forgo surgery.

The various conservative modalities for treating stress incontinence each aim at a different aspect of the continence mechanism. These modalities can thus be combined for optimal benefit.

Estrogen forms a cornerstone in the treatment of the menopausal woman. Estrogen has recognized physiologic effects on the lower urinary tract. Estrogen in conjunction with α-adrenergic medications appears to be effective in treating mild genuine stress incontinence by improving intrinsic urethral function.

The muscles of the pelvis promote continence through a supportive and sphincteric function. Loss of this function occurs with the denervation injury of childbirth and aging. Pelvic muscle training in the form of Kegel exercises or with weighted vaginal cones is effective in improving this function. Pelvic floor exercises can be optimized with biofeedback or with functional electrical stimulation, which has neuromodulating effects on the pelvic floor muscles.

REFERENCES

1. Wagner TH, Hu TW. Economic costs of urinary incontinence in 1995. *Urology* 1998;51:355–361.
2. Urinary Incontinence Guideline Panel. *Urinary incontinence in adults: clinical practice guidelines.* Rockville, MD: U.S. Department of Health and Human Services. AHCPR Publication no. 92-0038. March 1992.
3. Richardson DA. Conservative management of urinary incontinence: a symposium. *J Reprod Med* 1993;38:659–661.
4. Klarskov P, Belving D, Bischoff N, et al. Pelvic floor exercise versus surgery for female urinary incontinence. *Urol Int* 1986;41:129–132.
5. Delancy JO, Richardson AC. Anatomy of genital support. In: Benson JT, ed. *Female pelvic floor disorders, investigation and management.* New York: WW Norton, 1992:19–26.
6. Zacharin R. The suspensory mechanism of the female urethra. *J Anat* 1963;97:423–427.
7. Eriksen BC. Electrical stimulation. In: Benson JT, ed. *Female pelvic floor disorders, investigation and management.* New York: WW Norton, 1992:222.
8. Peterson I, Franksson C, Danielson GO. Electromyography of the pelvic floor and urethra in normal females. *Acta Obstet Gynecol Scand* 1955;34:273–285.
9. Snooks SJ, Badenoch DF, Tiptaft RC, et al. Perineal nerve damage in genuine stress urinary incontinence: an electrophysiologic study. *Br J Urol* 1985;57:422–426.
10. Kegel AH. Progressive resistance exercise in the functional restoration of the perineal muscles. *Am J Obstet Gynecol* 1948;56:238–248.
11. Bump RC, Hurt WG, Fantl JA, et al. Assessment of Kegel pelvic muscle exercises after brief verbal instruction. *Am J Obstet Gynecol* 1991;165:322–327.
12. Elia G, Bergman A. Pelvic muscle exercises: when do they work? *Obstet Gynecol* 1993;81:283–286.
13. Henalla SM, Kirwan P, Castleden CM, et al. The effect of pelvic floor exercises in the treatment of genuine urinary stress incontinence in women at two hospitals. *Br J Obstet Gynaecol* 1988;95:602–606.
14. Mouritsen L, Frimodt-Moller C, Moller M. Long-term effect of pelvic floor exercises on female urinary incontinence. *Br J Urol* 1991;68:32–37.
15. Hahn I, Milsom I, Fall M, et al. Long-term results of pelvic floor training in female stress urinary incontinence. *Br J Urol* 1993;72:421–427.
16. Peattie AB, Plevnik S, Stanton SL. Vaginal cones: a conservative method of treating genuine stress incontinence. *Br J Obstet Gynecol* 1988;95:1049–1053.
17. Olah KS, Bridges N, Denning J, et al. The conservative management of patients with symptoms of stress incontinence: a randomized, prospective study comparing weighted vaginal cones and interferential therapy. *Am J Obstet Gynecol* 1990;162:87–92.
18. Wilson PD, Borland M. Vaginal cones for the treatment of genuine stress incontinence. *Aust N Z J Obstet Gynaecol* 1990;30:157–160.
19. Kato K, Kondo A, Hasegawa S, et al. Pelvic floor muscle training as treatment of stress incontinence: the effectiveness of vaginal cones. *Nippon Hinyokika Gakkai Zasshi* 1992;88:498–504.
20. McIntosh LJ, Frahm JD, Mallett VT, et al. Pelvic floor rehabilitation in the treatment of incontinence *J Reprod Med* 1993;38:663–666.
21. Bors E. Effect of electric stimulation of the pudendal nerves on the vesical neck: its significance for the function of cord bladders. A preliminary report. *J Urol* 1952;67:925–935.
22. Caldwell KPS, Flack FC, Broad AF. Urinary incontinence following spinal injury treated by electronic implants. *Lancet* 1965;1:846–847.
23. Bazeed MA, Thuroff JW, Schmidt RA, et al. Effect of electrostimulation of the sacral roots on the striated urethral sphincter. *J Urol* 1982;128:1357–1358.
24. Sand PK, Richardson DA, Staskin DR, et al. Pelvic

floor electrical stimulation in the treatment of genuine stress incontinence: a multicenter, placebo-controlled trial. *Am J Obstet Gynecol* 1995;173:72–79.

25. Albright F, Smith PH, Richardson AM. Postmenopausal osteoporosis: its clinical features. *JAMA* 1941; 116:2465–2474.

26. Brincat M, Moniz CF, Kabalan S, et al. Decline in skin collagen content and metacarpal index after the menopause and its prevention with sex hormone replacement. *Br J Obstet Gynaecol* 1987;94:126–129.

27. Dube JY, Lesage RL, Tremblay RR. Androgen and estrogen binding in rat skeletal and perineal muscles. *Can J Biochem* 1976;54:50–55.

28. Dionne FT, Lesage RL, Dube JY. Estrogen binding proteins in rat skeletal and perineal muscles: in vitro and in vivo studies. *J Steroid Biochem* 1979;11:1073–1080.

29. Enhorning G. Simultaneous recording of intra urethral and intra vesical pressure: a study on urethral closure in stress incontinent women. *Scand J Urol Nephrol* 1978; 12:105–119.

30. Judge TG. The use of quinestradiol in elderly incontinent women. *Gerontol Clin* 1969;11:159–164.

31. Walter S, Wolf H, Barlebo H, et al. Urinary incontinence in postmenopausal women treated with oestrogens: a double blind clinical trial. *Urol Int* 1978;33:135–143.

32. Samsioe G, Jansson I, Mellstrom D, et al. Occurrence, nature and treatment of urinary incontinence in a 70 year old female population. *Maturitas* 1985;7:335–342.

33. Wilson PD, Faragher B, Butler B, et al. Treatment with oral piperazine oestrone sulphate for genuine stress incontinence in postmenopausal women. *Br J Obstet Gynaecol* 1987;94:568–574.

34. Foidart JM, Vervliet J, Buytaert PH. Efficacy of sustained-release vaginal estriol in alleviating urogenital and systemic climacteric complaints. *Maturitas* 1991;13: 99–107.

35. Fantl JA, Bump RA, Robinson D. Efficacy of estrogen supplementation in the treatment of urinary incontinence. *Obstet Gynecol* 1996;88:745–748.

36. Blaivas JG, Klutke CG, Raz S, et al. When sphincter failure is the cause of female stress incontinence. *Contemp Urol* 1993;1004;1–11.

37. Iosif S, Batra S, Ek A, et al. Estrogen receptors in the human female lower urinary tract. *Am J Obstet Gynecol* 1981;141:817–820.

38. Bergman A, Karram MM, Bhatia NN. Changes in urethral cytology following estrogen administration. *Gynecol Obstet Invest* 1990;29:211–213.

39. Salmon UJ, Walter RI, Geist SA. The use of estrogens in the treatment of dysuria and incontinence in postmenopausal women. *Am J Obstet Gynecol* 1941;42: 845–851.

40. Sarrel PM. Sexuality and menopause. *Obstet Gynecol* 1990;75:26S–32S.

41. Levin RM, Jacobowitz D, Wein AJ. Autonomic innervation of rabbit urinary bladder following estrogen administration. *Urology* 1981;17:449–453.

42. Hodgson BT, Dumas S, Bolling DR, et al. Effect of estrogen on sensitivity of rabbit bladder and urethra to phenylephrine. *Invest Urol* 1978;16:67–69.

43. Levin RM, Shofer FS, Wein AJ. Cholinergic, adrenergic and purinergic response of sequential strips of rabbit urinary bladder. *J Pharmacol Exp Ther* 1980;212:536–540.

44. Beisland HO, Fossberg E, Moer A, et al. Urethral sphincteric insufficiency in postmenopausal females: treatment with phenylpropanolamine and estriol separately and in combination. A urodynamic and clinical evaluation. *Urol Int* 1984;39:211–216.

45. Ek A, Andersson KE, Gullberg B, et al. Effects of oestradiol and combined norephedrin and oestradiol treatment on female stress incontinence. *Zentralbl Gynaekol* 1980;102:839–844.

46. Kinn A, Lindskog M. Estrogens and phenylpropanolamine in combination for stress urinary incontinence in postmenopausal women. *Urology* 1988;32:273–280.

47. Ahlstrom K, Sandahl B, Sjoberg B, et al. Effect of combined treatment with phenylpropanolamine and estriol, compared with estriol treatment alone, in postmenopausal women with stress urinary incontinence. *Gynecol Obstet Invest* 1990;30:37–43.

48. Brubaker L, Harris T, Gleason D, et al. The external urethral barrier for stress incontinence: a multicenter trial of safety and efficacy. *Obstet Gynecol* 1999;93:932–937.

49. Moore KH, Simons A, Dowell C, et al. Efficacy and user acceptability of the urethral occlusive device in women with urinary incontinence. *J Urol* 1999;162:464–468.

50. Sand PK, Staskin D, Miller J, et al. Effect of a urinary control insert on quality of life in incontinent women. *Int Urogynecol J Pelvic Floor Dysfunct* 1999;10: 100–105.

51. Choe JM, Staskin DR. Clinical usefulness of urinary control urethral insert devices. *J Urol* 1999;161: 1043–1044.

52. Moore KH, Foote A, Burton G, et al. An open study of the bladder neck support prosthesis in genuine stress incontinence. *Br J Obstet Gynaecol* 1999;106:42–49.

53. van Zon-Rabelink IJ, Laven VM. The bacteriological changes after re-using a vaginal continence guard. *Acta Obstet Gynecol Scand* 1999;78:722–727.

54. Bhatia N, Bergman A, Gunning J. Urodynamic effects of a vaginal pessary in women with stress urinary incontinence. *Am J Obstet Gynecol* 1983;147:876–879.

55. Nativ O, Moskowitz B, Issaq E, et al. A new intraurethral sphincter prosthesis with a self contained urinary pump. *ASAIO J* 1997;43:197–203.

56. Schurch B, Suter S, Dubs M. Intraurethral sphincter prosthesis to treat hyporeflexic bladder in women: does it work? *Br J Urol Int* 1999;84:789–794.

Ostergard's Urogynecology and Pelvic Floor Dysfunction, Fifth Edition. edited by A.E. Bent, et al.
Lippincott Williams & Wilkins, Philadelphia © 2003.

29

Surgical Correction of Stress Incontinence with Hypermobility

Joan Blomquist and Michelle M. Germain

Greater Baltimore Medical Center, Towson, Maryland

Advances in our understanding of pelvic floor anatomy and the dynamics of continence continue to improve the success rates of surgery for stress incontinence. The surgical success rate, however, declines with repeated attempts. It is thus imperative that precise preoperative diagnosis and careful surgical planning be carried out. Although the workup for stress incontinence with hypermobility has been previously described (see Chapter 7), the following points should be emphasized. The minimal evaluation should include a comprehensive history, physical examination, urinalysis, urine culture, and measurement of postvoid residual. Stress incontinence should be objectively documented with direct visualization of urine loss with stress. Hypermobility should be evident by Q-tip test, cystoscopy, cystogram, or ultrasound. Normal perineal nerve status should be documented. Finally, cystometrics should be performed in patients with a history suggestive of detrusor instability, mixed incontinence, prior incontinence surgery, or advanced age. Surgery should be reserved for those who decline or have failed conservative alternatives and, ideally, have completed childbearing (1).

The gold standard for treatment of stress incontinence with hypermobility is the Burch colposuspension or retropubic urethropexy. We now have the option of performing the procedure open or laparoscopically. Recently, there has been an increased interest in the use of primary suburethral slings, both traditional and with tension-free vaginal tape (TVT). Some still advocate the use of needle procedures. This chapter reviews the procedures mentioned including the historical perspective, technique, success rates, and complications.

RETROPUBIC PROCEDURES

The most commonly supported theory of continence requires proper urethral function and proximal urethral support within the abdominal cavity. Loss of anatomic support allows displacement of the urethra from its normal intraabdominal position during stress. An unequal transmission of pressure occurs so that bladder pressure exceeds maximal urethral pressure, and leakage results. The retropubic procedures are designed to reestablish the intraabdominal location of the proximal urethra by elevating the urethrovesical junction and proximal urethra into the retropubic space. The various techniques differ in what structures are used to achieve this elevation.

Marshall, Marchetti, and Krantz first described the retropubic approach to correction of stress incontinence in 1949, referred to as the Marshall-Marchetti-Krantz (MMK) procedure (2). The basic plan was designed from a study of voiding dysfunction in men after removal of the rectum. Voiding dysfunction occurred in those patients with marked mobility of the vesical base and outlet and could be

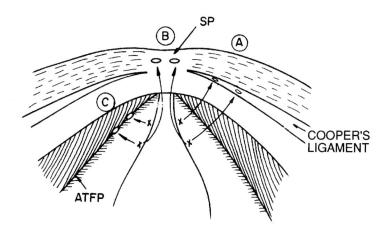

FIG. 29.1. Burch colposuspension with sutures attached to Cooper's ligament **(A)**. Marshall-Marchetti-Krantz procedure with sutures attached to the symphysis pubis (SP) **(B)**. Richardson paravaginal approach with sutures attached to the arcus tendineus fascia pelvis **(C)**.

relieved by firm upward pressure on the perineum. The first retropubic suspension of the vesical outlet was performed on one such 54-year-old man. Salient features of the original procedure include wide exposure of the retropubic space, double bites through the lateral urethral walls, attachment of the periurethral tissue to the periosteum of the symphysis pubis, and suturing of the bladder muscle to the posterior rectus fascia.

While attempting to perform an MMK procedure, Burch (3) noted that the sutures in the periosteum continued to pull out and that it was necessary to find another point of attachment. Using the arcus tendineus fascia pelvis (white line) created the most anatomically correct reattachment. Although normal anatomy was restored, the sutures held poorly. Cooper's ligament, the thick band of fibrous tissue running along the superior surface of the superior ramus of the pubic bone, proved to be ideal from the standpoint of both passing and holding a suture. Since Burch's original publication in 1961, there have been numerous modifications. We typically perform a modification proposed by Tanagho in 1976 (4). Tanagho's modification emphasizes placing the periurethral stitches 2 cm lateral to the urethra, thus avoiding damage to the sphincteric musculature.

As mentioned previously, the most anatomically correct repair of urethral hypermobility is elevation of the paravaginal fascia to the arcus tendineus fascia pelvis (white line). The paravaginal repair was originally described by Richardson to correct a cystourethrocele, not to correct stress incontinence. A prospective randomized trial showed a dismal 61% 1- to 3-year cure of stress incontinence for the paravaginal repair, compared with 100% for the Burch procedure (5). Although the paravaginal repair is anatomically correct, the supportive tissues involved in correction of stress incontinence are damaged with altered nerve function; therefore, a compensatory repair with an MMK or Burch procedure is needed (Fig. 29.1). One must take care that the overcorrection is not excessive because urinary retention or an overactive bladder may result.

Surgical Technique

Access to the Retropubic Space

The patient is positioned in either a modified dorsal lithotomy or frog-legged position to allow easy access to the vagina. The abdomen, perineum, and vagina are prepared and draped in a sterile fashion. A Foley catheter is placed and kept on the sterile field for easy access. One dose of an appropriate antibiotic is given intravenously for prophylaxis (6). A horizontal minilap or Pfannenstiel incision is made 2 cm above the symphysis, unless concurrent surgery dictates a larger or vertical incision. If intraperitoneal surgery is indicated, it is completed first, and the peritoneum is closed. The rectus abdominis muscles are carefully separated from the underlying transversalis fascia. Retractors are carefully placed under the rectus abdominis muscles, displacing them laterally. One must take care to avoid the inferior epigastric vessels. Self-retaining retractors are not used in minilap incisions.

The retropubic space is developed under direct visualization using blunt dissection. A lighted retractor or a headlamp is a valuable tool, especially with a minilap incision. The surgeon's hand is placed along the underside of the pubic bone to dissect bluntly the bladder and urethra medially away from the sidewall to allow identification of the endopelvic fascia. A sponge stick may aid in the dissection but must be used with caution. Cooper's ligament, the obturator notch, and the aberrant obturator vessels should be identified. Sharp dissection may be necessary if the patient has had prior incontinence surgery. The surgeon's nondominant hand is then placed in the vagina to elevate the pubocervical tissues and identify the urethrovesical junction. The urethrovesical junction (UVJ) is located by placing gentle traction on the catheter and palpating the lower edge of the balloon. A hemoclip can be placed at the UVJ to aid in later identification. Fat is removed from the pubocervical fascia using forceps or a peanut sponge pressing against the vaginal fingers. Removal of the fat facilitates identification of landmarks and promotes fibrosis. The midline area, including 2 cm lateral to the urethra on each side, is not dissected because of marked vascularity and small nerves in this area. Bleeding can be managed with hemoclips, cautery, or sutures.

An understanding of the vascular supply to the retropubic space is essential to prevent and control bleeding. A network of vessels exists in the midline behind the symphysis consisting of the anterior vesical and retrosymphysial vessels, both branches of the pudendal vessels. A rich venous plexus is located within the paravaginal fascia arising from the internal pudendal and vaginal arteries. Laterally, the vessels are frequently located within a fat pad. The aberrant obturator vessel joins the obturator and inferior epigastric systems and connects directly with the external iliac vessels (Fig. 29.2).

Marshall-Marchetti-Krantz Urethropexy

Entry into the retropubic space is as described previously. With the nondominant hand in the vagina elevating the pubocervical tissue, permanent or delayed absorbable sutures are placed at right angles to the urethra at the level of the UVJ. A double bite is taken, incorporating the full thickness of the vaginal wall except the epithelium. Cystotomy may be used to aid in identifying the UVJ. The sutures are then fixed to the fibrocartilage of the symphysis pubis. Marshall described bringing the superior surface of the urethra and vesical neck in direct opposition to the symphysis. To prevent overcorrecting, we recommend tying the sutures so that there is sufficient space for the operator to place a finger easily between the symphysis pubis and the endopelvic fascia (Fig. 29.1).

Burch Urethropexy

After entry into the retropubic space as described previously, Cooper's ligament is identified and cleared of all fat. Using permanent (e.g., polytetrafluoroethylene, silicone-treated polyester, polybutilate-coated polyester) suture, a figure-of-eight stitch is placed through the vaginal wall excluding the vaginal epithelium, 2 cm lateral to the UVJ. A second stitch is placed at the level of the midurethra, again 2 cm lateral to the midline. The procedure is repeated on the opposite side. Both ends of each suture are then secured to Cooper's ligament.

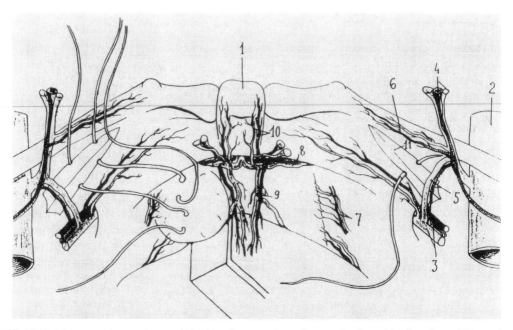

FIG. 29.2. The vascular anatomy of the Burch procedure. 1, symphysis pubis; 2, external iliac vein; 3, obturator artery and vein; 4, inferior epigastric artery and vein; 5, aberrant (accessory) obturator artery and vein; 6, pubic branch; 7, vaginal artery and vein; 8, internal pudendal artery and vein; 9, anterior vesical artery and vein; 10, retropubic artery and vein; 11, Cooper's ligament. (From Negura A, et al. Hemorrhagic risks in the burch procedure. *Int Urogynecol J Pelvic Floor Dysfunct* 1993;5:4, with permission.)

The midurethral stitch is attached 3 cm lateral to the symphysis, and the UVJ stitch is placed 1 cm more lateral. The needle should be directed upward and toward the midline to avoid injury to the aberrant obturator vessels. A piece of Gelfoam is placed at the lateral pelvic sidewall for hemostasis and to promote scarring. All four sutures are tied down with the assistant's hand in the vagina. The sutures should be tied without tension so that a finger can easily fit between the symphysis and the urethral catheter. Suture bridging exists because the fascia is not brought up to Cooper's ligament but is placed in apposition to the pelvic sidewall, where it will permanently fibrose (Fig. 29.1).

Adjuvant Procedures

A cul-de-sac repair, usually a Halban or Moschcowitz procedure, should be performed if an enterocele exists. Some advocate a prophylactic cul-de-sac repair because enterocele development is a known complication of

retropubic urethropexy (see later). In general, the repair should be performed before the urethropexy. There is no evidence that removing a normal, well-supported uterus improves the cure rate of incontinence. A cystoscopy should be performed at completion of the urethropexy to assess ureteral patency and integrity of the bladder and urethral walls. Suprapubic or transurethral catheters are used for postoperative bladder drainage. Voiding trials may begin on postoperative day 1 or 2 with postvoid residuals checked by suprapubic catheter, ultrasound, or intermittent self-catheterization.

Outcome

The MMK and Burch urethropexies have comparable outcomes, with success rates ranging from 85% to 90%. In a metaanalysis of 56 articles on the MMK procedure, Mainprize and Drutz (7) reported a 92% subjective continence rate if done as a primary procedure and 84.5% if performed after previous surgery. The largest long-term follow up series on MMK reported a subjective continence rate of 89.7% at 1 year, 85.7% at 5 years, and 75% at 15 years (8). A metaanalysis from retrospective and prospective studies on the Burch urethropexy showed an objective continence rate of 89.8% as a primary procedure and 82.5% in the presence of previous surgery (9). Ten-year cure rates are in excess of 70% (10,11).

Complications

The complications associated with MMK and Burch urethropexies are similar. Voiding dysfunction and *de novo* urge incontinence have been reported in 12.5% and 9.6% of patients, respectively, after the Burch procedure (9). Genitourinary prolapse (enterocele, cystocele, or rectocele) within 5 years of Burch colposuspension has been described in 13.6% (range, 2.5% to 26.7%) of patients (9). Lower abdominal or pelvic pain, possibly related to suture tension and referred to as the postcolposuspension syndrome, has been reported in 12% of patients (9). Voiding dysfunction and *de novo* urge incontinence have been reported in 11% to 12.5% and 9.6% of patients, respectively, after the MMK procedure (7). The MMK procedure is also associated with a 2.5% risk for osteitis pubis (7).

Direct surgical injury to the urinary tract has been reported in 1.6% of MMK and 2.7% of Burch urethropexy (12) cases. There are reports of ureteral obstruction through kinking or ligation after both procedures. We feel that these risks justify the routine intraoperative evaluation of ureteral and vesical integrity with both MMK and Burch urethropexies. Urinary retention and voiding dysfunction may require takedown of the surgery, usually performed by a vaginal approach.

LAPAROSCOPIC URETHROPEXY

Recent advances in minimally invasive surgery allow a laparoscopic approach to retropubic urethropexy. The advantages of a laparoscopic approach include shorter hospital stay, less patient discomfort, faster recovery, and better cosmesis. Some authors suggest that laparoscopy allows better visualization of the retropubic space because of laparoscopic magnification, insufflation effects, and better hemostasis. Disadvantages include cost of laparoscopic equipment, longer operative time, and the technical expertise required for proper dissection into the retropubic space and laparoscopic suturing.

Vancaillie and Schuessler described the first laparoscopic bladder neck suspension in 1991 (13). In their series of nine patients, an MMK was successfully performed in seven. Liu published a series of 58 laparoscopic Burch procedures using two to four sutures to suspend the UVJ to Cooper's ligament. The 3-month subjective cure rate was 95%. Various modifications have subsequently been developed to simplify the technical aspects of suturing. Techniques using staples, bone anchors, mesh, fibrin sealants, and various suturing devices have been described. It is our opinion that the suturing should be performed identically to that in the open retropubic urethropexy.

A transperitoneal or extraperitoneal approach may be used. Advantages of the transperitoneal approach include the ability to perform concomitant abdominopelvic surgery and a larger operative field. The extraperitoneal approach does not invade the peritoneal cavity and thus decreases the risk for vascular and bowel injuries, potentially decreases intraabdominal adhesion formation, and reduces symptoms associated with a pneumoperitoneum. Subcutaneous emphysema may occur with the extraperitoneal approach.

Procedure

The procedure is performed under general anesthesia. The patient is positioned in the dorsal lithotomy position using Allen stirrups to allow access to the urethra and vagina. The abdomen, perineum, and vagina are prepared, and the patient is draped in a sterile manner. A three-way Foley catheter is placed and left on the sterile field for easy access.

A conventional laparoscopic entry using a 10-mm trocar and laparoscope through an infraumbilical incision is used in the transperitoneal approach. A 5-mm port is then placed in each lower quadrant, 6 to 8 cm above the pubic rami and lateral to the inferior epigastric arteries (Fig. 29.3). The bladder is filled with 200 to 300 mL of fluid, distending the bladder to allow visualization of its contour. The retropubic space is entered by incising the anterior peritoneum 2 cm above the bladder reflection. As the dissection is carried caudal, the bladder drops inferiorly, allowing visualization of the urethra and paravaginal tissues. Dissection should avoid the midline owing to the rich vascular supply previously described.

The extraperitoneal approach involves an infraumbilical incision with dissection to the preperitoneal space. The dissection is carried caudal into the retropubic space using blunt dissection with the aid of Hegar dilators, hydrodistention, or a balloon dilator. Once the retropubic space is entered, a pneumoretzius is obtained, and the procedure is performed as described for the transperitoneal approach.

A 10-mm port is placed in the suprapubic region. The operator's or assistant's hand is placed in the vagina to elevate the pubocervical fascia. Fat is removed from the pubocervical fascia. A 2-0-polytetrafluorethylene suture on a CV2 needle is passed through the 10-mm port. The suture is passed down through Cooper's ligament, and a double-bite is taken through the pubocervical fascia 2 cm lateral to the UVJ. The suture is then brought back up through Cooper's ligament and tied with eight extracorporeal knots. A second suture is placed at the level of the midurethra. The procedure is repeated on the opposite side (Fig. 29.4). A cystoscopy is performed to assess ureteral patency and integrity of the bladder wall. The peritoneum of the retropubic space may be left open or closed with a running absorbable suture.

Outcome

If performed identically to the open retropubic urethropexy, the laparoscopic procedure should have similar cure rates. Analysis of the literature is difficult owing to variations in sur-

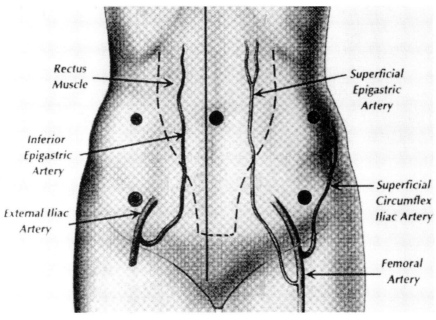

FIG. 29.3. Anatomy of the anterior abdominal wall with designated sites for port placement. (From Paraiso MFR, Falcone T. Laparoscopic surgery for genuine stress incontinence and pelvic organ prolapse. In: Walters MD, Karram MM, eds. *Urogynecology and reconstructive pelvic surgery,* 2nd ed. St Louis: Mosby, 1999, with permission.)

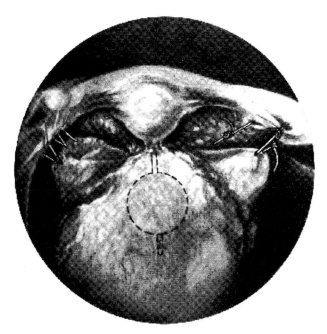

FIG. 29.4. Completed laparoscopic retropubic urethropexy. The appearance is identical to the result achieved by a transabdominal (open) approach.

gical technique and surgeon experience. Buller and Cundiff (14) reviewed 50 papers that collectively included 1,867 patients who underwent laparoscopic surgery for the treatment of genuine stress incontinence. At a mean follow-up of 17 months, a cure rate of 89% was observed. Thirty-five of the papers reviewed were case series. Only 30.8% of the studies reported objective outcome data, and a wide variety of laparoscopic techniques were used.

Three prospective, randomized, clinical trials compared open and laparoscopic retropubic urethropexies. Burton (15) showed lower objective and subjective cure rates for laparoscopic colposuspension, which decreased from 1 year (73% versus 97%) to 3 years (60% versus 93%). The use of absorbable suture in this study must be questioned. Su and colleagues (16) showed a lower 1-year objective cure rate for laparoscopic Burch colposuspension (80.4%), compared with the open group (95.6%); however, only one suture was placed bilaterally in the laparoscopic group, compared with two to three sutures placed bi-

laterally in the open group. Persson and associates (17) subsequently found a lower cure rate with the use of one suture bilaterally (58%), compared with two (83%). Summitt and co-workers (18) found similar objective cure rates for laparoscopic and transabdominal Burch procedures at 3 months (100% versus 97.06%) and 1 year (92.86% versus 88.24%). Two stitches were placed bilaterally in all patients using permanent sutures.

Postoperative urodynamic changes for laparoscopic Burch urethropexy are similar to those reported for laparotomy. In a prospective study of 48 patients who underwent laparoscopic Burch procedures for genuine stress incontinence, Ross (19) showed objective cure rates of 98%, 93%, and 89% at 6 weeks, 1 year, and 2 years, respectively. A decrease in urethral hypermobility and an increase in urethral pressure transmission ratios were found.

Studies on cost analysis are conflicting. Kung and colleagues (20) found lower costs associated with the laparoscopic Burch procedure ($2,398) compared with the open procedure ($5,692). Kohli and associates (21) found higher costs associated with the laparoscopic procedure ($4,960 versus $4,079). Shorter hospital stay and faster recovery must be weighed against the longer operative times and expensive laparoscopic equipment associated with the laparoscopic procedure.

Complications

Overall complication rates are 10% (range, 0% to 25%) (14). Complications are similar to those seen with the open urethropexy, with a few exceptions. Patients may void sooner after a laparoscopic approach. The laparoscopic approach is associated with a higher risk for major vascular injury, including inferior epigastric vessels, and bowel injury. Cystotomy is also more common with the laparoscopic approach, most likely related to the need for sharp dissection.

NEEDLE PROCEDURES

In 1959, Peyera described the first transvaginal needle suspension for the treatment of genuine stress incontinence. A specialized ligature carrier is used to secure the periurethral tissue to the rectus fascia. Numerous variations have been developed, including the Stamey, Raz, and Gittes procedures. The modifications differ in the extent of dissection and site of suture fixation. The American Urologic Association convened the Female Stress Urinary Incontinence Clinical Guidelines Panel to analyze published outcomes data on surgical procedures to treat female stress urinary incontinence and produced practice recommendations based primarily on outcomes evidence from the literature (22). Short-term and long-term (greater than 48 months) success rates were compared for the various procedures. Transvaginal suspensions (needle procedures) had a significantly lower long-term cure rate when compared with retropubic procedures and sling procedures (Table 29.1). The use of needle suspensions, thus, has little place in our current treatment of stress incontinence.

PRIMARY SLINGS

The suburethral sling has traditionally been considered a procedure for patients with intrinsic sphincter deficiency or for those who have failed primary procedures. Many surgeons now advocate the use of primary slings for genuine stress incontinence. The literature suggests an expected cure rate of 93.9% (95% confidence interval, 89.18% to 98.62%) when the sling is used as a primary procedure (9). Only one randomized trial has directly compared the sling (n = 14) to colposuspension (n = 36) for the treatment of primary genuine stress incontinence,

TABLE 29.1. *Comparative outcomes for stress incontinence surgery*

Outcomes	Retropubic suspensions, median CI (2.5%–97.5%)	Transvaginal suspensions, median CI (2.5%–97.5%)	Sling procedures, median CI (2.5%–97.5%)
Cure, dry:			
12–23 mo	84 (77–89)	79 (71–86)	82 (73–89)
24–47 mo	84 (80–88)	65 (50–77)	82 (73–89)
48 mo and longer	84 (79–88)	67 (53–79)	83 (75–88)
Cure, dry, improved:			
12–23 mo	86 (80–90)	82 (74–87)	91 (84–96)
24–47 mo	88 (85–91)	78 (71–83)	85 (77–91)
48 mo and longer	90 (87–92)	82 (73–89)	87 (80–92)

From American Urological Association. Female Stress Urinary Incontinence Clinical Guidelines Panel summary report on surgical management of female stress urinary incontinence. *J Urol* 1997;158(3):875–880, with permission.

showing comparable cure rates of 77% to 78% (23). The relatively high rate of *de novo* detrusor instability (16.6%) and postoperative voiding disorders (12.8%) reported in the literature must be considered (9). A large prospective randomized trial comparing colposuspension to suburethral sling for the treatment of primary genuine stress incontinence is in order. Sling procedures are extensively described in Chapter 30.

TENSION-FREE VAGINAL TAPE

The newest development in the treatment of genuine stress incontinence is the tension-free vaginal tape (TVT). The procedure was first described by Ulmsten and colleagues in 1996 (24) and involves placement of a suburethral support without repositioning the bladder neck. The basis for the procedure is "correction of inadequate urethral support from the pubourethral vesical ligaments and the suburethral vaginal wall." The TVT has four important features. The sling is placed under the midurethra, where, based on ure-thral pressure profilometry, the pubourethral ligaments are assumed to have their functional attachment. Second, no tension is applied to the sling. A suburethral support is developed, but the bladder neck is not repositioned. Third, a Prolene mesh is used. Although other synthetic materials are associated with a significant foreign-body reaction and tape rejection, Prolene causes a minimal inflammatory reaction without a significant change in collagen solubility (25). Finally, the procedure is meant to be ambulatory and performed under local anesthetic with appropriate intravenous sedation.

The TVT system (Gynecare, Somerville, NJ) consists of a reusable introducer to which two 5- to 6-mm metal disposable needles are attached. A Prolene mesh sling, (45 cm × 1.1 cm × 0.7 mm) covered with a removable plastic sheath is fixed to the needles (Fig. 29.5). The plastic sheath serves two purposes: it prevents contamination of the sling before insertion, and it enables the ends of the sling to be pulled up to the abdominal incision without trauma.

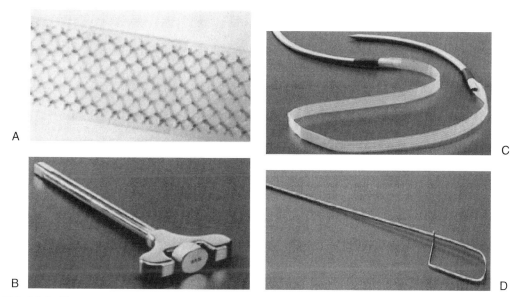

FIG. 29.5. The tension-free vaginal tape (TVT) device. Polypropylene mesh tape **(A)**, introducer **(B)**, protected mesh attached to introducer needles **(C)**, rigid catheter guide **(D)**. (Reproduced with permission from Gynecare, Somerville, NJ.)

Procedure

The procedure as described by Ulmsten colleagues is as follows (24). The patient is medicated with preoperative antibiotics. She is positioned in the dorsal lithotomy position, and the abdomen, perineum, and vagina are prepared. The bladder is emptied through a 16- to 18-French transurethral catheter. A total of about 100 mL of 0.25% lidocaine is used for local anesthetic: 60 to 70 mL is injected in the abdominal skin just above the pubis symphysis and downward along the back of the pubic bone to the space of Retzius, and 30 to 40 mL is injected into the vaginal wall suburethrally and paraurethrally. Two 1-cm incisions are made 6 cm apart just above the superior rim of the pubic bone. A 1.5-cm vertical incision is made in the anterior vagina beginning 0.5 to 1 cm inferior to the external urethral meatus. Dissection is carried out laterally for a distance of 1 cm on each side of the urethra. A rigid catheter guide is placed in the Foley catheter, and the bladder is deflected to the patient's left. The TVT needle with the introducer attached is inserted into the prepared right paraurethral incision. The urogenital diaphragm is perforated, and the tip of the needle is brought up to the abdominal incision by 'shaving' the back of the pubic bone (Fig. 29.6). The introducer is dis-

connected, cystoscopy is performed to confirm an intact bladder and urethra, and the needle with the attached tape is brought up through the abdominal incision. The procedure is repeated on the patient's left side while deviating the bladder to the patient's right side. The tape is positioned at the midurethra.

Adjustment of the tape is performed with the patient coughing repeatedly at a bladder volume of 250 to 300 mL. A few drops of urine may escape the external urethral meatus and indicates that the tension is not too tight, which should prevent postoperative retention. The needles are removed, and the plastic sheath is removed by pulling on both ends simultaneously. It is recommended that a blunt instrument be placed between the tape and urethra while removing the plastic sheath to ensure that the tape is not inadvertently tightened. The abdominal ends of the tape are cut below the skin surface, and the skin is closed. The vaginal wall is closed with an absorbable suture. The patient may have a Foley catheter overnight or may perform self-catheterization; most patients are voiding normally the day after surgery.

Outcome

Ulmsten's original paper reports 84% of patients dry, 8% improved, and 8% failed by

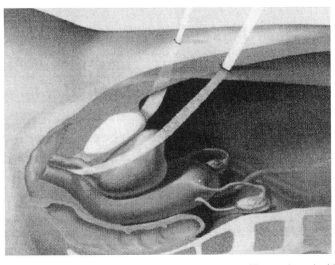

FIG. 29.6. Completed tension-free vaginal tape (TVT) procedure. (Reproduced with permission from Gynecare, Somerville, NJ.)

objective and subjective criteria (24). Subsequent reports show cure rates at 1 and 3 years of about 90% (26–28). A recent long-term case series reported 84.5% objective and subjective cure at 56 (range, 48 to 70) months (29). The patients included in these studies had genuine stress incontinence, and most procedures were primary. Although these cure rates are in line with retropubic urethropexy and traditional sling procedures, it should be noted that, to date, there are no prospective randomized comparative studies available.

The TVT has initially been recommended as a primary operation for patients with genuine stress incontinence due to hypermobility. Several recent case series investigate the use of the procedure for more complicated cases, such as patients with intrinsic sphincter deficiency, mixed incontinence, and failed primary procedures. Four-year (range, 3 to 5 years) objective and subjective cure rates of 74% for intrinsic sphincter deficiency, 85% for mixed incontinence, and 82% for recurrent stress incontinence have been reported (30–32). Again, no prospective randomized comparative studies are available.

Complications

Potential complications associated with the TVT include bleeding, infection, obturator nerve injury, bowel injury, sling rejection or erosion, cystotomy, and voiding dysfunction. Ulmsten reported no cases of intraoperative blood loss greater than 300 mL and two uncomplicated hematomas in 131 patients (26). A recent review of 404 TVT procedures reported retropubic bleeding requiring laparotomy and blood transfusion in 0.5% of patients and retropubic hematomas in 1.5% of patients (33). There has been a report of an external iliac vein perforation (34) with hemorrhage into the retropubic space, necessitating laparotomy and transfusion of 10 units of packed cells, and a case report of bleeding from vessels in the space of Retzius, also requiring laparotomy and 10 units of packed cells (35). Several cases of obturator nerve injury have been reported (33). According to industry standards, 24 vascular injuries, 12 vaginal mesh exposures, 5

urethral erosions, and 8 bowel perforations have occurred in 150,000 procedures (Gynecare, personal communication with Cheryl Bogardus, May 1, 2001). Cystotomy has been reported in 6% and postoperative voiding difficulties in 4% of TVT cases (33). If voiding dysfunction or urinary retention does develop, it is managed by self-catheterization or Foley drainage. If the problem does not resolve, the mesh should be cut within the first 4 weeks. This is performed under sedation and local anesthesia by opening the anterior vaginal wall over the tape and dividing the tape completely. The ends of the tape retract, but the mesh holds in the pubocervical fascia, and continence is generally maintained.

SUMMARY

Primary repair of stress incontinence has become a minimally invasive surgical procedure performed on an outpatient basis or as a one-day hospital stay. The choice of procedure may be dictated by the concurrent surgery. As a stand-alone surgery, the TVT or the laparoscopic approach may offer excellent cure rates with early ambulation.

REFERENCES

1. *Urinary incontinence.* ACOG technical bulletin No. 213, October 1995.
2. Marshall VF, Marchetti AA, Krantz KE. The correction of stress incontinence by simple vesicourethral suspension. *Surg Gynecol Obstet* 1949;88:509.
3. Burch JC. Urethrovaginal fixation to Cooper's ligament for correction of stress incontinence, cystocele, and prolapse. *Am J Obstet Gynecol* 1961;81:281–290.
4. Tanagho EA. Colpocystourethropexy: the way we do it. *J Urol* 1976;116:751–753.
5. Columbo M, Milate R, Vitobello D, et al. A randomized comparison of Burch colposuspension and abdominal paravaginal defect repair for female stress urinary incontinence. *Am J Obstet Gynecol* 1996;175(1):78–84.
6. Bhatia NN, Karram MM, Bergman A. Role of antibiotic prophylaxis in retropubic surgery for female stress urinary incontinence. *Obstet Gynecol* 1989;74(4):637–639.
7. Mainprize T, Drutz H. The Marshall-Marchetti-Krantz procedure: a critical review. *Obstet Gynecol Surv* 1988; 43(12):724–729.
8. McDuffie RW Jr, Litin RB, Blundon KE. Urethrovesical suspension (Marshall-Marchetti-Krantz): experience with 204 cases. *Am J Surg* 1981;141:297–298.
9. Jarvis GJ. Surgery for genuine stress incontinence. *Br J Obstet Gynecol* 1994;101:371–374.
10. Eriksen C, Hagen B, Eik-New SH, et al. Long-term effectiveness of the Burch colposuspension for female

urinary stress incontinence. *Acta Obstet Gynecol Scand* 1990;69:45–50.

11. Alcalay M, Monga A, Stanton S. Burch colposuspension: a 10–20 year follow-up. *Br J Obstet Gynaecol* 1995;102:740–745.

12. Demirce F, Yucel N, Ozden S, et al. A retrospective review of perioperative complications in 360 patients who had Burch colposuspension. *Aust N Z J Obstet Gynecol* 1999;39(4):472–452.

13. Vancaillie TG, Schuessler W. Laparoscopic bladder neck suspension. *J Laparoendosc Surg* 1991;1:169–173.

14. Buller JL, Cundiff GW. Laparoscopic surgeries for urinary incontinence. *Clin Obstet Gynecol* 2000;43(3):604–618.

15. Burton G. A three-year prospective randomized urodynamic study comparing open and laparoscopic colposuspension. *Neurourol Urodyn* 1997;16:353–354.

16. Su T, Want K, Hsu C, et al. Prospective comparison of laparoscopic and traditional colposuspensions in the treatment of genuine stress incontinence. *Acta Obstet Gynecol Scand* 1997;76:576–582.

17. Persson J, Wolner-Hanssen P. Laparoscopic Burch colposuspension for stress urinary incontinence: a randomized comparison of one or two sutures on each side of the urethra. *Obstet Gynecol* 2000;95:151–155.

18. Summitt RL, Lucente V, Karram MM, et al. Randomized comparison of laparoscopic and transabdominal Burch urethropexy for the treatment of genuine stress incontinence. *Obstet Gynecol* 2000;95(4S):2S(abst).

19. Ross JW. Multichannel urodynamic evaluation of laparoscopic Burch colposuspension for genuine stress incontinence. *Obstet Gynecol* 1998;91(1):55–59.

20. Kung R, Lie K, Lee P, et al. The cost effectiveness of laparoscopic versus abdominal Burch procedures in women with urinary stress incontinence. *J Am Assoc Gynecol Laparosc* 1996;3:537–544.

21. Kohli N. Open compared with laparoscopic approach to Burch colposuspension: a cost analysis. *Obstet Gynecol* 1997;90(3):411–415.

22. American Urological Association. Female stress urinary incontinence clinical guidelines panel summary report on surgical management of female stress urinary incontinence. *J Urol* 1997;158(3):875–880.

23. Lalos O, Gurglaund A, Bjerle P. Urodynamics in women with stress incontinence before and after surgery. *Eur J Obstet Gynecol Reprod Biol* 1993;48:197–205.

24. Ulmsten U, Henriksson L, Johnson P, et al. An ambulatory surgical procedure under local anesthesia for treatment of female urinary incontinence. *Int Urogynecol J* 1996;7:81–86.

25. Falconer C, Soderberg M, Blomgren B, et al. Influence of different sling materials on connective tissue metabolism in stress urinary incontinent women. *Int Urogynecol J Suppl* 2001;2:S19–S23.

26. Ulmsten U, Falconer C, Johnson P, et al. A multicenter study of tension-free vaginal tape (TVT) for surgical treatment of stress urinary incontinence. *Int Urogynecol J* 1998;9:210–213.

27. Olsson I, Kroon U. A three-year postoperative evaluation of tension-free vaginal tape. *Gynecol Obstet Invest* 1999;48:267–269.

28. Wang AC. An assessment of the early surgical outcome and urodynamic effects of the tension-free vaginal tape (TVT). *Int Urogynecol J* 2000;11:282–284.

29. Nilsson CG, Kuuva N, Falconer C, et al. Long-term results of the tension-free vaginal tape (TVT) procedure for surgical treatment of female stress urinary incontinence. *Int Urogynecol J Suppl* 2001;2:S5–S8.

30. Rezapour M, Falconer C, Ulmsten U. Tension-free vaginal tape (TVT) in stress incontinent women with intrinsic sphincter deficiency (ISD): a long-term follow-up. *Int Urogynecol J Suppl* 2001;2:S12–S14.

31. Rezapour M, Ulmsten U. Tension-free vaginal tape (TVT) in women with mixed urinary incontinence: a long-term follow-up. *Int Urogynecol J Suppl* 2001;2:S15–S18.

32. Rezapour M, Ulmsten U. Tension-free vaginal tape (TVT) in women with recurrent stress urinary incontinence: a long-term follow-up. *Int Urogynecol J Suppl* 2001;2:S9–S11.

33. Meschia M, Pifarotti P, Bernasconi F, et al. Tension-free vaginal tape: analysis of outcomes and complications in 404 stress incontinent women. *Int Urogynecol J Suppl* 2001;2:S24–S27.

34. Primicerio M, DeMatteis G, Montanino M, et al. Use of the TVT (tension-free vaginal tape) in the treatment of female urinary stress incontinence: preliminary results. *Minerva Ginecol* 1999;51:355–358.

35. Vierhout ME. Severe hemorrhage complicating tension-free vaginal tape (TVT): a case report. *Int Urogynecol J* 2001;12:139–140.

Ostergard's Urogynecology and Pelvic Floor Dysfunction, Fifth Edition. edited by A.E. Bent, et al. Lippincott Williams & Wilkins, Philadelphia © 2003.

30

Suburethral Sling Procedures and Treatment of Complicated Stress Incontinence

Kari Kubic and Nicolette S. Horbach

Department of Obstetrics and Gynecology, George Washington University, Annandale, Virginia

Until recently, suburethral sling procedures have been reserved for the treatment of recurrent stress incontinence, especially in women with urethral hypermobility or intrinsic sphincter deficiency (ISD). This is because of the technical difficulties of the procedure and the increased risk for postoperative complications after sling procedures. More recent evidence suggests that sling procedures may also be indicated in women with increased risk for failing primary incontinence procedures because of underlying medical or lifestyle risk factors. The current debate is whether sling procedures should be the primary approach in all women with genuine stress incontinence. The physician who undertakes the treatment of women with urinary incontinence must be cognizant of the indications, techniques, and management of complications of a suburethral sling procedure and consider this surgical option when designing a management plan.

HISTORICAL BACKGROUND

Suburethral sling procedures for the treatment of stress urinary incontinence were first introduced by von Giordano in 1907 using gracilis muscle flap (1). Since that time, numerous modifications of both the surgical approach and materials used as the sling have been published as summarized in Table 30.1. In 1910, Goebell described detaching the pyramidalis muscle and suturing it beneath the urethra. Frankenheim modified the technique in 1914 by attaching a vertical strip of rectus fascia to the pyramidalis muscle (2). The final alteration of the initial Goebell-Frankenheim-Stoekel procedure included securing the pyramidalis muscle and the rectus fascia beneath the urethra after plication of the periurethral fascia (3,4).

Musculature slings were ultimately abandoned owing to the difficulty in maintaining the muscle's blood supply and the mechanical problems associated with incorporating a bulky tissue beneath the urethra. To alleviate these problems, Aldridge chose to use two transverse strips of rectus fascia, which were detached at their lateral margins and then sutured below the urethra using a separate vaginal incision (5). Studdiford modified the Aldridge approach by passing a single continuous strip of rectus fascia attached at one lateral margin under the urethra (2). He then reattached the free end to the rectus fascia on the contralateral side. The Millin-Read procedure, published in 1948, was designed to decrease the risk for an ascending infection from the vaginal incision (6). A single strip of rectus fascia was insinuated between the urethra and the vaginal mucosa and elevated into the abdominal field without entry into the vagina. Unfortunately, this approach resulted in an increased incidence of bladder and urethral injury and thus is rarely used today. The last significant modification of the sling pro-

TABLE 30.1. *Historical review of suburethral sling procedures*

Year	Author	Tissue and technique
1907	Giordano	Double gracilis muscle sutured below and above urethra
1910	Goebell	Pyramidalis muscle split and sutures beneath the urethra
1914	Frankenheim	Pyramidalis muscle with attached strip of rectus fascia
1917	Stoekel	Pyramidalis muscle with attached strips of rectus fascia plus plication of urethra and bladder base
1942	Aldridge	Two strips of rectus fascia passed under the urethra with a vaginal incision and sutured together
1944	Studdiford	Single continuous strip to rectus fascia under urethra and reattached to rectus fascia
1947	Meigs	Plication of urethra plus rectus fascia sling
1948	Millin and Read	Single strip of rectus fascia tunneled under the urethra without vaginal incision
1962	Williams	Mersilene strips
1966	Ridley	Mersilene strips
1968	Moir	Mersilene gauze hammock
1970	Morgan	Marlex gauze hammock
1979	Raz	Patch of vaginal wall with helical sutures laterally and secured above rectus fascia
1983	Fainu	Vicryl absorbable mesh
1985	Jarvis	Porcine dermis
1985	Stanton	Silastic band
1988	Horbach	Gore-Tex soft tissue patch
1990	Ulmsten	Prolene tape
1996	Handa	Cadaveric fascia lata strip secured suburethrally and secured above rectus fascia
2000	Franks	Cadaveric dermal patch sutured under the urethra and secured above the rectus fascia

Data from references 1–13, 76, 79, and 95.

cedure by a proponent of autologous material was reported by Shaw, who employed fascia lata as the sling material (1).

Although organic tissues offer the advantages of being readily accessible and rarely rejected, mobilization of autologous fascia is at times difficult owing to poor tissue quality or inadequate fascial length. More recent research has been aimed at developing synthetic grafts. Nylon or Mersilene (polyethylene) strips, 0.5 cm in diameter, were initially chosen because they were thought to provide improved tensile strength compared with fascia (7). However, under tension, those grafts formed a taut, narrow cord, which resulted in urethral obstruction and a number of urethral transections (8).

Moir substituted Mersilene gauze, 2.5 cm in diameter, for the narrow Mersilene ribbon and showed a decreased incidence of postoperative complications (8). Marlex mesh (polypropylene) was preferred by Morgan because of its inert properties and its ability to be incorporated into the surrounding tissue without the extensive scarring associated with Mersilene gauze (9). In an attempt to use synthetic materials with less tissue incorporation and scarring, two studies using an inert Silastic band and a Gore-Tex (polytetrafluoroethylene) sling have been published (12,13). Theoretically, their porous nature makes these materials less prone to infection or rejection than the traditional synthetic meshes. The Silastic band prevents adhesion formation; this allows the sling tension to be adjusted on follow-up visits if necessary. Obviously, the ideal material—one that is easily accessible, provides adequate tensile strength, and carries no risk for infection, rejection, or excessive scarring—has yet to be discovered. The debate continues, therefore, whether organic or inorganic materials provide the optimal sling material.

MECHANISM

There are numerous theories regarding the etiology of genuine stress incontinence. Loss of anatomic support of the urethra (urethral hypermobility) may prevent normal transmission of increases in intraabdominal pressure to the proximal urethra during coughing, straining, or exercise (14). DeLancey has suggested that loss of anatomic integrity of the vaginal support tissue of the urethra creates a less rigid "hammock," which in turn fails to stabilize the urethra during increases in intraabdominal pressure (15). Failure of the normal intrinsic urethral sphincteric mechanism results in the most severe symptoms of stress incontinence.

Although the mechanism of action of the sling procedure is debated, the sling is thought to correct genuine stress incontinence by restoring normal urethrovesical junction support and mechanically compressing the urethra (16–20). In most sling procedures, the ends of the sling are fixed to the rectus fascia or are sutured together over the rectus fascia. During periods of increased abdominal pressure, the abdominal wall moves outward, and the sling is drawn upward. This compresses the urethra and increases intraurethral resistance. Variations of the sling procedure in which the ends of the sling are attached to an immovable tissue (Cooper's ligament or bone anchors in the pubic symphysis) do not allow upward displacement of the sling and urethra during straining. In these operations, the sling is thought to create a secure platform of urethral support (21). Increases in intraabdominal pressure press the urethra downward against the sling, thereby compressing the urethra from both above and below. It is this compression of the urethra that is believed to lead to increases in urethral resistance and a resolution of stress incontinence (15). However, the potential for excess compression of the urethra also contributes to the most common complications of the sling procedure—voiding dysfunction.

INDICATIONS

One of the most controversial aspects of incontinence surgery is the choice of the appropriate surgical candidate for a suburethral sling procedure. In the past, sling procedures were reserved for women with recurrent stress incontinence regardless of the etiology of the stress incontinence (20–22). Studies indicated reduced success rates in women who underwent repeat retropubic procedures compared with primary retropubic operations (23,24). In the mid-1980s, investigators recommended sling procedures for women with evidence of poor intrinsic urethral sphincter function, regardless of urethral support and prior incontinence surgery history. The sling was thought to restore continence by creating obstruction of the urethra. However, women with a scarred immobile urethra have been reported to have poor success rates or required intentional urethral obstruction with its inherent complications. Summit and colleagues reported only a 20% cure rate after sling procedures in women with low urethral pressure and an immobile urethra as determined by a straining Q-tip test of less than 30 degrees (25). The advent of periurethral bulking agents eliminated the need for slings in women with a scarred immobile urethra.

In an effort to reduce the number of women who experienced obstructive voiding dysfunction after slings, experts began to recommend that less tension be applied to the sling and that patients with a hypermobile urethra and poor intrinsic urethral tone were the most appropriate candidates for a sling (24–26). Limiting sling use to these women improved cure rates and reduced voiding complications. With improved outcomes after sling procedures, the appeal of these procedures has expanded. The current debate is whether sling procedures should be used as a primary incontinence procedure in all women.

Intrinsic Sphincter Deficiency

Numerous investigators have attempted to delineate those patients who may be at risk for failing primary retropubic incontinence operations so that an alternative surgical approach could be considered. McGuire compared the urodynamic and radiographic findings in 414 patients with primary stress incontinence with 234 patients with recurrent leakage who had failed one or more operative procedures (27). He found that 75% of patients who failed multiple surgeries for stress incontinence had evidence of poor intrinsic urethral function as indicated by low (<10 cm H_2O) urethral closure pressures. In 1978, McGuire reported surgical success in these patients with low urethral pressures following a fascial sling operation (24). Similarly, Sand and associates found women with low urethral pressures to be at high risk (28). In a retrospective study of 86 women, they reported a three-fold increased risk for failure of a Burch retropubic urethropexy in women with low preoperative urethral closure pressure (<20 cm H_2O) compared with those with normal pressure. A case-control study by Horbach and colleagues compared the objective cure rate in patients with primary or recurrent incontinence and a low urethral closure pressure treated with a sling procedure versus a Burch urethropexy (26). They found an 85% objective cure rate in the group of sling patients as opposed to 35% in the Burch group.

Given these data, one of the primary indications for a suburethral sling operation became genuine stress incontinence due to intrinsic urethral sphincter dysfunction (ISD). Patients with ISD appear to be at increased risk for failing standard retropubic operations (24,26–28). However, several recent reports suggest retropubic procedures may still provide relatively good cure rates in women with ISD. In a retrospective analysis of 45 women with low urethral pressure (<20 cm H_2O), Maher and co-workers compared the subjective and objective cure rates following Burch colposuspension and sling procedure (29). The subjective cure rate of the Burch group was superior to that of the sling group—90% and 71%, respectively; the objective success rates were 67% and 50%, respectively. Hsieh and associates found a 91.7% objective cure rate in 24 women following a Burch colposuspension for low Valsalva leak point pressure (VLPP, <60 cm H_2O) and normal urethral closure pressure (>20 cm H_2O) (30). Thus, ISD as the primary indication for sling procedures over retropubic operations remains somewhat controversial.

The difficulty is that no standard definition of ISD has been established and no single factor accurately predicts ISD (31,32). Maximum urethral closure pressure (MUCP) is the highest pressure generated along the length of the urethra above baseline intravesical pressure. Based on retrospective studies, low MUCP (<10 to 20 cm H_2O) has been used as one criteria for ISD. However, continent women also have MUCPs of less than 20 cm H_2O. Because of the inconsistencies with MUCP measurements and the more sophisticated equipment required to perform the test, the VLPP has been proposed as a more accurate indicator of intrinsic urethral function (33). The VLPP is defined as the lowest intraabdominal pressure needed to overcome the urethral sphincter resistance in the absence of detrusor activity. By convention, a VLPP of less than 60 cm H_2O is defined as ISD, and that between 60 and 90 cm H_2O is considered equivocal (34).

Other Indications

Other preoperative risks factor may predispose women to failure of traditional incontinence surgery. Any medical condition or lifestyle habit that repetitively causes increases in intraabdominal pressure may weaken the pelvic support tissues or contribute to suture failure following a retropubic procedure (35–38). Smoking, with its associated chronic bronchitis and coughing, has been shown to be a risk factor for stress incontinence (35). In epidemiologic studies, morbid obesity has been shown to be associated with all types of urinary incontinence. Mommsen and Foldspang surveyed 3,114 women and found that increased body mass index was an independent risk factor for all types of urinary incontinence (36). However, in studies on surgical outcome in these women, obesity was an inconsistent risk factor for failure of surgery (37). Nygaard and co-workers studied nulliparous, collegiate, competitive female athletes and found those who competed in high-impact sports such as gymnastics reported a 15-fold increase in stress incontinence compared with women participating in low-impact sports (38). They attributed their findings to the high intraabdominal pressures exerted on the bladder during their repetitive high-impact sport. These studies indicate that women with medical or lifestyle risk factors for stress incontinence and women who are at increased risk for failing surgical intervention may be candidates for a more aggressive surgical approach such as a sling operation.

The prevalence of ISD also appears to be higher in older women as intrinsic urethral sphincteric function declines with age. Although older women may be candidates for a sling procedure based on their diagnosis of ISD, some surgeons are hesitant to perform a sling in elderly patients. Surgeons fear increased postoperative voiding difficulties in older women who typically have less detrusor reserve for voiding and an increased likelihood of concomitant detrusor instability. However, these fears may be unfounded. Carr and associates recently reported subjective resolution of stress incontinence in all 19 geriatric women with a median age of 72 years who underwent a sling procedure (39). Griebling and colleagues found similar results in 26 women with a mean age of 67.6 years who had a sling operation (40). At a mean follow-up of 10.5 months, 65% were dry and 27% "significantly improved." Both groups of authors believe that age alone should not be a contraindication to a suburethral sling procedure.

Sling as a Primary Incontinence Procedure

One of the most controversial aspects of sling surgery is whether all patients with primary stress incontinence should undergo a suburethral sling regardless of the etiology of their incontinence. Appell and others have been strong proponents of this approach (41). According to the American Urologic Association Female Stress Urinary Incontinence Clinical Guidelines Panel (42), the sling is the most efficacious procedure for long-term successful treatment of genuine stress incontinence. Because many women with hypermobility of the bladder neck and proximal urethra do not have stress incontinence, some credence must be given to the thought that the presence of stress incontinence implies some deficiency in the bladder outlet function, not just an anatomic defect. It would appear that a sling procedure would benefit patients more because of its suburethral support during increases in intraabdominal pressure (41). All patients may have ISD to some extent. Because sling procedures have at least equivalent efficacy when compared with retropubic operations in primary stress incontinence and superior success rates in women with recurrent stress incontinence, and because the reported prevalence of complications with slings has diminished, Appell suggests that all women should undergo sling operations.

Ostergard in his corresponding editorial on the indications for primary sling procedure strongly disagreed (43). Although he concluded that the success rates of the two procedures are nearly equivalent, Ostergard reported a review of the literature totaling 1,771 sling patients and 551 Burch patients that showed a much higher incidence of complications in women having sling operations. There was an 11% versus 6% retention rate, 14% versus 5% *de novo* detrusor instability, and 15% versus 4% persistent detrusor instability in sling patients compared with Burch patients. Considering potential complications that may require further surgical intervention, there was a much greater likelihood in patients having sling operations than with a Burch procedure. Ostergard concluded that although success rates were comparable, complications were far more common in sling patients.

Weber and Walters published a recent report using a decision analytic model to compare the Burch and sling procedures for primary surgical treatment of genuine stress incontinence with urethral hypermobility regardless of intrinsic urethral function (44). Using the literature to determine the risks and benefits of the two procedures, they found the overall effectiveness of the Burch and sling to be equivalent in the percentage of women cured, 94.8% and 95.3%, respectively. In expanding their analytic model, they concluded that when the risk for retention from a sling was more than 9% or when the risk for *de novo* detrusor instability after sling was higher than 10.3%, the Burch procedure was more effective in balancing cure and risks. Thus, one area to be clarified with further research is the question of comprehensive versus selective use of sling procedures.

Sling as a Treatment of Mixed Incontinence

Considerable debate exists regarding the role of sling procedures in women with mixed urge and stress incontinence. McGuire found that 40% of patients with preoperative detrusor instability had resolution of their urge incontinence following surgery (23,45). He was unable to predict preoperatively on the basis of the degree of preoperative detrusor instability which patients would have a favorable outcome. He also found that in 10% to 15% of cases, the detrusor instability worsened postoperatively. Schrepferman and colleagues investigated 84 women who had a sling procedure and who had preoperative urge and stress incontinence (46). Patients were categorized as having motor urge incontinence or sensory urge incontinence based on the presence of demonstrable detrusor instability on videourodynamics. Urge incontinence symptoms were completely resolved in 39.3% of women and improved in 32.1%. In women with motor urge incontinence, the cure and improvement rates were 58.5% and 17.1%, respectively. The investigators then divided patients with motor urge incontinence into two groups based on the amplitude of the uninhibited detrusor contractions. The low-pressure contractions (≤ 15 cm H_2O) group had cure rates of 91.3%, compared with only 27.8% in the high-pressure contractions group.

The concern in patients with postoperative detrusor instability is the presence of detrusor contractions that occur against a partially obstructed urethra. This can lead to the development of a hypertrophic detrusor muscle and reduced bladder compliance. In women with severe ISD and detrusor instability who undergo a sling procedure, the tradeoff may be improved continence between voids but increased frequency of voiding or urge incontinence. By having the sling minimize the constant leakage that may occur between voids in women with severe ISD, the bladder reaches its maximum (but reduced) functional capacity more readily, leading to increased urinary frequency. This can be particularly bothersome at night, with significant nocturia due to reduced capacity, abnormal detrusor activity, and peripheral fluid mobilization. Finally, in women with a partially obstructed urethra and high-amplitude detrusor contractions (>40 cm H_2O) after surgery, ureteral reflux may occur, predisposing to pyelonephritis and renal damage.

For these reasons, all patients should be evaluated preoperatively for the presence of uninhibited detrusor contractions. If detrusor instability is diagnosed, it should be treated aggressively with medications or behavioral therapy before surgery. One also needs to consider that long-term anticholinergic therapy for detrusor instability may significantly exacerbate postoperative voiding dysfunction after slings. Some authors recommend that sling procedures should only be performed in patients with detrusor instability who experience low-amplitude, uninhibited contractions at greater than 200-mL bladder volume.

CONTRAINDICATIONS

A number of clinical conditions exist that are relative contraindications to sling procedures (23,47). The use of a sling is discouraged in women with a neurogenic bladder because of the potential for ureteral reflux from high amplitude uninhibited detrusor contractions. Patients with large atonic or areflexic bladders and high postvoid residuals may develop complete urinary retention after surgery. These patients should be counseled before surgery regarding the likelihood of requiring intermittent self-catheterization postoperatively. A patient at high risk for postoperative urinary retention who is unwilling or unable to perform self-catheterization may not be a good candidate for a sling operation. A history of pelvic irradiation or the presence of a urinary fistula may predispose the operative site to tissue breakdown. To prevent this, a Martius muscle flap may be mobilized and inserted between the urethra and vaginal mucosa at the time of the sling procedure.

PREOPERATIVE EVALUATION

It is essential that women complete a thorough preoperative assessment before surgery is contemplated to ensure that the diagnosis of genuine stress incontinence is correct. The specific etiology of a woman's stress incontinence must be determined. Is her stress incontinence due to urethrovesical junction hypermobility, ISD, or both? Other causes of urinary leakage that may not be amenable to surgery must be eliminated. These include detrusor instability, overflow incontinence due to a high postvoid residual, and urinary tract infections or anatomic abnormalities of the urinary tract such as fistulas or diverticula. A thorough history, physical examination, postvoid residual, urine culture, assessment of urethrovesical junction mobility, screening cystometry, and assessment of intrinsic urethral function by means of urethral pressure profile or leak point pressures should be performed in all patients before a sling procedure.

Preoperative assessment of women with ISD may be particularly challenging in patients with severe prolapse or detrusor instability. Urethral compression may occur in women with normal urethral support by compression of the urethra from a large cystocele, vaginal vault prolapse, or rectocele. The prolapse must be reduced manually or with a retractor, scopette, or pessary during urodynamic studies to assess intrinsic urethral function. Veronikis and colleagues examined 30 consecutive continent women with grade IV prolapse using four different techniques for reduction of the prolapse (48). The highest incidence of genuine stress incontinence was found using a scopette to reduce the prolapse. Eighty-three percent of women demonstrated

genuine stress incontinence, and 56% had a low-pressure urethra revealed with reduction of the prolapse. Chaikin and associates prospectively evaluated 24 continent women with severe urogenital prolapse using a vaginal pessary to reduce their prolapse (49). ISD, defined as a leak point pressure of less than 60 cm H_2O, was unmasked in 58% of women with prolapse. This subset of women underwent a sling procedure with an 86% success rate for incontinence, although 7% developed recurrent anterior compartment prolapse.

Severe ISD may compromise the ability to detect detrusor instability during urodynamic testing, and vice versa. Maximum cystometric capacity may appear reduced in women with spontaneous leakage during bladder filling as a result of severe ISD. To assess detrusor function properly, the urethra must be manually obstructed and filling continued until at least 300 to 350 mL bladder volume is obtained. If abnormal detrusor activity, such as uninhibited contractions or low compliance, is noted, surgery should be reconsidered. If a sling procedure is ultimately performed, the patient may experience significant postoperative problems with urgency, frequency, or urge incontinence. The detrusor instability should be addressed before performing a sling procedure.

Preoperative voiding pattern may assist the clinician in determining which patients are at risk for postoperative voiding difficulties and prolonged catheter usage. Studies indicate that women with a detrusor contraction of more than 10 cm H_2O during instrumented voiding studies are at minimal risk for postoperative retention (50,51). Women who void by straining should be taught correct voiding habits preoperatively. Some surgeons teach their patients intermittent self-catheterization preoperatively to ensure they are both able and willing to self-catheterize should the need arise after surgery.

SLING MATERIALS

Although the ideal sling material has yet to be discovered, the currently available materials used for sling procedures are summarized in Table 30.2. The ideal material would be in-

TABLE 30.2. *Summary of reported sling materials*

Nonsynthetic	Synthetic
Autologous rectus fascia	Mersilene strip
Autologous fascia lata	Mersilene gauze hammock
Cadaveric fascia lata	Marlex
Vaginal wall patch	Prolene
Dermal allograft	Gore-Tex
Porcine dermis	Silastic band
Porcine small intestinal submucosa	

expensive and easily obtained, have predictable and consistent strength, and be incorporated into the vaginal submucosal tissue without shrinkage, erosion, or rejection.

Organic Materials

Both autologous and allografts have been employed as organic sling materials. Autologous fascial grafts minimize the changes in tissue properties that may be seen in processed versus fresh tissue specimens and eliminate the risk for viral transmission from the donor. The grafts are harvested either from the rectus fascia or as fascia lata from the outer thigh. Aldridge originally described using rectus fascia as a sling material (5). Rectus fascia has also been advocated as a graft by recent authors (52–54). The advantage of this autologous tissue is the ability to obtain a long strip of tissue with a low incidence of rejection or autolysis. Fokaef and colleagues studied the fate of human rectus fascial strips implanted submucosally in the rabbit vagina animal model (55). The grafts were removed 3 months after implantation and examined using histologic and biochemical techniques. Although their results confirmed the viability of free fascial grafts, several changes in tissue properties were noted. All strips showed a loss of width (63%), length (37%) and strength (54%). Wider samples were found to maintain greater tissue strength over time. It is uncertain whether this animal model is indicative of what happens when human rectus

fascia is implanted in humans. Fitzgerald and co-workers analyzed a series of five women who underwent reexploration 3 weeks to 4 years after a rectus fascia sling (54). The fascia remained viable with fibroblastic proliferation, neovascularization, and remodeling of the graft. No evidence of graft infection or degeneration was noted. However, the use of rectus fascia requires a larger abdominal incision with more potential surgical morbidity and recovery time. The tissue quality may also be compromised in women with inherent tissue weakness and stress incontinence (56,57).

The use of autologous fascia lata was proposed to circumvent the problems associated with harvesting rectus fascia from a large abdominal incision (47,58–60). Using a fascial stripper, a fascial strip is harvested from the patient's outer thigh using a small incision just above the lateral femoral condyle. Although fascia lata is thicker and stronger than rectus fascia, operating time is prolonged because of the second operative site. Potential morbidity at the site of harvesting includes hematoma and seroma formation, incisional infections, and postoperative thigh pain (61).

The vaginal wall patch sling has been advocated by Raz and others as a readily available source of autologous material, without the need for a second operative site to harvest material (63–66). The vaginal wall patch may be left attached to the underlying submucosa. Alternatively, the vaginal mucosal patch is dissected off the underlying tissue and prepared as a free graft (64). The vaginal wall patch is ultimately covered by additional vaginal mucosa.

The primary disadvantage of vaginal wall patch slings is the propensity for tissue failure over time, leading to recurrent urethral hypermobility and stress incontinence. In an effort to evaluate the tissue properties of the vaginal wall, Winters examined the tensile strength and elongation propensity of vaginal wall specimens obtained from women undergoing surgery for pelvic organ prolapse (67). The maximum load to failure was 63.4 N (45.2). Full-thickness vaginal tissue was stronger than partial-thickness grafts, 87.1 N versus 58.9 N, respectively, but neither graft was as strong as Gore-Tex (140 N). Tissue elongation was 21.8 mm (7.2), more than either fascial strips or synthetic mesh. Given the structural properties of the vaginal wall, especially in women with stress incontinence due to urethral hypermobility, this is not unexpected.

The vaginal wall is designed to stretch when sustained forces are applied to it during vaginal childbirth. The submucosa and pubocervical fascia of the anterior vaginal wall may be disrupted by these forces, compromising tissue integrity and contributing in part to the development of the patient's stress incontinence due to urethral hypermobility (56,57). Over time, continued stress on the already compromised vaginal wall patch may lead to progressive loss of collagen and elastin from the endopelvic tissue. This finding explains the low long-term success rate reported with vaginal wall patch slings.

Allogenic Materials

Numerous studies regarding the successful use of allogenic grafts in orthopedic reconstruction have been published in the literature (68,69). The advantages of allogenic fascia lata grafts are accessibility, reduced operating time, and reduced postoperative morbidity from the harvesting site (70). One study compared the operating time and hospital stay for autologous and cadaveric fascia lata sling procedures. Operating room time was 24 minutes longer and 0.81 days longer hospital stay for autologous fascia lata (71). Despite the cost of cadaveric fascia lata, actual costs for the two materials may be equivalent. The theoretical disadvantages of donor fascia lata include the antigenicity of the material, the risk for transmission of viral infections, such as hepatitis and human immunodeficiency virus (HIV), and the potential loss of tissue integrity over time. To minimize these risks, specimens are either frozen or freeze-dried once they are harvested, reducing the graft to an acellular fibrous mesh (72). As a result, the risk for

HIV transmission is estimated to be 1 in 8 million (73).

Review of the orthopedic experience indicates variations in the strength of cadaveric fascia lata specimens depending on the method of tissue processing. Hinton and colleagues performed biomechanical testing on samples of commercially available donor fascia lata prepared using either solvent dehydration and gamma radiation, or freeze-dried specimens (74). Solvent dehydrated samples were superior to freeze-dried tissue in terms of maximum load (315 N versus 262.1 N), maximum load/graft width (31.6 N/mm versus 26.2 N/mm), and stiffness (188.2 N/mm versus 158.3 N/mm). Samples of lateral fascia lata were stronger than central fascial strips in both tissue preparations.

The fate of either cadaveric or autologous fascial strips has been investigated in a goat animal model (75). Necrosis of the graft was noted over the first 2 weeks, followed by significant neovascularization for the next 3 to 8 weeks. Neovascularization continued and was completed by 30 weeks. Cellular repopulation began at 12 weeks with collagen deposition and remodeling. No evidence of DNA from the graft specimens was noted after 4 weeks.

Handa and associates reported the first series of patients using cadaveric fascia lata in a suburethral sling procedure (76). Although most investigators report equivalent success rates for sling procedures using autologous or cadaveric fascia lata grafts, one recent author questioned the durability of cadaveric fascia lata. Fitzgerald and coauthors reported early sling failure in 6 of 35 women who underwent a sling procedure with cadaveric, freeze-dried, irradiated fascia lata (77). Failures occurred in a mean of 11.5 weeks (range, 1 to 20 weeks). At reexploration, four grafts appeared to have been reabsorbed and two were significantly softened and fragmented. The findings of Fitzgerald are not typical of the environmental reaction reported with the use of donor fascia lata in the orthopedic literature. This could be due to the use of freeze-dried, rather than solvent dehydrated, fascia lata in their series, or to the different biologic environment of the vagina. Although this is an isolated report, anecdotal experience confirms that there are isolated patients in whom the cadaveric graft does not maintain its integrity leading to sling failure owing to recurrent urethral hypermobility.

Based on the successful experience of other reconstructive surgeons using dermal allografts, several recent studies have reported 85% to 95% short-term subjective cure rates in women who underwent a suburethral sling procedure with cadaveric dermal grafts (78–80). Prior research has demonstrated that dermal grafts maintain their integrity and strength after implantation through neovascularization and host incorporation. Collagen fibrils are randomly oriented in dermal grafts that may improve suture retention (81,82).

One of the most recent materials investigated for use in reconstruction is porcine small intestine submucosa (83–85). Porcine small intestinal mucosa is harvested by removing the mucosa and muscularis externa from the intestinal wall. The remaining acellular, extracellular matrix is composed of 90% type I collagen without a fascial grain. The tissue is preserved in a freeze-dried state and sterilized with ethylene chloride. When prepared for use, the material is soft and pliable and has the consistency of cadaveric fascia lata. However, as opposed to cadaveric fascia lata, porcine small intestinal submucosa is biodegradable and resorbable. Experimental evidence in canine and murine models found that the graft acts as a scaffolding that allows ingrowth of host tissue before its total degradation. Kubricht and colleagues investigated the tensile strength of freeze-dried, irradiated cadaveric fascia lata and porcine small intestinal submucosa (83). They found that the mean suture pullout load for cadaveric fascia lata was slightly higher at 5.64 lb, compared with 3.36 lb for the porcine material. They concluded that further research was needed to determine whether porcine intestinal submucosa was a viable sling material. Table 30.3 summarizes the properties of nonsynthetic sling materials.

TABLE 30.3. *Summary of tissue properties of nonsynthetic sling materials*

	Histobiology	Tensile strength
Autologous rectus fascia	Graft persists; neovascularization, remodeling similar to noninflammatory scar tissue	Similar to solvent dehydrated cadaveric fascia lata and dermal grafts; in rabbit vagina model, graft constricts 30% and looses 50% of strength
Autologous fascia lata	Few data; slings appear intact when reexploration is done	Subjective studies showing increased tensile strength and improved collagen orientation compared with rectus fascia
Freeze-dried cadaveric fascia	In rabbit vagina model, graft was remodeled and replaced with parallel bundles of host collagen after 12 weeks	Less strength compared with autologous rectus fascia and solvent dehydrated cadaveric fascia
Solvent-dehydrated cadaveric fascia lata	No studies	Similar strength to autologous rectus fascia
Dermal allograft	Graft persists with neovascularization and host incorporation; collagen fibers oriented randomly compared to parallel, as with fascial grafts	Most consistent tensile strength; similar to autologous rectus fascia and solvent dehydrated cadaveric fascia lata; stronger than freeze-dried cadaveric fascia lata
Porcine small intestinal submucosa	Absorbable matrix composed of collagen, elastin, and growth factors	Suture pull-through occurs at less force than freeze-dried cadaveric fascia lata

Synthetic Materials

Much of the gynecologic experience with the use of synthetic mesh stems from the general surgery literature using these materials in abdominal wall reconstruction for hernia repair (86–90). Synthetic meshes provide a readily available source of inexpensive material with consistent biomechanical properties and without the risk for viral transmission from the donor. The use of these materials also reduces operating time and eliminates potential morbidity at the site of harvesting an autologous graft. The permanent meshes, Mersilene, Marlex, Prolene, and Gore-Tex, have all been shown to have high tensile strength up to 50 N. The construction of the meshes differs in their fiber components, weave, porosity, and flexibility. These properties affect tissue response and the ability to incorporate into the host tissue or fight infection. Numerous investigators have reported higher rates of infection and erosion with synthetic materials. In several series, erosion with reimplantation of the materials has been reported in 14% to 23% of patients (91–93).

The porosity of the mesh determines its ability to ward off infection and the development of tissue fibrosis (94). Multifilament materials, such as Mersilene and Gore-Tex, have small interstices (<10 μm) that allow bacteria into the spaces but prevent the host defense cells, macrophages and polymorphonuclear leukocytes, from entering the material to respond to infection. The number, size, and shape of the pores also affect tissue bonding and fibrosis. Marlex and Prolene are both derived from monofilament polypropylene but differ in pore size. Gore-Tex has the largest pore diameter (10- to 20-μm interstices) and produces minimal inflammatory reaction and low peritoneal fibrosis in a rabbit model (88). In humans, Gore-Tex is poorly incorporated into tissue. Research using Gore-Tex in abdominal wall hernia repair showed the formation of minimal, filmy adhesions that could be easily lysed if needed (90). Although this is an advantage in patients who need graft removal, failure to incorporate a graft may result in the repair being dependent only on suture integrity.

Marlex mesh has been shown to have the highest flexural rigidity (stiffness) compared with Mersilene or Gore-Tex (86). Marlex produces an intense inflammatory response with a dense, disorganized scar in animal models. This tendency in humans results in tissue rigidity and accounts for the propensity of Marlex to adhere to adjacent tissue, creating scarring and potential fistula formation (87). However, studies have shown that Marlex mesh is rarely involved when infection develops at the surgical site in inguinal or incisional hernia repairs (89).

Prolene mesh is a monofilament polypropylene double-woven mesh, similar to Marlex but with a larger pore size. This theoretically should lead to better tissue incorporation with deposition of collagen within the interstices. A Prolene tape is the basis for the currently popular tension-free vaginal tape (TVT) procedure advocated by Ulmsten and colleagues (95). The large pore structure of Prolene and the design of the tape enable the material to be placed without sutures to secure it into the correct position. Although the material has been used extensively, there are few data in the literature regarding complications with this mesh.

Although synthetic mesh materials clearly provide an alternative to harvesting autologous tissue or using a more expensive cadaveric graft, surgeons must be cautious with the use of synthetic materials in reconstructive surgery, especially because newer materials are marketed before extensive experience confirms their safety. Newer materials may have theoretical biologic advantages, such as the collagen-impregnated Protogen mesh, only to be found hazardous as a sling material when used in humans. Alternatively, some materials may function well as reconstructive materials in other parts of the body but be less advantageous in vaginal reconstructive surgery because of the thin vaginal mucosa, the contaminated environment, and the required functions of the vagina (Table 30.4).

TABLE 30.4. *Summary of the properties of synthetic materials*

Mesh	Trade name	Type of fiber	Pores shape	Pore size (μm)
Polyethylene terephthalate	Mersilene	Multifilament	Hexagonal	
Expanded polytetrafluoroethylene	Gore-Tex	Multifilament	Node and fibrils: macropore	800
Polypropylene	Marlex Prolene	Monofilament	Irregular Diamond	600 1,500
Polyglycolic acid	Dexon	Multifilament (absorbable)	Diamond	
Polyglactin	Vicryl	Multifilament (absorbable)	Diamond	

SURGICAL TECHNIQUES

The descriptions of sling procedures have undergone constant modifications in recent years in an attempt to achieve the following goals: select the "best" material for the sling, minimize the amount of material used, improve the quality of the attachment site for securing the sling, and minimize operative time, morbidity, and postoperative recuperation time. Some of the advances in techniques have been generated by surgeons' critical review and publication of their experience, but many changes have been industry driven. Before adopting new materials or instruments, each physician must critically weigh the peer-review data regarding new advances to ensure that women are truly informed of the risks of these new procedures.

The following description is one approach to a sling procedure using donor fascia lata. Other materials may be substituted, including autologous fascia lata or rectus fascial strips, allografts, or synthetic materials. Two strips of donor fascia lata measuring 3 cm wide by at least 15 cm long are used. Alternatively, a single, wider specimen (6 to 8 cm) may be used and divided into two narrower strips. The two 3-cm wide strips are overlapped longitudinally by 3 cm and sutured together in four points with permanent suture. The central portion of the sling that will be placed suburethrally is then double layered and 3 × 3 cm. The remaining tails are trimmed to 1 to 1.5 cm width. The graft is colored with a marking pen to facilitate visualization and minimize

twisting of the graft as it comes through the retropubic tunnels.

The patient is placed in dorsal lithotomy position with Allen stirrups, and the hip is flexed to 90 degrees. Care is taken not to hyperflex the hip beyond 90 degrees to prevent traction on the sciatic nerve and compression of the femoral nerve by the inguinal ligament. The abdominal–perineal–vaginal region is prepared, and a 16-French Foley catheter is inserted. A 4-cm incision is made just superior to the pubic symphysis and carried down to the rectus fascia. The incision is packed.

The vaginal mucosa is opened horizontally at least 2 cm above the urethrovesical junction and then longitudinally to within 0.5 cm of the urethral meatus. The vaginal mucosa is dissected from the underlying tissue laterally to the descending pubic ramus. The suburethral tissue is plicated with polyglycolic acid suture to increase the density of tissue between the sling and the urethra. Correction of any additional anterior midline defects should be completed at this time. The bladder is then drained. Transvaginal perforation through the endopelvic fascia is accomplished by blunt dissection along the posterior surface of the inferior pubic ramus using the surgeon's finger or with the aid of a tonsil clamp. The direction of perforation is toward the patient's ipsilateral shoulder. Care must be taken to remain lateral to the urethra as palpated by the catheter to avoid urethral trauma, but medial to the pubic tubercle to avoid injury to the ilioinguinal nerve. During perforation of the endopelvic fascia, bleeding may be encountered, which often responds to digital compression or compression by the sling once it is in place and temporary upward traction is applied to the sling ends.

The vaginal surgeon's finger is placed in the retropubic tunnel to indicate the appropriate location on the undersurface of the rectus muscle and fascia for perforation of the rectus fascia. The assistant proceeds abdominally and creates a stab wound in the rectus fascia overlying the tunnel. Uterine packing forceps are introduced through the fascial incision and guided through the retropubic tunnel by the vaginal surgeon's finger into the vaginal field. The end of the sling is grasped and transferred to the abdominal field. Once this is accomplished bilaterally, the sling is secured under the proximal urethra in four points using permanent suture. Cystoscopy with a 30- or 70-degree lens must be performed to rule out bladder or urethral injury. Upward traction on the sling during urethroscopy confirms correct placement suburethrally. A suprapubic catheter is placed under direct visualization. The vaginal mucosa is closed.

The most difficult aspect of the sling procedure is the art of determining how much tension to apply to the sling when securing it suprapubically. Numerous techniques have been advocated, including adjusting tension to create the appropriate Q-tip angle of urethral deflection, intraoperative urodynamic assessment of urethral pressures, or the placement of a cystoscopic sheath (13,45,58,59,96,97). Beck used intraoperative urethral pressure measurements to create an intraurethral pressure of 80 to 90 cm H_2O (59). McGuire and colleagues recommended adjusting sling tension by endoscopic visualization of mucosal coaptation (45), whereas Rovner and coauthors used a cystoscopic sheath placed transurethrally to stabilize the urethra as the sling was secured to rectus fascia (96). Govier described placing sutures at the sling ends and tying the sutures over rectus fascia, allowing one finger between the sutures and the rectus fascia (58). Most surgeons now advocate applying minimal tension on the sling because

excess tension is the most common cause of voiding dysfunction after sling procedures.

Our current technique is to adjust the sling tension based on the patient's body habitus and the degree of abdominal wall laxity. When the patient is in lithotomy position for surgery, there is minimal pressure on the abdominal wall from intraabdominal contents. As the woman assumes an upright position with sitting or standing, the intraabdominal contents settle into the lower abdomen, displacing the abdominal wall outward. Excess abdominal wall laxity and obesity result in more outward displacement of the abdominal wall and, thus, more upward traction on the sling. As such, each patient requires individualization for appropriate sling tension. Our approach has been not to suture the free ends of the sling to the perforation sites in the rectus fascia as previously advocated. Rather, the ends are sutured to each other using permanent suture, and the distance between the sutured sling and the rectus fascia is determined. In slender women with good abdominal wall tone, two finger breadths (about 3 cm) can just be inserted between the sling and the fascia, whereas in obese women or those with significant abdominal wall laxity, the sling may be as loose as 3 finger breadths distance. Using similar theoretical considerations, Choe recently published a novel approach to determining sling tension using a weight-adjusted nomogram (97). Fifty women underwent a Gore-Tex patch sling procedure, with a 94% cure rate. The mean catheter duration was 7 days (range, 1 to 21 days), and none of the women experienced urinary retention or urethral obstruction. Regardless of the techniques used to determine sling tension, remember the old adage "if you think it's too tight, it's probably just right."

Vaginal packing is placed for 24 hours. Voiding trials begin after 24 to 48 hours, once the patient's discomfort is minimal. The suprapubic catheter is removed once each void is more than 100 mL and each postvoid residual is less than 100 mL for 24 hours. All patients are taught intermittent self-catheterization preoperatively as an alternative management approach. Some surgeons do not place a suprapubic catheter and rely on either a regular Foley or intermittent self-catheterization for assurance of bladder emptying.

An alternative to using donor fascia lata is obtaining fascia lata from the patient (59,62). To identify the correct site for harvesting, a line can be drawn from the anterosuperior iliac crest to the lateral epicondyle of the knee. A 3- to 4-cm long incision is made just proximal to the lateral condyle and carried down to the fascia lata. Two small incisions are made in the fascia lata, parallel to the longitudinal axis of the leg. The distal end of the graft is mobilized, and a suture is placed. Using the fascial stripper, a 15 to 18 cm long and 1.5 to 2 cm wide strip of fascia lata is harvested. The subcutaneous tissue and skin are closed, and the leg is wrapped to provide hemostasis and minimize the chance of hematoma or seroma formation. Subcutaneous fluid collections can usually be managed conservatively but on occasion may required aspiration or drainage.

Modifications of the sling procedures usually differ in one of two ways: either the amount of material used for the sling is reduced, or the fixation point of the sling is different (21,98). Sling patches have been advocated in an attempt to limit the amount of material used for the sling. As opposed to a strip of material, it is far easier to harvest a 3 cm wide by 3 to 4 cm long patch of rectus fascia or fascia lata from a patient with less potential morbidity. Karram and Bhatia were the first to describe this technique in 1990 (98). Ten patients with severe, recurrent incontinence underwent a fascia lata patch sling with a 90% objective cure rate 1 to 2 years after surgery. The rationale for using a patch of synthetic material is to decrease the amount of material within the patient and, thus, decrease the potential of graft rejection. Reduced cost of the material is also a consideration. Once the patch is prepared, permanent sutures are placed at the lateral margins. These sutures are then brought through the opened retropubic tunnels as described previously or transferred from the vaginal field to the abdominal incision using a tra-

ditional Pereyra or Stamey needle. Newer devices are available that can be used to transfer the graft above the rectus fascia or secure the graft to bone anchors placed in the pubic symphysis through a vaginal or abdominal approach. Multiple manufacturers have introduced all inclusive kits containing the synthetic patch sling with sutures attached and disposable anchoring devices. The disadvantages of using sling patches and sutures tails in performing a sling procedure are the potential for suture pullout at the lateral attachment sites or breakage of the permanent suture.

A second variation in performing a sling procedure is the choice of attachment sites. Most surgeons prefer to bring the sling or suture tails through a perforation in the rectus fascia. The ends are then sutured to the rectus fascia at the perforation site or secured to each other in the midline over the rectus fascia. It is often more difficult to determine the correct amount of tension for the sling when suturing the sling to the rectus fascia openings. Some surgeons prefer to attach the sling ends to a fixed point. Strips of rectus fascia or fascia lata have been sutured to Cooper's ligament either through a transvaginal or transabdominal approach (21).

Bone anchors were introduced specifically to facilitate needle suspension procedures and operations using a patch sling and suture tails (99). The anchors are inserted into the pubic symphysis, and the surgeon secures the suture tails to the anchors. The theoretical advantage of this method was to provide a more secure superior attachment site and prevent suture pullout from the rectus fascia. However, the vulnerable locations in these operations are not the attachment site, but rather the suture or tissue integrity in the periurethral area. Biomechanical studies have also shown that suture breakage at the point of attachment of the suture to the anchor may occur, leading to surgical failure (99). Another disadvantage of bone anchors is the potential for postoperative pain or infection at the anchor sites. Treatment, including removal of the anchor, is often quite challenging.

RESULTS

The reported surgical success rate of sling procedures varies in the current literature between 63% and 97%. The recent American Urological Association Clinical Guidelines Panel summarized studies with at least 12 months of follow-up (42). The panel used the authors' definition of "cure/dry" and found an 82% "cure rate" for women, which remained consistent throughout the follow-up periods that were examined (12 to 23 months, 24 to 47

months, 48 months, and longer). The panel recognized that cure doesn't always equate with being dry. Some authors use cure to mean the patient was cured of stress incontinence. However, the patient herself may not consider that she is dry because she may still experience incontinence owing to postoperative urge incontinence. Table 30.5 summarizes the results of the currently reviewed series (17,20,22,24,53,66,71,93,100–115).

The wide variation of cure rates is due to multiple factors, and comparisons between

TABLE 30.5. *Summary of surgical results for suburethral sling procedures*

Lead author	No. of patients	Sling material	Length of follow-up	Subjective cure (%)		Objective cure (%)	
				Cure	Improvement	Cure	Improvement
McGuire, 1978	52	Rectus fascia	10 mo to 6 yr	96	—	—	—
Chaikin, 1998	251	Rectus fascia	1 yr to 15 yr	73	92	73[a]	92[a]
Hassouna, 1999	82	Rectus fascia	3.4 yr	49	78	—	—
Morgan, 2000	247	Rectus fascia	51 mo	88	92[b]	—	—
Richter, 2001	57	Rectus fascia, fascia lata	42 mo	84	88[b]	97	—
Parker, 1979	50	Fascia lata, autologous	—	84	—	84	—
Beck, 1988	170	Fascia lata, autologous	6 wk to 10 yr	92	—	—	—
Cross, 1998	150	Fascia lata, autologous	22 mo	93	—	—	—
Wright, 1998		Fascia lata					
	33	Autologous	16 mo	94	—	—	—
	59	Cadaveric	9 mo	98	—	—	—
Owens, 1999	24	Fascia lata	30	—	72	79	—
Elliot, 2000	26	Fascia lata, cadaveric	15 mo	77	96	—	—
Brown, 2000		Fascia lata					
	30	Autologous	44 mo	90	73	—	—
	104	Cadaveric	12 mo	84	77	—	—
Amundsen, 2000	104	Fascia lata	19 mo	—	—	63	84
Carbone, 2001	154	Fascia lata	10 mo	60	62	—	—
Juma, 1992	54	Vaginal wall	24 mo	91	94	91	94
Raz, 1996	163	Vaginal wall	17 mo	93	—	93	—
Kaplan, 2000	373	Vaginal wall	39 mo	96	—	—	—
Hilton, 1983	10	Marlex	6 mo to 9 yr	80	—	70	—
Morgan, 1985	274	Marlex	4 yr	77	—	—	—
Weinberger, 1995	108	Gore-Tex	38 mo	73	—	61	—
Barbalias, 1997	24	Gore-Tex	30 mo	—	—	83	100
Kersey, 1988	100	Mersilene mesh	Up to 5 yr	78	—	—	—
Young, 1995	67	Mersilene mesh	13 mo	95	—	93	—

[a]Objective data correlated to subjective results; however, subjective results used in event of discordance.
[b]Quality-of-life questionnaire.
Data from references 17, 20, 22, 24, 53, 66, 71, 93, and 100–114.

studies are almost impossible. Patient selection for a sling procedure varies widely in the literature. Most authors perform sling procedures in women with documented ISD but may use varying criteria for ISD. Reports may include both primary and recurrent incontinence and rarely control for other variables, such as underlying medical conditions that may affect cure rates. The definition of cure is not standardized between studies. Many authors perform telephone interviews or send questionnaires to patients with prior sling surgery to obtain subjective cure rates. A cure is considered to be the patient's report of an absence of stress urinary incontinence; however, in some cases, a cure may indicate a complete resolution of all urinary loss, including urge incontinence. Improvement usually signifies a greater than 50% alleviation of symptoms, but some studies report cure or improvement if the patient states she no longer wears pad protection. Some authors incorporate quality-of-life measurements or questionnaires that give a broader picture of improvement. Objective data are more accessible than in the past because sling procedures have become more common. Objective cure is based on one or more office studies showing no evidence of leakage. These studies may include a cough stress test, pad test, and urodynamics, although these tests are also poorly standardized.

Unlike women undergoing retropubic operations, patients who have a sling operation as a repeat procedure generally do as well as those in whom the procedure is the primary incontinence operation. Morgan reported a series of 281 women with recurrent incontinence with a 77.4% subjective cure rate 5 years after a Marlex sling procedure (22). Drutz and colleagues found a 95.3% objective cure rate in 65 women after a Marlex sling for recurrent incontinence (100). The results with Gore-Tex slings have been more disappointing, with Weinberger and co-workers reporting only a 61% objective cure in 108 women with recurrent stress incontinence (93). In his 1995 study on Mersilene slings, Young and associates described an objective cure rate of

97% in a subgroup of 33 women with recurrent incontinence (115). Although these findings are encouraging, the same concerns regarding the lack of standardization of patient selection, follow-up duration, and criteria for cure still exist.

A comparison of results for organic and synthetic slings reveals a slightly better cure rate for procedures in which synthetic sling materials are used. Choe and colleagues (64) compared the outcome in 40 consecutive patients randomized to an antimicrobial polytetrafluoroethylene mesh patch sling or a vaginal wall sling. After 22 months of mean follow-up, 95% of the synthetic mesh group were stress continent, whereas only 70% of the vaginal wall sling group were continent. The complication rate was not significantly different. Ogundipe and associates (116) found a 6-months objective cure rate of 100% for polytetrafluoroethylene versus 87% for autologous fascia lata slings in a nonrandomized group. Kuo (117) reported objective cure rates of 96% and subjective cure rates of 92% after two years of follow-up in patients randomized to polypropylene mesh or rectus fascia. A trend toward more urinary retention in patients after synthetic slings may contribute to decreased patient dryness in this group secondary to urge incontinence. Despite the small advantage of the synthetic material slings in resolving stress incontinence, the risk for complications with synthetic slings is still a cause for concern.

Few studies have compared autologous fascia with allograft fascia lata. Opponents of allograft fascia blame the process of sterilization and preservation of the cadaveric grafts for their presumed degradation *in vivo*. Carbone and colleagues, during repairs performed for sling failure, found their allograft patches to be attenuated and no other etiology for the failures (110). Others have shown good resilience of cadaveric tissue *in vivo* (107). Wright and colleagues (71) found that, after a mean follow-up of 11.5 months, autologous rectus fascia and cadaveric fascia lata were equally well tolerated and had subjective cure rates of 94% and 98%, respectively.

Another factor affecting cure rates is the type and severity of the preoperative incontinence. Mixed incontinence with postoperative persistent detrusor instability and urge incontinence leads to decreased patient dryness even when stress incontinence is cured. Historically, sling procedures have been performed for type III incontinence or ISD. With increase in surgical skill and subsequent decreased complication rates, sling procedures have been used for type II incontinence in greater numbers. In some studies, outcome varies based on indication. After a mean follow-up time of 51 months, the cure rate was 91% for women with type II incontinence versus 84% for women with type III incontinence in a study using rectus fascial slings by Morgan and co-workers (102). Two studies (66,112) looking at vaginal wall slings showed no difference in cure rates between women with type II incontinence and those with ISD even when Kaplan-Meier survival curves were employed to estimate long-term results. In a study of Mersilene mesh slings, Young and associates found that preoperative ISD decreased the objective cure rate from 97% to 84% after a mean of 13 months (115). Cure seen in women with the risk factor of chronically increased intraabdominal pressure showed very little difference at 95%. The cure rate seen for women with ISD treated with a polytetrafluoroethylene sling is comparable at 83% (113).

Postoperative detrusor instability, in some studies (112), is seen more commonly in women with preoperative ISD possibly because of advertent tighter sling placement. Again, urge incontinence may lead to overall less dryness in this group of women. Chaiken and colleagues divided their population of 251 incontinent women into those with simple incontinence (women who did not meet complex criteria and had type II or III incontinence, detrusor instability without leakage, and ISD) and those with complex incontinence (including urge incontinence, pipestem urethra, urethral or vesicovaginal fistula, urethral diverticulum, grade 3 or 4 cystocele, or neurogenic bladder) (53). After at least 1

year of follow-up, 98% of simple cases were objectively cured of their stress incontinence by a rectus fascia patch sling. Ninety three percent of complex cases were also cured of stress urinary incontinence. Kaplan-Meier survival curves showed a significant difference in cure rates between groups, however, most failures were due to persistent urge incontinence. Age alone has not been shown to be a risk factor for failure (39).

Patient satisfaction with the sling procedure is strongly associated with social dryness and inversely related to worsened detrusor instability and urge incontinence. In fact, patients often consider the surgery a failure if stress incontinence is relieved but urge incontinence is new or worsened (65,66,118). Therefore, it is important to record objective success or failure in a systematic and reproducible manner. It is also important to include subjective quality-of-life measures and overall satisfaction when evaluating the effectiveness of a procedure for any given patient.

URODYNAMIC CHANGES

Urodynamic studies have attempted to confirm the proposed mechanism of surgical cure of the sling procedure. Although the data are inconsistent, some authors have reported increases in functional urethral length or MUCP after sling procedures. Hilton and Stanton reported a decrease in functional urethral length postoperatively in 10 women who underwent a Marlex sling (17). This change was not substantiated in a larger series. Three studies found no change in functional urethral length after (18,119,120), but two others reported an increase in functional length after surgery (13,121). MUCP was noted to increase in Rottenberg's study (18), and Young and colleagues (115) reported an increase in both parameters in 110 women who underwent a Mersilene mesh sling. Three additional investigators have found an increase in MUCP postoperatively (13,23,121). However, surgical success could not be consistently predicted based on changes in these static parameters. Variations in the amount of tension applied to the sling may account for these discrepant finding.

The postoperative urodynamic changes that do appear to be consistent throughout the literature are an improvement in pressure transmission ratios and a reduction in peak flow during voiding. Three reports that have measured the differential changes in pressure transmission to the urethra and bladder have found a postoperative ratio of 100% or more compared with preoperative values of 70% to 90% (17–19). The improvement is seen primarily in the proximal one half to three quarters of the urethra and appears to be correlated with surgical success. In his study of 36 patients, Rottenberg found a significant increase in intraabdominal pressure transmission ratio from 81% to 104% in patients who achieved cure, compared with a decrease from 76% to 69% in the group of patients who failed surgery (18). Other investigators have found the increase in pressure transmission in the distal portion of the urethra. The location of the improved pressure transmission may be in part due to the final position of the sling along the urethra. The postoperative reduction in peak flow rate during voiding implies an increase in urethral outflow resistance following the sling operation (18,19). The observed increase in pressure transmission and reduction of flow rate in these studies correlates with the proposed mechanism of action of the sling procedure.

COMPLICATIONS

Historically, sling procedures have been associated with a greater incidence of intraoperative and postoperative complications than retropubic procedures. Some of these problems are seen more commonly with slings because of the indications and objectives of the surgery. Because many patients have had prior, failed procedures, the presence of scar tissue increases the surgical complication rate. Dissecting between the urethra and anterior vaginal wall and tunneling into the retropubic space without direct visualization may add to complications such as bleeding, cysto-

tomy, urethral injury, ilioinguinal nerve entrapment, or tracking of vaginal bacteria into the retropubic space. Use of a thin band of material for the sling, excess tension on the sling, or scarred, denuded vaginal mucosa may lead to sling erosion or urethral transection. The most common complications of sling operations are voiding dysfunction and irritative voiding symptoms.

Wide variations in the incidence of voiding dysfunction after slings have been reported. In his meta-analysis, Jarvis found a mean incidence of postoperative voiding disorders of 12.8% (range, 2% to 37%), including one series in which 28% of women required sling revision before voiding could take place (122). Factors that add to voiding dysfunction after slings may include an inadequate detrusor contraction and a loss of urethral relaxation owing to the obstructive nature of the sling (123). Problems associated with a partial obstruction of the urethra by the sling range from positional voiding to the need for episodic long-term intermittent self-catheterization. Unusual positions, such as bending forward, deep squatting, standing, or using the Credé maneuver to void may be necessary on a temporary or permanent basis in order to achieve complete bladder emptying (93). Prolonged postoperative catheterization is a well-recognized occurrence. Although its definition varies in length of time between studies, a need for catheterization past 90 days is considered prolonged. Obstruction of voluntary flow after a sling operation may be temporary and require prolonged postoperative catheterization or may be permanent and require lifelong catheterization or sling revision. Recurrent urinary tract infections are also a problem that can be exacerbated by elevated postvoid residuals (13,124).

Several authors have attempted to identify risk factors for postoperative voiding dysfunction and urinary retention. Many studies agree that preoperative voiding without a detrusor contraction increases the risk for post sling voiding dysfunction (124–126) and sling revision or removal (93). Valsalva voiding has been linked to early objective failures (54% versus

17% in non-Valsalva voiders) as well as a longer duration of postoperative catheterization (50). Other authors have found correlation, instead, with the type of procedure performed, age older than 65 years, additional procedures performed at the time of sling, and a preoperative urodynamic flow rate of less than or equal to 20 mL/sec (51,126). Therefore, the ability to predict postoperative voiding dysfunction, in most cases, is still conjectural.

Treatment of postoperative voiding dysfunction may be as simple as change of voiding habits or as aggressive as sling revision or removal. Unfortunately, pharmacologic management of urinary retention is notoriously unsuccessful. Cholinergic agents have proved to be no better than placebo for treating postoperative urinary retention in blinded, placebo-controlled studies. Occasionally, pharmacologic relaxation of the urethra may be helpful. Skeletal muscle relaxants, such as diazepam, appear to be more beneficial than α-adrenergic blockers. Partial or complete urinary retention can be treated by intermittent self-catheterization. In cases in which there is an inability to void and the patient is unable or does not wish to perform self-catheterization, a second procedure may be undertaken to alleviate the obstructed urethra.

Several authors have suggested methods of sling revision that have been successful in their population of patients (127–132). Most of these methods involve urethrolysis or dividing the sling material either abdominally or vaginally. Sling arm incision with or without a patch and with or without dissection to release arms from scar tissue is successful in 90% (range, 84% to 100%). Stress incontinence recurs in a limited number of women (mean, 15%; range, 0% to 23%), probably related to the extent of scar tissue that stabilizes the urethra even after sling revision.

The vaginal approach to sling revision is undertaken by initially making a single vertical incision or a U-shaped incision in the anterior vaginal mucosa under the sling. The sling is identified below the urethra and freed from surrounding fibrosis. The sling may be incised in the midline or laterally. Authors vary in their approach with the extent of lysis of scar tissue. Amundsen and colleagues reported the results of various strategies to treat voiding dysfunction in 32 women depending on the type of sling used (132). In women with autologous fascial slings, they were unable to identify discrete fascial tissue to divide. Thus, they primarily performed urethrolysis, at times high into the retropubic space. In patients with allograft fascia lata, the sling was identified and simply transected, whereas sling removal was required in patients with synthetics slings. Thirty of the 32 women (94%) were able to void adequately within 1 week of the revision. Stress incontinence returned in 9%.

Some authors have described attempts to place an additional patch of material into the sling versus simple excision. In two separate reports, McLennan and Bent (128) and Ghoniem and Elgamasy (129) described the approach to revision after a fascia lata sling by dividing the sling and inserting a patch of fascia lata between the two ends. The length of the inserted graft varied according to the amount of excess tension of the original sling. We have inserted an allograft fascia lata patch into women who underwent sling revision. All were voiding without the need for catheterization after 2 weeks.

Brubaker reported the results of an abdominal sling release technique (127). The abdominal incision is opened, and the location of the sling's perforation through the rectus fascia is identified. A section of rectus fascia surrounding the fascial perforation site is then mobilized to create a fascial plug. The plug is resutured below the rectus fascia once the tension has been adjusted.

Irritative voiding symptoms range from urgency and frequency without true voiding dysfunction to severe detrusor instability, and urge incontinence may occur in women after sling procedures (9,13). Although the data vary widely, these problems, when present before surgery, may persist or worsen postoperatively in 15% to 55%. *De novo* detrusor instability is also a common complication of the sling procedure, occurring in 7% of women, and must be discussed with patients preoperatively (42). Patients with worsened or new urge incontinence postoperatively are more likely to be dissatisfied despite full resolution of stress incontinence (65,118). Postoperative urgency, frequency, and urge incontinence are believed to be due to persistent failure of closure of the bladder neck at rest causing urine to escape into the proximal urethra and trigger a reflex detrusor contraction (118). *De novo* detrusor instability and urge incontinence are thought to result from postoperative obstruction to voiding, similar to that experienced in men with benign prostatic hypertrophy.

Several authors have attempted to correlate certain risk factors with persistent, postoperative urge symptoms (46,133). Schrepferman and Griebling found that more than 90% of patients with existing motor urge incontinence resulting from low-amplitude uninhibited detrusor contractions (<15 cm H_2O pressure) tended to see resolution of their urge symptoms. Women with pure sensory urge incontinence and women with high-amplitude motor detrusor instability fared much worse, with symptom resolution in only 39% and 28%, respectively (46). Risk factors associated with *de novo* detrusor instability are unclear.

Fortunately, medical management has been effective in treating many women (134,135). Although postoperative detrusor instability usually responds to anticholinergic medications, these agents may lead to worsened retention and elevated postvoid residuals and must be used cautiously. Behavioral therapy tends to be less effective in treating postoperative detrusor instability. At times, sling revision may be necessary to resolve irritative voiding complaints or detrusor instability (132).

Other, less common complications that are seen with the suburethral sling procedure can be subdivided into intraoperative or early postoperative complications and late postoperative complications. Examples of intraoperative or early postoperative complications include blood loss, cystotomy, and postoperative infections. Bleeding, when excessive, typically occurs from laceration of vessels in the retropubic plexus. If direct visualization with optimal lighting and ligation is ineffective, compression can usually be accomplished from below or by placing tension on the sling arms. Open dissection of the retropubic space from the abdominal route is rarely required but may be necessary in extreme cases. Cystotomy is visualized at the time of intraoperative cystoscopy following placement of the sling. It is essential that cystoscopy be performed in all patients undergoing a sling procedure to ensure that no trauma to the bladder or urethra has occurred. If the sling is visualized within the bladder, it should be removed and repositioned. The cystotomy often does not need to be closed; simple prolonged catheter drainage is usually sufficient.

Specific postoperative infections encompass vaginal wound infections, abdominal wound infections, abscesses, and urinary tract infections. Some authors maintain that soaking of the sling material in antibiotic solution and liberal use of the solution for wound irrigation during the procedure decrease the incidence of wound infections, although this has not been proved. Preoperative, intravenous, prophylactic antibiotics are widely used. Recurrent urinary tract infections are thought to occur because of elevated postvoid residuals, decreased immunity in the initial postoperative period, or foreign body (suture or sling) within the bladder because of failure to perform intraoperative cystoscopy or migration into the bladder or urethra over time. Treatment should address the underlying cause. At times, oral prophylactic antibiotics may be indicated for 3 to 6 months to decrease the incidence of urinary tract infections.

In addition to prolonged voiding dysfunction, late postoperative complications can include vaginal graft erosion, urethral erosion with or without urethral transection, postoperative pain syndromes, osteomyelitis pubis, and vaginal inclusion cysts. Vaginal erosion or poor healing of the vaginal epithelium is primarily a complication of synthetic slings (13, 21,92,100,115). Although the true incidence of graft erosion is difficult to determine because of its delayed presentation, the reported incidence is 3% to 23%, depending on the synthetic material. Patients may present with vaginal spotting or a malodorous discharge. The highest incidence of graft problems is reported with Gore-Tex soft tissue patch slings, with an incidence of 8% to 23% (13,92). Because of the open weave of Marlex and Mersilene, erosion or nonhealing of the vaginal epithelium is reported to occur in 3% to 7% of women (100,115). To prevent graft problems, overzealous dissection and devascularization of the vaginal mucosa should be avoided. Minor graft erosions or vaginal mucosal defects can be conservatively managed with excision of graft material and replication of the mucosa as an outpatient (136). Graft rejection may cause vaginal erosion, chronic inflammation, and abdominal sinus tract formation. Bent and associates found a 23% reaction or removal rate for the expanded polytetrafluoroethylene sling (92). Interestingly, the sling material was invariably colonized with gram-positive cocci, but it did not yield growth of organisms in culture. Silastic slings have been associated with a high rate of rejection as well. Surgical removal of the entire graft material is the only treatment for rejection.

Surgical removal also must be undertaken in cases of partial or complete urethral transection. In some cases, interpositioning allograft fascia or a Martius labial fat pad may be used, especially when a replacement sling is required or when incomplete urethral repair is undertaken (132). Although erosion into the urinary tract most commonly occurs with synthetic sling material, it has been reported with fascial slings as well (136–138). Other possibly associated risk factors for urethral erosion are slings that are too narrow or have too much tension placed on them and slings that are placed in patients with high intraabdominal pressures, such as patients with obesity or chronic pulmonary conditions (112,139).

Pain syndromes are uncommon yet may require sling revision or removal. The use of bone anchors in the pubic symphysis has led to chronic suprapubic pain. Pain over the mons and labia may be due to ilioinguinal nerve entrapment by the sling or a suture. Ilioinguinal nerve entrapment can be prevented during sling procedures by remaining medial to the pubic tubercle during transvaginal dissection and perforation through the endopelvic fascia into the retropubic space. After the diagnosis of ilioinguinal nerve entrapment is established, sling removal is indicated. However, not all women respond to sling removal. Miyazaki and Shook reported the results of managing nerve entrapment after needle suspension procedures (140). Despite suture removal, most women had persistent pain. If removal of the sling fails to resolve the pain, trigger-point injections using long-acting local anesthetics [bupivacaine (Marcaine)] and steroids may be helpful.

Vaginal wall inclusion cysts have been reported specifically in women after vaginal wall slings (141,142). Osteomyelitis remains a serious concern when using bone anchors to stabilize the sling (143), although the reported prevalence is only 0.6% (144). Resolution of the osteomyelitis may require intravenous antibiotics, surgical curettage, and débridement resulting in significant long-term morbidity.

SUMMARY

Suburethral sling procedures were one of the first types of operation described for stress incontinence, and their popularity has waxed and waned over the years. The improvements in sling materials and refinements in surgical techniques that have minimized postoperative complications have expanded the utility of the sling operation. Although the debate continues about whether all women with genuine stress incontinence due to urethral hypermobility should undergo a sling procedure regardless of the status of their intrinsic urethral sphincter, current efforts are being directed at discovering the ideal sling material. Sling procedures should be a part of the repertoire of all incontinence surgeons.

REFERENCES

1. Hofenfellner R, Petrie E. Sling procedures in surgery. In: Stanton SL, Tanagho E, eds. *Surgery of female incontinence,* 2nd ed. Berlin: Springer-Verlag, 1986: 105–113.

2. Studdiford WE. Transplantation of abdominal fascia for relief of urinary stress incontinence. *Am J Obstet Gynecol* 1944;47:764–775.

3. Ridley JG. Appraisal of the Goebell-Frankenheim-Stoekel sling procedure. *Am J Obstet Gynecol* 1966; 95:714.

4. Wheeless CR. Goebell-Stoeckel fascia lata sling operation for urinary incontinence. In: *Atlas of pelvic surgery.* Philadelphia: Lea & Febiger, 1988:125–135.

5. Aldridge AH. Transplantation of fascia for relief of urinary stress incontinence. *Am J Obstet Gynecol* 1942;44:398–411.

6. Millin T, Read C. Stress incontinence of urine in the female: Millin's sling operation. *Postgrad Med J* 1948; 24:51.

7. Williams TJ, Telinde RW. The sling operation for urinary incontinence using Mersilene ribbon. *Obstet Gynecol* 1962;19:243.

8. Moir JC. The gauze-hammock operation: a modified Aldridge sling procedure. *J Obstet Gynaecol Br Commonw* 1968;75:1.

9. Morgan JE. A sling operation using Marlex polypropylene mesh for treatment of recurrent stress incontinence. *Am J Obstet Gynecol* 1970;105:359.

10. Flanu S, Soderberg G. Absorbable polyglactin mesh for retropubic sling operations in female urinary stress incontinence. *Gynecol Obstet Invest* 1983;16:1.

11. Jarvis GJ, Fowlie A. Clinical and urodynamic assessment of the porcine dermis bladder sling in the treatment of genuine stress incontinence. *Br J Obstet Gynaecol* 1985;92:1189.

12. Stanton SL, Brindley GS, Holmes DM. Silastic sling for urethral sphincter incompetence in women. *Br J Obstet Gynaecol* 1985;92:747.

13. Horbach NS, Blanco JS, Ostergard DR, et al. A suburethral sling procedure with polytetrafluoroethylene for the treatment of genuine stress incontinence in patients with low urethral closure pressure. *Obstet Gynecol* 1988;71:648.

14. Enhorning G. Simultaneous recording of intraurethral and intravesical pressure: a study of urethral closure pressure and stress incontinence in women. *Acta Chir Scand* 1961;276[Suppl]:1.

15. DeLancey JOL. Structural support of the urethra as it relates to stress incontinence: the hammock hypothesis. *Am J Obstet Gynecol* 1994;170:1713–1720.

16. Henriksson L, Ulmsten U. A urodynamic evaluation of the effects of abdominal urethrocystopexy in women with stress incontinence. *Am J Obstet Gynecol* 1978; 113:78.

17. Hilton P, Stanton SL. Clinical and urodynamic evaluation of the polypropylene (Marlex) sling for genuine stress incontinence. *Neurourol Urodyn* 1983;2:145.

18. Rottenberg RD, Weil A, Brioschi PA, et al. Urodynamic and clinical assessment of the Lyodura sling operation for urinary stress incontinence. *Br J Obstet Gynaecol* 1985;92:829.

19. Hilton P. A clinical and urodynamic study comparing the Stamey bladder neck suspension and suburethral sling procedures in the treatment of genuine stress incontinence. *Br J Obstet Gynaecol* 1989;96:213.

20. Beck RP, McCormick RN, Nordstrom L. The fascia lata sling procedure for treating recurrent genuine stress incontinence of urine. *Obstet Gynecol* 1988;71;699.

21. Bryans FE. Marlex gauze hammock sling operation with Cooper's ligament attachment in the management of recurrent urinary incontinence. *Am J Obstet Gynecol* 1979;133:292.

22. Morgan JE, Furrow GA, Stewart FE. The Marlex sling operation for the treatment of recurrent stress urinary incontinence: a 16-year review. *Am J Obstet Gynecol* 1985;151:224.

23. McGuire EJ. Abdominal procedures for stress incontinence. *Urol Clin North Am* 1985;12:285.

24. McGuire EJ, Lytton B. Pubovaginal sling procedure for stress incontinence. *J Urol* 1978;119:82.

25. Summitt RL, Bent AE, Ostergard DR, et al. Stress incontinence and low urethral closure pressure: correlation of pre-operative urethral hypermobility with successful suburethral sling procedures. *J Reprod Med* 1990;35:877–880.

26. Horbach NS, Bent AE, Ostergard DR, et al. *A comparison of retropubic urethropexy and suburethral sling procedure for the treatment of genuine stress incontinence and low pressure urethra.* Presented at the 10th annual meeting of the American Uro-Gynecologic Society, 1989.

27. McGuire EJ. Uro-dynamic findings in patients after failure of stress incontinence operations. *Prog Clin Biol Res* 1981;78:351.

28. Sand PK, Bowen LW, Panganiban R, et al. The low pressure urethra as a factor in failed retropubic urethropexy. *Obstet Gynecol* 1987;69:399.

29. Maher CF, Dwyer PL, Carey MP, et al. Colposuspension or sling for low urethral pressure stress incontinence? *Int Urogynecol J* 1999;10:384–389.

30. Hsieh GC, Klutke JJ, Kobak WH. Low Valsalva leakpoint pressure and success of retropubic urethropexy. *Int Urogynecol J* 2001;12:46–50.

31. Bump RC, Coates KW, Cundiff GW, et al. Diagnosing intrinsic sphincter deficiency: comparing urethral closure pressure, urethral axis, and Valsalva leak point pressures. *Am J Obstet Gynecol* 1997;177: 303–310.

32. Swift SE, Ostergard DR. A comparison of stress leakpoint pressure and maximum urethral closure pressure in patients with genuine stress incontinence. *Obstet Gynecol* 1995;69:399–402.

33. Miklos JR, Sze EH, Karram MM. A critical appraisal of the methods of measuring leak-point pressures in women with stress incontinence. *Obstet Gynecol* 1995;86:349–352.

34. McGuire EJ, Fitzpatrick CC, Wan J. Clinical assessment of urethral sphincter function. *J Urol* 1993;15: 1452–1454.

35. Bump RC, McClish DK. Cigarette smoking and pure genuine stress incontinence of urine: a comparison of risk factors and determinants between smokers and nonsmokers. *Am J Obstet Gynecol* 1994;170:579–582.

36. Mommsen S, Foldspang A. Body mass index and adult female urinary incontinence. *World J Urol* 1994;12: 319–322.

37. Cummings JM, Rodning CB. Urinary stress incontinence among obese women: review of pathophysiology therapy. *Int Urogynecol J Pelvic Floor Dysfunct* 2000;11:41–44.

38. Nygaard IE, Thompson FL, Svengalis SL, et al. Urinary incontinence in elite nulliparous athletes. *Obstet Gynecol* 1994;84:183–187.

39. Carr LK, Walsh PJ, Abraham VE, et al. Favorable out-

come of pubovaginal slings for geriatric women with stress incontinence. *J Urol* 1997;157:125–128.

40. Griebling TL, Schrepferman CG, Nygaard IE, et al. Sling cystourethropexy for treatment of women with stress urinary incontinence: comparison of older and younger patients. *J Am Geriatr Soc* 1997;45:S42(abst P125).

41. Appell RA. Primary slings for everyone with genuine stress incontinence? The argument for. . . . *Int Urogynecol J* 1998;9:249–251.

42. Leach GE, Dmochowski RR, Appell RA, et al. Female Stress Urinary Incontinence Clinical Guidelines Pannel summary report on surgical management of female stress urinary incontinence. *J Urol* 1997;158:875–880.

43. Ostergard DR. Primary sling for everyone with genuine stress incontinence? The argument against. *Int Urogynecol J* 1998;8:321–322.

44. Weber AM, Walters MD. Burch procedure compared with sling for stress urinary incontinence: a decision analysis. *Obstet Gynecol* 2000;96:867–873.

45. McGuire EJ, Bennett CJ, Konnack JA, et al. Experience with pubovaginal slings for urinary incontinence at the University of Michigan. *J Urol* 1987;138:525–526.

46. Schrepferman AG, Griebling TL, Nygaard IE, et al. Resolution of urge symptoms following sling cystourethropexy. *J Urol* 2000;164:1628–1631.

47. Beck RP, McCormick S, Nordstrom L. The fascia lata sling procedure for treating recurrent genuine stress incontinence of urine. *Obstet Gynecol* 1978;72:699–703.

48. Veronikis DK, Nichols DH, Wakamatsu MM. The incidence of low-pressure urethra as a function of prolapse-reducing technique in patients with massive pelvic organ prolapse (maximum descent at all vaginal sites). *Am J Obstet Gynecol* 1997;177:1305–1314.

49. Chaikin DC, Grout A, Blaivas JG. Predicting the need for anti-incontinence surgery in continent women undergoing repair of severe urogenital prolapse. *J Urol* 2000;163:531–534.

50. Iglesia CB, Shott S, Fenner DE, et al. Effect of preoperative voiding mechanism on success rate of autologous rectus fascia suburethral sling procedure. *Obstet Gynecol* 1998;91:577–581.

51. McLennan MT, Melick CF, Bent AE. Clinical and urodynamic predictors of delayed voiding after fascia lata suburethral sling. *Obstet Gynecol* 1998;92:608–612.

52. Mason R, Roach M. Modified pubovaginal sling for the treatment of intrinsic sphincter deficiency. *J Urol* 1996;156:1991–1994.

53. Chaikin DC, Rosenthal J, Blaivas. Pubovaginal fascial sling for all types of stress urinary incontinence: long-term analysis. *J Urol* 1998;160:1312–1326.

54. Fitzgerald MP, Mollenhauer J, Brubaker L. The fate of rectus fascia suburethral slings. *Am J Obstet Gynecol* 2000;183:964–966.

55. Fokaef ED, Lampel A, Hofenfellner M, et al. Experimental evaluation of free versus pedicled fascial flaps for sling surgery for urinary stress incontinence. *J Urol* 1997;157:1039–1043.

56. Rechberger T, Postawski K, Jakowicki JA, et al. Role of fascial collagen in stress incontinence. *Am J Obstet Gynecol* 1998;179:1511–1514.

57. Falconer C, Ekman G, Malmstrom A, et al. Decreased collagen synthesis in stress incontinent women. *Obstet Gynecol* 1994;84:583–586.

58. Govier FE, Gibbons RP, Correa RJ, et al. Pubovaginal slings using fascia lata for the treatment of intrinsic sphincter deficiency. *J Urol* 1997;157:117–121.

59. Beck RP, Grove D, Arnusch D et al. Recurrent urinary stress incontinence treated by the fascia lata sling procedure. *Am J Obstet Gynecol* 1974;120:613–621.

60. Beck RP, Lai AR. Results in treating 88 cases of recurrent urinary stress incontinence with the Oxford fascia lata sling procedure. *Am J Obstet Gynecol* 1982;142:649–651.

61. McLennan MT, Bent AE. Fascia lata suburethral sling vs. Burch retropubic urethropexy: a comparison of morbidity. *J Reprod Med* 1998;43:488–494.

62. Kreder KJ, Nygaard IE. Fascia lata sling cystourethropexy. *J Urol* 1995;153:205A(abst V-7).

63. Raz S, Diegel AL, Short JL, Snyder JA. Vaginal wall sling. *J Urol* 1989;141:43.

64. Choe JM, Ogan K, Battino BS. Antimicrobial mesh versus vaginal wall sling: a comparative outcomes analysis. *J Urol* 2000;163:1829–1834.

65. Litwiller SE, Nelson RS, Fone PD, et al. Vaginal wall sling: long-term outcome analysis of factors contributing to patient satisfaction and surgical success. *J Urol* 1997;157:1279–1282.

66. Kaplan SA, Te AE, Young GPH, et al. Prospective analysis of 373 consecutive women with stress urinary incontinence treated with a vaginal wall sling: the Columbia-Cornell University experience. *J Urol* 2000;164:1623–1627.

67. Winters JC, Rackley RR, Kambic H, et al. *The biomechanical properties of the vaginal wall.* Proceedings of the American Urological Association 1995; 153:526A(abst 1191).

68. Cooper JL, Beck CL. History of soft tissue allografts in orthopedics. *Sports Med Arthrosc Rev* 1993;1:2–16.

69. Noyes FR, Barber SD, Mangine RE. Bone-patellar ligament–bone and fascia lata allografts for reconstruction of the anterior cruciate ligament. *J Bone Joint Surg Am* 1990;72:1125–1136.

70. Kaplan SA, Santarosa RP, Te AE. Comparison of fascial and vaginal wall slings in the management of intrinsic sphincter deficiency. *Urology* 1996;47:885–889.

71. Wright EJ, Iselin CE, Carr LK, et al. Pubovaginal sling using cadaveric allograft for the treatment of intrinsic sphincter deficiency. *J Urol* 1998;160:759–762.

72. Buck BE, Malinin TI. Human bone and tissue allografts: preparation and safety. *Clin Orthop* 1994;303: 8–17.

73. Buck BE, Resnick L, Shah SM, et al. Human immunodeficiency virus cultured from bone: implications for transplantation. *Clin Orthop* 1990;251:249–253.

74. Hinton R, Jinnah RH, Johnson C, et al. A biomechanical analysis of solvent-dehydrated and freeze-dried human fascia lata allografts. *Am J Sports Med* 1992; 20:607–612.

75. Deleted in proofs.

76. Handa VL, Jensen JK, Germain MM, et al. Banked human fascia lata for the suburethral sling procedure: a preliminary report. *Obstet Gynecol* 1996;88:1045–1049.

77. Fitzgerald MP, Mollenhauer J, Brubaker L. Failure of allograft suburethral slings. *Br J Urol Int* 1999;84: 785–788.

78. Smith JJ, Bresette JF, Wang D. Early experience with acellular dermal allograft for pubovaginal slings. *Issues Incontinence* 2001;Spring:1–11.

79. Chung SY, Franks M, Smith CP, et al. Technique of

combined pubovaginal sling and cystocele repair using a single piece of cadaveric dermal graft. *Urology* 2002;59:538–541.

80. Mangel JM, Spurlock JW. Suburethral sling using cadaveric dermis as a treatment for complicated stress urinary incontinence. *Obstet Gynecol* 2001;97S:143.

81. Kridel RW, Foda H, Lunde KC. Septal perforation repair with acellular dermal allograft. *Arch Otolaryngol* 1998;124:73–78.

82. Wainwright D, Madden M, Luterman A, et al. Clinical evaluation of an acellular allograft dermal matrix in full-thickness burns. *J Burn Care Rehabil* 1996;17:124–136.

83. Kubricht WS, Williams BJ, Eastham JA, et al. Tensile strength of cadaveric fascia lata compared to SIS using suture pull through analysis. *J Urol* 2001;165:486–490.

84. Vecchia LD, Engum S, Kogan B, et al. Evaluation of small intestine submucosa and acellular dermis as diaphragmatic prostheses. *J Pediatr Surg* 1999;34:167–171.

85. Cobb MA, Badylak SF, Janas W, et al. Porcine small intestine submucosa as a dural substitute. *Surg Neurol* 1999;51:99–104.

86. Chu CC, Welch L. Characterization of morphologic and mechanical properties of surgical mesh fabrics. *J Biomed Mater Res* 1985;19:903–916.

87. Voyles CR, Richardson JD, Bland KI, et al. Emergency abdominal wall reconstruction with polypropylene mesh: short term benefits versus long-term complications. *Ann Surg* 1981;194:219–223.

88. Elliot MP, Juler GL. Comparison of Marlex mesh and microporous Teflon sheets when used for hernia repair in the experimental animal. *Am J Surg* 1979;137:342–344.

89. Usher FC. The repair of incisional and inguinal hernias. *Surg Gynecol Obstet* 1970;131:525–530.

90. Brown GL, Richardson D, Malangoni MA, et al. Comparison of prosthetic material for abdominal wall reconstruction in the presence of contamination and infection. *Ann Surg* 1985;201:705–711.

91. Ghoniem GM, Shaaban A. Suburethral slings for the treatment of stress urinary incontinence. *Int Urogynecol J* 1994;5:228–239.

92. Bent AE, Ostergard DR, Zwick-Zafuto M. Tissue reaction to expanded polytetrafluoroethylene suburethral sling for urinary incontinence: clinical and histologic study. *Am J Obstet Gynecol* 1993;169:1189–1204.

93. Weinberger MW, Ostergard DR. Long-term clinical and urodynamic evaluation of polytetrafluoroethylene sling for treatment of genuine stress incontinence. *Obstet Gynecol* 1995;86:92–96.

94. Pourdeyhimi B. Porosity of surgical mesh fabrics: new technology. *J Biomed Mater Res* 1989;23:145–152.

95. Ulmsten U, Henriksson L, Johnson P, et al. An ambulatory surgical procedure under local anesthesia for treatment of female urinary incontinence. *Int Urogynecol J* 1996;7:81–86.

96. Rovner ES, Ginsberg DA, Raz S. A method for intraoperative adjustment of sling tension: prevention of outlet obstruction during vaginal wall sling. *Urology* 1997;50:273–276.

97. Choe JM. Preventing urethral obstruction using the 6-point fixation and weight-adjusted spacing nomogram during sling surgery. *Int Urogynecol J* 2001;12:122–128.

98. Karram MM, Bhatia NN. Patch procedure: modified transvaginal fascia lata sling for recurrent or severe stress urinary incontinence. *Obstet Gynecol* 1990;75:461–463.

99. Schulthesis D, Jonas U. Do we need bone anchors in urogynecology? *Int Urogynecol J* 1999;10:153–154.

100. Drutz HP, Buckspan M, Flax S, et al. Clinical and urodynamic re-evaluation of combined abdominovaginal Marlex sling operations for recurrent stress urinary incontinence. *Int Urogynecol J* 1990;1:70–73.

101. Hassouna ME, Ghoniem GM. Long-term outcome and quality of life after modified pubovaginal sling for intrinsic sphincter deficiency. *Urology* 1999;53:287–291.

102. Morgan TO Jr, Westney OL, McGuire EJ. Pubovaginal sling: 4-year outcome analysis and quality of life assessment. *J Urol* 2000;163:1845–1848.

103. Richter HE, Varner RE, Sanders E, et al. Effects of pubovaginal sling procedure on patients with urethral hypermobility and intrinsic sphincter deficiency: would they do it again? *Am J Obstet Gynecol* 2001;184:14–19.

104. Parker RT, Addison WA, Wilson CJ. Fascia lata urethrovesical suspension for recurrent stress urinary incontinence. *Am J Obstet Gynecol* 1979;135:843–852.

105. Cross, CA, Cespedes RD, McGuire EJ. Our experience with pubovaginal slings in patients with stress urinary incontinence. *J Urol* 1998;159:1195–1198.

106. Owens RG, Kohli N, Wynne J, et al. Long-term results of a fascia lata suburethral patch sling for severe stress urinary incontinence. *J Pelvic Surg* 1999;5(4):196–202.

107. Amundsen CL, Visco AG, Ruiz H, et al. Outcome in 104 pubovaginal slings using freeze-dried allograft fascia lata from a single tissue bank. *Urology* 2000;56[Suppl 6A]:2–8.

108. Brown SL, Govier FE. Cadaveric versus autologous fascia lata for the pubovaginal sling: surgical outcome and patient satisfaction. *J Urol* 2000;164:1633–1637.

109. Elliott DS, Boone TB. Is fascia lata allograft material trustworthy for pubovaginal sling repair? *Urology* 2000;56:772–776.

110. Carbone JM, Kavaler E, Hu JC, et al. Pubovaginal sling using cadaveric fascia and bone anchors: disappointing early results. *J Urol* 2001;165:1605–1611.

111. Juma S, Little NA, Raz S. Vaginal wall sling: four years later. *Urology* 1992;39(5):424–428.

112. Raz S, Stothers L, Young GPH, et al. Vaginal wall sling for anatomical incontinence and intrinsic sphincter dysfunction: efficacy and outcome analysis. *J Urol* 1996;156:166–170.

113. Barbalias GA, Liatsikos EN, Athanasopoulos A. Gore-Tex sling urethral suspension in type III female urinary incontinence: clinical results and urodynamic changes. *Int Urogynecol J* 1997;8:344–350.

114. Kersey J, Martin MR, Mishra P. A further assessment of the gauze hammock operation for recurrent stress incontinence. *Br J Obstet Gynaecol* 1988;95:382–385.

115. Young SB, Rosenblatt PL, Pingeton DM, et al. The Mersilene mesh suburethral sling: a clinical and urodynamic evaluation. *Am J Obstet Gynecol* 1995;173:1719–1726.

116. Ogundipe A, Rosenzweig BA, Karram MK, et al. Modified suburethral sling procedure for treatment of recurrent or severe stress urinary incontinence. *Surg Gynecol Obstet* 1992;175:173–176.

117. Kuo H-C. Comparison of video urodynamic results after the pubovaginal sling procedure using rectus fascia and polypropylene mesh for stress urinary incontinence. *J Urol* 2001;165:163–168.

118. Fulford SCV, Flynn R, Barrington J, et al. An assessment of the surgical outcome and urodynamic effects of the pubovaginal sling for stress incontinence and the associated urge syndrome. *J Urol* 1999;162:135–137.

119. Obrink A, Bunne G. The margin of incontinence after three types of operation for stress incontinence. *Scand J Urol Nephrol* 1978:12:209–214.

120. Henriksson L, Ulmsten U. A urodynamic evaluation of the effects of abdominal urethrocystopexy in women with stress incontinence. *Am J Obstet Gynecol* 1978; 113:78–82.

121. Poliak A, Daniller AI, Liebling RW. Sling operation for recurrent stress incontinence using the tendon of the palmaris longus. *Obstet Gynecol* 1984;63:850–854.

122. Jarvis GJ. Surgery for genuine stress incontinence. *Br J Obstet Gynecol* 1994;101:371–374.

123. Fitzgerald MP, Brubaker L. The etiology of urinary retention after surgery for genuine stress incontinence. *Neurourol Urodyn* 2001;20:13–21.

124. Beck RP. The sling operation. In: Buchsbaum HJ, Schmidt JD, eds. *Gynecologic and obstetric urology,* 2nd ed. Philadelphia: WB Saunders, 1982:285–306.

125. Bhatia NN, Bergman A. Use of preoperative uroflowmetry and simultaneous urethrocystometry for predicting risk of prolonged postoperative bladder drainage. *Urology* 1986;28:440–445.

126. Sze EH, Miklos JR, Karram MM. Voiding after Burch colposuspension and effects of concomitant pelvic surgery: correlation with preoperative voiding mechanism. *Obstet Gynecol* 1996;88:564–567.

127. Brubaker, L. Suburethral sling release. *Obstet Gynecol* 1995;86:686–688.

128. McLennan MT, Bent AE. Sling incision with associated vaginal wall interposition for obstructed voiding secondary to suburethral sling procedure. *Int Urogynecol J* 1997;8:168–172.

129. Ghoniem G, Elgamasy A. A simplified approach to bladder outlet obstruction following pubovaginal sling. *J Urol* 1995;154:181–183.

130. Cross CA, Cespedes RD, English SF, et al. Transvaginal urethrolysis for urethral obstruction after anti-incontinence surgery. *J Urol* 1998;159:1199–1201.

131. Goldman HB, Rackley RR, Appell RA. The efficacy of urethrolysis without re-suspension for iatrogenic urethral obstruction. *J Urol* 1999;161:196–199.

132. Amundsen CL, Guralnick ML, Webster GD. Variations in strategy for the treatment of urethral obstruction after a pubovaginal sling procedure. *J Urol* 2000;164: 434–437.

133. Jorgensen L, Lose G, Molsted-Pedersen L. Vaginal repair in female motor urge incontinence. *Eur Urol* 1987;13:382–385.

134. Eriksen BC, Hagen B, Eik-Nes SH, et al. Long-term effectiveness of Burch colposuspension in female urinary stress incontinence. *Acta Obstet Gynecol Scand* 1990;69:45–50.

135. Sand PK, Bowen LW, Ostergard DR, et al. The effect of the retropubic urethropexy on detrusor stability. *Obstet Gynecol* 1988;71:818–822.

136. Myers DL, LaSala CA. Conservative surgical management of Mersilene mesh suburethral sling erosion. *Am J Obstet Gynecol* 1998;179:1424–1429.

137. Handa VL, Stone A. Erosion of a fascial sling into the urethra. *Urology* 1999;54:923.

138. Clemens JQ, DeLancey JO, Faerber GJ, et al. Urinary tract erosions after synthetic pubovaginal slings: diagnosis and management strategy. *Urology* 2000;56: 589–595.

139. Colhan HJ, Stevenson KR. Sling transection of urethra: a rare complication. *Int Urogynecol J* 1996;7: 331–334.

140. Miyazaki F, Shook G. Ilioinguinal nerve entrapment during needle suspension for stress incontinence. *Obstet Gynecol* 1992;80:246–248.

141. Mikhail MS, Rosa H. Vaginal wall inclusion cyst formation following a modified vaginal wall patch sling technique for patients with genuine stress incontinence. *Obstet Gynecol* 2000;95[4 Suppl 1]:535.

142. Woodman PJ, Davis GD. The relationship of the in-situ advancing vaginal wall sling to vaginal epithelial inclusion cysts. *Int Urogynecol J* 2000;11:124–126.

143. Franks ME, Lavelle JP, Yokoyama T, et al. Metastatic osteomyelitis after pubovaginal sling using bone anchors. *Urology* 2000;56:330.

144. Rackley RR, Abdelmalak JB, Madjar S, et al. Bone anchor infections in female pelvic reconstructive procedures: a literature review of series and case reports. *J Urol* 2001;165:1975–1978.

Ostergard's Urogynecology and Pelvic Floor Dysfunction, Fifth Edition. edited by A.E. Bent, et al. Lippincott Williams & Wilkins, Philadelphia © 2003.

31

Periurethral Injections

Michael Gross* and Rodney A. Appell**

*Department of Urology, Haifa University; and Female Urology and Voiding Dsyfunction Unit, Department of Urology, Bnei Zion Medical Center, Haifa, Israel
**Scott Department of Urology, Baylor College of Medicine, Houston, Texas

Selection of patients appears crucial to the outcome of the periurethral injection of bulking agents. The ideal candidate for this procedure has good anatomic support; a normal, compliant, stable bladder; and a malfunctioning urethra with a low leak point pressure. Other subsets of patients who may benefit from the procedure are patients with high leak point pressure and minimal hypermobility and elderly women with bladder base mobility who are less active and are a poor surgical risk for other interventions.

INJECTABLE MATERIALS

The desirable injectable material should be biocompatible, nonimmunogenic, and hypoallergenic. The material should retain its bulking characteristics for an extended period of time and neither degrade nor migrate. The material should be easily targeted and injected. As yet, there is no bulking agent that meets all these criteria, and the search for the ideal bulking agent continues.

Most agents attain satisfactory results only after repeated treatments. Currently, there is no method to predict how many injections a given patient will need. The position, volume, and operator's impression of tissue coaptation have not been correlated with clinical outcome, and the optimal timing between injections has not been determined.

The outcomes for procedures using bulking agents vary considerably depending on the method of assessment. Currently, there is no standardized regimen for evaluating the procedural result. The definition of cure may vary from absolute dryness to acceptable social comfort. Any assessment of results should include the information about the patients' selection, the number of injections required, volume of each injection, and the timing of assessment since the last treatment. Definitions of cure, improvement, and failure should be explicitly outlined. The gold standard for assessment of outcome should incorporate physical examination, urodynamic study, and a subjective assessment.

Cross-linked Bovine Collagen

Currently, the most commonly used injectable is a sterile bovine dermal collagen (Contigen) that is cross-linked with glutaraldehyde and is dispersed in phosphate-buffered saline that composes about 65% of the total injectable volume. The U.S. Food and Drug Administration (FDA) approved the material in 1993 for male and female intrinsic sphincteric deficiency (ISD). This collagen is both biocompatible and biodegradable. The glutaraldehyde cross-linking reduces the antigenicity of the material and makes it less degradable by collagenase. In the early period after collagen injection, the buffered saline vehicle is reabsorbed. The collagen begins to degrade about 3 months after the injection and is completely degraded within a period of about 10 to 20 months (1). There are no reports of particle migration (2). The material achieves part of its bulking effect from neovascularization and fibroblast ingrowth into the implant.

Technique

Collagen may be injected either transurethrally through a cystoscope (2,3) or periurethrally using a spinal needle inserted percutaneously with simultaneous viewing through a cystoscope for material positioning and effect. Another technique available is percutaneous injection with assessment of localization by ultrasonography (4). The optimal depth of collagen placement appears to be into the superficial urethral muscle adjacent to the submucosa (5). No matter which technique is used, precise placement of the material is of paramount importance. To facilitate placement in the periurethral area, Neal and co-workers introduced a technique of injecting methylene blue into the suburethral tissue, making localization more easily accomplished (6).

Injection of bulking agents may be done as an office procedure. The patient is placed in lithotomy position. The introitus is anesthetized with 20% topical benzocaine, and the urethra is anesthetized with 2% lidocaine jelly.

A local injection of 1% lidocaine is performed periurethrally at the 3- and 9-o'clock positions with a total volume of 2 to 4 mL on each side.

When using the periurethral approach, urethroscopy is performed with a 0- or 30-degree lens. A 20-French spinal needle with the obturator in place is positioned periurethrally at the 4- or 8-o'clock position, with the bevel of the needle directed towards the lumen. The needle's tip can be seen bulging toward the urethral lumen. The needle is advanced under vision into the muscle just lateral to the lamina propria in a zone just below the bladder neck, and the material is injected. Before injecting, the cystoscope is aimed such that the bladder neck and bladder can be observed simultaneously. During injection, swelling is visible protruding toward the lumen. If, while injecting, the mucosal surface becomes blanched or the collagen is visible under the mucosal surface, then the material has been injected too superficially and the needle needs to be repositioned. After occlusion of about 50% of the lumen, the needle is withdrawn and reinserted on the opposite side. After the injection of the second side, the bladder neck may resemble the appearance of two "kissing" lateral prostatic lobes (Fig. 31.1A,B).

Correlation of the position and volume of collagen injected with success rates has not

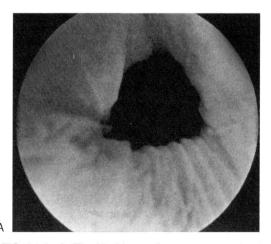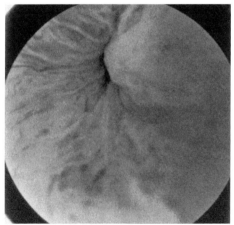

A B

FIG. 31.1. A: The bladder neck as appears prior to injection. **B:** The bladder neck as appears with good coaptation postinjection.

TABLE 31.1. *Collagen injection series*

Lead author	No. of patients	Mean volume injected	Mean number of procedures	Mean follow-up (mo)	Cure	Improvement	Fail
Herschorn (35)	31	12.7	2	12	48	42	10
Stricker (36)	50	14.4	1.9	11	42	40	14
Winters (37)	160	NS	NS	24	—	78	22
Monga (38)	60	19	1.6	24	47	20	32
Richardson (39)	42	28.3	2	46	40	43	17
Swami (40)	111	NS	NS	39	25	40	0
Corcos (41)	40	9	2.2	48	30	40	30

NS, not significant.

been examined (7). In most cases, 2 to 5 injection sessions are required per patient to attain satisfactory results, and subsequent injections are needed to maintain the continence acquired. The improved/cure rate is 70% to 90%, whereas the actual cure rate is about 40% to 60% (Table 31.1).

Complications associated with collagen injections include *de novo* urgency, which occurs in about 13% of patients; urinary retention, which is brief and resolves by itself in 2%; urinary tract infection in 1% to 4%; and hematuria in 5%. An early hypersensitivity reaction may present in up to 3.5% (8,9) and a delayed hypersensitivity reaction in about 1% (10). Another, less common complication is the formation of a sterile abscess (11).

Carbon Particles

Durasphere pyrolytic zirconium oxide beads, coated with carbon in the size range of 200 to 500 μm, were approved by the FDA in September 1999. The Durasphere particles are suspended in a water-based β-glucan vehicle (Fig. 31.2). The material is intended for injection submucosally at the bladder neck using an 18-g needle through the cystoscope. More recently, a periurethral needle has also been introduced. As yet, there is very limited literature concerning this injectable. However, a randomized, multicenter, double blind study conducted for FDA approval comparing collagen to Durasphere showed similar outcomes (12). In that study, adverse reactions attributed to Durasphere treatment were acute re-

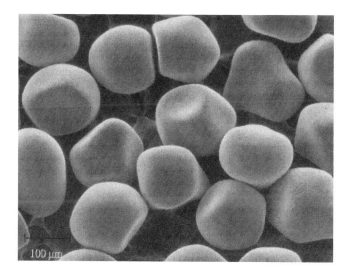

FIG. 31.2. A hundred-fold magnification of Durashere pyrolytic zirconium oxide beads.

TABLE 31.2. *Injectable agents and manufacturers*

Agent	Marketed name	Manufacturer
Bovine crossed-linked collagen	Contigen	CR Bard, Convington, GA
Carbon particles	Durasphere	Carbon Medical Technologies, St. Paul, MN
Polytetrafluoroethylene	Polytef	Mentor Medical Systems, Santa Barbara, CA
Human collagen	Urologen	Collagenesis, Minneapolis, MN
Autologous cartilage		Reprogenesis, Boston, MA
Crossed-linked hyaluronic acid	Hylagel	Biomatrix, New York City
Silicone	Macroplastique	Uroplasty, Minneapolis, MN
Ethylene vinyl alcohol copolymers	Uryx	Genyx, San Diego, CA
Hyaluronic acid and dextranomer microspheres	Deflux	Q-Med, Upppsala, Sweden
Myoblasts		Departments of Urology, Pharmacology and Orthopedics, University of Pittsburgh, School of Medicine, Pittsburgh, PA.

tention (<7 days' duration) in 16%, dysuria in 12%, urinary tract infection in 9%, and irritative symptoms in 15% of patients. Durasphere is more viscous than collagen; therefore, its injection is technically more demanding.

The following injectable substances (Table 31.2) are not currently available in the United States but are involved in investigational studies to seek FDA approval.

Polytetrafluoroethylene

Polytetrafluoroethylene (PTFE) was used for treatment of urinary incontinence as early as the 1970s (13,14), with cure rates of 54% and improvement rates of another 18%. Other studies of incontinent women demonstrated equivalent results with cure rates of 55% to 61%. The mean volume of PTFE injected was 18.9 mL with 1.5 injection sessions (15). PTFE is a paste of micropolymeric particles 50 μm in size. Particles smaller than 110 μm may be phagocytosed and may migrate to distant organs. The material was taken off the market because of migration and formation of granulomas in the lymph nodes, lung, brain, and kidneys of experimental animals (16,17). Several case reports have documented migration of PTFE and alveolitis in humans. Two cases of cancer adjacent to PTFE have been reported (18). Other complications with PTFE injections include a noninfectious febrile disorder, urethral fibrosis, formation of granu-loma in urethral walls, and formation of periurethral abscesses. Recently, Herschorn and Glazer (19) used small-volume periurethral PTFE injections in 46 women, with a cure rate of 30.4% and improvement in 41.3% and with the probability of remaining dry at 90% at 1 year and 60% at 2 years. At a mean follow-up of 28 months, no significant long-lasting complications were noted.

Human Collagen

Intact human collagen may be harvested from cadaveric dermal skin specimens. The extracted dermis is mechanically separated from the epidermis and is suspended in a buffered phosphate solution. Collagen concentration may vary from 25 to 100 mg/mL; however, because of the material's viscosity, high-concentration solutions are difficult to inject through small-bore needles. Experience with human collagen has already been obtained in the fields of ophthalmology, otolaryngology, and dermatology, and the material has proved to be stable, producing only a minimal inflammatory response and enabling ingrowth of vascular vessels and fibroblasts (20,21).

Autologous Ear Chondrocytes

Autologous chondrocytes are harvested from the pinna of the ear of a patient, and the cells can then be grown in tissue culture and suspended with polysaccharides in hydrogel suspension. The gel that enables the material to be injected is absorbed. The volume is maintained by the extracellular matrix secreted by the chondrocytes. In a single study, 32 women with ISD were treated once with an average injected volume of 5.9 mL (22). Sixteen patients were cured, and 10 more improved, with an overall 81.3% cure or improvement rate at a follow-up of 12 months. No major tolerability issues were encountered. This type of process brings to mind fears of the mix-up of tissue, resulting in the chondrocytes of one patient returned for injection into the wrong patient.

Crossed-linked Hyaluronic Acid

Hyaluronic acid is an insoluble glycosamine glycan composed of disaccharide units that can be dissolved in saline. Hyaluronic acid is already in use in the fields of ophthalmology, orthopedics, and rheumatology and has been proved to be a biocompatible and safe (23). The suspended material has significant elasticity and viscosity to be used as a soft tissue–bulking agent. To date, only preliminary industry-initiated studies have been done with hyaluronic acid as a bulking material. The results were 53% objective improvement rate and 83% rate of improvement of quality of life (24).

Hyaluronic Acid and Dextranomer Microspheres

Dextranomer, a crossed-linked dextran and hyaluronic acid, had been used in combination as a bulking agent for vesicourethral reflux and stress incontinence (24). Both materials are biocompatible, nonimmunogenic, and biodegradable. No migration was noted in animal models (25). The hyaluronic acid is the vehicle material in the admixture, whereas the dextranomer particles are the bulking agent. The hyaluronic acid is degradable in about 2 weeks, whereas the Dextranomer microspheres remain in the injection site for about 4 years. In theory, collagen ingrowth into the injected material later acts as a bulk-

ing agent when the injected material has been degraded. The injection is performed with standard cystoscopic equipment under local anesthesia. Because of the material's low viscosity, very little pressure is necessary to position and deploy the material. Short-term follow-up of a group of 20 women with GSUI showed objective cure or improvement in 85%. Apart from transient urinary retention observed in 4 women, no other adverse effects were observed (26).

Silicone

Silicone has been used as a bulking agent for more than 5 years. The material is a 60/40 mixture of hydrophilic povidone gel that serves as the vehicle, and solid dimethylsiloxane elastomer that serves as the bulking agent. Mean fragment size is 160 µm, but 25% of the particles are less than 50 µm in size. Animal studies have revealed migration of small particles to distant organs (27,28). The material causes minimal inflammatory response, with collagen ingrowth and encapsulation of the material. The reported short-term outcome is that 10% of patients are cured, 42% have improvement, and 52% have no improvement. With a 31-month follow-up, 19% were classified as dry, 29% improved, and 52% failed (29). Other studies have reported a success rate of 48% at 2-year follow-up (30). The most common reason for failure is retrograde extravasation of the material. To eliminate extravasation, there should be adequate distance from the injection puncture site and the deployment site.

Ethylene Vinyl Alcohol Copolymers

Ethylene vinyl alcohol copolymer suspended in dimethyl sulfoxide (DMSO) has been used as an embolic material (31). When exposed to physiologic temperature and tissue water, the DMSO diffuses and the ethylene vinyl alcohol solidifies (becomes a gel) at the injected site. Human trials are currently in progress (Fig. 31.3).

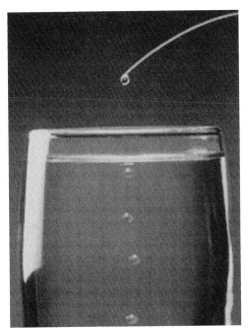

FIG. 31.3. Liquid ethylene vinyl alcohol copolymers (Uryx) transformed to gel when exposed to water at physiologic temperature.

Synthetic Calcium Hydroxylapatite

Synthetic calcium hydroxylapatite is identical to the material found in human bones and teeth. The injectable is composed of hydroxylapatite spheres of a uniform smooth shape in an aqueous gel composed of sodium carboxylmethylcellulose, and it can be seen on radiograph or ultrasound, which may be useful in some cases. Injection is carried out with a 21-gauge needle with standard endoscopy equipment. A pilot trial demonstrated efficacy, stability, and minimal discomfort at the injection site (32). A multicenter study in the United States is currently underway.

Myoblast Injection

Injection of periurethral myoblasts, proposed by Chancellor and colleagues (33) as a different way to restore continence is based on the concept that myoblasts can be injected, not as a bulking agent, but as a vehicle to restore muscular activity and function. Myoblasts, transduced by different viral vectors, can be used as gene delivery vehicles to produce required proteins and to differentiate into multinucleated muscle fibers capable of muscle contraction (Fig. 31.4). Myoblasts that were

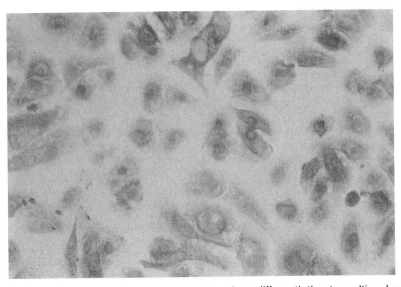

FIG. 31.4. Myoblasts injected to rats' proximal urethra show differentiation to multinucleated muscle fibers.

transduced with adenovirus were injected into rat bladders and proximal urethral submucosa with subsequent successful formation of myotubes in the smooth muscles of the lower urinary tract. A different technique to restore muscle activity was introduced by Furness and associates (34). Regeneration of smooth muscle formulations was evaluated after injections of harvested intestinal submucosa to the urethral submucosa in dogs. Time will tell whether either of the proposed techniques will become applicable as a treatment option in humans.

CONCLUSIONS

Periurethral bulking agents are a therapeutic modality to restore continence in women who suffer from urinary stress incontinence. The currently available agents in the United States include cross-linked bovine collagen and the carbon-coated zirconium beads. With either of these agents, the cure rates are reasonable; however, most patients require repeated injections to attain continence and to maintain continence. The ability to inject most patients under local anesthesia as an office procedure facilitates the treatment and reduces cost.

Each of the periurethral bulking agents currently in use or pending approval for use has its advantages and disadvantages. One should be familiar with the unique characteristics of each bulking material before initiating treatment. Some of the new promising bulking agents have been discussed because they are in the process of clinical trials, which will add to the armamentarium of injectable treatment in the not-too-distant future.

REFERENCES

1. Stegman SJ, Chu S, Bensch K, et al. A light and electron microscopic evaluation of Zyderm collagen and Zyplast implants in aging human facial skin: a pilot study. *Arch Dermatol* 1987;123:1644–1649.
2. Remacle M, Marbaix E. Collagen implants in the human larynx: pathological examinations of two cases. *Arch Otorhinolaryngol* 1988;245:203–209.
3. O'Connell HE, McGuire EJ, Aboseif S, et al. Transurethral collagen therapy in women. *J Urol* 1995;154:1463–1465.
4. Kageyama S, Kawabe K, Suzuki K, et al. Collagen implantation for post-prostatectomy incontinence: early experience with a transrectal ultrasonographically guided method. *J Urol* 1994;152:1473–1475.
5. Appell RA. Collagen injection therapy for urinary incontinence. *Urol Clin North Am* 1994;21:177–182.
6. Neal DE Jr, Lahaye ME, Lowe DC. Improved needle placement technique in periurethral collagen injection. *Urology* 1995;45:865–866.
7. Carr LK, Herschorn S, Leonhardt C. Magnetic resonance imaging after intraurethral collagen injected for stress urinary incontinence. *J Urol* 1996;155:1253–1255.
8. Elson ML. Adverse reactions to tretinoin and collagen injections. *J Am Acad Dermatol* 1989;20:861–862.
9. Elson ML. The role of skin testing in the use of collagen injectable materials. *J Dermatol Surg Oncol* 1989;15:301–303.
10. Stothers L, Goldenberg SL. Delayed hypersensitivity and systemic arthralgia following transurethral collagen injection for stress urinary incontinence. *J Urol* 1998;159:1507–1509.
11. Sweat SD, Lightner DJ. Complications of sterile abscess formation and pulmonary embolism following periurethral bulking agents. *J Urol* 1999;161:93–96.
12. Lightner D, Calvosa C, Andersen R, et al. A new injectable bulking agent for treatment of stress urinary incontinence: results of a multicenter, randomized, controlled, double-blind study of Durasphere. *Urology* 2001;58:12–15.
13. Politano VA, Small MP, Harper JM, et al. Periurethral Teflon injection for urinary incontinence. *Trans Am Assoc Genitourin Surg* 1973;65:54–57.
14. Politano VA, Small MP, Harper JM, et al. Periurethral Teflon injection for urinary incontinence. *J Urol* 1974;111:180–183.
15. Lopez AE, Padron OF, Patsias G, et al. Transurethral polytetrafluoroethylene injection in female patients with urinary continence. *J Urol* 1993;150:856–858.
16. Malizia AA Jr, Dewanjee MK, Reiman HM, et al. Polytef (Teflon) migration after periurethral injection: tracer and x-ray microanalysis techniques in experimental study. *Trans Am Soc Artif Intern Organs* 1984;30:330–334.
17. Malizia AA Jr, Reiman HM, Myers RP, et al. Migration and granulomatous reaction after periurethral injection of polytef (Teflon). *JAMA* 1984;251:3277–3281.
18. Hakky M, Kolbusz R, Reyes CV. Chondrosarcoma of the larynx. *Ear Nose Throat J* 1989;68:60–62.
19. Herschorn S, Glazer AA. Early experience with small volume periurethral polytetrafluoroethylene for female stress urinary incontinence. *J Urol* 2000;163:1838–1842.
20. Ford CN, Staskowski PA, Bless DM. Autologous collagen vocal fold injection: a preliminary clinical study. *Laryngoscope* 1995;105:944–948.
21. Cendron M, DeVore DP, Connolly R, et al. The biological behavior of autologous collagen injected into the rabbit bladder. *J Urol* 1995;154:808–811.
22. Bent AE, Tutrone RT, McLennan MT, et al. Treatment of intrinsic sphincter deficiency using autologous ear chondrocytes as a bulking agent. *Neurourol Urodyn* 2001;20:157–165.
23. *Formal report of feasibility study of Hyalagel Uro.* Ridgefield, NJ, Biomatrix Corporation.
24. Joyner BD, Atala A. Endoscopic substances for the treatment of vesicoureteral reflux. *Urology* 1997;50:489–494.

25. Stenberg AM, Sundin A, Larsson BS, et al. Lack of distant migration after injection of a ^{125}iodine labeled dextranomer based implant into the rabbit bladder. *J Urol* 1997;158:1937–1941.

26. Stenberg A, Larsson G, Johnson P, et al. DiHA Dextran Copolymer, a new biocompatible material for endoscopic treatment of stress incontinent women: short term results. *Acta Obstet Gynecol Scand* 1999;78:436–442.

27. Henly DR, Barrett DM, Weiland TL, et al. Particulate silicone for use in periurethral injections: local tissue effects and search for migration. *J Urol* 1995;153: 2039–2043.

28. Smith DP, Kaplan WE, Oyasu R. Evaluation of polydimethylsiloxane as an alternative in the endoscopic treatment of vesicoureteral reflux. *J Urol* 1994;152: 1221–1224.

29. Barranger E, Fritel X, Kadoch O, et al. Results of transurethral injection of silicone micro-implants for females with intrinsic sphincter deficiency. *J Urol* 2000; 164:1619–1622.

30. Sheriff MK, Foley S, McFarlane J, et al. Endoscopic correction of intractable stress incontinence with silicone micro-implants. *Eur Urol* 1997;32:284–288.

31. Lylyk P, Vinuela F, Vinters HV, et al. Use of a new mixture for embolization of intracranial vascular malformations: preliminary experimental experience. *Neuroradiology* 1990;32:304–310.

32. Mayer R, Lightfoot M, Jung I. Preliminary evaluation of calcium hydroxylapatite as a transurethral bulking agent for stress urinary incontinence. *Urology* 2001; 57:434–438.

33. Chancellor MB, Yokoyama T, Tirney S, et al. Preliminary results of myoblast injection into the urethra and bladder wall: a possible method for the treatment of stress urinary incontinence and impaired detrusor contractility. *Neurourol Urodyn* 2000;19:279–287.

34. Furness PD 3rd, Kolligian ME, Lang SJ, et al. Injectable small intestinal submucosa: preliminary evaluation for use in endoscopic urological surgery. *J Urol* 2000;164: 1680–1685.

35. Herschorn S, Radomski SB, Steele DJ. Early experience with intraurethral collagen injections for urinary incontinence. *J Urol* 1992;148:1797–1800.

36. Stricker P, Haylen B. Injectable collagen for type 3 female stress incontinence: the first 50 Australian patients. *Med J Aust* 1993;158:89–91.

37. Winters JC, Appell R. Periurethral injection of collagen in the treatment of intrinsic sphincteric deficiency in the female patient. *Urol Clin North Am* 1995;22:673–678.

38. Monga AK, Robinson D, Stanton SL. Periurethral collagen injections for genuine stress incontinence: a 2-year follow-up. *Br J Urol* 1995;76:156–160.

39. Richardson TD, Kennelly MJ, Faerber GJ. Endoscopic injection of glutaraldehyde cross-linked collagen for the treatment of intrinsic sphincter deficiency in women. *Urology* 1995;46:378–381.

40. Swami S, Batista JE, Abrams P. Collagen for female genuine stress incontinence after a minimum 2-year follow-up. *Br J Urol* 1997;80:757–761.

41. Corcos J, Fournier C. Periurethral collagen injection for the treatment of female stress urinary incontinence: 4-year follow-up results. *Urology* 1999;54:815–818.

Ostergard's Urogynecology and Pelvic Floor Dysfunction, Fifth Edition. edited by A.E. Bent, et al.
Lippincott Williams & Wilkins, Philadelphia © 2003.

32

Prevention and Management of Complications after Continence Surgery

Kenneth S. Leffler* and Geoffrey W. Cundiff**

Department of Gynecology and Obstetrics, The Johns Hopkins Medical Institutions, Baltimore, Maryland
**Department of Gynecology and Obstetrics, Johns Hopkins School of Medicine; and Department of Obstetrics and Gynecology, Johns Hopkins Bayview Medical Center, Baltimore, Maryland*

Every surgeon recognizes that any surgical procedure can result in immediate and delayed postoperative complications. Many of the most severe complications are related to the patient's preexisting medical disorders, to anesthetic risks and reactions, and to restrictions in mobility imposed by postoperative discomfort or paraphernalia. Procedures performed to restore urinary continence are not spared these surgical risks. The prevalence of perioperative complications in reconstructive pelvic surgery was noted by Lambrou and colleagues to be 45% (1). The prevalence of intraoperative complications was 12%, primarily due to injury to the urinary tract and bowel. The prevalence of postoperative complications was 33%, including infectious, pulmonary, gastrointestinal, cardiac, neurologic, and hematologic complications. The readmission rate for complications was 8%. Comparing the rate of complications from this study to the CREST (calcinosis, Raynaud's phenomenon, esophageal dysmotility, sclerodactyly, and telangiectasia) study (2), which described complications in a cohort of 1,851 women undergoing hysterectomy, there was an increase in urinary tract injuries, thromboembolic events, paralytic ileus, and pneumonia. This rate of perioperative complications is higher than that of general gynecologic surgery and is comparable to the rate described for gynecologic oncology surgery.

This chapter is primarily concerned with complications specific to individual continence procedures. These include retropubic space hematoma, infectious and inflammatory complications, lower urinary tract injuries, postoperative urinary retention, suprapubic catheter complications, and detrusor instability (DI) after continence surgery.

RETROPUBIC SPACE HEMATOMA

The retropubic space is a potential space that extends from the muscular floor of the pelvis to the level of the umbilicus. It is bounded anteriorly by the posterior lamina of the rectus sheath, the pubic bones, and medial portions of the pubic rami. The posterior boundaries are the prevesical fascia and the lateral pillars of the bladder. Above the bladder, the vesicoumbilical fascia and peritoneum make up the posterior wall of the space. The space is closed laterally by fascia, which fuses to the deep inferior epigastric vessels (3). The floor of the space is bounded by the anterior vaginal wall, urethra, and bladder. The space is occupied by varying amounts of fatty and areolar tissue in loose apposition to the surrounding structures. A

TABLE 32.1. *Retropubic hematoma*

Prevention
  Careful dissection
  Meticulous hemostasis
  Drains
Management
  Observation
  Drainage

rich, thin-walled perivesical venous plexus is found under the fat, overlying the bladder and vaginal wall.

In surgery, during the performance of transabdominal incontinence procedures such as the Burch colposuspension, the space is developed and exposed predominantly by blunt dissection. During needle urethropexy, suburethral sling, and tension-free vaginal tape (TVT) procedures, the space is less extensively developed because it is entered from the vagina by perforating the pubocervical fascia lateral to the urethra. The major complications encountered as a result of these incursions include bleeding and hematoma formation. Given the potential for bacterial contamination, particularly when using a vaginal approach, the presence of a hematoma predisposes to development of a retropubic abscess. Less common postoperative complications include clinically significant accumulations of serum or urine. Table 32.1 outlines the approach to retropubic hematoma.

Prevention

Hemorrhage from the rich perivesical venous plexus can be considerable during an abdominal colposuspension. This is particularly true if extensive defatting of the paravaginal fascia is performed in an effort to promote fibrosis and fixation of the vaginal wall. It has been hypothesized that the use of permanent rather than absorbable suture material may obviate the need for such extensive defatting. Prevention of a hematoma requires meticulous dissection, meticulous hemostasis, and occasional drainage.

Dissection of the retropubic space requires knowledge of the potential vascular hazards.

Examples include the dorsal vein of the clitoris, which lies directly posterior to the symphysis pubis, and the accessory or aberrant obturator vessels. The obturator artery is connected to the deep inferior epigastric artery in 25% to 80% of individuals through an arcade, which has been variably termed the aberrant or accessory obturator artery. A wide degree of variation is present. The obturator artery or its accessory artery may also send branches medially coursing across Cooper's ligament in 10% of individuals. These vessels are commonly well hidden by overlying fat and lymphatics, making them particularly vulnerable to damage by dissection or retractors. The resulting hemorrhage can be nearly impossible to control if the lacerated vessel retracts into the obturator canal. Accessory obturator veins are even more common and can present a problem during laparoscopic surgery in the form of delayed hemorrhage after the pressure of the pneumoperitoneum has been released (3).

Knowledge of the pelvic vasculature used when exposing the retropubic space recommends a dissection technique that begins lateral to the pubic symphysis but medial to the obturator notch and immediately posterior to Cooper's ligament. Blunt dissection from lateral to medial carried posteriorly to the arcus tendineus fascia pelvis usually eliminates vascular disruption and significant bleeding during these procedures. Using this lateral to medial approach, it is often possible to isolate and ligate the vessels if disruption is unavoidable.

Careful hemostasis is as important as the dissection technique in minimizing retropubic space hematomas. An extended electrocautery tip is indispensable, especially for veins that run along the inner surface of the superior pubic ramus (4). Hemostatic vascular clips may also prove invaluable in avoiding or controlling troublesome bleeding. Hemostasis is further aided by placing figure-of-eight sutures in the periurethral tissue when performing a Burch colposuspension because tying them down to Cooper's ligament generally controls minor venous bleeding from the periurethral plexus. Similarly, encircling the vaginal vessels when placing paravaginal stitches can prevent bleeding when they are tied.

The use of these techniques maximizes hemostasis in the retropubic space. As a result, in recent years, we have largely abandoned the routine use of retropubic drainage. However, if residual oozing of blood is observed after all suspending sutures are tied, retropubic placement of a pliable suction drainage system is a wise precaution (5). An active drainage system is less likely to serve as a wick to contaminate the space and also evacuates blood more efficiently than a passive drain. We advocate the use of sterile dressings, antiseptic ointment, and sterile technique when manipulating the drain sites. Finally, the drain should be removed promptly when drainage becomes negligible and serous. Using these techniques during and after an exclusive abdominal route continence procedure, a retropubic hematoma should be an unusual complication (5). Because accumulation of blood is the major risk factor for retropubic abscess formation after these procedures, these techniques should render abscess formation a rare occurrence as well.

With combined abdominovaginal needle and sling procedures, direct attempts at hemostasis and retropubic space drainage are not possible because of the blind, although limited, dissection of the space. As long as the retropubic dissection is performed intimately against the pubis, significant disruption of the venous plexus is unlikely. However, contamination of the space with vaginal organisms is unavoidable during dissection and ligature passage. This bacterial contamination, along with the accumulation of blood, is the major risk factor for retropubic cellulitis and abscess after these procedures. Measures to minimize these risks are considered in the section on infectious complications.

Management

The most effective management technique for a retropubic hematoma is prevention. Small, noninfected collections of blood are probably quite common and likely reabsorb

TABLE 32.2. *Indications for evacuation of a retropubic space hematoma*

Hemodynamic instability
Symptoms of compression
Evidence of infection
Evidence of expansion

spontaneously. If a hematoma is large or enlarging, symptoms of compression may occur. This can manifest as pelvic discomfort, pain, or weakness in the distribution of the obturator nerve, or as a dropping hematocrit with symptoms of hemodynamic instability. A pelvic ultrasound or abdominal imaging study such as computed tomography or magnetic resonance imaging can characterize the hematoma. Serial imaging studies and serial hematocrit levels can detect expansion. Hemodynamic instability or evidence of expansion of a hematoma mandates exploration for an uncontrolled arterial source. Expectant management is reasonable in the case of a stable hematoma without evidence of infection or symptoms of compression. If symptoms of compression or infection indicate the need for evacuation, this can be accomplished by exploration or percutaneous drainage in consultation with an interventional radiologist. The management of infected hematoma or abscess is considered in the next section. Table 32.2 outlines the indications for drainage of a hematoma.

INFECTIOUS AND INFLAMMATORY COMPLICATIONS

Retropubic Abscess

The development of a postoperative abscess has two basic prerequisites: an accumulation of blood or serum to serve as a culture medium, and the introduction of bacteria into the culture medium (6). Tactics developed to prevent abscess formation are aimed at eliminating the prerequisites. This includes maximizing hemostasis during the procedure, draining the operative site to prevent accumulation of the culture medium if hemostasis is not optimal, and eliminating or minimizing bacterial contamination of the operative site, usually through the use of short courses of prophylactic antibiotics. Both drainage and prophylaxis have proved successful in reducing the incidence of cuff infections after hysterectomy (7). Although neither approach has been prospectively validated in continence surgery, each tactic is used, either alone or in combination. Techniques for the control of retropubic space bleeding and for postoperative drainage of the space have already been considered. Although studies demonstrating the efficacy of antibiotic prophylaxis during continence surgery are lacking, we generally favor single-dose perioperative antibiotic prophylaxis with a first-generation cephalosporin (cefazolin, 1 g given intravenously), the same prophylaxis we use with vaginal hysterectomy (8). Other elements of operative technique may diminish contamination of the abdominal operative site. These include the use of a separate clean instrument set for the abdominal incision and closure and use of a clean ligature carrier or fascial clamp for each passage through the rectus fascia and retropubic space when performing a suburethral sling procedure. Operators should change gloves to avoid contamination of the abdominal incision after operating in the vaginal field (9). Finally, we recommend only monofilament permanent suture material for needle suspensions because of concerns about the ability of multifilament braided suture to harbor a larger inoculum of vaginal bacteria. Removal of such suture had previously been necessary in several patients because of chronic, refractory infections and foreign-body reactions as late as 2 years after surgery.

Despite best efforts at prevention, there is still a small risk for retropubic abscess formation after abdominal and abdominovaginal colposuspension. The incidence of this complication is difficult to estimate because most reports of surgical procedures that enumerate operative complications do not specifically mention retropubic space abscess or infection among their complications. Consequently, it would seem that such occurrences are extremely rare using the preventative techniques described above. Stanton (5) reported one

retropubic abscess among 40 women (2.3%) undergoing Burch colposuspension.

An abscess should be suspected when persistent fever, tenderness, pain, and irritative voiding symptoms are encountered postoperatively. The bimanual pelvic-abdominal examination often reveals a tender mass in the retropubic area. Purulent drainage may be noted around a suprapubic bladder catheter. An abdominal or vaginal ultrasound examination should be able to confirm the lesion. Once the diagnosis is established, prompt surgical drainage and broad-spectrum antibiotic coverage should be instituted. As discussed in the next section, the decision to retain or remove a permanent foreign body used to perform the surgery is difficult and must be individualized.

Foreign-body Complications

Complications resulting from the presence of a permanent foreign body in an operative site are related either to enhanced invasiveness and persistence of infections or to noninfectious foreign-body reactions. The foreign bodies most commonly left permanently in place after continence surgery include suture material, synthetic bands for some sling procedures, synthetic endopelvic fascia bolsters and anterior rectus fascia pledgets for various needle procedures, artificial urinary sphincters, and various materials used for periurethral injection. The significant problem of a bacterial infection in an operative site occupied by a foreign body has already been mentioned. When the bulk of the material and the magnitude of the infection are both substantial, effective management involves the removal of the foreign body in addition to appropriate drainage and antibiotic therapy. This is particularly true with the artificial sphincter and most synthetic sling materials.

Foreign-body reactions represent a chronic, granulomatous inflammatory response to a nondigestible irritant. Such reactions can occur in response to any of the permanent materials already described. Table 32.3 lists various materials that have been used for pelvic

TABLE 32.3. *Synthetic materials used in pelvic reconstructive surgery requiring removal due to erosion*

Stamey procedure
  Dacron rectus fascia pledgets
  Marlex pledgets
Pubovaginal sling procedures
  Polyethylene (Mersilene gauze)
  Polypropylene (Marlex mesh)
  Silastic
  Polytetrafluorethylene (Gore-Tex patch)
  Pressure-injected bovine collagen (ProteGen)

TABLE 32.4. *Management options for erosion of synthetic graft material*

Local drainage and antibiotic therapy
Conservative removal of exposed mesh and primary
  closure
Complete excision of all graft material

reconstructive procedures and have subsequently required removal because of erosion or infection. Because the foreign body is incorporated into the granulomatous reaction, resolution of the reaction requires removal of the foreign body.

Pubovaginal sling procedures for stress incontinence can be performed with autologous fascia (most commonly, anterior rectus fascia or fascia lata) or with synthetic, inorganic materials listed in Table 32.3. Proposed advantages of organic slings over synthetic slings include the avoidance of infection, better wound healing, and absence of erosion necessitating sling removal (10). Rejection rates of up to 21% have been reported for synthetic slings (11). Organic slings are not exempt from complications of erosion, however. Case reports of urethral erosion of fascia lata slings appear in the literature citing excessive tension on the sling as the likely etiology (12). In contrast, series that have followed women for up to 16 years after surgery revealed no synthetic sling removals for infection (13,14). Polypropylene (Prolene) mesh is currently used in the TVT procedure. Histologic study shows that it does not generate the typical granulomatous reaction in surrounding tissue, which may explain the rarity of rejection of this material (15). Animal experiments comparing polytetrafluoroethylene (Gore-Tex) with Marlex mesh in the reconstruction of infected abdominal walls suggest that the porous structure of Gore-Tex should allow infected slings to be treated, *in situ,* with antibiotics (16). However, histologic studies of Gore-Tex slings removed for tissue rejection have revealed gram-positive cocci in

the patch interstices (11). Certainly, if an acute infection does not respond rapidly to or recurs after antibiotic therapy, removal of the sling would seem most prudent.

Erosion can occur in the vagina, urethra, or bladder, and symptoms include vaginal and urethral pain, irritative voiding symptoms, vaginal discharge or bleeding, and recurrent urinary tract infections (17). Diagnosis is usually made by physical examination and cystoscopy; however, vaginoscopy through the flexible cystoscope has been described as a valuable adjunct (18). Fortunately, removal of a sling does not necessarily compromise the success of the original procedure. A continence rate of 74% has been reported after removal of 23 Gore-Tex slings for tissue reaction (11), and a rate 50% has been seen after removal of "synthetic" slings (17). Conservative management of Mersilene mesh sling erosion was described, but continence rates were not stated (19). Table 32.4 summarizes a stepwise management approach to erosion of synthetic graft material.

Osteitis Pubis and Pyogenic Arthritis

Osteitis pubis is a self-limiting nonbacterial inflammation of the symphysis pubis that can follow trauma, childbirth, prolonged running and kicking exercise, and pelvic surgery (20). Although it can occur in any of these circumstances, in urogynecology, it most commonly follows the Marshall-Marchetti-Krantz procedure, with an overall frequency of 2.5%, presumably due to the placement of the suspending sutures into the periosteum of the superior pubic ramus or the perichondrium of the pubic symphysis. Although self-limiting, the syndrome can be quite distressing to the patient, resulting in incapacitating symptoms for weeks to months (21,22). Table 32.5 summa-

TABLE 32.5. *Osteitis pubis*

Symptoms
　Abrupt onset of burning pelvic or groin pain
　Aggravated by walking, coughing, climbing stairs,
　　getting out of bed
Signs
　Tenderness of the pubic symphysis
　Pain on pelvic compression
　Adductor spasm, limitation of abduction
　Waddling gait
Diagnosis
　Elevated erythrocyte sedimentation rate
　Radiographs show "moth-eaten" lytic lesions
　　appearing after several weeks
Management
　Bed rest
　Nonsteroidal antiinflammatory drugs
　Corticosteroid injection
　Heparinization
　Physical therapy with diathermy or hydrotherapy
　Differentiation from osteomyelitis or pyogenic
　　arthritis

rizes the symptoms, signs, diagnosis, and management of this condition. Antibiotics are not part of therapy if there is no evidence of frank infection. However, differentiating osteitis pubis from the rare conditions of pyogenic arthritis and osteomyelitis may be difficult. Needle biopsy of the symphysis and culture of aspirate may be necessary to distinguish the two conditions. One report of three patients described dramatic responses to heparinization and suggested that pubic thrombosis may be involved in the pathogenesis of the condition (22).

Pyogenic arthritis and pubic bone osteomyelitis can also occur after pelvic operations and have been described after the Marshall-Marchetti-Krantz procedure. As noted previously, signs, symptoms, and radiographic findings are virtually identical to those of osteitis pubis except for signs of overt bacterial infection. If the diagnosis is made immediately, intravenous antibiotic therapy may be adequate, although consideration should be given to removal of suture material used for the urethropexy. In chronic or advanced cases, surgical drainage and débridement are required in addition to antibiotic therapy (20).

Of particular interest is the increasing use of bone anchors in treatment of urinary in-

continence. A variety of devices have been developed to facilitate placement of bone anchors using either a transvaginal or suprapubic approach to attach a variety of sling designs (23). Success rates have been reported that are comparable with those of the more traditional procedures, although randomized trials are lacking. Case reports of pubic osteomyelitis requiring bone anchor removal and pubic bone débridement are appearing in the literature. *Pseudomonas aeruginosa* and methicillin-resistant *Staphylococcus aureus* are among the organisms grown on culture (24). Metastatic osteomyelitis has also been reported (25).

Urinary Tract Infections

Significant bacteriuria after continence surgery is quite common. The risks of bacteriuria, if allowed to progress to a frank infection, include febrile morbidity, bacteremia, pyelonephritis, perinephric abscess, and sepsis. Independent risk factors for bacteriuria have been shown to include duration of catheterization, absence of prophylactic antibiotics, colonization of the drainage bag, female patient, diabetes mellitus, and periurethral colonization. In a catheterized patient, a meticulously maintained closed drainage system can reduce the rate of bacteriuria to 5% to 10% per day, compared with 100% at 4 days with an open drainage system. This underscores the importance of intraluminal entry of organisms into the bladder. However, the fact that even a closed system cannot prevent infections confirms that extraluminal entry is ultimately unavoidable. The most effective way of preventing catheter-associated urinary tract infection is to avoid prolonged, continuous transurethral catheterization (26,27). If such catheterization cannot be avoided, efforts should be directed toward postponement of the inevitable bacteriuria, treatment of symptomatic bacteriuria, and surveillance for the management of significant complications of bacteriuria. Trying to preserve fastidiously a closed system can postpone the inevitable with chronic catheterization and avoid many infections in acute, short-term catheterization. Table 32.6 outlines important aspects of such a system.

One technique that has been primarily employed to avoid continuous transurethral catheterization is suprapubic catheterization. This technique has been shown to decrease significantly the risk for bacteriuria when the duration of catheterization exceeds 5 days (28). These data would appear to indicate that suprapubic catheterization is the preferred method of managing postoperative bladder drainage for incontinence surgery. However, if the duration of catheterization can reasonably be expected to be less than 5 days, the advantage in reduction of bacteriuria is not so clear. Infection rates are similar when voiding trials are initiated early in the postoperative course, and more complications have been seen with suprapubic catheters than with a transurethral catheter (29,30). The issue of complications of suprapubic catheterization are addressed in a subsequent section, but the previous discussion of infection rates would seem to indicate that if the routine postoperative management of patients involves early voiding trials, either suprapubic or transurethral bladder catheterization is reasonable.

When it becomes obvious that the postoperative patient will require bladder drainage for a prolonged period of time, intermittent catheterization is the preferred technique. Even with prolonged use, the proportion of patients able to maintain sterile urine with aseptic intermittent catheterization varies between 45% and 90%. With clean, intermittent self-catheterization, the proportion is 39% to 65% (27). The

incidence of urinary tract infection with the latter technique is less than half that observed with indwelling catheters (26).

Prevention

Two controversial methods to prevent bacteriuria are bladder irrigation and the use of systemic antibiotics. The sum of evidence regarding antibiotic or antiseptic irrigation of indwelling catheters does not support the value of the practice in postponing bacteriuria. The irrigation appears to represent yet another breach of the closed system. Systemic antibiotic therapy can postpone infections but is likely of value only if the catheter is removed after a relatively short period of time. The advantage of this effect is diminished by the fact that, in many patients, short-term, catheter-associated bacteriuria resolves spontaneously once the catheter is removed. Although short courses of antibiotics can clear catheter-associated bacteriuria, infections typically recur a few days after discontinuing antibiotics if the catheter is still in place. Long-term therapy in the face of long-term catheterization does not prevent bacteriuria, but it does favor the emergence of resistant organisms (26,28).

Any treatment scheme of catheter-associated urinary tract infection must acknowledge that sterile urine cannot be maintained indefinitely with the catheter in place. Thus, there is no rationale for the treatment of asymptomatic bacteriuria. Antibiotic therapy is indicated only if the patient becomes symptomatic. Systemic evidence of infection, such as high fever or signs of pyelonephritis or bacteremia, should prompt a search for other infectious complications and for catheter or ureteral obstruction. Bacteremia is relatively uncommon, occurring in only 2% to 4% of catheterized bacteriuric patients. However, if such signs are due to infection of the urinary tract, parenteral antibiotic therapy is appropriate (26). Symptoms of localized bladder infection, most commonly lower abdominal pain and bladder spasms (DI), often respond to short courses of oral antibiotics. The requi-

TABLE 32.6. *Maintenance of a closed urinary drainage system*

- Avoid disconnecting the catheter from the drainage bag for any reason.
- Use a drainage bag with an incorporated urometer.
- Avoid touching the distal end of the drainage tube to other surfaces.
- Keep the drainage bag below the level of the bladder to prevent retrograde flow of urine.
- Never clamp a transurethral catheter and only clamp a suprapubic catheter as part of a voiding trial before anticipated catheter removal.

site adjunct to antibiotic therapy in the cure of all such infections is discontinuation of the indwelling catheter as soon as possible.

URINARY TRACT INJURIES

Surgical injury to the lower urinary tract is described with virtually every continence procedure. Such injuries have been described with 3% to 6% of Burch colposuspensions, with 1% to 7% of needle-type urethropexies, with 1.6% of Marshall-Marchetti-Krantz procedures, and with as many as 6% of TVT procedures. The risk for injury can be minimized but not eliminated with experience and attention to the details of the technique. More importantly, the risk for unrecognized injury can be virtually eliminated with cystoscopic assessment of the integrity of the lower urinary tract during and after the performance of the procedure.

Injury to the bladder and urethra can occur during the dissection of these structures from the overlying rectus muscles and pubic bone as the space of Retzius is developed during abdominal retropubic procedures. It can also occur when the space is entered or when the ligature carrier is passed during Pereyra-Stamey–type or TVT procedures. Such injuries are especially likely when there is extensive scarring in the retropubic space because of previous continence surgery. Ureteric injuries are a particular concern with the Burch colposuspension procedure. They are most likely to occur during placement of suspending sutures at or just above the urethrovesical junction if the lateral edge of the bladder has been inadequately dissected and defined (5). The risk for ureteric injuries during laparoscopic Burch colposuspension remains to be clearly defined, but the rate of injury to the lower urinary tract has been reported to be lower than that reported for an open Burch procedure (31). Ureteric injury, especially kinking and obstruction, is also a concern during surgical correction of severe degrees of uterovaginal prolapse. The ureter is at greatest risk during the closure of the cul-de-sac and plication of the uterosacral ligaments (32).

There are several techniques that can help prevent unrecognized urinary tract injuries. The instillation of a small amount of contrast material (30 to 50 mL) into the bladder at the start of the dissection will make any breach of the bladder obvious. Appropriate fluids include irrigation fluid stained with indigo carmine or methylene blue dye, or sterile infant's formula. The latter is readily available in any hospital with a newborn nursery, is easily distinguishable from normal body fluids, and will not stain tissues. Finally, reserving blue dye for systemic administration, renal excretion, and ureteric evaluation facilitates separate evaluation of bladder and ureteric integrity during surgery.

The performance of a controlled, high extraperitoneal cystotomy during abdominal retropubic procedures is another excellent technique to avoid more serious bladder, ureteral, or urethral injuries. Some authorities advocate cystotomy to avoid injury and to ensure proper suture placement in every retropubic procedure (33). Certainly, such a cystotomy is invaluable as the initial step in repeat retropubic procedures, in which significant scarring is often encountered.

We advocate examination of the urethra, bladder, and ureters at the conclusion of every surgery for incontinence or prolapse. This can be done either by cystotomy, cystourethroscopy, or suprapubic telescopy. When continence surgery is performed in the supine position, valuable operative time is lost by repositioning and preparing for transurethral cystoscopy. In this situation, if significant cystoscopic findings are encountered, the abdomen must be reopened for surgical correction. Suprapubic telescopy avoids these disadvantages and provides an excellent view of the bladder and ureters. In terms of operating time and morbidity, suprapubic telescopy compares favorably to the alternatives of open cystotomy, dissection of ureters, or transurethral cystoscopy (34).

Inserting a three-way transurethral catheter during preparation for the supine procedure in anticipation of telescopy allows convenient bladder distention for the procedure. The technique is described in detail elsewhere. Alternatively, positioning the patient in the low lithotomy position using Allen universal stirrups allows access to the perineum to perform transurethral cystourethroscopy. This eliminates the need to reposition the patient. If suture perforation is visualized, the suture can be immediately removed and replaced. Ureteral integrity is assessed by the administration of indigo carmine only after all suspension or plication sutures have been tied. Excretion of dye should be observed from both ureteral orifices. In the absence of ureteral efflux, management decisions are complicated by the absence of preoperative demonstration of bilateral ureteric competence (by intravenous pyelography, ultrasonography, or cystoscopy).

Ureteral visualization is usually not possible with a zero-degree endoscope and is difficult with a 30-degree telescope owing to elevation of the urethrovesical junction after sutures are tied. We have found a 70-degree telescope with a 17-French diagnostic sheath ideal in this situation. It has the added advantage of simplicity and ready availability in most gynecologic operating rooms. If bilateral spill is not observed, a reasonable first step is to pass a 6-French whistle-tip ureteral catheter by means of an operative cystoscope. Passing the catheter 20 cm places the tip above the level of any sutures or dissection from the procedure and rules out obstruction. In our experience, this has also resulted in free flow of indigo carmine–stained urine from the ureteral orifice. If kinking or obstruction of the ureter halts the passage of the stent, the level of the obstruction is identified. The corresponding sutures should be removed and ureteral function reassessed. If spill is observed and ureteric or ureterovesical kinking was due only to imperfect suture placement, no further intervention is necessary. Ureteral catheterization with a double J stent for 7 to 14 days should be considered if the ureter itself has been damaged (35). If a more extensive injury is suspected, or if spill is not observed, ureteral dissection and direct ureteral inspection are necessary. If the injury has extensively damaged and devitalized the ureter (an extremely

uncommon occurrence with continence surgery), excision of the damaged section and ureteroneocystostomy should be performed (36). Intraoperative evaluation of the lower urinary tract has demonstrated a previously unrecognized injury in between 1.5% and 4% of urogynecologic procedures (32).

When bladder injury and laceration are identified, careful two-layer closure should be performed. Only absorbable suture material should be used for any suture line that is likely to be in contact with urine, owing to the risk for stone formation. Chromic catgut suture is still considered the material of choice because the brevity of absorption minimizes stone formation. Knots should be tied on the extraluminal surface, and bladder decompression should be maintained for 5 to 10 days after injury. This can be accomplished with a transurethral catheter or a suprapubic tube. If significant intravesical bleeding is anticipated, a 30- to 32-French suprapubic Malecot catheter is desirable to prevent obstruction with clots (37). When a controlled surgical cystotomy is performed extraperitoneally and repair is accomplished without tension, such prolonged decompression is not necessary. As long as the retropubic space is drained adequately, the catheter in such cases can often be managed as it is after comparable continence procedures without cystotomy, and voiding trials can begin 5 to 7 days postoperatively.

POSTOPERATIVE URINARY RETENTION

Immediate postoperative retention, an inability to empty the bladder effectively on the initial attempt to void after surgery, is the most common of all complications after continence surgery. The precise incidence of this complication is difficult to determine because there is no standard definition for acute retention and because many authors omit reference to this particular complication when reporting their results. It would appear that retention depends on the procedure and the way it is performed as well as on the patient and her preoperative voiding mechanism.

No continence procedure is immune to the risk for immediate postoperative retention. The risk after various procedures varies among reports citing the same procedure. Pereyra-Stamey–type procedures, the Marshall-Marchetti-Krantz procedure, the Burch colposuspension, and suburethral sling procedures all have reported postoperative voiding dysfunction rates approaching 25%. With sling procedures performed in patients with recurrent genuine stress incontinence (GSI) with irreparably poor local support tissues and in patients with low urethral closure pressure, short-term retention is nearly universal. Time required for postoperative catheterization can be 1 to 2 months. It is clear that sling procedures in such patients must significantly increase urethral resistance if they are to cure disabling incontinence. This attempt to increase urethral resistance often results in functional obstruction.

Successful continence surgery permanently reconstructs anatomic relationships between the bladder and urethra, resulting in a unique stress continence mechanism whereby the urethra and urethrovesical junction (UVJ) are compressed during increases in abdominal pressure by the momentary descent of more mobile posterior and superior pelvic viscera (38). This stress-activated, obstructive sphincteric mechanism may be activated by variable degrees of stress, depending on the degree of correction or overcorrection of UVJ support. Thus, the surgeon who aggressively elevates the UVJ by design for whatever reason is more likely to create retention than one who is less aggressive. Studies of acute (6 weeks to 6 months) and chronic (up to 12 years) postcontinence surgery voiding dysfunction have demonstrated that procedures that aggressively support the bladder neck and result in extreme preferential stress pressure transmission to the urethra are more likely to cause new voiding-phase dysfunction (39). Likewise, the patient whose preoperative voiding mechanism depends heavily on Valsalva, with minimal detrusor activity, will activate her new sphincteric mechanism when she employs her former voiding mechanism. Thus, women who have normal preoperative uroflowmetry parameters are less likely to experience postoperative retention. The risk for prolonged retention is particularly significant after surgery to correct incontinence or severe degrees of prolapse in elderly women, many of whom have deceptively precarious lower urinary tract function before surgery. An evaluation of urodynamic and clinical parameters in women undergoing fascia lata sling procedures showed that women older than 65 years of age, those who underwent additional procedures, and those with a preoperative urine flow rate of less than 20 mL/s had prolonged return of normal voiding, whereas preoperative voiding mechanism was independent of time to normal voiding.

A number of techniques can facilitate management of postoperative urinary retention. These are summarized in Table 32.7 and include the use of a suprapubic catheter, intermittent self-catheterization, and instruction on new voiding mechanisms.

Even more important than these postoperative management techniques is preoperative anticipation of the problem in a particular patient. This allows a realistic and frank discussion of the complication and enables the patient to make an informed decision regarding the proposed surgery. Some high-risk patients are unwilling or unable to trade self-catheterization for protective garments, and they should be given the option of sharing in this decision.

It is important to explain to the patient that successful voiding after surgery may require a change in her voiding mechanism. She should understand that the process of bearing down to urinate actually activates her new sphincter mechanism. Alternatively, she should be encouraged to initiate voiding by relaxing the pelvic floor. This process can be facilitated if the patient attempts to void in a

TABLE 32.7. *Management strategies for postoperative urinary retention*

Preoperative anticipation and patient education
Suprapubic catheter
Intermittent self-catheterization
Instruction on new voiding mechanisms

warm sitz bath. When we anticipate retention in a given patient to be prolonged beyond 1 or 2 weeks, we train the patient in the technique of clean, intermittent self-catheterization. Patients whose preoperative sphincteric status demands frankly obstructive surgery (i.e., low-pressure urethra with apparently good support and immobile anatomy but with inefficient stress pressure transmission) are instructed in self-catheterization preoperatively.

Pharmacologic manipulation is sometimes beneficial in some cases of postoperative retention. Diazepam (Valium) has a relaxant effect on striated muscle through its polysynaptic inhibitory action. In addition, its well-known anxiolytic effect through its depressant action on the brain-stem reticular system can also benefit many patients who are unable to void after surgery. Diazepam in doses of 2 to 10 mg, one to three times daily, has been shown to be more effective than bethanechol (Urecholine) in these circumstances (40). Bethanechol in high doses can increase bladder tone but does not generally stimulate a coordinated voiding pattern. The muscarinic action of systemically administered bethanechol can enhance detrusor contractions, but its nicotinic activity simultaneously stimulates preganglionic sympathetic as well as parasympathetic activity. This results in increased α-adrenergic activity of the urethra and bladder neck (smooth muscle contraction) when these agents are used to stimulate detrusor activity. The intravesical instillation of Prostaglandin F_{2a} has been shown to decrease acute urinary retention after vaginal hysterectomy. It has also been shown to improve voiding function on the day of instillation in women who were unable to micturate 3 days after continence surgery. The role of such instillations in the management of postoperative retention is not yet established.

The most dramatic management approach to prolonged postoperative retention is surgical takedown and revision of the surgical repair, often with extensive urethrolysis. This is an infrequent occurrence, being performed in only 2.9% of 170 consecutive fascia lata sling procedures in the series reported by Beck and colleagues (10). Indications for urethrolysis include obstructive or irritative voiding symptoms, *de novo* urge incontinence, frank obstruction, or elevated postvoid residual (>100 mL). Specific urodynamic parameters cited include flow of less than 12 to 15 mL/s and peak detrusor pressure during voiding of more than 20 to 50 cm H_2O; however, multiple authors caution that no such parameter is predictive of successful outcome, and a low percentage of patients with symptoms actually meet such criteria preoperatively (41,42).

The surgical approach to urethrolysis can be retropubic (43), transvaginal (44), or suprameatal (infrapubic) (45). Success of urethrolysis, defined as resolution of irritative or obstructive voiding symptoms and lack of stress urinary incontinence, was reported by Carr and Webster as 86% for retropubic procedures, 73% for vaginal procedures, and 25% for epiurethral or infrapubic procedures (41). Nitti and Raz reported overall benefit of 80% from a transvaginal approach with concurrent modified Pereyra suspension (42). Petrou and associates noted 65% reduction of urinary retention and 67% reduction in urgency symptoms after the suprameatal approach (45). Another option is interposition of a vaginal patch to lengthen a pubovaginal sling, which was successful in relieving obstruction in 4 of 4 cases and maintained continence in 3 of 4 cases (46).

The need for concurrent bladder neck resuspension at the time of urethrolysis is controversial. Although some series have included a concurrent bladder neck suspension in all patients, Goldman and co-workers evaluated 31 patients undergoing transvaginal urethrolysis without concurrent bladder neck suspension (47). Eighty-four percent had improvement in their obstructive voiding symptoms. Nineteen percent of those patients had recurrent stress incontinence, most cases of which were treated successfully with periurethral collagen injections, giving an overall success of 77%. Moreover, Foster and McGuire reported a series of 48 patients undergoing transvaginal urethrolysis alone with no cases of recurrent stress urinary incontinence (48).

COMPLICATIONS OF SUPRAPUBIC CATHETERIZATION

Suprapubic catheterization is an excellent option for postoperative bladder drainage, having been shown by some to lower risk for infection and improve resumption of normal voiding. In addition, many patients who have had both types of bladder drainage prefer the suprapubic route. However, as with any other invasive procedure, suprapubic catheters and their insertion are not completely free of complications. Relatively minor though aggravating complications include kinking and obstruction of the tubes, dislodging of the catheter because of difficulty in fixation to the abdominal skin, breakage of the catheter, and catheter-associated DI.

The most serious complication is bowel perforation at the time of insertion of the catheter, which can occur both with suprapubic stab and transurethral insertion techniques. This risk can be minimized by distention of the bladder with at least 400 mL of fluid and by placing the patient in steep Trendelenburg position before insertion. A further margin of safety is realized by inserting the catheter no more than 3 cm above the pubic symphysis, with the trocar directed 30 degrees to the plane of the rectus abdominis muscles in a caudal direction. We usually insert the suprapubic catheter under direct cystoscopic visualization when the bladder and ureters are examined at the conclusion of the continence procedure. Visualization of the insertion helps to confirm proper orientation and final positioning of the catheter. During insertion, attention to the pressure on the trocar and depth of trocar insertion is important to avoid bladder-base damage. Nonetheless, perforations have been described despite such precautions, especially in cases in which bowel was fixed in the anterior pelvis as a result of prior surgery.

Bowel perforation should be suspected if the patient has unexplained lower abdominal pain, fever, or peritoneal signs after surgery. Third spacing and regression of bowel function have been reported as subtle signs of bowel perforation. Radiographic evidence of a pneumoperitoneum after vaginal repair without opening of the cul-de-sac is pathognomonic for bowel perforation. Occasionally, the diagnosis is entertained only after bowel contents drain around the catheter site. A further risk to transperitoneal insertion of the catheter, even if bowel injury does not occur, is intraperitoneal leakage of urine after the catheter is removed. Finally, an extremely rare but life-threatening complication of suprapubic catheter use is necrotizing fasciitis in high-risk (diabetic) patients who develop inflammation at the insertion site. Immediate and extensive surgical débridement to well-vascularized margins is the foundation of therapy for this condition. Broad-spectrum antibiotic coverage is also standard.

DETRUSOR INSTABILITY AFTER CONTINENCE SURGERY

The complication of persistent or recurrent GSI after continence surgery is addressed elsewhere. Equally distressing to the patient and the surgeon alike is the development of urgency-associated incontinence or DI postoperatively. Six to 20% of women with pure GSI develop DI for the first time after continence surgery (49). Women who have mixed incontinence (combined GSI and DI) have a 40% to 45% risk for persistent DI postoperatively (50). In most cases, the continence procedure has been a technical success, achieving both stabilization of the anatomy and correction of the pressure transmission defects. However, the woman who exchanges the loss of a spurt of urine with physical activity before surgery for the loss of a stream of urine with the sensation of uncontrollable urgency after surgery understandably does not consider her surgery successful. There are four major circumstances that can result in DI after continence surgery: the original incontinence was due to DI; the development of DI is unrelated to the surgery or to preexisting DI; local irritative lesions are created by the surgery; and surgery overcorrected UVJ support. Etiology and evaluation of postoperative DI are summarized in Table 32.8.

TABLE 32.8. *Postoperative detrusor instability (DI)*

Etiology
  Original incontinence was due to DI
  DI unrelated to surgery (mixed incontinence)
  Irritative lesions created by the surgery
  Obstruction due to overcorrected urethrovesical
    junction
Evaluation
  Preoperative urodynamics and documentation of
    symptoms and diagnosis
  Infection surveillance
  Cystourethroscopy
Management
  Removal of drainage catheter
  Antimicrobial therapy
  Anticholinergic therapy
  Bladder retraining
  Urethrolysis

An indefensible but avoidable cause of DI after continence surgery is the failure to establish the correct cause of the patient's incontinence before surgery. The presence of mixed incontinence should be appreciated before therapy is started. In such a situation, it is usually best to attempt nonsurgical treatment of the DI component first. Although there are individual situations in which surgery may be performed as initial therapy, the mixed nature of the problem should be known. If an increased risk for postoperative DI exists, this should be clearly acknowledged by the surgeon and the patient. On the other hand, continence surgery plays no role in treatment of incontinence caused by pure DI. It is always incumbent on the physician to prove that the patient does not have DI before surgery. The fact that there is a 6% to 20% *de novo* risk for DI after surgery makes this particularly important. When a patient develops DI after surgery, the only way to prove it was not present before surgery is to have specifically tested for it preoperatively. Surgery for GSI does not prevent the later, unrelated development of DI. For this prospect to be tenable, the onset of the DI should be temporally distant from the surgery. In addition, urinary control should have been acceptable during the interim.

Local irritative lesions in and around the lower urinary tract can result in the loss of volitional suppression of detrusor activity. As already noted in this chapter, a number of acute and chronic irritations can result from continence surgery. These include acute inflammation related to surgical trauma, suture material, and the drainage catheter, in addition to bacterial infections of the bladder. A careful assessment for infection is always the initial step in the management of postoperative DI. When instability and infection persist despite adequate antimicrobial therapy, the bladder should be examined for the presence of a foreign body (suture material or stone) as an ongoing source of the irritation. Examination of the bladder and urethra at the conclusion of surgery obviates this complication. When pharmacologic therapy of DI is necessary, a variety of long-acting preparations are available, such as extended-release tolterodine or oxybutynin. These agents are cholinergic blockers and direct smooth muscle relaxants that also have local anesthetic activity. This last characteristic makes them particularly useful in patients with discomfort and DI due to surgical irritation, infection, or catheters.

There is accumulating evidence that surgical overcorrection of anatomic support of the UVJ can cause DI. Women who develop persistent DI after continence surgery have been shown to have pressure transmission ratios (PTRs) substantially above 100%, a finding associated with significant stress-induced obstruction of the urethra (39). Such women also have significantly higher PTRs than women who have normal continence after surgery and women who develop DI without prior surgery. Surgeons who achieve PTRs of more than 100% with the Burch colposuspension report much higher *de novo* DI rates than surgeons who achieve PTRs of less than 100% with the same procedure (27% versus 6%). If a surgical procedure overcorrects UVJ support, as manifested by preferential urethral pressure transmission (PTRs higher than 100%) rather than equal pressure transmission, urethral obstruction is likely more profound and may not require significant stress activation. This high degree of relative obstruction may result in DI. Further support for the role of partial obstruction in the genesis of postoperative DI is the demonstration of decreased urine flow rates and increased residual urine volumes in such women. The development of DI in men with partial bladder obstruction from prostatic enlargement and in animals after experimental outflow obstruction also supports this hypothesis.

It has been our experience that postoperative DI due to overcorrection is more refractory to bladder retraining than DI that does not follow surgery. The former women nearly always require pharmacologic suppression of their detrusor activity. Furthermore, they often need to remain on such therapy indefinitely. Anticholinergic and smooth muscle relaxant therapy does pose some risk for urinary retention in these circumstances, and patients should be instructed in intermittent self-catheterization before starting such agents. Just as is the case with patients who develop prolonged retention after continence surgery, women with prolonged DI that is refractory to tolerable medical therapy may need takedown and revision of their surgical repair. In our limited experience, this has resulted in the reversal of DI-associated symptoms.

FUTURE RESEARCH

The subject of antibiotic prophylaxis has received considerable attention in the case of vaginal and abdominal hysterectomy. It seems reasonable that when performing incontinence procedures in which a hysterectomy is part of the planned procedure, antibiotic prophylaxis should be commensurate with the most invasive component of the procedure. However, respected authorities differ in their use and recommendations of antibiotics in these cases. Future research in this area would be well directed at determining the need and most appropriate antibiotic regimen both in abdominal cases in which the vagina is not entered and in cases performed through the vagina.

As noted in this chapter, bone anchors are a component of many innovative procedures for urinary incontinence. Success rates of these procedures are often quoted to be comparable with those of the more established procedures, such as the Burch colposuspension. It should be emphasized that randomized trials evaluating these procedures are lacking, not only in terms of the success rates of curing incontinence, but also in evaluation of both the short- and long-term complications of these procedures. Glowacki and Wall reviewed the various bone anchor procedures and noted that decreased operative time, possible avoidance of an abdominal incision, and a "more anatomic" point of fixation are potential benefits of these procedures (51). However, the complications of the bone anchor procedures mandate that well-designed prospective randomized controlled trials demonstrate a benefit to the patient over traditional incontinence procedures before their adoption into general practice.

Laparoscopic surgery has increased in popularity as one of the standard options of approach when performing incontinence surgery. Significant time and energy must be expended on the part of the surgeon who wishes to become proficient at this approach. Potential advantages to the patient include less postoperative pain and recovery time, less hospitalization with the possibility of lower cost, and a more cosmetically pleasing result. Disadvantages can include longer operative time with associated increased anesthetic risk and increased operating room expense. Studies have compared the success rates of open procedures with those of laparoscopic procedures, and at least one study has evaluated complication rates of laparoscopic procedures (31). What seems to be lacking is a clear understanding of relative risk of injury or complication to the patient and the experience required of a laparoscopic surgeon to bring the risk to the patient in line with that of an open procedure.

Finally, the TVT procedure is rapidly increasing in popularity. It has been used for more than 5 years in Europe and has been reported on extensively in the international literature. Success rates appear to be similar to those of the Burch colposuspension, and complication rates appear to be low. Postoperative urinary retention has been reported to follow the TVT procedure at a rate of 2% to 4%. Simple immediate postoperative adjustment of the UVJ elevation has been successful in relieving this obstruction; however, more long-term data on this device are needed. A multicenter randomized clinical trial comparing the TVT procedure with the Burch colposuspension to evaluate all of these issues would be an invaluable aid in counseling patients of their options for incontinence surgery.

REFERENCES

1. Lambrou NC, Buller JL, Thompson JR, et al. Prevalence of perioperative complications among women undergoing reconstructive pelvic surgery. *Am J Obstet Gynecol* 2000;183(6):1355–1358.

2. Dicker RC, Greenspan JR, Strauss LT, et al. Complications of abdominal and vaginal hysterectomy among women of reproductive age in the United States: the collaborative review of sterilization. *Am J Obstet Gynecol* 1982;144:841–848.

3. Kingsnorth AN, Skandalakis PN, Colborn GL, et al. Embryology, anatomy, and surgical applications of the preperitoneal space. *Surg Clin North Am* 2000;80(1): 1–24.

4. Shull BL. How I do the abdominal paravaginal repair? *J Pelvic Surg* 1995;1:43–49.

5. Stanton SL. Surgery of urinary incontinence. *Clin Obstet Gynecol* 1978;5:83–108.

6. Swartz WH, Tanaree P. Suction drainage as an alternative to prophylactic antibiotics for hysterectomy. *Obstet Gynecol* 1975;45:305–310.

7. Swartz WH, Tanaree P. T-Tube suction drainage and/or prophylactic antibiotics: a randomized study of 451 hysterectomies. *Obstet Gynecol* 1976;69:879–882.

8. Soper DE, Yarwood RL. Single-dose antibiotic prophylaxis in women undergoing vaginal hysterectomy. *Obstet Gynecol* 1987;69:879–882.

9. Elser DM, Tomezsko JE. A randomized prospective comparison of changing gloves during abdomino-vaginal pelvic reconstructive surgery [Abstract]. Society of Gynecologic Surgeons, 27th Scientific Meeting, Lake Buena Vista, Fl. Mar 5–7, 2001.

10. Beck RP, McCormick S, Nordstrom L. The fascia lata sling procedure for treating recurrent genuine stress incontinence of urine. *Obstet Gynecol* 1988;72:699–703.

11. Bent AE, Ostergard DR, Zwick-Zaffulo M. Tissue reaction to expanded polytetrafluoroethylene suburethral sling for urinary incontinence: clinical and histological study. *Am J Obstet Gynecol* 1993;169:1198–1204.

12. Golomb J, Groutz A, Mor Y, et al. Management of urethral erosion caused by a pubovaginal fascial sling. *Urology* 2001;57:159–160.

13. Horbach NS, Blanco JS, Ostergard DR, et al. A suburethral sling procedure with polytetraflurorethylene for the treatment of genuine stress incontinence in patients with low urethral closure pressure. *Obstet Gynecol* 1988;71:648–652.

14. Morgan JE, Farrow GA, Stewart FE. The Marlex sling operation for the treatment of recurrent stress urinary

15. Falconer C, Söderberg M, Blomgren B, et al. Influence of different sling materials on connective tissue metabolism in stress urinary incontinent women. *Int Urogynecol J* 2001;12 [Suppl 2]:S19–S23.

16. Brown GL, Richardson JE, Malangoni MA, et al. Comparison of prosthetic materials and abdominal wall reconstruction in the presence of contamination and infection. *Ann Surg* 1985;201:705–711.

17. Clemens JQ, DeLancey JOL, Faerber GJ, et al. Urinary tract erosions after synthetic pubovaginal slings: diagnosis and management strategy. *Urology* 2000;56: 589–594.

18. Chai TC, Sklar GN. Use of the flexible cystoscope as a vaginoscope to aid in the diagnosis of artificial sling erosion. *Urology* 1999;53:617–618.

19. Myers DL, LaSala CA. Conservative surgical management of Mersilene mesh suburethral sling erosion. *Am J Obstet Gynecol* 1998;179:1424–1428.

20. Gamble JG, Simmons SC, Freedman M. The symphysis pubis: anatomic and pathologic considerations. *Clin Orthop* 1986;203:261–272.

21. Mainprize TC, Drutz HP. The Marshall-Marchetti-Krantz procedure: a critical review. *Obstet Gynecol Surv* 1988;43:724–729.

22. Merimsky E, Canetti R, Firstater M. Osteitis pubis: treatment by heparinization. *Br J Urol* 1981;53:154–156.

23. Winters JC, Scarpero HM, Appell RA. Use of bone anchors in female urology. *Urology* 2000;56[6 Suppl 1]: 15–22.

24. Fitzgerald MP, Gitelis S, Brubaker L. Pubic osteomyelitis and granuloma after bone anchor placement. *Int Urogynecol J Pelvic Floor Dysfunct* 1999; 10(5):346–348.

25. Franks ME, Lavelle JP, Yokoyama T, et al. Metastatic osteomyelitis after pubovaginal sling using bone anchors. *Urology* 2000;56:330–331.

26. Warren JW. Catheter-associated urinary tract infections. *Infect Dis Clin North Am* 1987;1:823–854.

27. Khanna OP. Nonsurgical therapeutic modalities. In: Krane RJ, Siroky MB, eds. *Clinical neuro-urology.* Boston: Little Brown, 1979:159–196.

28. Sethia KK, Selkon JB, Turner CM, et al. Prospective randomized controlled trial of urethral versus suprapubic catheterization. *Br J Surg* 1987;74:624–625.

29. Schiotz HA, Malme PA, Tanbo TG. Urinary tract infections and asymptomatic bacteriuria after vaginal plastic surgery: a comparison of suprapubic and transurethral catheters. *Acta Obstet Gynecol Scand* 1989;68:453–455.

30. Theofrastous J, Cobb D, VanDyke A, et al. *A randomized trial of suprapubic vs. transurethral catheter drainage following Burch urethropexy* [Abstract]. The Society of Gynecologic Surgeons 26th Scientific Meeting, New Orleans, LA, February 28 to March 1, 2000.

31. Speights SE, Moore RD, Miklos JR. Frequency of lower urinary tract injury at laparoscopic Burch and paravaginal repair. *J Am Assoc Gynecol Laparosc* 2000;7:515–518.

32. Harris RL, Cundiff GW, Theofrastous JP, et al. The value of intraoperative cystoscopy in urogynecologic and reconstructive pelvic surgery. *Am J Obstet Gynecol* 1997;177:1367–1371.

33. Lee RA, Symmonds RE, Goldstein RA. Surgical complications and results of modified Marshall-Marchetti-

Krantz procedure for urinary incontinence. *Obstet Gynecol* 1979;53:447–450.

34. Timmons MC, Addison WA. Suprapubic teloscopy: extraperitoneal intraoperative technique to demonstrate ureteral patency. *Obstet Gynecol* 1990;75:137–139.

35. Pettit PD. Double-J ureteral catheters in gynecologic surgery. *Obstet Gynecol* 1989;75:536–540.

36. Podratz KC, Angerman NS, Symmonds RE. Complications of ureteral surgery in the nonradiated patient. In: Delgada G, Smith JP, eds. *Management of complications in gynecologic oncology.* New York: Wiley, 1982:113–149.

37. Maxted W. Complications of bladder surgery and cystoscopy. In: Delgado G, Smith JP, eds. *Management of complications in gynecologic oncology.* New York: Wiley, 1982:151–162.

38. Hertogs K, Stanton SL. Mechanism of urinary continence after colposuspension: barrier studies. *Br J Obstet Gynaecol* 1985;92:1184–1188.

39. Bump RC, Fantl JA, Hurt WG. Dynamic urethral pressure profilometry pressure transmission ratio determinations after continence surgery: understanding the mechanism of success, failure, and complications. *Obstet Gynecol* 1988;72:870–877.

40. Stanton SL, Cardozo LD, Kerr-Wilson R. Treatment of delayed onset of spontaneous voiding after surgery for incontinence. *Urology* 1979;13:494–496.

41. Carr LK, Webster GD. Voiding dysfunction following incontinence surgery: diagnosis and treatment with retropubic or vaginal urethrolysis. *J Urol* 1997;157:821–823.

42. Nitti VW, Raz S. Obstruction following anti-incontinence procedures: diagnosis and treatment with transvaginal urethrolysis. *J Urol* 1994;152:93–98.

43. Webster GD, Kreder KJ. Voiding dysfunction following cystourethropexy: its evaluation and management. *J Urol* 1990;144:670.

44. Zimmern PE, Hadley HR, Leach GE, et al. Female urethral obstruction after Marshall-Marchetti-Krantz operation. *J Urol* 1987;138:517.

45. Petrou SP, Brown JA, Blaivas JG. Suprameatal transvaginal urethrolysis. *J Urol* 1999;161:1268–1271.

46. McLennan MT, Bent AE. Sling incision with associated vaginal wall interposition for obstructed voiding secondary to suburethral sling procedure. *Int Urogynecol J Pelvic Floor Dysfunct* 1997;8:168–172.

47. Goldman HB, Rackley RR, Appell RA. The efficacy of urethrolysis without re-suspension for iatrogenic urethral obstruction. *J Urol* 1999;161:196–198.

48. Foster HE, McGuire EJ. Management of urethral obstruction with transvaginal urethrolysis. *J Urol* 1993;150:1448–1451.

49. Cardozo LD, Stanton SL, Williams JE. Detrusor instability following surgery for genuine stress incontinence. *Br J Urol* 1979;51:204–207.

50. Sand PK, Bowen LW, Ostergard DR, et al. The effect of retropubic urethropexy on detrusor stability. *Obstet Gynecol* 1988;71:818–822.

51. Glowacki CA, Wall LL. Bone anchors in urogynecology. *Clin Obstet Gynecol* 2000;43:659–669.

SUGGESTED READINGS

Awad SA, Flood HD, Acker KL. The significance of prior anti-incontinence surgery in women who present with urinary incontinence. *J Urol* 1988;140:514–517.

Crane JK, Bump RC. Drug therapy for urologic disorders. In: Rayburn WF, Zuspan FP, eds. *Drug therapy in obstetrics and gynecology,* 2nd ed. Norwalk, CT: Appleton-Century-Crofts, 1986:419–433.

Jaschevatzky OE, Anderman S, Shalit A, et al. Prostaglandin F2a for prevention of urinary retention after vaginal hysterectomy. *Obstet Gynecol* 1985;66:244–247.

McLennan MT, Melick CF, Bent AE. Clinical and urodynamic predictors of delayed voiding after fascia lata suburethral sling. *Obstet Gynecol* 1998;92:608–612.

Rackley RR, Abdelmalak JB, Tchetgen MB, et al. Tension-free vaginal tape and percutaneous vaginal tape sling procedures. *Tech Urol* 2001;7:90–100.

Romanzi LJ, Blaivas JG. Protracted urinary retention necessitating urethrolysis following tension-free vaginal tape surgery. *J Urol* 2000;164:2022–2023.

Tammela T, Kontturi M, Kaar K, et al. Intravesical prostaglandin F2 for promoting bladder emptying after surgery for female stress incontinence. *Br J Urol* 1987; 60:43–46.

Wang AC, Lo TS. Tension-free vaginal tape. A minimally invasive solution to stress urinary incontinence in women. *J Reprod Med* 1998;43:429.

Appendices

Ostergard's Urogynecology and Pelvic Floor Dysfunction, Fifth Edition. edited by A.E. Bent, et al. Lippincott Williams & Wilkins, Philadelphia © 2003.

Appendix I

The Standardisation of Terminology of Lower Urinary Tract Function: Report from the Standardisation Sub-committee of the International Continence Society

Paul Abrams, Linda Cardozo, Magnus Fall, Derek Griffiths, Peter Rosier, Ulf Ulmsten, Philip van Kerrebroeck, Arne Victor, and Alan Wein

This report presents definitions of the symptoms, signs, urodynamic observations and conditions associated with lower urinary tract dysfunction (LUTD) and urodynamic studies (UDS), for use in all patient groups from children to the elderly.

The definitions restate or update those presented in previous International Continence Society (ICS) Standardisation of Terminology reports (see references) and those shortly to be published on Urethral Function [Lose et al., in press] and Nocturia [van Kerrebroeck et al., 2002]. The published ICS report on the technical aspects of urodynamic equipment [Rowan et al., 1987] will be complemented by the new ICS report on urodynamic practice to be published shortly [Schäfer et al., 2002]. In addition there are four published ICS outcome reports [Fonda et al., 1998; Lose et al., 1998; Mattiasson et al., 1998; Nordling et al., 1998].

New or changed definitions are all indicated; however, recommendations concerning technique are not included in the main text of this report.

The definitions have been written to be compatible with the World Health Organization (WHO) publication ICIDH-2 [International Classification of Functioning, Disability and Health] published in 2001 and ICDIO, the International Classification of Diseases. As far as possible, the definitions are descriptive of observations, without implying underlying assumptions that may later prove to be incorrect or incomplete. By following this principle, the ICS aims to facilitate comparison of results and enable effective communication by investigators who use urodynamic methods. This report restates the ICS principle that symptoms, signs and conditions are separate categories, and adds a category of urodynamic observations. In addition, terminology related to therapies is included [Andersen et al., 1992].

When a reference is made to the whole anatomical organ the vesica urinaria, the correct term is the bladder. When the smooth muscle structure known as the m. detrusor urinae is being discussed, then the correct term is detrusor.

It is suggested that acknowledgement of these standards in written publications be indicated by a footnote to the section "Methods and Materials" or its equivalent, to read as follows:

"Methods, definitions and units conform to the standards recommended by the International Continence Society, except where specifically noted."

The report covers the following areas:

LOWER URINARY TRACT SYMPTOMS (LUTS)

Symptoms are the subjective indicator of a disease or change in condition as perceived by the patient, carer or partner and may lead him/her to seek help from health care professionals. (NEW)

Symptoms may either be volunteered or described during the patient interview. They are usually qualitative. In general, Lower Urinary Tract Symptoms cannot be used to make a definitive diagnosis. Lower Urinary Tract Symptoms can also indicate pathologies other than lower urinary tract dysfunction, such as urinary infection.

SIGNS SUGGESTIVE OF LOWER URINARY TRACT DYSFUNCTION (LUTD)

Signs are observed by the physician including simple means, to verify symptoms and quantify them. (NEW)

For example, a classical sign is the observation of leakage on coughing. Observations from frequency volume charts, pad tests and validated symptom and quality of life questionnaires are examples of other instruments that can be used to verify and quantify symptoms.

URODYNAMIC OBSERVATIONS

Urodynamic observations are observations made during urodynamic studies. (NEW)

For example, an involuntary detrusor contraction (detrusor overactivity) is a urodynamic observation. In general, a urodynamic observation may have a number of possible underlying causes and does not represent a definitive diagnosis of a disease or condition and may occur with a variety of symptoms and signs, or in the absence of any symptoms or signs.

CONDITIONS

Conditions are defined by the presence of urodynamic observations associated with characteristic symptoms or signs and/or non-urodynamic evidence of relevant pathological processes. (NEW)

TREATMENT

Treatment for lower urinary tract dysfunction: these definitions are from the 7th ICS report on Lower Urinary Tract Rehabilitation Techniques [Andersen et al., 1992].

1. LOWER URINARY TRACT SYMPTOMS (LUTS)

Lower urinary tract symptoms are defined from the individual's perspective, who is usually, but not necessarily a patient within the healthcare system. Symptoms are either volunteered by, or elicited from, the individual or may be described by the individual's caregiver.

Lower urinary tract symptoms are divided into three groups: storage, voiding, and post micturition symptoms.

1.1 **Storage symptoms** are experienced during the storage phase of the bladder, and include daytime frequency and nocturia. (NEW)

- *Increased daytime frequency* is the complaint by the patient who considers that he/she voids too often by day. (NEW) This term is equivalent to pollakisuria used in many countries.
- *Nocturia* is the complaint that the individual has to wake at night one or more times to void. (NEW)[1]
- *Urgency* is the complaint of a sudden compelling desire to pass urine, which is difficult to defer. (CHANGED)
- *Urinary incontinence* is the complaint of any involuntary leakage of urine. (NEW)[2]

---

[1]The term night-time frequency differs from that for nocturia; it includes voids that occur after the individual has gone to bed, but before he/she has gone to sleep, and voids which occur in the early morning which prevent the individual from getting back to sleep as he/she wishes. These voids before and after sleep may need to be considered in research studies, for example, in nocturnal polyuria. If this definition were used then an adapted definition of daytime frequency would need to be used with it.

[2]In infants and small children the definition of Urinary Incontinence is not applicable. In scientific communications the definition of incontinence in children would need further explanation.

In each specific circumstance, urinary incontinence should be further described by specifying relevant factors such as type, frequency, severity, precipitating factors, social impact, effect on hygiene and quality of life, the measures used to contain the leakage, and whether or not the individual seeks or desires help because of urinary incontinence.[3]

Urinary leakage may need to be distinguished from sweating or vaginal discharge.

- *Stress urinary incontinence* is the complaint of involuntary leakage on effort or exertion, or on sneezing or coughing. (CHANGED)[4]
- *Urge urinary incontinence* is the complaint of involuntary leakage accompanied by or immediately preceded by urgency. (CHANGED)[5]
- *Mixed urinary incontinence* is the complaint of involuntary leakage associated with urgency and also with exertion, effort, sneezing or coughing. (NEW)
- *Enuresis* means any involuntary loss of urine. (ORIGINAL) If it is used to denote incontinence during sleep, it should always be qualified with the adjective "nocturnal."
- *Nocturnal enuresis* is the complaint of loss of urine occurring during sleep. (NEW)
- *Continuous urinary incontinence* is the complaint of continuous leakage. (NEW)
- *Other types of urinary incontinence* may be situational, for example the report of incontinence during sexual intercourse, or giggle incontinence.

- *Bladder sensation* can be defined, during history taking, by five categories.

  Normal: the individual is aware of bladder filling and increasing sensation up to a strong desire to void. (NEW)

  Increased: the individual feels an early and persistent desire to void. (NEW)

  Reduced: the individual is aware of bladder filling but does not feel a definite desire to void. (NEW)

  Absent: the individual reports no sensation of bladder filling or desire to void. (NEW)

  Non-specific: the individual reports no specific bladder sensation, but may perceive bladder filling as abdominal fullness, vegetative symptoms, or spasticity. (NEW)[6]

1.2 Voiding symptoms are experienced during the voiding phase. (NEW)

- *Slow stream* is reported by the individual as his or her perception of reduced urine flow, usually compared to previous performance or in comparison to others. (NEW)
- *Splitting or spraying* of the urine stream may be reported. (NEW)
- *Intermittent stream (Intermittency)* is the term used when the individual describes urine flow, which stops and starts, on one or more occasions, during micturition. (NEW)
- *Hesitancy* is the term used when an individual describes difficulty in initiating micturition resulting in a delay in the onset of voiding after the individual is ready to pass urine. (NEW)
- *Straining* to void describes the muscular effort used to initiate, maintain or improve the urinary stream. (NEW)[7]
- *Terminal dribble* is the term used when an individual describes a prolonged final part

---

[3]The original ICS definition of incontinence, "Urinary incontinence is the involuntary loss of urine that is a social or hygienic problem," relates the complaint to quality of life (QoL) issues. Some QoL instruments have been, and are being, developed in order to assess the impact of both incontinence and other LUTS on QoL.

[4]The committee considers the term "stress incontinence" to be unsatisfactory in the English language because of its mental connotations. The Swedish, French and Italian expression "effort incontinence" is preferable, however, words such as "effort" or "exertion" still do not capture some of the common precipitating factors for stress incontinence such as coughing or sneezing. For this reason the term is left unchanged.

[5]Urge incontinence can present in different symptomatic forms, for example, as frequent small losses between micturitions, or as a catastrophic leak with complete bladder emptying.

[6]These non-specific symptoms are most frequently seen in neurological patients, particularly those with spinal cord trauma and in children and adults with malformations of the spinal cord.

[7]Suprapubic pressure may be used to initiate or maintain urine flow. The Credé manoeuvre, used by some spinal cord injury patients, and girls with detrusor underactivity sometimes press suprapubically to help empty the bladder.

of micturition, when the flow has slowed to a trickle/dribble. (NEW)

1.3 Post micturition symptoms are experienced immediately after micturition. (NEW)

- *Feeling of incomplete emptying* is a self-explanatory term for a feeling experienced by the individual after passing urine. (NEW)
- *Post micturition dribble* is the term used when an individual describes the involuntary loss of urine immediately after he or she has finished passing urine, usually after leaving the toilet in men, or after rising from the toilet in women. (NEW)

1.4 Symptoms Associated with Sexual Intercourse

Dyspareunia, vaginal dryness and incontinence are amongst the symptoms women may describe during or after intercourse. These symptoms should be described as fully as possible. It is helpful to define urine leakage as: during penetration, during intercourse, or at orgasm.

1.5 Symptoms Associated with Pelvic Organ Prolapse

The feeling of a lump ("something coming down"), low backache, heaviness, dragging sensation, or the need to replace the prolapse digitally in order to defaecate or micturate, are amongst the symptoms women may describe who have a prolapse.

1.6 Genital and Lower Urinary Tract Pain[8]

Pain, discomfort and pressure are part of a spectrum of abnormal sensations felt by the individual. Pain produces the greatest impact on the patient and may be related to bladder filling or voiding, may be felt after micturition, or may be continuous. Pain should also be characterised by type, frequency, duration, precipitating and relieving factors and by location as defined below:

- *Bladder pain* is felt suprapubically or retropubically, usually increases with bladder filling, and may persist after voiding. (NEW)
- *Urethral pain* is felt in the urethra and the individual indicates the urethra as the site. (NEW)
- *Vulval pain* is felt in and around the external genitalia. (NEW)
- *Vaginal pain* is felt internally, above the introitus. (NEW)
- *Scrotal pain* may or may not be localised, for example to the testis, epididymis, cord structures or scrotal skin. (NEW)
- *Perineal pain* is felt: in the female, between the posterior fourchette (posterior lip of the introitus) and the anus, and in the male, between the scrotum and the anus. (NEW)
- *Pelvic pain* is less well defined than, for example, bladder, urethral or perineal pain and is less clearly related to the micturition cycle or to bowel function and is not localised to any single pelvic organ. (NEW)

1.7 Genito-Urinary Pain Syndromes and Symptom Syndromes Suggestive of LUTD

Syndromes describe constellations, or varying combinations of symptoms, but cannot be used for precise diagnosis. The use of the word syndrome can only be justified if there is at least one other symptom in addition to the symptom used to describe the syndrome. In scientific communications the incidence of individual symptoms within the syndrome should be stated, in addition to the number of individuals with the syndrome.

The syndromes described are functional abnormalities for which a precise cause has not been defined. It is presumed that routine

---

[8]The terms "strangury," "bladder spasm," and "dysuria" are difficult to define and of uncertain meaning and should not be used in relation to lower urinary tract dysfunction, unless a precise meaning is stated. Dysuria literally means "abnormal urination," and is used correctly in some European countries; however, it is often used to describe the stinging/burning sensation characteristic of urinary infection. It is suggested that these descriptive words should not be used in future.

assessment (history taking, physical examination, and other appropriate investigations) has excluded obvious local pathologies, such as those that are infective, neoplastic, metabolic or hormonal in nature.

1.7.1 Genito-urinary pain syndromes are all chronic in their nature. Pain is the major complaint but concomitant complaints are of lower urinary tract, bowel, sexual or gynaecological nature.

- *Painful bladder syndrome* is the complaint of suprapubic pain related to bladder filling, accompanied by other symptoms such as increased daytime and night-time frequency, in the absence of proven urinary infection or other obvious pathology. (NEW)[9]
- *Urethral pain syndrome* is the occurrence of recurrent episodic urethral pain usually on voiding, with daytime frequency and nocturia, in the absence of proven infection or other obvious pathology. (NEW)
- *Vulval pain syndrome* is the occurrence of persistent or recurrent episodic vulval pain, which is either related to the micturition cycle or associated with symptoms suggestive of urinary tract or sexual dysfunction. There is no proven infection or other obvious pathology. (NEW)[10]
- *Vaginal pain syndrome* is the occurrence of persistent or recurrent episodic vaginal pain which is associated with symptoms suggestive of urinary tract or sexual dysfunction. There is no proven vaginal infection or other obvious pathology.
- *Scrotal pain syndrome* is the occurrence of persistent or recurrent episodic scrotal pain

which is associated with symptoms suggestive of urinary tract or sexual dysfunction. There is no proven epididimo-orchitis or other obvious pathology.

- *Perineal pain syndrome* is the occurrence of persistent or recurrent episodic perineal pain, which is either related to the micturition cycle or associated with symptoms suggestive of urinary tract or sexual dysfunction. There is no proven infection or other obvious pathology. (NEW)[11]
- *Pelvic pain syndrome* is the occurrence of persistent or recurrent episodic pelvic pain associated with symptoms suggestive of lower urinary tract, sexual, bowel or gynaecological dysfunction. There is no proven infection or other obvious pathology. (NEW)

1.7.2. Symptom syndromes suggestive of lower urinary tract dysfunction

In clinical practice, empirical diagnoses are often used as the basis for initial management after assessing the individual's lower urinary tract symptoms, physical findings and the results of urinalysis and other indicated investigations.

- *Urgency,* with or without urge incontinence, usually with frequency and nocturia, can be described as the *overactive bladder syndrome, urge syndrome or urgency-frequency syndrome.* (NEW)

These symptom combinations are suggestive of urodynamically demonstrable detrusor overactivity, but can be due to other forms of urethro-vesical dysfunction. These terms can be used if there is no proven infection or other obvious pathology.

- *Lower urinary tract symptoms suggestive of bladder outlet obstruction* is a term used when a man complains predominately of voiding symptoms in the absence of infection or obvious pathology

---

[9]The ICS believes this to be a preferable term to "interstitial cystitis." Interstitial cystitis is a specific diagnosis and requires confirmation by typical cystoscopic and histological features. In the investigation of bladder pain it may be necessary to exclude conditions such as carcinoma in situ and endometriosis.

[10]The ICS suggests that the term vulvodynia (vulva—pain) should not be used, as it leads to confusion between single symptom and a syndrome.

[11]The ICS suggests that in men, the term prostatodynia (prostate—pain) should not be used as it leads to confusion between a single symptom and a syndrome.

other than possible causes of outlet obstruction. (NEW)[12]

2. SIGNS SUGGESTIVE OF LOWER URINARY TRACT DYSFUNCTION (LUTD)

2.1 Measuring the Frequency, Severity and Impact of Lower Urinary Tract Symptoms

Asking the patient to record micturitions and symptoms[13] for a period of days provides invaluable information. The recording of micturition events can be in three main forms:

- *Micturition time chart:* this records only the times of micturitions, day and night, for at least 24 hours. (NEW)
- *Frequency volume chart (FVC):* this records the volumes voided as well as the time of each micturition, day and night, for at least 24 hours. (CHANGED)
- *Bladder diary:* this records the times of micturitions and voided volumes, incontinence episodes, pad usage and other information such as fluid intake, the degree of urgency and the degree of incontinence. (NEW)[14]

The following measurements can be abstracted from frequency volume charts and bladder diaries:

- *Daytime frequency* is the number of voids recorded during waking hours and includes the last void before sleep and the first void after waking and rising in the morning. (NEW)
- *Nocturia* is the number of voids recorded during a night's sleep: each void is preceded and followed by sleep. (NEW)
- *24-hour frequency* is the total number of daytime voids and episodes of nocturia during a specified 24-hour period. (NEW)
- *24-hour production* is measured by collecting all urine for 24 hours. (NEW)

This is usually commenced *after* the first void produced after rising in the morning, and is completed by including the first void on rising the following morning.

- *Polyuria* is defined as the measured production of more than 2.8 litres of urine in 24 hours in adults. It may be useful to look at output over shorter time frames [van Kerrebroeck et al., 2002]. (NEW)[15]
- *Nocturnal urine volume* is defined as the total volume of urine passed between the time the individual goes to bed with the intention of sleeping and the time of waking with the intention of rising. (NEW) Therefore, it excludes the last void before going to bed but includes the first void after rising in the morning.
- *Nocturnal polyuria* is present when an increased proportion of the 24-hour output occurs at night (normally during the 8 hours whilst the patient is in bed. (NEW) The night-time urine output excludes the last void before sleep but includes the first void of the morning.[16]
- *Maximum voided volume* is the largest volume of urine voided during a single micturition and is determined either from the frequency/volume chart or bladder diary. (NEW)

---

[12]In women voiding symptoms are usually thought to suggest detrusor underactivity rather than bladder outlet obstruction.

[13]Validated questionnaires are useful for recording symptoms, their frequency, severity and bother, and the impact of LUTS on QoL The instrument used should be specified.

[14]It it useful to ask the individual to make an estimate of liquid intake. This may be done precisely by measuring the volume of each drink or crudely by asking how many drinks are taken in a 24-hour period. If the individual eats significant quantities of water containing foods (vegetables, fruits, salads) then an appreciable effect on urine production will result. The time that diuretic therapy is taken should be marked on a chart or diary.

---

[15]The causes of polyuria are various and reviewed elsewhere but include habitual excess fluid intake. The figure of 2.8 is based on a 70-kg person voiding >40 mL/kg.

[16]The normal range of nocturnal urine production differs with age and the normal ranges remain to be defined. Therefore, nocturnal polyuria is present when greater than 20% (young adults) to 33% (over 65 years) is produced at night. Hence the precise definition is dependant on age.

The maximum, mean and minimum voided volumes over the period of recording may be stated.[17]

2.2 Physical examination is essential in the assessment of all patients with lower urinary tract dysfunction. It should include abdominal, pelvic, perineal and a focussed neurological examination. For patients with possible neurogenic lower urinary tract dysfunction, a more extensive neurological examination is needed.

2.2.1 Abdominal: the bladder may be felt by abdominal palpation or by suprapubic percussion. Pressure suprapubically or during bimanual vaginal examination may induce a desire to pass urine.

2.2.2 Perineal/genital inspection allows the description of the skin, for example the presence of atrophy or excoriation, any abnormal anatomical features and the observation of incontinence.

- *Urinary incontinence (the sign)* is defined as urine leakage seen during examination: this may be urethral or extraurethral.
- *Stress urinary incontinence* is the observation of involuntary leakage from the urethra, synchronous with exertion/effort, or sneezing or coughing. (CHANGED)[18]

Stress Leakage is presumed to be due to raised abdominal pressure.

- *Extra-urethral incontinence* is defined as the observation of urine leakage through channels other than the urethra. (ORIGINAL)
- *Uncategorised incontinence* is the observation of involuntary leakage that cannot be classified into one of the above categories on the basis of signs and symptoms. (NEW)

2.2.3 Vaginal examination allows the description of observed and palpable anatomical abnormalities and the assessment of pelvic floor muscle function, as described in the ICS report on Pelvic Organ Prolapse. The definitions given are simplified versions of the definitions in that report. [Bump et al., 1996]

- *Pelvic organ prolapse* is defined as the descent of one or more of: the anterior vaginal wall, the posterior vaginal wall, and the apex of the vagina (cervix/uterus) or vault (cuff) after hysterectomy. Absence of prolapse is defined as stage 0 support; prolapse can be staged from stage I to stage IV. (NEW)

  Pelvic organ prolapse can occur in association with urinary incontinence and other lower urinary tract dysfunction and may on occasion mask incontinence.
- *Anterior vaginal wall prolapse* is defined as descent of the anterior vagina so that the urethrovesical junction (a point 3 cm proximal to the external urinary meatus) or any anterior point proximal to this is less than 3 cm above the plane of the hymen. (CHANGED)
- *Prolapse of the apical segment of the vagina* is defined as any descent of the vaginal cuff scar (after hysterectomy) or cervix, below a point which is 2 cm less than the total vaginal length above the plane of the hymen. (CHANGED)
- *Posterior vaginal wall prolapse* is defined as any descent of the posterior vaginal wall so that a midline point on the posterior vaginal wall 3 cm above the level of the hymen or any posterior point proximal to this, is less than 3 cm above the plane of the hymen. (CHANGED)

---

[17]The term "functional bladder capacity" is no longer recommended as "voided volume" is a clearer and less confusing term, particularly if qualified, e.g., "maximum voided volume." If the term bladder capacity is used, in any situation, it implies that this has been measured some way, if only by abdominal ultrasound. In adults, voided volumes vary considerably. In children, the "expected volume" may be calculated from the formula [30 + (age in years × 30) in mL]. Assuming no residual urine this will be equal to the "expected bladder capacity."

[18]Coughing may induce a detrusor contraction, hence the sign of stress incontinence is only a reliable indication of urodynamic stress incontinence when leakage occurs synchronously with the first proper cough and stops at the end of that cough.

2.2.4 Pelvic floor muscle function can be qualitatively defined by the tone at rest and the strength of a voluntary or reflex contraction as strong, weak or absent or by a validated grading system (e.g. Oxford 1–5). A pelvic muscle contraction may be assessed by visual inspection, palpation, electromyography or perineometry. Factors to be assessed include strength, duration, displacement, and repeatability.

2.2.5 Rectal examination allows the description of observed and palpable anatomical abnormalities and is the easiest method of assessing pelvic floor muscle function in children and men. In addition, rectal examination is essential in children with urinary incontinence to rule out faecal impaction.

- *Pelvic floor muscle function* can be qualitatively defined, during rectal examination, by the tone at rest and the strength of a voluntary contraction, as strong, weak or absent. (NEW)

2.3 Pad testing may be used to quantify the amount of urine lost during incontinence episodes, and methods range from a short provocative test to a 24-hour pad test.

3. URODYNAMIC OBSERVATIONS AND CONDITIONS

3.1 Urodynamic Techniques

There are two principal methods of urodynamic investigation:

- *Conventional urodynamic studies* normally take place in the urodynamic laboratory and usually involve artificial bladder filling. (NEW)
- *Artificial bladder filling* is defined as filling the bladder, via a catheter, with a specified liquid at a specified rate. (NEW)
- *Ambulatory urodynamic studies* are defined as a functional test of the lower urinary tract, utilising natural filling, and reproducing the subject's every day activities.[19]
  - *Natural filling* means that the bladder is filled by the production of urine rather than by an artificial medium.

Both filling cystometry and pressure flow studies of voiding require the following measurements:

- *Intravesical pressure* is the pressure within the bladder. (ORIGINAL)
- *Abdominal pressure* is taken to be the pressure surrounding the bladder. In current practice it is estimated from rectal, vaginal or, less commonly from extraperitoneal pressure or a bowel stoma. The simultaneous measurement of abdominal pressure is essential for the interpretation of the intravesical pressure trace. (ORIGINAL)
- *Detrusor pressure* is that component of intravesical pressure that is created by forces in the bladder wall (passive and active). It is estimated by subtracting abdominal pressure from intravesical pressure. (ORIGINAL)

3.2 Filling Cystometry

The word "cystometry" is commonly used to describe the urodynamic investigation of the filling phase of the micturition cycle. To eliminate confusion the following definitions are proposed.

- *Filling cystometry* is the method by which the pressure/volume relationship of the bladder is measured during bladder filling. (ORIGINAL)

The filling phase starts when filling commences and ends when the patient and urodynamicist decide that "permission to void" has been given.[20]

---

[19]The term Ambulatory Urodynamics is used to indicate that monitoring usually takes place outside the urodynamic laboratory, rather than the subject's mobility using natural filling.

[20]The ICS no longer wishes to divide filling rates into slow, medium and fast. In practice almost all investigations are performed using medium filling rates which have a wide range. It may be more important during investigations to consider whether or not the filling rate used during conventional urodynamic studies can be considered physiological.

Bladder and urethral function, during filling, need to be defined separately.

The rate at which the bladder is filled is divided into:

- *Physiological filling rate* is defined as a filling rate less than the predicted maximum - predicted maximum body weight in kg divided by 4, expressed as mL/mm (17) (CHANGED)
- *Non-physiological filling rate* is defined as a filling rate greater than the predicted maximum filling rate minus predicted maximum body weight in kg divided by 4 expressed as mL/mm [Klevmark, 1999]. (CHANGED)

Bladder storage function should be described according to bladder sensation, detrusor activity, bladder compliance and bladder capacity.[21]

3.2.1 Bladder sensation during filling cystometry

- *Normal bladder sensation* can be judged by three defined points noted during filling cystometry and evaluated in relation to the bladder volume at that moment and in relation to the patient's symptomatic complaints.
- *First sensation of bladder filling* is the feeling the patient has, during filling cystometry, when he/she first becomes aware of the bladder filling. (NEW)
- *First desire to void* is defined as the feeling, during filling cystometry, that would lead the patient to pass urine at the next convenient moment, but voiding can be delayed if necessary. (CHANGED)
- *Strong desire to void* is defined, during filling cystometry, as a persistent desire to void without the fear of leakage. (ORIGINAL)
- *Increased bladder sensation* is defined, during filling cystometry, as an early first sensation of bladder filling (or an early desire to void) and/or an early strong desire to

void, which occurs at low bladder volume and which persists (NEW)[22]
- *Reduced bladder sensation* is defined, during filling cystometry, as diminished sensation throughout bladder filling. (NEW)
- *Absent bladder sensation* means that, during filling cystometry, the individual has no bladder sensation. (NEW)
- *Non-specific bladder sensations,* during filling cystometry, may make the individual aware of bladder filling, for example, abdominal fullness or vegetative symptoms. (NEW)
- *Bladder pain,* during filling cystometry, is a self-explanatory term and is an abnormal finding. (NEW)
- *Urgency,* during filling cystometry, is a sudden compelling desire to void. (NEW)[23]
- *The vesical/urethral sensory threshold* is defined as the least current which consistently produces a sensation perceived by the subject during stimulation at the site under investigation [Andersen et al., 1992]. (ORIGINAL)

3.2.2 Detrusor function during filling cystometry

In everyday life the individual attempts to inhibit detrusor activity until he or she is in a position to void. Therefore, when the aims of the filling study have been achieved, and when the patient has a desire to void, normally the "permission to void" is given (see Filling Cystometry). That moment is indicated on the urodynamic trace and all detrusor activity before this "permission" is defined as "involuntary detrusor activity."

- **Normal detrusor function:** allows bladder filling with little or no change in pressure.

---

[21]Whilst bladder sensation is assessed during filling cystometry the assumption that it is sensation from the bladder alone, without urethral or pelvic components may be false.

[22]The assessment of the subject's bladder sensation is subjective and it is not, for example, possible to quantify "low bladder volume" in the definition of "increased bladder sensation."

[23]The ICS no longer recommends the terms "motor urgency" and "sensory urgency." These terms are often misused and have little intuitive meaning. Furthermore, it may be simplistic to relate urgency just to the presence or absence of detrusor overactivity when there is usually a concomitant fall in urethral pressure.

No involuntary phasic contractions occur despite provocation. (ORIGINAL)

- **Detrusor overactivity** is a urodynamic observation characterised by involuntary detrusor contractions during the filling phase which may be spontaneous or provoked. (CHANGED)[24]

There are certain patterns of detrusor overactivity:

- *Phasic detrusor overactivity* is defined by a characteristic wave form, and may or may not lead to urinary incontinence. (NEW)[25]
- *Terminal detrusor overactivity* is defined as a single involuntary detrusor contraction occurring at cystometric capacity, which cannot be suppressed, and results in incontinence usually resulting in bladder emptying (voiding). (NEW)[26]
- *Detrusor overactivity incontinence* is incontinence due to an involuntary detrusor contraction. (NEW)

In a patient with normal sensation urgency is likely to be experienced just before the leakage episode.[27]

Detrusor overactivity may also be qualified, when possible, according to cause; for example:

- *Neurogenic detrusor overactivity* when there is a relevant neurological condition. This term replaces the term "detrusor hyperreflexia." (NEW)

Idiopathic detrusor overactivity when there is no defined cause. This term replaces "detrusor instability." (NEW) [28]

In clinical and research practice, the extent of neurological examination/investigation varies. It is likely that the proportion of neurogenic-to-idiopathic detrusor overactivity will increase if a more complete neurological assessment is carried out.

Other patterns of detrusor overactivity are seen, for example, the combination of phasic and terminal detrusor overactivity, and the sustained high-pressure detrusor contractions seen in spinal cord injury patients when attempted voiding occurs against a dyssynergic sphincter.

- *Provocative manoeuvres* are defined as techniques used during urodynamics in an effort to provoke detrusor overactivity, for example, rapid filling, use of cooled or acid medium, postural changes and hand washing. (NEW)

3.2.3. Bladder compliance during filling cystometry

- *Bladder compliance* describes the relationship between change in bladder volume and change in detrusor pressure. (CHANGED)[29]

Compliance is calculated by dividing the volume change (ΔV) by the change in detrusor pressure (Δpdet) during that change in bladder volume ($C = V. \Delta$pdet). It is expressed in mL/cm H_2O.

A variety of means of calculating bladder compliance has been described. The ICS rec-

---

[24]There is no lower limit for the amplitude of an involuntary detrusor contraction but confident interpretation of low-pressure waves (amplitude smaller than 5 cm H_2O) depends on "high-quality" urodynamic technique. The phrase "which the patient cannot completely suppress" has been deleted from the old definition.

[25]Phasic detrusor contractions are not always accompanied by any sensation, or may be interpreted as a first sensation of bladder filling, or as a normal desire to void.

[26]"Terminal detrusor overactivity" is a new ICS term: it is typically associated with reduced bladder sensation, for example in the elderly stroke patient when urgency may be felt as the voiding contraction occurs. However, in complete spinal cord injury patients there may be no sensation whatsoever.

[27]The ICS recommends that the terms "motor urge incontinence" and "reflex incontinence" should no longer be used as they have no intuitive meaning and are often misused.

---

[28]The terms "detrusor instability" and "detrusor hyperreflexia" were both used as generic terms, in the English speaking world and Scandinavia, prior to the first ICS report in 1976. As a compromise they were allocated to idiopathic and neurogenic overactivity, respectively. As there is no real logic or intuitive meaning to the terms, the ICS believes they should be abandoned.

[29]The observation of reduced bladder compliance during conventional filling cystometry is often related to relatively fast bladder filling; the incidence of reduced compliance is markedly lower if the bladder is filled at physiological rates, as in ambulatory urodynamics.

ommends that two standard points should be used for compliance calculations: the investigator may wish to define additional points. The standards points are:

1. the detrusor pressure at the start of bladder filling and the corresponding bladder volume (usually zero), and
2. the detrusor pressure (and corresponding bladder volume) at cystometric capacity or immediately before the start of any detrusor contraction that causes significant leakage (and therefore causes the bladder volume to decrease, affecting compliance calculation). Both points are measured excluding any detrusor contraction.

3.2.4. Bladder capacity: during filling cystometry

* *Cystometric capacity* is the bladder volume at the end of the filling cystometrogram, when "permission to void" is usually given. The end point should be specified, for example, if filling is stopped when the patient has a normal desire to void. The cystometric capacity is the volume voided together with any residual urine. (CHANGED)[30]
* *Maximum cystometric capacity,* in patients with normal sensation, is the volume at which the patient feels he/she can no longer delay micturition (has a strong desire to void). (ORIGINAL)
* *Maximum anaesthetic bladder capacity* is the volume to which the bladder can be filled under deep general or spinal anaesthetic and should be qualified according to the type of anaesthesia used, the speed of filling, the length of time of filling, and

the pressure at which the bladder is filled. (CHANGED)

3.2.5 Urethral function during filling cystometry

The urethral closure mechanism during storage may be competent or incompetent.

* *Normal urethral closure mechanism* maintains a positive urethral closure pressure during bladder filling even in the presence of increased abdominal pressure, although it may be overcome by detrusor overactivity. (CHANGED)
* *Incompetent urethral closure mechanism* is defined as one which allows leakage of urine in the absence of a detrusor contraction. (ORIGINAL)
* *Urethral relaxation incontinence* is defined as leakage due to urethral relaxation in the absence of raised abdominal pressure or detrusor overactivity. (NEW)[31]
* *Urodynamic stress incontinence* is noted during filling cystometry, and is defined as the involuntary leakage of urine during increased abdominal pressure, in the absence of a detrusor contraction. (CHANGED)

Urodynamic stress incontinence is now the preferred term to "genuine stress incontinence."[32]

3.2.6. Assessment of urethral function during filling cystometry

* *Urethral pressure measurement*
  – *Urethral pressure* is defined as the fluid pressure needed to just open a closed urethra. (ORIGINAL)

---

[30]In certain types of dysfunction, the cystometric capacity cannot be defined in the same terms. In the absence of sensation the cystometric capacity is the volume at which the clinician decides to terminate filling. The reason(s) for terminating filling should be defined, e.g., high detrusor filling pressure, large infused volume or pain. If there is uncontrollable voiding, it is the volume at which this begins. In the presence of sphincter incompetence the cystometric capacity may be significantly increased by occlusion of the urethra, e.g., by Foley catheter.

[31]Fluctuations in urethral pressure have been defined as the "unstable urethra." However, the significance of the fluctuations and the term itself lack clarity and the term is not recommended by the ICS. If symptoms are seen in association with a decrease in urethral pressure a full description should be given.

[32]In patients with stress incontinence, there is a spectrum of urethral characteristics ranging from a highly mobile urethra with good intrinsic function to an immobile urethra with poor intrinsic function. Any delineation into categories such as "urethral hypermobility" and "intrinsic sphincter deficiency"' may be simplistic and arbitrary, and requires further research.

– The *urethral pressure profile* is a graph indicating the intraluminal pressure along the length of the urethra. (ORIGINAL)

– The *urethral closure pressure profile* is given by the subtraction of intravesical pressure from urethral pressure. (ORIGINAL)

– *Maximum urethral pressure* is the maximum pressure of the measured profile. (ORIGINAL)

– *Maximum urethral closure pressure (MUCP)* is the maximum difference between the urethral pressure and the intravesical pressure. (ORIGINAL)

– *Functional profile length* is the length of the urethra along which the urethral pressure exceeds intravesical pressure in women.

– *Pressure "transmission" ratio* is the increment in urethral pressure on stress as a percentage of the simultaneously recorded increment in intravesical pressure.

• *Abdominal leak point pressure* is the intravesical pressure at which urine leakage occurs due to increased abdominal pressure in the absence of a detrusor contraction. (NEW)[33]

• *Detrusor leak point pressure* is defined as the lowest detrusor pressure at which urine leakage occurs in the absence of either a detrusor contraction or increased abdominal pressure. (NEW)[34]

3.3 Pressure Flow Studies

Voiding is described in terms of detrusor and urethral function and assessed by measuring urine flow rate and voiding pressures.

• *Pressure flow studies* of voiding are the method by which the relationship between pressure in the bladder and urine flow rate is measured during bladder emptying. (ORIGINAL)

The voiding phase starts when "permission to void" is given or when uncontrollable voiding begins, and ends when the patient considers voiding has finished.

3.3.1 Measurement of urine flow

Urine flow is defined either as continuous, that is without interruption, or as intermittent, when an individual states that the flow stops and starts during a single visit to the bathroom in order to void. The continuous flow curve is defined as a smooth arc-shaped curve or fluctuating when there are multiple peaks during a period of continuous urine flow.[35]

• *Flow rate* is defined as the volume of fluid expelled via the urethra per unit time. It is expressed in mL/s. (ORIGINAL)

• *Voided volume* is the total volume expelled via the urethra. (ORIGINAL)

• *Maximum flow rate* is the maximum measured value of the flow rate after correction for artefacts. (CHANGED)

• *Voiding time* is total duration of micturition, including interruptions. When voiding is completed without interruption, voiding time is equal to flow time. (ORIGINAL)

• *Flow time* is the time over which measurable flow actually occurs. (ORIGINAL)

• *Average flow rate* is voided volume divided by flow time. The average flow should be interpreted with caution if flow

---

[33]The leak pressure point should be qualified according to the site of pressure measurement (rectal, vaginal or intravesical) and the method by which pressure is generated (cough or Valsalva). Leak point pressures maybe calculated in three ways from the three different baseline values which are in common use: zero (the true zero of intravesical pressure), the value of pves measured at zero bladder volume, or the value of pves immediately before the cough or Valsalva (usually at 200 or 300 mL bladder capacity). The baseline used and the baseline pressures should be specified.

[34]Detrusor leak point pressure has been used most frequently to predict upper tract problems in neurological patients with reduced bladder compliance. ICS has defined it "in the absence of a detrusor contraction" although others will measure DLPP during involuntary detrusor contractions.

---

[35]The precise shape of the flow curve is decided by detrusor contractility, the presence of any abdominal straining and the bladder outlet (11).

is interrupted or there is a terminal dribble. (CHANGED)

- *Time to maximum flow* is the elapsed time from onset of flow to maximum flow. (ORIGINAL)

3.3.2. Pressure measurements during pressure flow studies (PFS)

The following measurements are applicable to each of the pressure curves: intravesical, abdominal and detrusor pressure.

- *Premicturition pressure* is the pressure recorded immediately before the initial iso-volumetric contraction. (ORIGINAL)
- *Opening pressure* is the pressure recorded at the onset of urine flow (consider time delay). (ORIGINAL)
- *Opening time* is the elapsed time from initial rise in detrusor pressure to onset of flow. (ORIGINAL)

This is the initial isovolumetric contraction period of micturition. Flow measurement delay should be taken into account when measuring opening time.

- *Maximum pressure* is the maximum value of the measured pressure. (ORIGINAL)
- *Pressure at maximum flow* is the lowest pressure recorded at maximum measured flow rate. (ORIGINAL)
- *Closing pressure* is the pressure measured at the end of measured flow. (ORIGINAL)
- *Minimum voiding pressure* is the minimum pressure during measurable flow. This is not necessarily equal to either the opening or closing pressures.
- *Flow delay* is the time delay between a change in bladder pressure and the corresponding change in measured flow rate.

3.3.3. Detrusor function during voiding

- *Normal detrusor function*

Normal voiding is achieved by a voluntarily initiated continuous detrusor contraction that leads to complete bladder emptying within a normal time span, and in the absence of obstruction. For a given detrusor contraction, the magnitude of the recorded pressure rise will depend on the degree of outlet resistance. (ORIGINAL)

- *Abnormal detrusor activity* can be subdivided:
  - *Detrusor underactivity* is defined as a contraction of reduced strength and/or duration, resulting in prolonged bladder emptying and/or a failure to achieve complete bladder emptying within a normal time span. (ORIGINAL)
  - *Acontractile detrusor* is one that cannot be demonstrated to contract during urodynamic studies. (ORIGINAL)[36]
  - *Post void residual (PVR)* is defined as the volume of urine left in the bladder at the end of micturition. (ORIGINAL)[37]

3.3.4. Urethral function during voiding

During voiding, urethral function may be:
Normal urethra function is defined as urethra that opens, and is continuously relaxed to allow the bladder to be emptied at a normal pressure. (CHANGED)
Abnormal urethra function may be due to either obstruction to urethral overactivity, or a urethra that cannot open due to anatomic abnormality, such as an enlarged prostate or a urethral stricture.

- *Bladder outlet obstruction* is the generic term for obstruction during voiding and is characterised by increased detrusor pressure and reduced urine flow rate. It is usually diagnosed by studying the synchronous values of flow rate and detrusor pressure. (CHANGED)[38]

---

[36]A normal detrusor contraction will be recorded as: a high pressure if there is high outlet resistance, normal pressure if there is normal outlet resistance, or low pressure if urethral resistance is low.

[37]If after repeated free flowmetry no residual urine is demonstrated, then the finding of a residual urine during urodynamic studies should be considered an artifact, due to the circumstances of the test.

[38]Bladder outlet obstruction has been defined for men but as yet, not adequately in women and children.

- *Dysfunctional voiding* is defined as an intermittent and/or fluctuating flow rate due to involuntary intermittent contractions of the peri-urethral striated muscle during voiding, in neurologically normal individuals. (CHANGED)[39]
- *Detrusor sphincter dyssynergia* is defined as a detrusor contraction concurrent with an involuntary contraction of the urethral and/or periurethral striated muscle. Occasionally flow may be prevented altogether. (ORIGINAL)[40]
- *Non-relaxing urethral sphincter obstruction* usually occurs in individuals with a neurological lesion and is characterised by a non-relaxing, obstructing urethra resulting in reduced urine flow. (NEW)[41]

4. CONDITIONS

- *Acute retention of urine* is defined as a painful, palpable or percussable bladder, when the patient is unable to pass any urine. (NEW)[42]

---

[39]Although dysfunctional voiding is not a very specific term it is preferred to terms such as "non-neurogenic neurogenic bladder." Other terms such as "idiopathic detrusor sphincter dyssynergia," or "sphincter overactivity voiding dysfunction" may be preferable. However, the term dysfunctional voiding is very well established. The condition occurs most frequently in children. Whilst it is felt that pelvic floor contractions are responsible, it is possible that the intra-urethral striated muscle may be important.

[40]Detrusor sphincter dyssynergia typically occurs in patients with a supra-sacral lesion, for example after high spinal cord injury, and is uncommon in lesions of the lower cord. Although the intraurethral and periurethral striated muscles are usually held responsible, the smooth muscle of the bladder neck or urethra may also be responsible.

[41]Non-relaxing sphincter obstruction is found in sacral and infra-sacral lesions such as meningomyelocoele, and after radical pelvic surgery. In addition there is often urodynamic stress incontinence during bladder filling. This term replaces "isolated distal sphincter obstruction."

[42]Although acute retention is usually thought of as painful, in certain circumstances pain may not be a presenting feature, for example when due to prolapsed intervertebral disc, post partum, or after regional anaesthesia such as an epidural anaesthetic. The retention volume should be significantly greater than the expected normal bladder capacity. In patients after surgery, due to bandaging of the lower abdomen or abdominal wall pain, it may be difficult to detect a painful, palpable or percussable bladder.

- *Chronic retention of urine* is defined as a non-painful bladder, which remains palpable or percussable after the patient has passed urine. Such patients may be incontinent. (NEW)[43]
- *Benign prostatic obstruction* is a form of *bladder outlet obstruction* and may be diagnosed when the cause of outlet obstruction is known to be benign prostatic enlargement, due to histologic benign prostatic hyperplasia. (NEW)
- *Benign prostatic hyperplasia* is a term used (and reserved for) the typical histological pattern which defines the disease. (NEW)
- *Benign prostatic enlargement* is defined as prostatic enlargement due to histologic benign prostatic hyperplasia. The term "prostatic enlargement" should be used in the absence of prostatic histology (NEW)

5. TREATMENT

The following definitions were published in the 7th ICS report on Lower Urinary Tract Rehabilitation Techniques (3) and remain in their original form.

5.1 Lower urinary tract rehabilitation is defined as non-surgical, non-pharmacological treatment for lower urinary tract function and includes:

- *Pelvic floor training,* defined as repetitive selective voluntary contraction and relaxation of specific pelvic floor muscles.
- *Biofeedback* is the technique by which information about a normally unconscious physiological process is presented to the patient and/or the therapist as a visual, auditory or tactile signal.

---

[43]The ICS no longer recommends the term "overflow incontinence." This term is considered confusing and lacking a convincing definition. If used, a precise definition and any associated pathophysiology, such as reduced urethral function, or detrusor overactivity/low bladder compliance, should be stated. The term chronic retention excludes transient voiding difficulty, for example after surgery for stress incontinence, and implies a significant residual urine; a minimum figure of 300 mL has been previously mentioned.

- *Behavioural modification* is defined as the analysis and alteration of the relationship between the patient's symptoms and his or her environment for the treatment of maladaptive voiding patterns.

This may be achieved by modification of the behaviour and/or environment of the patient.

5.2 Electrical stimulation is the application of electrical current to stimulate the pelvic viscera or their nerve supply.

The aim of electrical stimulation may be to induce directly a therapeutic response or to modulate lower urinary tract, bowel or sexual dysfunction.

5.3 Catheterisation is a technique for bladder emptying employing a catheter to drain the bladder or a urinary reservoir.

5.3.1 Intermittent (in/out) catheterisation is defined as drainage or aspiration of the bladder or a urinary reservoir with subsequent removal of the catheter.

The following types of intermittent catheterisation are defined:

- *Intermittent self-catheterisation* is performed by the patient himself/herself
- *Intermittent catheterisation* is performed by an attendant (e.g., doctor, nurse or relative)
- *Clean intermittent catheterisation:* use of a clean technique. This implies ordinary washing techniques and use of disposable or cleansed reusable catheters.
- *Aseptic intermittent catheterisation:* use of a sterile technique. This implies genital disinfection and the use of sterile catheters and instruments/gloves.

5.3.2 Indwelling catheterisation: an indwelling catheter remains in the bladder, urinary reservoir or urinary conduit for a period of time longer than one emptying.

5.4 Bladder Reflex Triggering comprises various manoeuvres performed by the patient or the therapist in order to elicit reflex detrusor contraction by exteroceptive stimuli.

The most commonly used manoeuvres are suprapubic tapping, thigh scratching and anal/rectal manipulation.

5.5 Bladder Expression comprises various manoeuvres aimed at increasing intravesical pressure in order to facilitate bladder emptying.

The most commonly used manoeuvres are abdominal straining, Valsalva manoeuvre and Credé manoeuvre.

ACKNOWLEDGEMENTS

The authors of this report are very grateful to Vicky Rees, Administrator of the ICS, for her typing and editing of numerous drafts of this document.

ADDENDUM

Formation of the ICS Terminology Committee

The terminology committee was announced at the ICS meeting in Denver 1999. Expressions of interest were invited from those who wished to be active members of the committee, and these people were asked to comment in detail on the preliminary draft (the discussion paper published in *Neurourology and Urodynamics*). The nine authors replied with a detailed critique by 1st April 2000 and constitute the committee: Paul Abrams, Linda Cardozo, Magnus Fall, Derek Griffiths, Peter Rosier, Ulf Ulmsten, Philip van Kerrebroeck, Arne Victor, and Alan Wein.

We thank other individuals who later offered their written comments: Jens Thorup Andersen, Walter Artibani, Jerry Blaivas, Linda Brubaker, Rick Bump, Emmanuel Chartier-Kastler, Grace Dorey, Clare Fowler, Kelm Hjalmas, Gordon Hosker, Vik Khullar, Guus Kramer, Gunnar Lose, Joseph Macaluso, Anders Mattiasson, Richard Millard, Rien Nijman, Arwin Ridder, Werner Schäfer, David Vodusek, and Jean Jacques Wyndaele.

A half-day workshop was held at the ICS Annual Meeting in Tampere (August 2000) and a two-day meeting in London, January 2001, which produced draft 5 of the report which was then placed on the ICS website (*www.icsoffice.org*). Discussions on draft 6 took place at the ICS meeting in Korea, September 2001, draft 7 then remained on the ICS website until final submission to journals in November 2001.

REFERENCES

Abrams P (Chair), Blaivas JG, Stanton S, Andersen T. 1988. ICS standardisation of terminology of lower urinary tract function. Neurourol Urodyn 7:403–26.

Abrams P, Blaivas JG, Stanton SL, Andersen J. 1992. ICS 6th report on the standardisation of terminology of lower urinary tract function. Neurourol Urodyn 11:593–603.

Andersen JT, Blaivas JG, Cardozo L, Thüroff J. 1992. ICS 7th report on the standardisation of terminology of lower urinary tract function: lower urinary tract rehabilitation techniques. Neurourol Urodyn 11:593–603.

Bump RC, Mattiasson A, Bo K, Brubaker LP, DeLancey JOL, Klarskov P, Shull BL, Smith ARB. 1996. The standardisation of terminology of female pelvic organ prolapse and pelvic floor dysfunction. Am J Obstet Gynecol 175:10–1.

Fonda D, Resnick NM, Colling J, Burgio K, Ouslander JG, Norton C, Ekelund P, Versi K, Mattiasson A. 1998. Outcome measures for research of lower urinary tract dysfunction in frail and older people. Neurourol Urodyn 17:273–81.

Griffiths D, Höfner K, van Mastrigt R, Rollema HJ, Spangberg A, Gleason D. 1997. ICS report on the standardisation of terminology of lower urinary tract function: pressure-flow studies of voiding, urethral resistance and urethral obstruction. Neurourol Urodyn 16:1–18.

International Classification of Functioning, Disability and Health. ICIDH-2 website http://www.who.int/icidh.

Klevmark B. 1999. Natural pressure: volume curves and conventional cystometry. Scand J Urol Nephrol Suppl 201:1–4.

Lose G, Fantl JA, Victor A, Walter S, Wells TL, Wyman J, Mattiasson A. 1998. Outcome measures for research in adult women with symptoms of lower urinary tract dysfunction. Neurourol Urodyn 17:255–62.

Lose G, Griffiths D, Hosker G, Kulseng-Hanssen S, Perucchini D, Schäfer W, Thind P, Versi E. Standardisation of urethral pressure measurement: report from the standardisation sub-committee of the International Continence Society. Neurourol Urodyn (In press).

Mattiasson A, Djurhuus JC, Fonda D, Lose G, Nordling J, Stöhrer M. 1998. Standardisation of outcome studies in patients with lower urinary dysfunction: a report on general principles from the standardisation committee of the International Continence Society. Neurourol Urodyn 17:249–53.

Nordling J, Abrams P, Ameda K, Andersen JT, Donovan J, Griffiths D, Kobsyashi S, Koyanagi T, Schäfer W, Yalla S, Mattiasson A. 1998. Outcome measures for research in treatment of adult males with symptoms of lower urinary tract dysfunction. Neurourol Urodyn 17:263–71.

Rowan D, James ED, Kramen AEJL, et al. 1987. Report on urodynamic equipment, technical aspects. J Med Eng Technol 11(2):57–64.

Stöhrer M, Goepel M, Kondo A, Kramer G, Madersbacher H, Millard R, Rossier A, Wyndaele JJ. 1999. ICS report on the standardisation of terminology in neurogenic lower urinary tract dysfunction. Neurourol Urodyn 18:139–58.

Schäfer W, Sterling AM, Liao L, Spangberg A, Pesce F, Zinner NR, van Kerrebroeck P, Abrams P, Mattiasson A. 2002. Good urodynamic practice: report from the standardisation sub-committee of the International Continence Society. Neurourol Urodyn (In press).

van Waalwijk, van Doorn K, Anders K, Khullar V, Kulseng-Hansen S, Pesce F, Robertson A, Rosario D, Schäfer W. 2000. Standardisation of ambulatory urodynamic monitoring: report of the standardisation sub-committee of the International Continence Society for ambulatory urodynamic studies. Neurourol Urodyn 19:113–25.

van Kerrebroeck P, Abrams P, Chaikin D, Donovan J, Fonda D, Jackson S, Jennum P, Johnson T, Lose G, Mattiasson A, Robertson G, Weiss J. 2002. ICS standardisation report on nocturia: report from the standardisation sub-committee of the International Continence Society. Neurourol Urodyn 21:193–99.

wan D, James ED, Kramer AEJI, Sterling AM, Suhel PF. 1987. ICS report on urodynamic equipment technical aspects. J Med Eng Technol 11(2):57–64.

Ostergard's Urogynecology and Pelvic Floor Dysfunction, Fifth Edition. edited by A.E. Bent, et al.
Lippincott Williams & Wilkins, Philadelphia © 2003.

Appendix II

The Standardisation of Terminology in Nocturia: Report from the Standardisation Sub-Committee of the International Continence Society

Philip van Kerrebroeck,[1] Paul Abrams,[2] David Chaikin,[3] Jenny Donovan,[4] David Fonda,[5] Simon Jackson,[6] Poul Jennum,[7] Theodore Johnson,[8] Gunnar Lose,[9] Anders Mattiasson,[10] Gary Robertson,[11] Jeff Weiss[12]

[1]*Chairman of the International Continence Society Standardisation Committee, Department of Urology, University Hospital Maastricht, The Netherlands*
[2]*Bristol Urological Institute, Southmead Hospital, Bristol, United Kingdom*
[3]*Morristown Memorial Hospital, Morristown, New Jersey, and Department of Urology, Weill Medical College of Cornell University, New York, New York*
[4]*Department of Social Medicine, University at Bristol, Bristol, United Kingdom*
[5]*Aged Care Services, Caulfield General Medical Centre, Victoria, Australia*
[6]*Department of Gynaecology, John Radcliffe Hospital, Oxford, United Kingdom*
[7]*Department of Clinical Neurophysiology, University of Copenhagen and Sleep Laboratory, Glostrup, Denmark*
[8]*Rehabilitation Research and Development Center, Atlanta VA Medical Centre, Atlanta, Georgia*
[9]*Department of Obstetrics and Gynaecology, Glostrup County Hospital, University of Copenhagen, Denmark*
[10]*Department of Urology, Lund University Hospital, Lund, Sweden*
[11]*Northwestern University Medical School, Chicago, Illinois*
[12]*Department of Urology, Weill Medical College of Cornell University and The New York Presbyterian Hospital, New York, New York*

1. INTRODUCTION

Nocturia is the complaint that the individual has to wake at night one or more times to void. (International Continence Society Definition from IGS Standardisation of Terminology Report 2002).

Nocturia is a condition that has only recently begun to be recognised as a clinical entity in its own right rather than a symptom of some other disorder, or classed as one of many lower urinary tract symptoms. Studies that have investigated nocturia have varied in their definitions of the condition and its surrounding terminology, and these discrepancies have been highlighted in the literature [Robertson et al., 2000; Weiss & Blaivas, 2000; van Kerrebroeck & Weiss, 1999]. However it is defined, prevalence studies show that nocturia is reported to be a very common condition, affecting particularly older age groups [Chute et al., 1993; Malmsten et al., 1997; Swithinbank et al., 1998].

Four per cent of children aged 7–15 years were reported to experience habitual nocturia [Mattsson, 1994], whereas the prevalence has been reported to be 58% and 66% in women and men of 50–59 years, and 72% and 91% in women and men over 80 years [Middlekoop, 1996]. It is evident that nocturia may not only present to the urologist, but that the gynaecologist, geriatrician, neurologist, sleep expert, endocrinologist and general practitioner will all be consulted by patients with this problem. Each specialty is likely to approach their patients from a different perspective, and it is important that some of the basic terms surrounding nocturia have specific definitions so that each individual physician is referring to the same condition and managing it appropriately.

In order to further the discussion on nocturia and in particular, how it should be defined and investigated, a series of meetings were held to facilitate discussion and to reach consensus on definitions [Mattiasson, 1999]. These discussions were finalised in March 2000, and are presented here as an aid to primary and secondary care clinicians involved in assessing and treating patients who suffer from nocturia, and to aim towards standardisation in future clinical study design.

These are the first recommendations for the diagnosis of nocturia. Most of the terms used are listed in Table A.1, along with their existing or newly agreed definitions. When considering "normal" measurements, an average 70-kg individual who sleeps 8 hours a night is the basis for these values, and ranges are generally considered to be within 2 standard de-

viations of this. It must be noted that, while these guidelines aim to provide help with diagnosis, each physician must be prepared to use his or her clinical judgement in individual cases, as the boundaries of the categories presented are not fixed, and a person's nocturia may have mixed aetiology.

2. CLINICAL ASSESSMENT

The assessment of nocturia can be described by a simple algorithm, which is outlined in Fig. A.1. This considers the possibility that the patient may present to the physician specifically because of nocturia, or may present with another condition, whilst also suffering from nocturia. It is possible that a physician will be able to determine nocturia as one cause of distress if the correct questions are asked, which enables further investigation as to the course of nocturia. Of course, there will be a proportion of the population with nocturia, who are not bothered by their condition and who do not present to a clinician at all. However, by definition, these individuals should still be classified as having nocturia. Initial screen-

TABLE A.1. *Definitions of terms associated with nocturia and derived from the frequency volume chart*

Terms	Definition
Nocturia	Is the number of voids recorded during a night's sleep: each void is preceded and followed by sleep
Nocturnal urine volume	Total volume of urine passed during the night including the first morning void (see definition)[a]
Rate of nocturnal urine production	Nocturnal urine volume/time asleep (i.e., night). Measured in mL/min[a]
Nocturnal polyuria	Nocturnal urine volume > 20–30% of total 24 hour urine volume (age dependent)[a]
24-hour voided volume	Total volume of urine voided during a 24-hour period (1st void to be discarded; 24 hours begins at the time of the next void)
Polyuria	24-hour voided volume in excess of 2800 mL (in 70 kg person, i.e., >40 mL/kg)
Night[b]	The period of time between going to bed with the intention of sleeping and waking with the intention of arising
Night-time frequency[b]	Is the number of voids recorded from the time the individual goes to bed with the intention of going to sleep, to the time the individual wakes with the intention of rising[a]
First morning void	The first void after waking with the intention of rising
Maximum voided volume	The largest single voided volume measured in a 24-hour period[a]

[a]In the new ICS terminology report these are signs as their derivation is from the frequency volume chart. Symptoms are defined as complaints.

[b]These terms are from the definition of nocturia but may be useful in research studies, for example in urine production rate, related to posture.

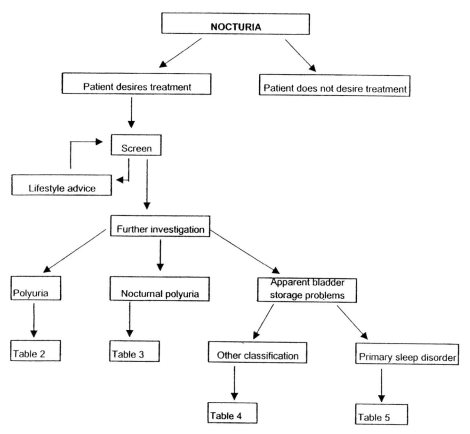

FIG. A.1. Patients without any bother may present with different conditions, when noccturia is identified.

ing can lead to lifestyle advice or to further investigations, which will enable the aetiology to be determined and an appropriate management strategy developed.

2.1 Nocturia

Nocturia is waking at night to void. This applies to any number of voids at any time during the night, as long as the person is awake before voiding. When voiding occurs during sleep, this is nocturnal enuresis. Both conditions can be referred to as night-time voiding, although the distinction between the two is clearly determined by the state of wakefulness.

The first morning void is not included as a night-time void since this is a natural expulsion of the urine produced during the night. In addition, although many people may consider one night-time void to be normal, they are still considered to have nocturia. For some individuals, the trigger for waking may not be a desire to void, yet voiding is perceived to be necessary once awake; however, these individuals are still considered to have nocturia. Those (e.g., the infirm or frail elderly) who wake with the need to void, but are unable to reach the bathroom before voiding, have a mixture of nocturia and incontinence, not nocturnal enuresis. Patients experiencing nocturia may or may not be bothered by this condition, and it is the level of bothersomeness that will determine their help-seeking behaviour.

2.2 Night

Night-time is the period of time between going to bed with the intention of sleeping and waking with the intention of arising. It must be noted that this varies with age, and elderly people often spend longer periods of time in bed than younger people. It is important that the sleeping time is considered, not the actual time in bed.

Shift workers may have a variation in their night-time, and the same definition exists for them. The same is true for people who split their sleeping time into two or more periods during the day. Jetlag and varied shift patterns may disrupt the natural circadian rhythm, and this can lead to poor sleeping patterns, disrupted sleep and nocturia.

2.3 Screen

An initial screen should include a detailed history, including questions relevant to voiding behaviour, medical and neurological abnormalities and sleep disturbance, as well as information on relevant surgery or previous urinary infections. A simple urine test, such as dipstick or urinalysis, should be performed to exclude any relevant pathology. A physical examination should also be performed.

2.4 Advice

General lifestyle advice, such as reducing caffeine and alcohol intake, and limiting excessive liquid/food volume intake prior to bedtime can, in some cases, be sufficient to elicit a satisfactory response. However, care should be taken not to impose a general fluid restriction as this could have serious consequences in patients with undiagnosed diabetes insipidus. Patients should be encouraged to return to their doctor for further evaluation if they are not content with the results following their initial advice.

2.5. Further Evaluation

This should begin by asking the patient to keep a frequency/volume chart. The chart should also include a record of the volume and type of fluid ingested as well as the volume and time of each voided urine for 24 to 72 hours. It also should include the time of retiring to bed,

time of rising and subjective evaluation of whether each night measured was good, bad or normal in terms of their usual sleeping pattern. In research studies, the impact on quality of life should also be measured using questionnaires such as ICS male [Donovan et al., 1996] or the DAN-PSS in men [Hald et al., 1991] and the BFLUTS in women [Jackson et al., 1996], which allow the assessment of the occurrence of nocturia and the degree of problem or bother that it causes. No specific measure has yet been devised to evaluate the full impact of nocturia on aspects of everyday life, although one is currently under development.

If a sleep disorder is suspected, a nocturnal polysomnograph should be considered. Examples of sleep disorders with a potential relation to nocturia are presented in Table V (see later). The pathophysiological causes of these disorders are not fully clarified and may be due to polyuria (e.g., obstructive sleep apnoea syndrome) or arousals with voiding (e.g., insomnia) [Thorpy, 1990].

2.6 Polyuria

A patient with urine output exceeding 40 mL/kg body weight during a 24-hour period should be considered to be suffering from polyuria. This should be investigated further to determine if the polyuria is due to a solute diuresis (e.g., diabetes mellitus) or diabetes insipidus and, if it is the latter, which type of diabetes insipidus is present (Table A.2). These distinctions can be made by measuring the glucose, specific gravity and osmolality of a 24-hour urine collection, followed by a variety of more specialized tests best undertaken by the appropriate subspecialist [Robertson, 1995].

TABLE A.2. *Causes of polyuria*

Diabetes mellitus
  Insulin dependent (type I)
  Insulin independent (type II)
Diabetes insipidus
  Pituitary
  Renal
  Gestational
  Primary polydipsia (psychogenic, dipsogenic or
    iatrogenic)

2.7 Nocturnal Polyuria

Nocturnal polyuria [Asplund, 1995; Carter, 1992] is defined as the production of an abnormally large volume of urine during sleep. The measurement should include all the urine produced after going to bed and the first void after arising. It can be expressed in several different ways [Robertson, 1999]. If the 24-hour urine volume is normal, the output during sleep can be expressed as a percentage of the total. This value varies considerably from person to person and normally increases with age. Healthy young adults from 21 to 35 years of age excrete around 14% ± 4% or their total urine between the hours of 11 p.m. and 7 a.m. (95% CI, 10%–19%) [Robertson et al., 1999], whereas older people excrete an average of 34% ± 15% (95% CI, 30%–36%) [Rembratt et al., 2000; Kirkland et al., 1983]. Thus, nocturnal polyuria may be defined as an output greater than of 20% of the daily total in the young and 33% [Carter, 1992] in the elderly with the value for middle age probably falling somewhere between these two extremes. Exceptions to this rule are patients with diabetes insipidus, and those whose sleeping patterns vary greatly from the normal 8-hour nighttime pattern. There are many causes of nocturnal polyuria that should be considered when carrying out further investigations (Table A.3).

2.8 Bladder Storage Problems

Patients with nocturia, who do not have either polyuria or nocturnal polyuria according

TABLE A.3. *Causes of nocturnal polyuria*

Water diuresis
Circadian defect in secretion or action of antidiuretic hormone
Primary (idiopathic)
Secondary (excessive evening intake of fluid, caffeine, alcohol)
Solute/water diuresis
Congestive heart failure
Autonomic dysfunction
Sleep apnoea syndrome
Renal insufficiency
Oestrogen deficiency

TABLE A.4. *Causes of problems related to bladder storage*

Reduced functional bladder capacity (e.g., significant post void residual)
Reduced nocturnal bladder capacity
Detrusor overactivity
Neurogenic (e.g., multiple sclerosis)
Non-neurogenic
Bladder hypersensitivity
Bladder outlet obstruction with post-void residual urine
Urogenital ageing

to the above criteria, will most likely have a reduced voided volume or a sleep disorder. The former can be determined from the frequency/volume chart by comparing the nighttime voided volume with the maximal bladder capacity that occurs at any time; however, a definite range of normal or abnormal volumes is currently lacking, and it is for the physician to evaluate the patient based on the frequency/volume charts and clinical judgement. Some mathematical indices have been suggested in the literature to describe this situation; measurements of the nocturia index (mean measured nocturnal urine volume/functional bladder capacity*) and nocturnal polyuria index (mean measured nocturnal urine volume/24-hour voided volume) may be very useful in a clinical trial situation, although an explanation of these is beyond the scope of this document and can be found in other publications [Weiss et al., 1998; Weiss & Blaivas, 2000; van Kerrebroeck & Weiss, 1999]. For patients exhibiting signs of bladder storage problems, further urological investigation should be carried out to determine the classification of the problem (Table A.4).

Some patients will have been categorised as having bladder storage problems, which is borne out by their frequency/volume chart, yet their real problem is one of sleep disturbance. Patients who are constantly waking at night for other reasons may feel the need to

---

*The term functional bladder capacity, deduced from frequency/volume charts, has been superceded by "voided volume" in the latest ICS Terminology Report.

TABLE A.5. *Sleep disorders potentially related to nocturia*

Insomnia
Obstructive and central apnoea syndrome
Periodic legs syndrome
Restless legs syndrome
Parasomnias
Sleep disorders related to medical diseases, e.g., chronic obstructive lung disease, cardiac diseases, etc.
Sleep disorders related to neurological diseases, e.g., Alzheimer's, Parkinson's, and epileptic seizures

void at each waking stage, and void a small volume. This might appear to the physician to be a problem with bladder storage, especially if the patient is unaware of the sleep problem. Further investigation in a sleep laboratory may be necessary to determine the cause of nocturia in these patients (Table A.5).

REFERENCES

Asplund R. 1995. The Nocturnal Polyuria Syndrome (NPS). Gen Pharmacol 26(6):1203.

Carter PG. 1992. The role of nocturnal polyuria in nocturnal urinary symptoms in healthy elderly males. MD thesis, Bristol.

Chute CG, Panser LA, Girman CJ, et al. 1993. The prevalence of prostatism: a population based survey of urinary symptoms. J Urol 150:85–9.

Donovan JL, Abrams P, Peters TJ et al. 1996. The ICS 'BPH' Study: the psychometric validity and reliability of the ICS male questionnaire. Br J Urol 77:554–62.

Hald T, Nordling J, Andersen JT, Bilde T, Meyhoff HH, Walter S. 1991. A patient weighted symptom score system in the evaluation of uncomplicated benign prostatic hyperplasia. Scand J Urol Nephrol Suppl 138:59–62.

Jackson S, Donovan J, Brookes S, Eckford S, Swithinbank L, Abrams P. 1996. The Bristol Female Lower Urinary Tract Symptoms questionnaire: development and psychometric testing. Br J Urol 77:805–12.

Kirkland JL, Lye M, Levy DW, Banerjee AK. 1983. Patterns of urine flow and electrolyte excretion in healthy elderly people. BMJ 287(6406):1665–7.

Malmsten UG, Milsom I, Molander U, Norlen LJ. 1997. Urinary incontinence and lower urinary tract symptoms: an epidemiological study of men aged 45 to 99 years. J Urol 158:1733–7.

Mattiasson A. 1999. Nocturia towards a consensus. BJU Suppl 1; Vol 84.

Mattsson S. 1994. Urinary incontinence and nocturia in healthy schoolchildren. Acta Paediatr 83:950–54.

Middlekoop HA, Smilde van den Doel DA, Neven AK, Kamphuisen HA, Springer CP. 1996. Subjective sleep characteristics of 1485 males and females aged 50–93: effects of sex and age, and factors related to self evaluated quality of sleep. J Gerontol A Biol Sci Med Sci 51:108–15.

Rembratt Å, Robertson GL, Nøgaard JP, Andersson KE. 2000. Pathogenic aspects of nocturia in the elderly Differences between nocturics and nonnocturics. ICS meeting.

Robertson G, Rembratt A, Eriksson KE. 2000. Desmopressin in the Treatment of Disorders of Urine Output in Humans. Arch Intern Med (In Press).

Robertson GL. 1995. Diabetes insipidus. Endocrinol Metab Clin North Am 24(3):549–72.

Robertson GL. 1999. Br J Urol 84(Suppl 1):17–9.

Robertson GL, Rittig S, Kovacs L, Gaskill MB, Zee P, Naninga J. 1999. Scand J Urol Nephrol Suppl 202:36–9.

Swithinbank LV, Donovan J, James MC, Yang Q, Abrams P. 1998. Female urinary symptoms: age prevalence in a community dwelling population using a validated questionnaire. Neurourol Urodyn 16:432–4.

Thorpy MJ. 1990. International classification of sleep disorders: diagnostic and coding manual. Rochester MN, American Sleep Disorders Association (Chairman).

van Kerrebroeck P, Weiss JP. 1999. Standardisation and terminology of nocturia. In: Mattiasson A (ed): "Nocturia towards a consensus." BJU Suppl I Vol 84:1–4.

Weiss JP, Blaivas JG. 2000. Nocturia. J Urol 163:5–12.

Weiss JP, Blaivas JG, Stember DS, Brooks MM. 1998. Nocturia in adults: etiology and classification. Neurourol Urodyn 17:467–72.

Ostergard's Urogynecology and Pelvic Floor Dysfunction, Fifth Edition. edited by A.E. Bent, et al. Lippincott Williams & Wilkins, Philadelphia © 2003.

Appendix III

Urogynecology and the Internet

Joseph M. Montella

The Internet and the World Wide Web have changed the practice of medicine dramatically. Information that was once available to a select few in the field of medicine is now available to anyone with access to a computer and questions to be answered. Physicians are now more inclined to see patients who come prepared with information (at times inaccurate) and address these issues. The purpose of this appendix is to guide the reader to web sites containing information pertinent to the field of urogynecology and female pelvic floor medicine. The following list of web sites is by no means exhaustive because the World Wide Web is fluid, and there are bound to be several more sites related to the field by the time of publication of this text. The reader can use one of the variety of search engines on the web (e.g., Yahoo, Excite, Alta Vista) to explore the various physician- and patient-oriented web sites. Also, each site has links to other sites that may be useful to the reader. Keep in mind that there are many sites with erroneous information, and it is incumbent on the physician to sort out the facts for the patients and correct any misconceptions.

GOVERNMENT SITES

www.nlm.nih.gov

The United States National Library of Medicine provides an excellent resource for Medline, research funding opportunities, and library services.

www.niddk.nih.gov

The link to the National Institute of Diabetes, Digestive, and Kidney Diseases provides a resource in government funding for research into urinary incontinence and pelvic floor disorders.

clinicaltrials.gov

The U.S. National Institutes of Health, through its National Library of Medicine, has developed ClinicalTrials.gov to provide patients, family members, and members of the public with current information about clinical research studies.

www.niddk.nih.gov/health/kidney/nkudic.html

The National Kidney and Urologic Diseases Information Clearinghouse (NKUDIC) is an information dissemination service established in 1987 to increase knowledge and understanding about diseases of the kidneys and urologic system among people with these conditions and their families, health care professionals, and the general public.

www.nichd.nih.gov

The National Institute of Child Health and Development (NICHD) administers a multidisciplinary program of research, research training, and public information, nationally and within its own facilities, on reproductive biology and population issues; on prenatal development as well as maternal, child, and family health; and on medical rehabilitation. The Institute supports and conducts basic, clinical, and epidemiologic research in the reproductive sciences.

www.ahcpr.gov

The Agency for Healthcare Research and Quality (formerly the Agency for Healthcare Policy and Research) offers information on government programs and grants.

www.hcfa.gov

The web site of the Health Care Financing Administration (HCFA), the federal agency that administers Medicare, Medicaid, and the State Children's Health Insurance Program (SCHIP) includes information on reimbursement, statistics, and publications.

PROFESSIONAL SOCIETIES

www.augs.org

The American Urogynecologic Society, founded in 1979, is dedicated to research and education in urogynecology and to improved care for women with lower urinary tract disorders. This site provides both physician and patient education materials, research funding opportunities, links to government and congressional web sites, and information on postgraduate fellowship training programs in urogynecology.

www.acog.org

The American College of Obstetrics and Gynecology provides resources for physicians and patients as well as information on postgraduate courses in urogynecology.

www.auanet.org

The American Urologic Association provides a wide range of services, including publications, the Annual Meeting, continuing medical education, and health policy advocacy.

www.continet.org

The primary mission of the International Continence Society is to study the storage and voiding function of the lower urinary tract, its diagnosis, and the management of lower urinary tract dysfunction and to encourage research into pathophysiology, diagnostic techniques, and treatment.

www.iuga.org

The International Urogynecological Association is an international organization committed to promoting and exchanging knowledge regarding the care of women with urinary and pelvic floor dysfunction.

sgsonline.org

The goal of the Society of Gynecologic Surgeons is to promote the acquisition of knowledge and the improvement of skills in gynecologic surgery, to enhance the understanding of gynecology and gynecologic surgery through basic and clinical research, and to be a source of public and professional information.

www.nafc.org

The National Association for Continence (NAFC), formerly Help for Incontinent People (HIP), is a not-for-profit organization established in 1982 dedicated to improving the quality of life of people with incontinence. NAFC's purpose is to be the leading source of education, advocacy, and support to the public and to health professionals about the causes, prevention, diagnosis, treatments, and management solutions for incontinence.

www.simonfoundation.org

The work of the Simon Foundation includes aid to patients with incontinence, aid to the families of those patients, creating public awareness, reviewing relevant legislation, and encouraging the medical professions' interest in incontinence and pelvic floor dysfunction.

MEMBERSHIP AND PATIENT-ORIENTED SITES

www.obgynlinx.com

ObGynLinx.com is designed to keep obstetrics and gynecology professionals up to date with the latest medical developments by aggregating the top obstetrics and gynecology articles from hundreds of premiere medical journals and categorizing the information into 14 subspecialties, including urogynecology.

womenshealth.medscape.com

Medscape offers access to abstracts from conferences in all medical specialties, including gynecology, and offers continuing medical education (CME) credits as well as access to journal articles.

www.centerwatch.com

This CenterWatch site is a comprehensive guide to clinical trials underway in every region of the United States, listed by disease or condition as well as research centers and additional resources specifically for each disease entity.

www.obgyn.net

OBGYN.net includes such features as current clinical news, original articles, CME, cases of the month, an events locator and other interactive tools, professional forums in English and Spanish, and free procedure videos viewable online.

www.mybladder.com

MyBladder is an online community dedicated to encouraging people with bladder control problems to seek help while promoting an understanding of bladder control problems and awareness of the latest treatment options.

Subject Index

Page numbers followed by italic *f* or *t* denote figures or tables, respectively.